Foundations of Clinical Neuropsychology

Foundations of Clinical Neuropsychology

Edited by

Charles J. Golden
University of Nebraska Medical Center
Omaha, Nebraska

and

Peter J. Vicente
Industrial Commission of Ohio
Columbus, Ohio

PLENUM PRESS • NEW YORK AND LONDON

Library of Congress Cataloging in Publication Data

Main entry under title:

Foundations of clinical neuropsychology.

Bibliography: p.
Includes index.
1. Brain — Diseases — Diagnosis. 2. Neuropsychology. 3. Psychometrics. I. Golden,
Charles J., 1949–   . II. Vicente, Peter J., 1947–
RC386.2.F68   1983   616.89′075   83-16097
ISBN 0-306-41286-1

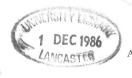

© 1983 Plenum Press, New York
A Division of Plenum Publishing Corporation
233 Spring Street, New York, N.Y. 10013

Printed in the United States of America

Contributors

Russell L. Adams Center for Alcohol and Drug Related Studies, Department of Psychiatry and Behavioral Science, University of Oklahoma Health Sciences Center, Oklahoma City, Oklahoma

Rona Ariel Department of Psychology, Indiana State University, Terre Haute, Indiana

Richard A. Berg Division of Neurology/Psychology, Saint Jude Children's Research Hospital, Memphis, Tennessee

Richard J. Browne Neuropsychology Laboratory, McGuire Veterans Administration Medical Center, Richmond, Virginia

Robert L. Brunner Department of Pediatrics, Children's Hospital Medical Center, Cincinnati, Ohio

Nick A. DeFilippis Clinical Psychologist, Independent Practice, Augusta, Georgia

Charles J. Golden Department of Psychiatry, University of Nebraska Medical Center, Omaha, Nebraska

Gerald Goldstein Research, Veterans Administration Medical Center, Pittsburgh, Pennsylvania

Lawrence C. Hartlage Department of Neurology, Medical College of Georgia, Augusta, Georgia

Henry Leland Psychological Services, Nisonger Center for Mental Retardation, Ohio State University, Columbus, Ohio

William J. Lynch Brain Injury Rehabilitation Unit, Palo Alto Veterans Administration Medical Center, Palo Alto, California

Elizabeth A. McMahon Private Practice, Gainesville, Florida

Manfred J. Meier Neuropsychology Laboratory, Department of Neurosurgery, University of Minnesota Medical School, Minneapolis, Minnesota

James A. Moses, Jr. Psychology Services, Palo Alto Veterans Administration Medical Center, Palo Alto, California, and Department of Psychiatry and Behavioral Sciences, Stanford University School of Medicine, Stanford, California

David C. Osmon Department of Psychology, University of Wisconsin-Milwaukee, Milwaukee, Wisconsin

Oscar A. Parsons Center for Alcohol and Drug Related Studies, Department of Psychiatry and Behavioral Sciences, University of Oklahoma Health Sciences Center, Oklahoma City, Oklahoma

Mark Schachter Robert Warner Rehabilitation Center, Children's Hospital, Department of Pediatrics and Department of Psychology, State University of New York at Buffalo, Buffalo, New York

Steven D. Sherrets Director of Day Hospital, Bradley Hospital, Section of Psychiatry and Human Behavior, Brown University, East Providence, Rhode Island

Mary Ann Strider Department of Psychiatry, University of Nebraska Medical Center, Omaha, Nebraska

Michael G. Tramontana Psychology Department, Bradley Hospital, Section of Psychiatry and Human Behavior, Brown University, East Providence, Rhode Island

Preface

In the last decade, neuropsychology has grown from a small subspecialty to a major component in the practice of clinical and medical psychology. This growth has been caused by advances in psychological testing (such as the Halstead–Reitan neuropsychological battery, as discussed in Chapter 5) that have made evaluation techniques in the field available to a wider audience, by advances in neuroradiology and related medical areas that have enabled us to better understand the structure and function of the brain in living individuals without significant potential harm to those individuals, and by increased interest by psychologists and other scientists in the role that the brain plays in determining behavior. Many disorders that were believed by many to be caused purely by learning or environment have been shown to relate, at least in some cases, to brain dysfunction or damage.

With the growth of the field, there has been increased interest in the work of neuropsychologists by many who are not in the field. This interest has come from several major groups: first, from graduate and undergraduate students in psychology and related areas who are considering neuropsychology as a possible profession; second, from allied health professionals, rehabilitation workers, physicians, and others who are interested in the possible role that neuropsychology might play in their patients or setting; third, from the lay public about the role of neuropsychology in the assessment, understanding, and treatment of brain-injured children and adults; and finally, from students enrolled in classes in clinical psychology and neuropsychology in which there is an attempt to teach the role of the neuropsychologist within the health delivery system.

At present, there are few references (if any) available for these individuals. There is a plethora of books on how the brain functions, but most of these assume too much knowledge and background to be of interest to many readers not in the field. Furthermore, these books do not focus on what the neuropsychologist actually does, but on other more academic or clinical issues. While these are important, they most often offer at best a vague impression of the role of the neuropsychologist and the role of the field.

The purpose of the present volume is to remedy these problems. The volume begins with a discussion on the history of neuropsychology, followed by chapters on assessment approaches and techniques commonly used in the field. The subsequent chapters, comprising the bulk of the volume, then examine the role of the neuropsychologist in a variety of populations, in several different settings, and in relationship to several major issues. Thus, these sections explore such topics as the role of the neuropsychologist in neurology, psychiatry, and medical populations, and with such populations as children and adults. The chapters also cover such issues as the role of the neuropsychologist in rehabilitation and in forensic (law) work, as well as such issues as the influence of a person's sex on neuropsychological performance. The final chapter is on the question of training and credentialing in neuropsychology, an issue growing in importance as the field expands.

There are several things that this book is not. Although there are numerous references throughout the book, this book is not intended as a comprehensive research review of the areas covered. Neither is it intended to break new theoretical ground in each area. The chapters are attempts to acquaint the individual not currently trained in neuropsychology with the field, how it has developed, what it does, and how it goes about performing its activities. It is our hope that the reader will acquire a balanced presentation of typical activities (although not all approaches to such activities or all tests related to these activities) and instruments associated with neuropsychology. The reader should come away with a feel for what the neuropsychologist does and how neuropsychology fits into the more general areas of psychological and medical care.

We have attempted to minimize as much as possible the use of jargon and vocabulary peculiar to neuropsychology. However, we have found that some basic minimum of neuroanatomy is necessary as well as some familiarization with the functions of the brain. For those with absolutely no familiarity with basic neuroanatomy, we have included an Appendix, which is a short (and somewhat oversimplified) view of this area. Several of the chapters (e.g., Chapter 7) also present some basic introductory material on such topics as hemispheric specialization.

In general, we have attempted to avoid most duplication among chapters, although sometimes we have left such material in to make each chapter more readable. Furthermore, because of the general attempt to avoid duplication, the book is intended to be read in the order in which the chapters are written. For example, later chapters may refer in examples to specific tests that are explained in Chapters 2 through 6.

We are highly appreciative of each author's contribution to this book. We are grateful also for the coordinating secretarial contributions of Ms. Paula Dinkel. And finally, we are most appreciative of the encouragement and forbearance shown to us throughout this effort by our family members, Ellen, Peg, Sean, Brian, and Kevin.

Charles J. Golden
Peter J. Vicente

Contents

Chapter 13

Chapter 14

Chapter 15

Chapter 16

Chapter 17

History of Neuropsychological Assessment

LAWRENCE C. HARTLAGE and NICK A. DeFILIPPIS

Although there is evidence of interest in neuropsychological processes from a very early period in recorded history, credit for first attempting to localize cognitive facilities in the ventricles is generally attributed to Herophilius around 300 B.C. (Mann, 1979). Subsequently, Erasistratus (310–250 B.C.) was the first to postulate localization of function within the substance of the brain, and Galen (130–200 A.D.) assigned imagination to the "forebrain" and sensation to the "hindbrain" (Riese, 1959). Because Galen considered the interconnecting chambers of the ventricles as a reservoir that integrated psychological functions, Luria (1966) describes him as a ventricular localizationist, and subsequent medieval theorists such as Albertus Magnus (1193–1280) and da Vinci (1452–1519) further developed these ventricular localization concepts. Shortly after the death of da Vinci, Huarte (1529–1588) first proposed a localizationist position involving both ventricles and brain tissue (Hunt, 1869), and a century later Willis (1620–1675) made the complete translation of localization of function to the cerebrum (McHenry, 1969). Localization attempts during this period almost universally focused on finding a single area of the brain underlying all mental functions (Luria, 1966).

Localization of specific functions by specific cortical areas was recognized early in the eighteenth century, and de Petit (1644–1771) demonstrated contralateral innervation in both man and dogs (Tizard, 1959). Further work on con-

LAWRENCE C. HARTLAGE ● Department of Neurology, Medical College of Georgia, Augusta, Georgia 30902. NICK A. DeFILIPPIS ● Clinical Psychologist, Independent Practice, Augusta, Georgia 30901.

tralateral innervation of motor function was reported by Saucerotte (1741–1814), but contemporary neurologists tended to regard these findings as being of no relevance to clinical neurology, in part because they did not derive from any specific theory or systematic line of research (Mann, 1979).

It was in such a context that Gall (1758–1828) introduced his theory relating skull contours to behavioral functions. Gall described this as the science of craniology, although it is better known as phrenology, a term applied by Spurzheim (Mann, 1979). The scientific bases of his theory grew from Gall's observations that his schoolmates who had good memories also had bulging eyes (Spoerl, 1936). Gall's theory was rejected by both fellow neurologists (e.g., Flourens, Magendie, Rolando) and physiologists (e.g., Mueller), and in the 1860s the standard physiology texts of the day reiterated the concept of the cortex as a unitary organ (Mann, 1979).

Gall's writings were not totally without influence, however, especially those having to do with the localization of speech functions. In papers published in 1807 and 1813, he localized speech in the convolutions of the interior aspect of the frontal lobes (Head, 1963), and in 1825 Bouillaud (1796–1881) offered a prize to anyone who could show him the brain of a patient with a confirmed diagnosis of loss of speech without a lesion in the frontal lobes (Head, 1963). Even though the prize was never awarded, this was not regarded as necessarily supporting Gall's position, and for a number of decades, the generally accepted view was, as expressed by Gratiolet in 1861, that the total volume of the brain was related to intelligence, and that the functions of all parts of the brain were the same (Lee, 1981).

Although aphasia had been described more than a century earlier by Genner, a French physician named Paul Broca (1824–1880) was the first (1861) to report detailed autopsy findings demonstrating the localization of speech in the third frontal convolution. In the April 4, 1861, meeting of the Société d'Anthropoligie, its founder and first Secretary, Broca, proposed a patient he called "Tan" as a test case of Bouillaud's wager. "Tan," who in reality was a man named Leborgne, had died from gangrene shortly after admission to Broca's surgical service. He had been a patient at Broca's hospital for 21 years, ever since he lost his speech, and Broca presented "Tan's" brain to the society to demonstrate the pathological alteration in what came to be known as "Broca's area" (Mann, 1979). By 1863 Broca and his colleagues had collected 19 cases of aphasia which all showed lesions in the third frontal convolution of the left cerebral hemispheres.

Although Broca's impressive findings did not fully convert the critics of localization of function, they were influential in shaping the course of research of a number of important scientists of the day. In 1870, for example, Fritsch and Hitzig reported, on the basis of their research with dogs, that motor functions are more anteriorly located, with nonmotor functions more posterior, and that electrical stimulation of motor areas produces contractions on the contralateral side of the body. Even more important than their findings was their introduction of careful operative procedures in the study of localization research done during the remainder of the nineteenth century.

Subsequently, Ferrier (1876) located a vision center in the occipital lobe, and by the mid-1870s the literature on brain localization was so voluminous that researchers of the time began simply listing references (Mann, 1979). Notable among the findings of this decade were those of Wernicke (1874), who demonstrated receptive aphasia from a lesion of the posterior third of the left hemisphere superior temporal gyrus.

NEUROPSYCHOLOGY: DEVELOPMENT OF MODERN BASES (1900–1945)

The developments pertinent to neuropsychology occurring between 1900 and 1945 included significant advancements in several content areas that had either been delineated earlier or become increasingly important to rapidly changing societal conditions. These inlcude: (1) development of the equipotentiality versus cortical specialization controversy; (2) investigations into the functions of the right or "silent" hemisphere; (3) the relationship between brain impairment and academic performance; (4) increased interest in the influence of brain damage; and (5) development of standardized measures of intelligence.

It is natural to end this period with the end of the Second World War because it was at this time that the field of clinical psychology began to apply its techniques to an increasingly varied array of medical and social problems. The advances made during this era set the stage for postwar clinical psychologists to develop clinical procedures to be used in the diagnosis and treatment programming of organically based disorders. Although there were scattered case reports of the utilization of test instruments in the diagnosis or description of brain-damaged patients (Mahan, 1980), these largely dealt with the use of intelligence tests in isolation. Also, when more specialized test instruments were used, they usually lacked the psychometric sophistication that current neuropsychological instruments display. For example, Hanfmann's (1939) report of the use of Vigotsky's (1934) test of concept formation was entirely qualitative to the point of omitting test scores.

Equipotentiality versus Cortical Specialization

After Broca and Wernicke demonstrated differential effects on speech following specific types of damage to the left frontal and temporal areas of the cerebral cortex, it seemed as if even the most complex psychological processes of man could be localized in various specific cortical areas. The search for specialized areas of the cerebrum particularly concerned with intelligence, abandoned after the rejection of Gall's phrenology, began again in earnest. One of the first of these resurgents was Hitzig, who localized abstract thinking in the frontal lobes (Hitzig, 1884).

Anatomical evidence for Hitzig's belief came from the work of Bolton (1903a, 1903b), who examined histologically the brains of a number of cases of mental retardation and dementia. He reported a reduction in the thickness of the cerebral cortex in these cases, particlarly in the area of the prefrontal region. This work was, however, not supported by others (Hammarberg, 1895), and Bolton himself admitted that the techniques for measuring cortical thickness were not very accurate.

Bianchi (1922) reported on a series of experiences in which lesions in the frontal lobes resulted in serious loss of learning abilities in various animals. He ascribed to the frontal lobes the specialized ability of cortical organization. He also attributed to the temporal lobes the ability to utilize language for the formation of intellect. Unfortunately, Bianchi's experimental methodologies were quite deficient, lacking experimental controls in most studies.

Hughlings Jackson (1931–1932) put forth the idea that a disturbance of higher cortical functions should be regarded as a regression of functional organization, rather than as the result of lesions of circumscribed areas of the brain, and that the interpretation of all symptoms evoked by brain damage must be regarded from this more integrative and dynamic position. Munk (1909) and Monakow (1914) held similar positions and believed that the evidence was inadequate to establish any special intellectual functions in the association areas. They believed that while simple sensory and motor functions may be localized, the more complex processes of the mind involve the coordination of many diverse sensory and motor processes individually localized in various sections of the cortex, and hence incapable of inclusion within any circumscribed area. An analogous position was held by the prominent neurologist, Kurt Goldstein (1939) who repeatedly emphasized that disturbance of complex forms of mental activity may occur in the presence of damage in practically any area of the brain.

Flouren's (1824) early theory that intelligent behavior is an indivisible function of the activity of the entire cerebrum, or the theory of cortical function, was reintroduced by Loeb (1902), who believed the existing evidence did not support the restriction of intelligence to any part of the cerebrum. He evolved a theory that cerebral integration consists of the establishment of functional periodicities among the parts of the cortex, such that associations are called out by resonance. Lashley's (1929) work with rats provided experimental support to this notion of "mass action," which has served as the basic objection to theories ascribing specialized functions to areas of the cortex. Though a classic, Lashley's work is also not without its methodological problems, as has been recently pointed out by Thomas (1970).

This controversy continues to exist, in modified form, even today. For the most part, it has not had many practical implications for the field of clinical neuro-psychology since it is, in a sense, a controversy without any possible resolution. Luria (1966) pointed out that a higher mental function might suffer as a result of the destruction of any link which is part of the structure of a complex functional system and consequently may be disturbed even when centers differ greatly in localization. However, when one or another link has been lost, the whole functional system will be disturbed in a particular way. Thus, although it may be true that a lesion in almost any area of the cortex will result in a decrement in intellect, this finding does not negate the possibility of localized functions, nor does it imply the fruitlessness of diagnostic investigations of specific behavioral impairments following destruction of different areas of the brain.

The "Silent" Hemisphere

Since the time of Broca, the left hemisphere has been thought to be of considerable importance, although at first its importance was thought to be true only for speech functions. It was soon noted, however, that aphasic patients often seemed to suffer from intellectual difficulties as well. Thus, Hughlings Jackson (1874), Pierre Marie (1906), and Kurt Goldstein (1927) spoke of the loss of abstract reasoning and the use of symbols in thought in aphasics. The abilities of ideomotor apraxia (Liepmann, 1900), visuoconstructive ability (Kleist, 1923), and finger agnosia (Gerstmann, 1924) were also later ascribed to be the domain of the left hemisphere. These observations, taken together, emphasized the importance and "dominance" of the left hemisphere in mediating those distinctly human capacities for language as well as reasoning, symbolic thinking, and higher level praxis and orientation to one's body. This designation of the left hemisphere as dominant or "major" implied that the right hemisphere was "minor."

Benton (1972) described the general trend of scientific thought on the workings of the right hemisphere during this period. He pointed out that although the right hemisphere was not thought to be totally uninvolved with language, its functions were mainly limited to the storage of duplicate verbal engrams learned during the acquisition of speech and called forth when the left hemisphere sustained damage. This notion was supported by the observations of aphasics who were able to produce perfectly intelligible speech at certain times, usually when under stress. This theory was also used to explain recovery from aphasia; that is, the assumption that the right hemisphere takes over the functions of the left.

Hughlings Jackson (1874) was one of the first investigators in this area to ascribe separate functions to the right hemisphere in a study of a tumor that produced deficits in visual recognition and visual memory. Rieger (1909) and his student Reichardt (1923) advanced the idea, supported by clinicopathological observations, that a spatial–practical ability was localized in the posterior right hemisphere. During this same period, observations in the field of opthalmology pointed to the possibility that the right hemisphere played a role in subserving certain aspects of visual perception. Disturbances in spatial orientation were noted in patients with right hemisphere damage who had intact central visual acuity, indicating that the deficit was not sensory or intellectual in nature (Benton, 1969; Critchley, 1953).

Babinski (1914) added to the spatial functions subserved by the right hemisphere when he described a case of agnosia in the form of unawareness of left hemiplegia. He and other authors suggested that the right hemisphere might contain a center for the integration of somatosensory information with somesthetic images.

Kleist (1923) described constructional apraxia as being a disorder that is neither visual nor motoric in nature, but arises out of an inability to translate intact visual perceptions of forms into appropriate motor actions. He attributed this function, as noted previously, to the left hemisphere. Later workers in the field tended to ignore Kleist's formulation of the "connectional" nature of the disorder, and noted that the impairment seemed to occur at least as frequently in patients with right hemisphere lesions as with lesions in the dominant hemisphere. Other visuospatial disabilities were also noted to occur frequently in patients with right hemisphere disease (Lange, 1936).

Dide (1938) further emphasized the importance of the right hemisphere in the mediation of perceptual and motor performances, and allied himself with a group of clinicians who felt that musical abilities depended upon the integrity of the superior temporal gyrus of the right hemisphere, in analogy to Wernicke's area in the left hemisphere. Vignolo (1969) outlines the evidence presented during this period for the existence of the disability of auditory agnosia as separate from language disturbances, and the limited but provocative evidence presented suggesting right hemisphere mediation of this function. Others also presented experimental evidence in support of the right hemisphere being responsible for the mediation of specific, nonverbal abilities (Brain, 1941; Hebb, 1939; Weisenberg & McBride, 1935). Donald Hebb's report (1939) was of particular relevance since it involved the description of test performance of a patient who underwent a large excision of the right temporal lobe and later exhibited defective visuoperceptive and visuoconstructive abilities, but maintained superior verbal intelligence.

Although most authors still refer to the left hemisphere as being dominant, the reports cited above had a definite effect on the investigations of the 1940s and 1950s, and no doubt spurred the development of several psychometric instruments designed to measure right hemisphere functions (Benton, 1955, 1963; Benton & Fogel, 1962; Graham & Kendall, 1960; Reitan, 1955). This further led to the development of the concept of test "scatter" profiles indicating significant discrepancies in performance on measures of right versus left hemisphere functions, as a sign of cerebral dysfunctioning.

Neuropsychological Implications for Academic Performance

Although Benton and Meyers (1956) credit Badal, a French opthalmologist, with the first detailed report of a case of finger agnosia in 1888, it was Gerstmann (1924) who called this disability in naming and differentiating individual fingers "Finger agnosia." By 1930, Gerstmann had linked this disability with right–left disorientation, agraphia, and acalulia as the components of a neurological syndrome resulting from damage to the parieto-occipital region of the left hemisphere. He also felt that finger agnosia, as the central defect in the syndrome, was due to disintegration of the body schema as it pertained to the fingers (Gerstmann, 1940). Strauss and Werner (1938) also implicated body schema disturbance as the cause of finger localization problems, but Stengel (1944) argued early on that constructional apraxia and the symptoms of the Gerstmann syndrome resulted from a loss of spatial orientation. Stengel later received substantial support for his contentions by the research of Ettlinger (1963). The status of the symptoms Gerstmann outlined as a "syndrome" has since been questioned by numerous authors, but the "Gerstmann syndrome" continues to focus attention on finger agnosia and other related disturbances as precursors of learning disabilities (Croxen & Lytton, 1971; Hemann, 1964; Peters, Romine, & Dykman, 1975; Sparrow & Satz, 1970).

Orton's (1928) theory of cerebral dominance evolved from clinical observations of the coincidence of letter reversals and inconsistent laterality in reading disability cases. He attributed this reversal tendency to poorly defined cerebral dominance, which he thought was evidenced in these children by mixed eye–hand dominance and ambidexterity (Orton, 1937). On the basis of these observations, he theorized that incomplete cerebral dominance may account for reading disability in general. Orton hypothesized that the two hemispheres of the brain store visual information in the form of mirror images of one another, and he therefore attributed this condition of strephosymbolia to the neurological condition in which neither hemisphere asserted complete dominance over the other in the recall of graphic symbols.

While the term strephosymbolia has fallen into disuse, Orton's theory of cerebral dominance continues to stimulate a great deal of interest. Although the first part of his theory (i.e., concerning mirror images) remains untested, many researchers have studied the relationship of reading ability to cerebral dominance, which has been conventionally considered to be manifest in eyedness, handedness, or consistency of eye–hand preference. Unfortunately for Orton's thesis, most of these investigations have proven to be negative. For example, the vast majority of studies have reported no difference between poor versus good readers in terms of inconsistent or left-eyedness, left-handedness, ambidexterity, or crossed dominance (Belmont and Birch, 1965; Gates & Bennett, 1933; Wolfe, 1939). Actually, Orton's assertion that eyedness is relevant to the assessment of cerebral dominance is quite unsound on a purely anatomical basis, since each eye has bilateral cortical representation (Money, 1969).

Despite the succession of negative findings, the role of cerebral dominance in reading disability continues to attract research interest. The reasons for this appear to lie in the consistent finding of a weak relationship between more deviant lateral organization and poor reading and general intelligence. Also, the early studies usually assessed laterality by subjects' self-report, or in younger subjects by demonstrations of hand preference, which could be confounded by imitation. Today, both of these methods appear to have questionable validity and have been replaced in neuropsychological laboratories by more systematized procedures. For example, current evidence suggests that it is more accurate to define handedness in terms of a continuous rather than a dichotomous variable (Benton, Myers, & Polder, 1962).

Brain Damage and Personality

The name most closely associated with this area during this period is that of Kurt Goldstein (1878–1965). Goldstein was born in Germany and received his M.D. at the University of Breslau in 1903. He became director of the Neurological Institute at the University of Frankfurt and during World War I conducted a number of intensive long-term studies of brain-injured soldiers, on which many of his theoretical personality concepts are based. He later taught at several universities in the United States while maintaining a private practice. His early involvement with Gestalt psychology, phenomenology, and existentialism reflects an interest in philosophical issues that he retained throughout his career. As mentioned previously, Goldstein is associated with the equipotentiality school of thought in neurology. He believed that the personality structure of the patient is disturbed particularly by lesions of the frontal lobes, the parietal lobes, and the insula Reili; but he also felt that diffuse damage to the cortex, as in alcoholism and metabolic disturbances, affected personality. Goldstein (1939) theorized that the personality structure of the individual is a complex function of the brain, which is the same for all its parts.

Specifically, Goldstein presented seven areas in which brain-damaged individuals are unable to perform. These included: (1) taking initiative; (2) shifting from one aspect of a situation to another; (3) accounting to oneself one's actions; (4) keeping in mind more than one aspect of a given situation; (5) grasping a whole from its parts; (6) abstracting and planning ahead; and (7) doing something that necessitates detaching the ego from the outer world or from inner experiences. He summarized all these defects in terms of one general impairment: failure to maintain an "abstract attitude" (Goldstein & Scheerer, 1941).

Goldstein (1939) also outlined the phenomenon of the "catastrophic reaction." He felt that this response occurred when a patient was not able to fulfill a task set before him. When confronted with a failure, the brain-damaged patient would often react by becoming dazed, agitated, unfriendly, and evasive. His capacity to react in subsequent situations would also be impaired for some time after the reaction. Goldstein explained this reaction as something that is intrinsic to the organism in failing, and not a reaction to the failure. He believed that for the brain-damaged patient any failure meant the impossibility of self-realization and existence, and thus a minor failure could result in a dramatic reaction. Goldstein also related the occurrence of anxiety to the same sort of failure situations that produce catastrophic reactions in brain-damaged people; that is, there is a discrepancy between the individual's capacities and the demands made on him, and this discrepancy makes self-realization impossible. In order to protect himself against catastrophic reactions and anxiety, Goldstein felt that the brain-damaged patient developed a characteristic mode of behavior that included withdrawal, maintaining familiar surroundings, extreme orderliness, and keeping himself busy with things he was able to do (Goldstein, 1939). By adopting these behaviors, the brain-damaged person is usually able, without the aid of special treatment, to diminish catastrophic reactions and anxiety even though the defect caused by damage to the brain remains.

Goldstein also offered the interesting hypothesis concerning the observations that brain-damaged patients are sometimes unaware of their obvious defects, such as hemiplegias or hemianopsias. He proposed that this unawareness was not hysterical, but due to the brain-damaged person's tendency to stick to what he is able to do. That is, he compensates for his defect to the extent that self-realization is not essentially disturbed. For example, the aphasic patient will utter a word that is only vaguely related to the correct word he needs to produce, and will believe he is correct. This false belief represents a form of denial that defends the patient's ego from the potentially devastating realization of failure. Goldstein's observations on the adaptive responses of brain-damaged individuals have generally been incorporated into rehabilitation programs for organically impaired patients (e.g., the recognized need to incorporate orderliness and sameness into rehabilitation settings, and the typical building of new skills onto existing abilities).

A particularly important development during this period concerned the emerging conception of "minimal brain damage," which is minimal in the sense that it is not detectable through ordinary neurological diagnostic procedures. Nonetheless, it produces considerable changes in personality even years after the damage is sustained. This conception began with the early publications by physicians reporting behavioral characteristics they considered to be sequelae of lethargic encephalitis that had been contracted by children during the epidemic of World War I (Ebaugh, 1923; Hohman, 1922). These reports focused on symptoms of antisocial behavior, irritability, impulsiveness, emotional lability, and overactivity associated with a minimal loss of intelligence. This condition was further defined and supported by reports on the effects of head trauma in which the symptoms of overactivity, impulsiveness, antisocial behavior, and disturbances in motility and emotionality were increased and cognitive deficiencies were minimized (Strother, 1973).

Somewhat later, Strauss and his associates published a series of reports of behavioral characteristics that differentiated groups of brain-injured from non-brain-injured mentally retarded children (Strauss, 1939; Strauss & Lehtinen, 1955). The behaviors of the brain-injured children were quite similar to those noted in the observations of children who contracted encephalitis. After identifying these characteristics, Strauss offered the hypothesis that all children showing these symptoms were probably brain-damaged. This conclusion was based on the admittedly circular reasoning that if a set of symptoms are known to be the result of brain damage in one group of children, then these symptoms are indicative of brain damage whenever they are found in other children. This interpretation of a set of behaviors was made even though the neurological examinations did not demonstrate cerebral insult.

The lack of convincing neurological evidence of brain damage in most of the children who demonstrated Strauss' brain damage symptom complex led to the use of the term "minimal brain damage" to describe these children. Justification for the use of the adjective "minimal" was the fact that the behavioral deficiencies associated with the syndrome, although readily observable, were much less severe than the results of gross brain damage. Thus, minimal brain damage was set forth as a possible cause of some behavior disorders of children. Tregold (1908) and others had previously asserted that mild cases of brain injury during birth could cause deficiencies that would be noticeable only years later when the child attended school and when highly complex behaviors were required of him. Additional support for the concept of minimal brain damage was provided by studies on humans, which indicated a significant relationship between birth anoxia and subsequent developmental deviations (Preston, 1945; Rosenfeld & Bradley, 1948).

Considerable controversy has been generated by the work of Strauss and his associates and their contention that minimal brain damage can cause a particular behavioral syndrome in children. For example, Benton (1973) points out that a large amount of animal research and some work with humans suggests that young animals as well as humans can sustain quite severe brain injuries and still not show gross behavioral disturbances. Also, the relationship between brain damage and later behavioral disturbance in children has been found to be quite variable (Ernhardt, Graham, Eichman, Marshall, & Thurston, 1963; Pond, 1961). In spite of these difficulties, the concept of minimal brain damage or dysfunction continues to generate a good deal of research and clinical interest, and has contributed to the view that brain damage in childhood can result in extensive behavioral disturbances (Black, Jeffries, Blumer, Wellner, & Walker, 1969; Rutter, Graham, & Yale, 1970).

HALSTEAD AND THE MODERN ERA OF NEUROPSYCHOLOGY

Chronologically paralleling David Wechsler's development of measurement procedures for assessment of mental ability, Ward Halstead (1908–1969) established at the University of Chicago the first laboratory for the study of behavioral correlations of brain damage in humans. Halstead's academic preparation and prior work having been in animal rather than clinical studies, he proceeded to observe the behavior of persons with known brain damage to determine how they differed from non-brain-damaged persons in the performance of various activities at home, on the job, and in leisure settings. By the mid 1940s, drawing from his first-hand observations of many adults with various types of brain damage, Halstead had developed a fairly comprehensive battery of standardized tests of cortical function (Halstead, 1947). Like the majority of brain behavior researchers of his time, his focus was on differentiation of organic from normal populations, and the classifications of organicity used relatively loose criteria. Working closely with his neurosurgical colleagues, Doctors Percival Bailey and Paul Bucy, Halstead was able to conceptualize, develop, and validate a number of psychological measures that correlated with surgical verification of actual brain pathology. Thus, even though there was considerable heterogeneity among those classified as brain-injured, the accuracy of his tests in differentiating organic from nonorganic patients demonstrated both the inherent soundness in his choices of test items and the power of his combined battery.

During the same era as Halstead's development of his laboratory, other pioneers of the modern era of neuropsychology were developing single tests for the differentiation of organically impaired from unimpaired patients. The primary focus of single diagnostic test research tended to be on short-term memory for nonverbal stimuli, typically geometric figures. In 1943, Hunt produced the Hunt–Minnesota Test (Hunt, 1943), Benton and Ackerly carefully standardized the Benton Visual Retention Test (Benton, 1955), and Graham and Kendall produced their Memory for Designs Test (Graham & Kendall, 1960). Although perhaps appearing somewhat simplistic when examined in light of current neuropsychological knowledge, one cannot help but be impressed by their robustness in differentiating loosely categorized, organically impaired patients from normal controls (i.e., hit rates ranging from 75% to 90%: Korman & Blumberg, 1963; Yates, 1954).

A somewhat different approach was taken by Shipley, who developed a brief "hold–don't hold" type of scale that was a precursor of Wechsler's subsequent and more complicated formula for the Wechsler–Bellevue subtest comparison (Hunt, 1949; Shipley, 1940; Wechsler, 1939). Wechsler's formula, based on his clinical observations that (heterogenously) brain-damaged adults tended to do poorly on subtests requiring immediate memory, concentration, abstraction, and speed of responding, involved a comparison of "hold" tests, which were considered unlikely to decrease with organic impairment, with "don't hold" tests, involving those abilities least resistant to decline. Thus Wechsler compared vocabulary, information, object assembly, and picture completion with digit span, similarities, digit symbol, and block design subscales to derive his deterioration index. Correct classification with this method ranged to 75% (Yates, 1954). Hewson (1949) reclassified subtest scores to yield a ratio reported as 91% successful in identifying brain tumor patients (Smith, 1962).

It is interesting that, although clinical neurologists and neurosurgeons of the time were well aware of lateralization of brain functions, the neuropsychology of the day was concerned with global measures of organic integrity. In 1951, Ralph Reitan, a Halstead student, opened a neuropsychology laboratory at Indiana University Medical Center, and pursued a research strategy that produced psychometric evidence of certain differential effects of right and left cerebral hemisphere lesions (Reitan, 1955). To the extent that the development of knowledge is determined by available methodological approaches (Reitan, 1974), clinical neuropsychology in the decade of the 1950s and beyond must attribute a good deal of its progress to Halstead's seminal contributions and Reitan's refinement of his thinking into an impressive methodology for studying brain-behavior relationships.

Reitan himself pursued many of the potential applications of the battery he refined and augmented it with a number of his own tests, relating test findings to such conditions as site lesion, causal effects, age at onset, premorbid condition, and severity and extent of lesion (Doehring & Reitan, 1962; Klove & Fitzhugh, 1962; Reitan, 1958; Reitan & Davison, 1974; Reitan & Fitzhugh, 1971). By the late 1950s, neuropsychological research was proliferating, to a large extent reflecting the refinements in available measurement procedures (e.g., Benton & Joynt, 1959; Chapman & Wolff, 1959; Fitzhugh, Fitzhugh, & Reitan, 1961; Heimburger & Reitan, 1961; Reitan, 1958), and the foci of the research were becoming much more sophisticated. Although many clinical psychologists continued to treat organically impaired patients as a homogeneous entity, serious neuropsychologists were much more molecular in their studies of brain-behavior relationships.

Lateralization of brain function was an important feature of much research during the decade of the 1960s (e.g., Bakker, 1966; Benton, 1967; Benton & Hecaen, 1970; Costa, Vaughan, Levita, & Farber, 1963; DeRenzi & Faglioni, 1965; Doehring & Reitan, 1962; Gazzaniga, 1965; Geschwind & Levitsky, 1968; Hecaen, 1962; Heimburger & Reitan, 1961; Klove & White, 1963; Lansdell, 1968, 1969; Matthews, Folk, & Zerfas, 1966; McFie & Zangwill, 1960; Meier & French, 1965; Parsons, Vega, & Burn, 1969; Reed, 1967; Reed & Reitan, 1969; Reitan, 1967; Semmes, 1968; Smith, 1966; Sperry, 1961; Spreen & Benton, 1967; von Bonin, 1962; Warrington, James, & Kinsbourne, 1966). An approach to the measurement of lateralization, which became a popular research area during this decade, involved dichotic listening tasks, which was the focus of a fairly wide variety of research attempting to measure asymmetries in the processing of different types of auditory stimuli. Research during this period, with its continued emphasis on basic neurological processes, served an important function in providing a scientific translation on which subsequent clinical research was to be based (e.g., Bryden, 1967, 1969; Curry, 1967; Kimura, 1961, 1964, 1967; Milner, 1962; Milner, Taylor, & Sperry, 1968; Satz, 1968; Sparks & Geschwind, 1968). Such investigatory activity was exemplified in Sperry's Nobel Prize winning research (1981) on split brain behavior.

During the 1960s, Reitan and his coworkers expanded their work with children (Reed & Fitzhugh, 1966; Reed, Reitan, & Klove, 1965; Reitan, 1964), and neurological correlates of various types of learning and behavior problems in children were investigated. Ayres (1963), Bender (1961, 1963), Birch (1964), Frostig, Lefever, and Whittlesey (1961), and Cruickshank and Dolphin (1951) addressed motor problems, and attentional deficits were studied by Chalfant and Scheffelin (1969), Clements (1966), and Cruse (1962). Behavior problems were studied by Sabatino and Cramblett (1968), Doris and Solnit (1963), and Rapin (1964). Neuropsychological correlates of hyperactivity was an area of considerable interest, and Anderson (1963), Buddenhagen and Sickler (1969), Cromwell, Baumeister, and Hawkins (1963), and Werry (1968) were among the researchers focusing on different brain-behavior relationships in this syndrome. Near the end of the decade, Connors (1969) published a scale for the objective measurement of hyperactivity in recognition of the problems resultant from each investigator's use of a different approach to measurement of this condition.

The fruition of the basic research concerning cerebral lateralization was reached in a proliferation of clinically applicable research from the beginning of the 1970s. Russell, Neuringer, and Goldstein's (1970) neuropsychological key approach to integration and interpretation of procedures was developed by Halstead and expanded by Reitan, Klove and James Reed, and other colleagues of Reitan. Small (1973) published a book relating neuropsychodiagnosis to psychotherapy, and Reitan's long-awaited book appeared (Reitan & Davison, 1974). Lezak subsequently published a comprehensive sourcebook in neuropsychology (Lezak, 1976), and Golden (1978) published a book relating neuropsychology to rehabilitation.

Methodological sophistication related cerebral asymmetry reflected in neuropsychological test findings to such newer neurosurgical procedures as angiographic venous patterns (DiChiro, 1972); electrophysiological measures (Grabow & Elliott, 1974; Hartlage & Green, 1972, 1973); amino acid analyses (Hansen, Perry, & Wada, 1972); and regional cerebral blood flow (Ingvar & Schwartz, 1974; Risberg, Halsey, Wills, & Wilson, 1975). Also, the considerable works in split brain research were summarized by Levy (1976). Increasing attention was devoted to developmental cortical asymmetries (Chi, Dooling, & Gilles, 1977;

Galaburda, LeMay, Kemper, & Geschwind, 1978; Yeni-Komishian & Benson, 1976), computerized axial tomography (Golden, Graber, Blose, Berg, Coffman, & Bloch, 1981; Golden, Graber, Coffman, Berg, & Bloch, 1980; Golden, Graber, Moses, & Zatz, 1979, 1980; Golden, Moses, Zelazowski, Graber, Zatz, Horvath, & Berger, 1980) and sex differences (McGlone & Kertesz, 1973; Witelson & Pallie, 1973).

Hemispheric specialization was related to educational programming (Bogen, 1975; Hartlage & Hartlage, 1977, 1978) and psychiatric diagnosis (Galin, 1974) and precipitated vigorous research activities pursuing these lines of inquiry. Special acceleration in research relating neuropsychological processes to learning disabilities began to appear (Hartlage, 1975, 1979; Rourke, 1975).

The burgeoning research in neuropsychology was reflected in the emergence of new journals devoted exclusively to the topic, such as the research-oriented *Journal of Clinical Neuropsychology* and the more practice-oriented *Clinical Neuropsychology*. The increasing numbers of researchers identified with neuropsychology resulted in the formation of the International Neuropsychological Society, and those more concerned with professional practice issues established the National Academy of Neuropsychologists (1975). The American Psychological Association approved a new division of Clinical Neuropsychology (1979), and other professional groups, such as the Association for the Advancement of Behavior Therapy, established neuropsychology special interest groups.

Although a prolific researcher whose work had been published internationally for many years, the Russian psychologist–neurologist A. R. Luria became an important influence on research in the United States in the 1970s. While Christensen's translations of some of his diagnostic approaches into a standardized battery (Christensen, 1975a, 1975b) helped contribute to this influence, it was largely the work of Golden in developing, standardizing, and publicizing a neuropsychological assessment battery based on Luria's concepts that awakened neuropsychologists to the potential of his approach (Golden, 1978; Golden, Hammeke, & Purisch, 1978; Luria & Majovski, 1977; Purisch, Golden, & Hammeke, 1978).

REPRISE

In 1980, surveys of all neuropsychologists in the National Academy of Neuropsychologists and all members of the American Psychological Association Division of Clinical Neuropsychology were conducted. In both surveys, respondents were asked to indicate: (1) the tests they used for neuropsychological assessment; (2) whom they thought had been most influential in U.S. neuropsychology since the 1950s; and (3) such practice-related items as where they practiced, the number of neuropsychological examinations done each month, and whether they used a technician. In the initial survey, Hartlage and Telzrow (1980) found that 89% of respondents included the age-appropriate Wechsler Intelligence scale in a neuro-psychological battery, with 56% including portions of the Reitan Battery, 52% including the Wide Range Achievement Test, 49% including the Bender Gestalt, with 38%, 32%, and 31% respectively including the Entire Reitan Battery, the Benton Visual Retention Test, and the Luria–Nebraska Battery. Named as most influential was Reitan (71%), followed by Halstead (42%) and Benton (31%), with Luria, Golden, Teuber, Geschwind, Hartlage, Milner, and K. Goldstein all named by more than 10% of respondents. Typical neuropsychological practitioners average 15 neuropsychological evaluations per month, with a range of 1 to 84 evaluations per month; 59% used a technician. In the second survey (Hartlage, Chelune, & Tucker, 1981), responses were very similar in most respects, except that this group averaged slightly fewer evaluations per month, and slightly fewer respondents used a technician. The data suggest considerable similarity in perception of appropriate tests and of individuals influencing the profession, and may be viewed as indications of an emerging professional identity among practitioners.

Neuropsychology has evolved from a theoretical approach to discovering whether individuals with brain injury differed from those without such injury, to a highly sophisticated methodologically oriented approach to determining discrete neuropsychological substrates of behavior. Concurrent with the development of a refined methodology has evolved a range of application of findings relative to brain-behavior relationships in such diverse practice areas as medical psychology, neurology, neurosurgery, pediatrics, psychiatry, special education, and rehabilitation. Neuropsychologists are now found in greater numbers in applied rather than academic settings. Far from compromising a research emphasis, however, the affiliation with practitioners in applied settings has led to increased research activity involving correlative studies with computerized tomography, evoked potential, positron emission, and regional cerebral blood flow, and prognostic studies of rehabilitation outcome following a variety of surgical, medical, and social intervention approaches to ameliorating the impact of brain injury.

The progression of neuropsychology into applied areas contains a number of implications for the future of the field. To some extent, reflecting the current *zeitgeist* in health care, neuropsychological research will likely become focused on issues that have more applied foci. This will most likely expand in the areas of neuropsychological processes in the aged; legal matters related to effects of head trauma on residual functional capacities; and the evaluation of the efficacy of given medical and surgical regimens. Less obvious but nonetheless important emphasis areas in neuropsychology will involve its role in educational and vocational planning, involving both neurologically handicapped and normal populations. Practicing psychologists will increasingly perceive the neurological substrates of behavior as being relevant to their practice, and will seek advanced training in neuropsychology as part of their continuing education.

University training in neuropsychology can be expected to expand, primarily in the form of emphasis on neuropsychology as an adjunct to traditional graduate programs in clinical and school psychology, although a few universities will inaugurate formal graduate programs with a terminal focus on neuropsychology. Thus, by the end of the present decade, neuropsychology will be recognized both as a discrete speciality area of professional practice, and as an academic field with implications for a variety of traditional psychological research foci.

The placing in focus of the major historical antecedents of current neuropsychological theory and practice should enable emerging psychologists, independent of area of expertise, to appreciate the contributions of the leaders in the field, and should provide these new professionals with the challenge to build on the work of these pioneers for the better understanding of human neurological assets for dealing with the complexities of this world.

REFERENCES

Anderson, W. The hyperkinetic child: A neurological appraisal. *Neurology*, 1963, *13*, 317–382.

Ayres, A. J. The development of perceptual–motor abilities: A theoretical basis for treatment of dysfunction. *American Journal of Occupational Therapy*, 1963, *17*, 221–225.

Babinski, J. Contribution à l'étude des troubles mentaux dans l'hémiplégré organique cérébrale (amosognosie). *Revue Nuerologie*, 1914, *22*, 845–848.

Bakker, D. J. Sensory dominance in normal and backward readers. *Perceptual and Motor Skills*, 1966, *23*, 1055–1058.

Belmont, L., & Birch, H. G. Lateral dominance, lateral awareness and reading disability. *Child Development*, 1965, *36*, 57–72.

Bender, L. The brain and child behavior. *Archives of General Psychiatry*, 1961, *4*, 531–548.

Bender, L. The concept of plasticity from a neurological and psychiatric point of view. *American Journal of Orthopsychiatry*, 1963, *33*, 305–307.

Benton, A. L. Development of finger-localization capacity in school children. *Child Development*, 1955, *26*, 225–230.

Benton, A. L. *The revised visual retention test.* New York: Psychological Corporation, 1963.

Benton, A. L. Constructional apraxia and the minor hemisphere. *Confinia Neurologica*, 1967, *29*, 1–16.

Benton, A. L. Constructional apraxia: Some unanswered questions. In A. L. Benton (Ed.), *Contributions to Clinical Neuropsychology.* New York: Aldine, 1969.

Benton, A. L. The minor hemisphere. *Journal of the History of Medicine and Allied Sciences*, 1972, *27*, 5–14.

Benton, A. L. *Test of three-dimensional constructional praxis (Manual).* Neurosensory Center Publications No. 286., University of Iowa, 1973.

Benton, A. L., & Fogel, M. L. Three-dimensional constructional praxis: A clinical test. *Archives of Neurology*, 1962, *7*, 347.

Benton, A. L., & Hecaen, H. Stereoscopic vision in patients with unilateral cerebral disease. *Neurology*, 1970, *20*, 1084–1088.

Benton, A. L., & Joynt, R. J. Reaction time in unilateral cerebral disease. *Confinia Neurologica*, 1959, *19*, 247.

Benton, A. L., & Meyers, R. An early definition of the Gerstmann syndrome. *Neurology*, 1956, *6*, 838–842.

Benton, A. L., Meyers, R., & Polder, G. Some aspects of handedness. *Psychiatric Neurology*, 1962, *144*, 321–337.

Bianchi, L. *The mechanism of the brain and the function of the frontal lobes*. New York: Livingston, 1922.

Birch, H. G. (Ed.). *Brain damage in children: The biological and social aspects*. Baltimore: Williams & Wilkins, 1964.

Black, P., Jeffries, J. J., Blumer, D., Wellner, A. M., & Walker, A. E. The post-traumatic syndrome in children: Characteristics and incidence. In A. E. Walker, W. F. Caveness, and M. Critchley (Eds.), *The late effects of head injury*. Springfield, Ill.: Charles C Thomas, 1969.

Bogen, J. E. Some educational aspects of hemisphere specialization. *UCLA Educator*, 1975, *17*, 24–32.

Bolton, J. S. The function of the frontal lobes. *Brain*, 1903a, *26*, 215–241.

Bolton, J. S. The histological basis of amentia and dementia. *Archives of Neurology*, 1903b, *2*, 424–620.

Brain, W. R. Visual disorientation with special reference to lesions of the right cerebral hemisphere. *Brain*, 1941, *64*, 244–272.

Bryden, M. P. An evaluation of some models of laterality effects in dichotic listening. *Acta Oto Laryngolgica*, 1967, *63*, 595–604.

Bryden, M. P. Binaural competition and division of attention as determinants of the laterality effects in dichotic listening. *Canadian Journal of Psychology*, 1969, *23*, 101–113.

Buddenhagen, R., & Sickler, P. Hyperactivity: A forty-eight hour sample plus a note on etiology. *American Journal of Mental Deficiency*, 1969, *73*, 580.

Chalfant, J. C., & Scheffelin, M. A. *Central processing dysfunctions in children: A review of research*. NINDS Monograph No. 9. Bethesda, Md.: U.S. Department of HEW, 1969.

Chapman, L. F., & Wolff, H. G. The cerebral hemispheres and the highest integrative functions of man. *Archives of Neurology*, 1959, *1*, 357–424.

Chi, J. G., Dooling, E. C., & Gilles, F. H. Gyral development of the human brain. *Annals of Neurology*, 1977, *1*, 86.

Christensen, A.L. *Luria's neuropsychological investigation*. New York: Spectrum, 1975a.

Christensen, A. L. *Luria's neuropsychological investigation: Text cards and manual*. New York: Spectrum, 1975b.

Clements, S. D. *Minimal brain dysfunction in children—Technology and identification*. NINDB Monograph No. 3. Washington D.C.: U.S. Public Health Service, 1966.

Connors, K. A teacher rating scale for use in drug studies with children. *American Journal of Psychiatry*, 1969, *126*, 884–888.

Costa, L. D., Vaughan, H. G., Levita, E., & Farber, N. Purdue pegboard as a predictor of the presence of the laterality of cerebral lesions. *Journal of Consulting Psychology*, 1963, *27*, 133–137.

Critchley, M. *The parietal lobes*. Baltimore: Williams & Wilkins, 1953.

Cromwell, R. L., Baumeister, A., & Hawkins, W. F. Research in activity level. In N. Ellis (Ed.), *Handbook of mental retardation*. New York: McGraw-Hill, 1963.

Croxen, M. E., & Lytton, H. Reading disability and difficulties in finger localization and right–left discrimination. *Developmental Psychology*, 1971, *5*, 256–262.

Cruickshank, W. M., & Dolphin, J. E. The educational implications of psychological studies of cerebral palsied children. *Exceptional Children*, 1951, *18*, 3–11.

Cruse, D. B. The effects of distraction upon the performance of brain-injured and familial retarded children. In E. P. Trapp & P. Himelstein (Eds.), *Readings on the Exceptional Child*. New York: Appleton-Century-Crofts, 1962.

Curry, F. K. W. A comparison of left-handed and right-handed subjects on verbal and nonverbal dichotic listening tasks. *Cortex*, 1967, *3*, 343–352.

DeRenzi, E., & Faglioni, P. The comparative efficiency of intelligence and vigilance tests in detecting hemispheric damage. *Cortex,* 1965, *1,* 410–433.

DiChiro, G. Venous patterns of cerebral dominance. *New England Journal of Medicine,* 1972, *287,* 933–934.

Dide, M. Les désorientations temporo-spatiales et la preponderance de l'hemisphere droit dans les agnoso-akinesies proprioceptives. *Encephale,* 1938, *33,* 276–294.

Doehring, D. G., & Reitan, R. M. Concept attainment of human adults with lateralized cerebral lesions. *Perceptual and Motor Skills,* 1962, *14,* 27–33.

Doris, J., & Solnit, A. J. Treatment of children with brain damage and associated school problems. *Journal of the Academy of Child Psychiatry,* 1963, *2,* 618–635.

Ebaugh, F. G. Neuropsychiatric sequelae of acute epidemic encephalitis in children. *American Journal of Diseases of Children,* 1923, *25,* 89–97.

Ernhardt, C., Graham, F., Eichman, P., Marshall, J., & Thurston, D. Brain injury in the preschool child: Some developmental considerations: 11 comparisons of brain-injured and normal children. *Psychological Monographs,* 1963, *77,* 17–33.

Ettlinger, G. Defective identification of fingers. *Neuropsychologia,* 1963, *1,* 39–45.

Ferrier, D. *The functions of the brain.* London: Smith, Elder, 1876.

Fitzhugh, K. B., Fitzhugh, L. C., & Reitan, R. M. Psychological deficits in relation to acuteness of brain dysfunction. *Journal of Consulting Psychology,* 1961, *25,* 61–66.

Flourens, P. Recherches expérimentales sur les propriétés et les fonctions du systeme nerveux dans les animaux vertebres. Paris: Cervot, 1824.

Frostig, M., Lefever, D. W., & Whittlesey, J. R. B. A developmental test of visual perception for evaluating normal and neurologically handicapped children. *Perceptual and Motor Skills,* 1961, *12,* 383–394.

Galaburda, A. M., LeMay, M., Kemper, T. L., & Geschwind, N. Left–right asymmetries in the brain. *Science,* 1978, *199,* 852–856.

Galin, D. Implications for psychiatry of left–right cerebral specialization. *Archives of General Psychiatry,* 1974, *31,* 440–443.

Gates, A. I., & Bennett, C. C. *Reversal tendencies in reading.* New York: Bureau of Publications, Teachers College, Columbia University, 1933.

Gazzaniga, M. S. Psychological properties of the disconnected hemispheres in man. *Science,* 1965, *150,* 372.

Gerstmann, J. Fingeragnosie. Eine umschriebene Störung der Orientierung am eigenen körper. *Wiener Klinische Wochenschrift,* 1924, *37,* 1010–1012.

Gerstmann, J. Syndrome of finger agnosia, disorientation for right and left, agraphia, and acalculia. *Archives of Neurology and Psychiatry,* 1940, *44,* 398–408.

Geschwind N., & Levitsky, W. Human brain: Left–right asymmetries in temporal speech regions. *Science,* 1968, *161,* 186–187.

Golden, C. J. *Diagnosis and rehabilitation in clinical neuropsychology.* Springfield, Ill.: Charles C Thomas, 1978.

Golden, C. J., Graber, B., Blose, I., Berg, R., Coffman, J., and Bloch, S. Difference in brain densities between chronic alcoholic and normal control patients. *Science,* 1981, *211,* 508–510.

Golden, C. J., Graber, B., Coffman, J., Berg, R., & Bloch, S. Brain density deficits in chronic schizophrenia. *Psychiatry Research,* 1980, *3,* 179–184.

Golden, C. J., Graber, B., Moses, J. A., & Zatz, L. N. Relationships of neuropsychological test scores to ventricular enlargement in schizophrenic patients. *Journal of Computer Assisted Tomography,* 1979, *3,* 563.

Golden C. J., Graber, B., Moses, J. A., Jr., & Zatz, L. Differentiation of chronic schizophrenics with and without ventricular enlargement by the Luria–Nebraska Neuropsychological Battery. *International Journal of Neuroscience,* 1980, *11,* 131–138.

Golden, C. J., Hammeke, T. A., & Purisch, A. D. Diagnostic validity of a standardized neuropsychological battery derived from Luria's neuropsychological tests. *Journal of Consulting and Clinical Psychology,* 1978, *46,* 1258-1265. (Reprinted in *Clinical Neuropsychology,* 1979, *1,* 1-6.)

Golden, C. J., Moses, J. A., Jr., Zelazowski, R., Graber, B., Zatz, L. M., Horvath, T. B., & Berger, P. A. Cerebral ventricular size and neuropsychological impairment in young chronic schizophrenics. *Archives of General Psychiatry,* 1980, *37,* 619-623.

Goldstein, K. Die Lokalisation in der Grosshirnrinde. In A. Bethe, G. von Bergman, G. Embden, & A. Ellingsi (Eds.), *Handbuch der Normalen und Pathologischen Physiologie (Vol. 10).* Berlin: Springer, 1927.

Goldstein, K. *The organism: A holistic approach to biology.* New York: American, 1939.

Goldstein, K., & Scheerer, M. Abstract and concrete behavior. *Psychological Monographs,* 1941, *53*(2), 1-151.

Grabow, J. D., & Elliott, F. W. The electrophysiological assessment of hemispheric asymmetries during speech. *Journal of Speech and Hearing Research,* 1974, *17,* 64-72.

Graham, F., & Kendall, B. Memory for designs test: Revised general manual. *Perceptual & Motor Skills,* 1960, *11,* 147-188.

Halstead, W. C. *Brain and intelligence.* Chicago: University of Chicago Press, 1947.

Hammarberg, C. *Studien über Klinik und Pathologie der Idiotie.* Upsala, Sweden: E. Berling, 1895.

Hanfmann, E. Thought disturbances in schizophrenia as revealed by performance on a picture completion test. *Journal of Abnormal and Social Psychology,* 1939, *34,* 249-284.

Hansen, S., Perry, T. L., & Wada, J. A. Amino acid analysis of speech areas in human brain: Absence of left–right asymmetry. *Brain Research,* 1972, *45,* 318-320.

Hartlage, L. C. Neuropsychological approaches to predicting outcome of remedial educational strategies for learning disabled children. *Pediatric Psychology,* 1975, *3,* 23.

Hartlage, L. C. Current states and future directions in clinical neuropsychology. *Gramma,* 1979, *3,* 1-2.

Hartlage, L. C., & Green, J. B. EEG abnormalities and WISC subtest differences. *Journal of Clinical Psychology,* 1972, *28,* 170-171.

Hartlage, L. C., & Green, J. B. The EEG as a predictor of intellective and academic performance. *Journal of Learning Disabilities,* 1973, *6,* 42-45.

Hartlage, L. C., & Hartlage, P. L. Relationships between neurological, behavioral, and academic variables. *Journal of Clinical Psychology,* 1977, *6,* 52-53.

Hartlage, L. C., & Hartlage, P. L. Clinical consultation to Pediatric Neurology and Developmental Pediatrics. *Journal of Clinical Child Psychology,* 1978, *7,* 52-53.

Hartlage, L. C., & Telzrow, C. F. The practice of clinical neuropsychology in the U.S. *Clinical Neuropsychology,* 1980, *2,* 200-202.

Hartlage, L. C., Chelune, G., & Tucker, D. Survey of professional issues in the practice of clinical neuropsychology. Paper presented at American Psychological Association, Los Angeles, California, 1981.

Head, H. *Aphasia and kindred disorders of speech.* New York: Hafner, 1963.

Hebb, D. O. Intelligence in man after large removals of cerebral tissue. Defects following right temporal lobectomy. *Journal of General Psychology,* 1939, *21,* 437-446.

Hecaen, H. Clinical symptomatology in right and left hemisphere lesions. In V. B. Mountcastle (Ed.), *Interhemispheric Relations and Cerebral Dominance.* Baltimore: Johns Hopkins University Press, 1962.

Heimburger, R. F., & Reitan, R. M. Easily administered written test for lateralizing brain lesions. *Journal of Neurosurgery,* 1961, *18,* 301-312.

Hemann, K. Specific reading disability. *Danish Medical Bulletin,* 1964, *11,* 34-40.

Hewson, L. The Wechsler–Bellevue Scale and the substitution test as aids in neuropsychiatric diagnosis. *Journal of Nervous and Mental Disease,* 1949, *109,* 158-183.

Hitzig, F. Zur physiologie des grosshirms. *Archiv fur Psychiatrie und Nervenheilkrankheit,* 1884, *15,* 270–275.

Hohman, L. B. Post encephalitic behavior disorders in children. *Johns Hopkins Hospital Bulletin,* 1922, *33,* 372–375.

Hunt, H. F. A practical clinical test for organic brain damage. *Journal of Applied Psychology,* 1943, *27,* 375–386.

Hunt, J. On the localization of the functions of the brain with special reference faculty of language (Part II). *The Anthropological Review,* 1949, *7,* 100–116.

Hunt, W. L. The relative rates of decline of Wechsler–Bellevue "hold–don't hold" tests. *Journal of Consulting Psychology,* 1949, *13,* 440–443.

Ingvar, D. H., & Schwartz, M. S. Blood flow patterns induced in the dominant hemisphere by speech and reading. *Brain,* 1974, *97,* 278–288.

Jackson, J. H. On the nature of the duality of the brain. *Medical Press,* 1874, *17.* (Reprinted in *Brain,* 1915, *38,* 80–103.)

Jackson, J. H. *Selected writings of John Hughlings Jackson* (2 vols.). London: Hodder, 1931–1932.

Kimura, D. Cerebral dominance and the perception of verbal stimuli. *Canadian Journal of Psychology,* 1961, *15,* 166–171.

Kimura, D. Left–right differences in the perception of melodies. *Quarterly Journal of Experimental Psychology,* 1964, *16,* 355–358.

Kimura, D. Functional asymmetry of the brain in dichotic listening. *Cortex,* 1967, *3,* 163–178.

Kleist, K. Kriegsverletzungen des Gehirns in ihrer Bedeutung für Hirnlokalisation und Hirnpathologie. In O. von Scherning (Ed.), *Handbuch der ärtzlichen Erfahrung im Weltkriege, 1914–1918* (Vol. 4). *Geistes- und Nervenkrankheiten.* Leipzig: Barth, 1923.

Klove, H., & Fitzhugh, K. B. Relationship of differential EEG patterns to the distribution of Wechsler–Bellevue scores in a chronic epileptic population. *Journal of Clinical Psychology,* 1962, *18,* 334–337.

Klove, H., & White, P. T. The relationship of degree of electroencephalographic abnormality to the distribution of Wechsler–Bellevue scores. *Neurology,* 1963, *13,* 423–430.

Korman, M. A., & Blumberg, S. Comparative efficiency of some tests of cerebral damage. *Journal of Consulting Psychology,* 1963, *27,* 303–309.

Lange, J. Agnosien und apraxien. In O. Bunke & O. Foerster (Eds.), *Handbuch der Neurologie* (Vol. 6). Berlin: Springer, 1936.

Lansdell, H. C. Effect of context of temporal lobe ablations on two lateralized deficits. *Physiology & Behavior,* 1968, *3,* 271–273.

Lansdell, H. C. Verbal and nonverbal factors in right hemisphere speech: Relation to early neurological history. *Journal of Comparative and Physiological Psychology,* 1969, *69,* 734–738.

Lashley, K. S. *Brain mechanisms and intelligence.* Chicago: University of Chicago Press, 1929.

Lee, D. A. *Paul Broca and the history of aphasia* (Roland McKay Award Essay, 1980). *Neurology,* 1981, *31,* 600–602.

Levy, J. Cerebral asymmetries as manifested in split-brain man. In M. Kinsbourne & W. L. Smith (Eds.). *Hemispheric disconnection and cerebral function.* New York: Spectrum, 1976.

Lezak, M. D. *Neuropsychological assessment.* New York: Oxford University Press, 1976.

Leipmann, H. Das Krankheitsbild der Apraxie. *Monatsschrift für Psychiatrie und Neurologie,* 1900, *8,* 15–44, 102–132, 182–197.

Loeb, J. *Comparative physiology of the brain and comparative psychology.* New York: Putnam, 1902.

Luria, A. R. *Higher cortical function in man.* New York: Basic Books, 1966.

Luria, A. R., & Majovski, L. V. Basic approaches used in American and Soviet clinical neuropsychology. *American Psychologist,* 1977, *32,* 959–968.

Mahan, H. C. Early quantitative studies of neuropsychological impairment, 1899–1939. *Clinical Neuropsychology*, 1980, *2*, 38–45.

Mann, L. *On the trail of process*. New York: Grune & Stratton, 1979.

Marie, P. Revision de la question de l'aphasie: La troisième circonvolution frontale gauche ne joue aucun rôle spécial dans la fonction du language. *Semaine Medicale*, 1906, *26*, 241–247.

Matthews, C. G., Folk, E. D., & Zerfas, P. G. Lateralized finger localization deficits and differential Wechsler–Bellevue results in retardates. *American Journal of Mental Deficiency*, 1966, *70*, 695–702.

McFie, L., & Zangwill, O. Visual-constructive disabilities associated with lesions of the left cerebral hemisphere. *Brain*, 1960, *83*, 243–260.

McGlone, J., & Kertesz, A. Sex differences in cerebral processing of visuo-spatial tasks. *Cortex*, 1973, *9*, 313–320.

McHenry, L. C. *Garrison's history of neurology*. Springfield, Ill.: Charles C Thomas, 1969.

Meier, M. J., & French, L. A. Lateralized deficits in complex visual discrimination and bilateral transfer of reminiscence following unilateral temporal lobectomy. *Neuropsychologia*, 1965, *3*, 261–273.

Milner, B. Laterality effects in audition. In V. B. Mountcastle (Ed.), *Interhemispheric relations and cerebral dominance*. Baltimore: Johns Hopkins University Press, 1962.

Milner, B., Taylor, L., & Sperry, R. W. Lateralized suppression of dichotically presented digits after commissural section in man. *Science*, 1968, *161*, 185–186.

Monakow, C. von. *Die Lokalisation im Grosshirn und der Abbau der Funktionen durch Corticale Herde*. Wiesbaden: Bergmann, 1914.

Money, J. Developmental dyslexia. In P. J. Vinren & G. W. Bruyn (Eds.), *Handbook of Clinical Neurology* (Vol. 4). New York: Wiley, 1969.

Munk, H. *Über die Funktionen von Hirn und rückenmark*. Berlin: A. Hirschwald, 1909.

Orton, S. T. Specific reading disability—strephosymbolia. *Journal of the American Medical Association*, 1928, *90*, 1095–1099.

Orton, S. T. *Reading, writing and speech problems in children*. London: Chapman Hall, 1937.

Parsons, O. A., Vega, A., & Burn, J. Different psychological effects of lateralized brain damage. *Journal of Consulting & Clinical Psychology*, 1969, *33*, 551–557.

Peters, J. E., Romine, J. S., & Dykman, R. A. A special neurological examination of children with learning disabilities. *Developmental Medicine and Child Neurology*, 1975, *17*, 63–78.

Pond, D. Psychiatric aspects of epileptic and brain-damaged children. *British Medical Journal*, 1961, *2*, 1377–1382, 1454–1459.

Preston, M. I. Late behavioral effects found in cases of prenatal, perinatal, and postnatal anoxia. *Journal of Pediatrics*, 1945, *26*, 353–366.

Purisch, A. D., Golden, C. J., & Hammeke, T. A. Discrimination of schizophrenic and brain damaged patients by a standardized version of Luria's neuropsychological tests. *Journal of Consulting and Clinical Psychology*, 1978, *46*, 1266–1273.

Rapin, I. Brain damage in children. In J. Brennemann (Ed.), *Practice of pediatrics* (Vol. 4). Hagerstown, Md.: Prior Publications, 1964.

Reed, J. C. Lateralized finger agnosia and reading achievement at ages 6 and 10. *Child Development*, 1967, *38*, 213–220.

Reed, H. B. C., Jr., & Fitzhugh, K. B. Patterns of deficits in relation to severity of cerebral dysfunction in children and adults. *Journal of Consulting and Clinical Psychology*, 1966, *30*, 98–102.

Reed, J. C., & Reitan, R. M. Verbal performance differences among brain-injured children with lateralized mortor deficits. *Perceptual and Motor Skills*, 1969, *29*, 747–752.

Reed, H. B. C., Jr., Reitan, R. M., & Klove, H. The influence of cerebral lesions on psychological test performances of older children. *Journal of Consulting Psychology*, 1965, 29, 247–251.

Reichardt, M. *Allgemeine und spezielle Psychiatric. Ein Lehrbuch für Studierinde und Arzte.* Jena: G. Fisher, 1923.

Reitan, R. M. Certain differential effects of left and right cerebral lesions in human adults. *Journal of Comparative Physiological Psychology,* 1955, *48,* 474–484.

Reitan, R. M. Validity of the Trail Making Test as an indicator of organic brain damage. *Perceptual and Motor Skills,* 1958, *8,* 271–276.

Reitan, R. M. *Manual for administering and scoring the Reitan–Indiana neuropsychological battery for children (aged 5 through 8).* Indianapolis: University of Indiana Medical Center, 1964.

Reitan, R. M. Psychological assessment of deficits associated with brain lesions in subjects with normal and subnormal intelligence. In J. L. Khanna (Ed.), *Brain damage and mental retardation: A psychological evaluation.* Springfield, Ill.: Charles C Thomas, 1967.

Reitan, R. M. Methodological problems in clinical neuropsychology. In Reitan, R. M., & Davison, L. A. (Eds.), *Clincial neuropsychology: Current status and applications.* Washington, D.C.: V. H. Winston & Sons, 1974.

Reitan, R. M., & Davison, L. A. *Clinical neuropsychology: Current status and applications.* Washington, D.C.: V. H. Winston & Sons, 1974.

Reitan, R. M., & Fitzhugh, K. B. Behavioral deficits in groups with cerebral vascular lesions. *Journal of Consulting and Clinical Psychology,* 1971, *37,* 215–223.

Rieger, C. Über Apparate in dem Hirn. *Arb Psychatriche Klinik Wuerzburg,* 1909, *5,* 176–197.

Riese, W. *A history of neurology.* New York: M. D. Publications, 1959.

Risberg, J., Halsey, J. H., Wills, E. L., & Wilson, E. M. Hemispheric specialization in normal man studied by bilateral measurements of the regional cerebral blood flow: A study with the 133-Xe inhalation technique. *Brain,* 1975, *98,* 511–524.

Rosenfeld, G. B., & Bradley, C. Childhood behavior sequelae of asphyxia in infancy. *Pediatrics,* 1948, *12,* 486–494.

Rourke, B. P. Brain-behavior relationships in children with learning disabilities. *The American Psychologist,* 1975, *30,* 911–920.

Russell, E. W., Neuringer, C., & Goldstein, G. *Assessment of brain damage.* New York: Wiley, 1970.

Rutter, M., Graham, P., & Yale, W. *A neuropsychiatric study in childhood.* Philadelphia: Lippincott, 1970.

Sabatino, D., & Cramblett, H. Behavioral sequelae of California encephalitis virus infection in children. *Developmental Medicine and Child Neurology,* 1968, *10,* 331–337.

Satz, P. Laterality effects in dichotic listening. *Nature,* 1968, *218,* 277–78.

Semmes, J. Hemispheric specialization: A possible clue to mechanism. *Neuropsychologia,* 1968, *6,* 11–26.

Shipley, W. C. A self administering scale for measuring intellectual impairment and deterioration. *New England Journal of Medicine,* 1940, *293,* 113–118.

Small, L. *Neuropsychodiagnosis in psychotherapy.* New York: Brunner/Mazel, 1973.

Smith, A. Psychodiagnosis of patients with brain tumors. *Journal of Nervous and Mental Diseases,* 1962, *135,* 513–533.

Smith, A. Certain hypothesized hemispheric differences in language and visual functions in human adults. *Cortex,* 1966, *2,* 109–126.

Sparks, R., & Geschwind, N. Dichotic listening in man after section of neocortical commissures. *Cortex,* 1968, *4,* 3–16.

Sparrow, S., & Satz, P. Dyslexia, laterality, and neuropsychological development. In D. J. Bakker & P. Satz (Eds.), *Specific reading disability.* Rotterdam: Rotterdam University Press, 1970.

Sperry, R. W. Cerebral organization and behavior. *Science,* 1961, *133,* 1749.

Spoerl, H. Faculties versus traits: The solution of Franz Joseph Gall. *Character and Personality,* 1936, *4,* 216–231.

Spreen, O., & Benton, A. L. Comparative studies of some psychological tests for cerebral damage. *Journal of Nervous and Mental Disease*, 1967, *140*, 323-333.

Stengel, E. Loss of spatial orientation, constructional apraxia, and Gerstmann's syndrome. *Journal of Mental Science*, 1944, *90*, 753-760.

Strauss, A. A. Typology in mental deficiency. *Proceedings of the American Association of Mental Deficiency*, 1939, *44*, 85-90.

Strauss, A. A., & Lehtinen, L. E. *Psychopathology and education of the brain-injured child* (Vol. 2). New York: Grune and Stratton, 1955.

Strauss, A. A., & Werner, H. Deficiency in the finger schema in relation to arithmetic disability (finger agnosia and acalculia). *American Journal of Orthopsychiatry*, 1938, *8*, 719-724.

Strother, C. R. Minimal cerebral dysfunction: A historical overview. *Annals of the New York Academy of Science*, 1973, *205*, 6-17.

Thomas, R. K. Mass function and equipotentiality: A reanalysis of Lashley's retention data. *Psychological Reports*, 1970, *27*, 899-902.

Tizard, B. Theories of brain localization from Flourens to Lashley. *Medical History*, 1959, *3*, 132-145.

Tregold, A. F. *Mental deficiency (amentia)*. New York: William Wood, 1908.

Vignolo, L. A. Auditory agnosia: A review and report of recent evidence. In A. L. Benton (Ed.), *Contributions to clinical neuropsychology*. Chicago: Aldine, 1969.

Vigotsky, L. S. Thought in schizophrenia (J. Kasanin, trans.). *Archives of Neurology and Psychiatry*, 1934, *31*, 1063-1077.

von Bonin, G. Anatomical asymmetries of the cerebral hemispheres. In V. B. Mountcastle (Ed.), *Interhemispheric relations and cerebral dominance*. Baltimore: Johns Hopkins University Press, 1962.

Warrington, E. K., James, M., & Kinsbourne, M. Drawing disability in relation to laterality of cerebral lesion. *Brain*, 1966, *86*, 53-82.

Wechsler, D. *Measurement of adult intelligence*. Baltimore: Williams and Wilkins, 1939.

Weisenberg, T., & McBride, K. *Aphasia: A clinical and psychological study*. New York: Commonwealth Fund, 1935.

Wernicke, K. *Das aphasische Symptomekomplex*. Breslau, Poland: Cohn and Weigart, 1874.

Werry, J. Studies on the hyperactive child. IV. Empirical analysis of the Minimum Brain Dysfunction syndrome. *Archives of General Psychiatry*, 1968, *19*, 9-16.

Witelson, S. F., & Pallie, W. Left hemisphere specialization for language in the newborn. *Brain*, 1973, *96*, 641-646.

Wolfe, L. S. An experimental study of reversals in reading. *American Journal of Psychology*, 1939, *52*, 533-561.

Yates, A. J. The validity of some psychological tests of brain damage. *Psychological Bulletin*, 1954, *51*, 359-379.

Yeni-Komishian, G. H., & Benson, D. A. Anatomical study of cerebral asymmetry in the temporal lobe of humans, chimpanzees, and rhesus monkeys. *Science*, 1976, *192*, 387-389.

2

Assessment of Visual–Motor Skills

JAMES A. MOSES, JR.

The neuropsychological assessment of visual–motor functioning often seems to be a simple matter to the novice. One has the patient copy or recall a few simple line drawings or block or stick constructions, and the quality of these is compared to some objective standard for accuracy, speed, and/or quality of performance. The processes underlying these seemingly simple behaviors are, however, very complex. The variety of apraxias and agnosias known to clinical neurologists and neuropsychologists attests to the numerous ways in which voluntary action and perception may be impaired. The whole cerebral cortex must be mobilized in an integrated fashion to smoothly complete drawing, construction, and/or perceptual processes routinely (Luria, 1966, 1973). It is only after long practice through a childhood developmental sequence that these processes become automatized and hence seemingly simple to the adult with normal brain functioning, in whom they have become overlearned.

If the patient draws the necessary figures accurately or otherwise performs the tasks provided in an unimpaired way, we need not necessarily concern ourselves as clinicians with the complexities of the response process. The normal performance usually is passed off as elementary. If, however, there is distortion, omission, or rotation of the figures drawn, then one must begin to analyze the complex visual–motor encoding and decoding processes involved to find the point or points

JAMES A. MOSES, JR. ● Psychology Services, Palo Alto Veterans Administration Medical Center, Palo Alto, California 94304, and Department of Psychiatry and Behavioral Sciences, Stanford University School of Medicine, Stanford, California 94305.

at which the patient experiences difficulty. Is s/he able to perceptually recognize the figures to be drawn? If not, then the motor output apparatus alone cannot yield an adequate reproduction by itself. On the other hand, a patient may be able to perceptually recognize the stimulus but s/he may be unable to motorically reproduce the figure. Another patient with prefrontal lobe dysfunction or damage may be unable to form an integrated plan to execute the task and thus may make impulsive guesses at solution or perseverative reproductions of simpler, more elementary figures when s/he cannot cope with the complexities of the more difficult items. Such a patient may have intact perceptual and motor skills but still make errors on a reproduction or recall task. When errors are made, one must consider further what has gone awry. The same performance can occur for a variety of reasons. It is possible and necessary to test these alternatives with relatively simple drawing and constructional tasks in the case of visual–motor dysfunction.

Visual–motor tasks should be chosen to highlight the central entity of a perceptual or motoric process. They can be graded in level of difficulty so that one can determine at what level and in what sensory modality the performance deficit emerges. Here we will be considering only visual input and motor output. There are, of course, many other input–output sensorimotor feedback loops through which we process information. Auditory–verbal, visual–verbal, and haptic–motor are a few examples of these cross-modal transfer pathways. We will be considering only the visual–motor sphere in detail to understand assessment of this input–output system more thoroughly.

The patient who has sustained cerebral injury experiences a breakdown of the integrated, automatized mode of problem-solving that is characteristic of the visual–motor performance of the adult. Visual–motor regression ensues and there emerges a more elementary, piecemeal attempt at feature analysis. Thus an adult who has already learned to automatically recognize the difference between the lower case letters "b" and "d" will write them spontaneously without difficulty. If this individual sustains a left posterior parietal lobe injury, however, there will be great laboring to distinguish the differences in orientation of the bottom part of these letters and their common vertical line element (Conley, Moses, & Helle, 1980). A child who is learning to write for the first time experiences the same sort of difficulty because the relevant portion of the association cortex has not yet been programmed to perform the feature analysis and recognition routinely. An adult learning a foreign language with a different alphabet would experience similar difficulty. The more severe the decompensation in the adult, the more elementary and piecemeal his or her attempts at task solution tend to become. This reversal of the developmental progression in the adult with cerebral disease or dysfunction is seen clearly in impaired adult performance on the Bender–Gestalt Test, which has a well understood developmental sequence and an established set of norms for children and adults (cf. Bender, 1938; Koppitz, 1964; Pascal & Suttell, 1951).

BENDER VISUAL MOTOR GESTALT TEST

The Bender Visual Motor Gestalt Test (more commonly known as the Bender–Gestalt, after its creator Lauretta Bender and the Gestalt school of psychology from which she drew her basic ideas) was introduced as a clinical technique to investigate visual–motor functioning of adults and children (Bender, 1938). It consists of nine geometric designs that were taken from figures originally employed in experimental studies of visual perception by Wertheimer (1923). The rationale advanced by Bender in support of her technique followed directly from the Gestalt school's theory that perception is a holistic integrative function of the central nervous system (CNS). The ability to carry out a visual–motor task thus should require intact CNS functioning, and impairment of visual–motor functioning on copying tasks of graded complexity should be sensitive to the effects of cerebral dysfunction. This position has been confirmed and extended by a wide variety of studies since the test was introduced (cf. Golden, 1978; Lacks, 1979; Lacks & Newport, 1980; and Lezak, 1976, for reviews). Today the Bender–Gestalt remains the most widely used screening test in psychiatric settings for the evaluation of cerebral dysfunction. Its usage is reported by 73.7% of clinicians in a recent survey (Craig, 1979).

The usual administration procedure involves placing each figure to be copied before the patient on a card with the request that s/he copy it on a blank sheet of paper as well as possible. Some examiners advocate an incidental memory task after the subject is allowed to copy each of the figures. Each card is placed on top of the previous one as it is copied. In this way each figure is exposed only once, for as long as the patient requires to copy it. When all of the figures have been copied, the cards and the patient's reproductions of them are removed and a new sheet of blank paper is provided. Then the patient is told to draw as many of the designs as s/he can recall. Normal individuals with intact cerebral functioning typically can recall five or more of the nine designs with this procedure or the Wepman modification (Lezak, 1976; Van Couvering, 1970).

Lezak (1976) cites a more detailed procedure for Bender–Gestalt administration that was suggested by Wepman. He advocates a three-step procedure. The patient first is shown each card for 5 seconds to memorize the pattern, after which the card is removed and s/he reproduces it from immediate memory. After all nine designs have been recalled in this manner, the drawing sheet is removed and a new blank piece of paper is provided. The cards are again shown one at a time to the patient, who is asked to copy each of them with the card in full view for the entire copying period. Each new figure is presented only once by placing the subsequent card on top of it. Thereafter the sheet with the copied designs and the cards are removed, and the patient is given another sheet of blank paper. Without previous warning s/he then is asked to reproduce as many of the designs as s/he can recall. Small (1973) advocates another procedure with presentation of only the designs A, 3, and 4 for a 5-second interval for immediate reproduction from memory. He follows this with the usual copying task. This procedure seems less satisfactory because only three of the nine designs are evaluated on the immediate memory task, and even with the nine-design procedure there is a relatively small behavioral sample.

Winter (1969) suggests a useful testing-the-limits procedure when the patient has produced a poor copying performance on the Bender–Gestalt. He presents the patient with the copied designs and the stimulus cards a second time, one card at a time, and asks if the patient's reproductions of the designs are just the same as the stimulus figures. If the patient notes that s/he has made copying errors, a red pencil is provided and the patient is asked to make corrections on the copies of the original figures. No erasures are allowed. The patient is then asked to redraw the corrected figures on a new sheet of paper from the stimulus cards after the corrected figures have been removed. This provides an opportunity to observe whether the patient can benefit from experience and self-correction. The examiner does not offer suggestions as to how the figures should be improved or corrected when they are redrawn, since it is the patient's awareness of the errors that is of prime interest. Inability to recognize gross errors between the reproduction and the stimulus card suggests a perceptual problem. Inability to correct errors on the drawing correction phase but intact ability to recognize errors that require correction suggests a problem in motor output.

Analysis of specific errors on the Bender–Gestalt is of prime interest because these errors tend to fall into predictable and specific categories. The most thorough interpretive system for analysis of adult Bender–Gestalt protocols has been advanced by Pascal and Suttell (1951). They operationalized criteria for 106 drawing features and provided a formal scoring system for them. Based upon a review of the major scoring systems for adults with the Bender–Gestalt, Lezak (1976) concluded that a formal scoring system is necessary for use of the test in research work, but that inspection of the protocol for significant errors usually is sufficient for clinical screening applications. There are a number of useful, easily recognized features of Bender–Gestalt performance in adults that are characteristic of visual–motor regression. Such errors are typical in the protocols of children before age 9 years. At that age most children are able to copy the Bender–Gestalt figures "without serious errors" (Koppitz, 1964), but Bender (1938) observed that the child's performance does not fully approximate the normal adult performance on the Bender–Gestalt until age 11 years. After that age difficulty with copying of the figures suggests a developmental lag, learning disability, psychiatric disturbance, and/or cerebral dysfunction (cf. Bender, 1938; Hutt, 1969; Koppitz, 1964, 1975). See Figure 1 for illustrative examples.

Hutt (1969) and Hutt and Briskin (1960) have noted a number of important qualitative errors in the adult Bender–Gestalt protocol. The drawing of discrete

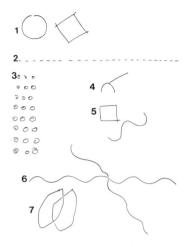

Figure 1. Common Bender–Gestalt errors. Note the closure difficulty on designs numbered 1, 3, 5; the dashes for dots and perseveration on design numbered 2; the rotation of design numbered 3; the distortion on designs numbered 4, 5; the angulation difficulty on design numbered 7; and the crossing difficulty on designs numbered 6, 7.

dots on several of the Bender–Gestalt figures, for instance, requires a modicum of visual–motor coordination. In particular, fine motor coordination of the small muscles of the hand is necessary to make a discrete dot. The younger child and the regressed adult show a similar pattern of making *circles or loops for dots*. These circles may be filled in to create enlarged dots. Difficulty making a discrete dot may also lead to the substitution of *dashes for dots*. *Rotation* is another commonly seen error, and it is particularly notable if the figure is rotated by 45 to 90 degrees or if it is mirror imaged. Perseveration of a motor sequence once initiated is commonly seen in younger children and adults with prefrontal cerebral dysfunction. *Distortion* in which the shape of the figure is partially or totally lost may lead to *confabulation* of a new design or *perseveration* of a previous figure with some similar elements. *Overdrawing* or sketching repeatedly over some design elements may be part of an attempt at analysis of elements and reinforcement of what is recognized in piecemeal fashion by a patient with an intact left hemisphere but right hemispheric dysfunction. *Simplification* through omission of elements may also be seen.

Angulation, closure, and curvature difficulties also are significant errors. Obtuse angles are the most difficult to reproduce accurately, since they usually become rounded or flattened rather than angled when distortions occur. *Closure difficulty* refers to overlapping of the ends of a vertex or failure to close the vertex. *Curvature difficulty* may be seen in flattening of a sinusoidal curve or replacement of the smooth curvature pattern with a pointed peak series, in picket-fence fashion.

Overlapping or collision of discrete figures is a serious sign of visual–motor dysfunction in the adult. Attention to these errors in the Bender–Gestalt protocol of the dysfunctional adult will provide a valid means of inspection screening.

The persistence or reemergence of errors on the Bender–Gestalt protocol of an adult, therefore, is a sign of significant visual–motor regression that was recognized by Bender (1938) in her original monograph. This early observation has received new clinical application in the assessment of retarded adults with the Koppitz developmental scoring system (Koppitz, 1964), even though it was developed for evaluation of visual–motor functioning in young children. This system has been renormed for the three standard AAMD retardation categories with an adult resident retardate population (Andert, Dinning, & Hustak, 1976). It has also been shown to provide a reliable measure of perceptual–motor functioning for retarded adults (Hustak, Dinning, & Andert, 1976).

Bender (1938) included a variety of patients with proven organic brain damage in her original validation studies of the Bender–Gestalt Test. She presented test protocols of patients with mental subnormality, sensory aphasia, dementia paralytica, Korsakoff's psychosis, cerebral malaria, alcoholic psychoses, head injury, and acute confusional states. There have been many subsequent case reports in the literature of brain-damaged subjects, and attempts have been made to develop Bender–Gestalt scoring systems that would be sensitive to brain dysfunction or damage (cf. Hain, 1964; Hutt & Briskin, 1960; Pauker, 1976). The Hain system is based on a weighted error scoring system for inspection of the protocol. The Pauker system is a simplified inspection system that can be completed in only 20 seconds by an experienced scorer (Pauker, 1976). Details of Hutt and Briskin's scoring system already have been presented.

Lacks and Newport (1980) evaluated the validity of these three scoring systems and a fourth system based on the number of figure rotations as indicators of brain dysfunction in a mixed psychiatric and brain-damaged population. They concluded that the Hutt–Briskin system was a useful diagnostic tool with an 84% hit rate, and that the Pauker system was also promising with a 79% hit rate but that it was in need of cross-validation with an independent sample. The Hain system produced a hit rate of 71%, and the presence of rotated figures produced a hit rate of only 63% when the best cutting score points were used for this sample. Use of the standard cutoff suggested by Hain (1964), however, produced only a 42% hit rate for organic diagnosis, with a 73% hit rate for functional cases. Level of experience among scorers ranged from expert to novice and showed no effect on diagnostic accuracy.

The sensitivity of the Bender–Gestalt to visual–motor dysfunction in adult patients with focal brain lesions was demonstrated in a study by Black and Strub (1976). They studied patients with focal lesions in each of the four quadrants of the brain for evidence of constructional difficulty. The order of groups from most to least impaired performance level was: right posterior, left posterior, right anterior, left anterior. The anteriorly wounded groups performed at a higher level than did the posteriorly wounded groups, and patients with left hemispheric lesions performed at a higher level than did patients with right hemispheric lesions. The Koppitz (1964) developmental scoring criteria were used for this study; the total error score was the criterion score for group comparison.

Lyle and Quast (1976) studied patients with proven Huntington's disease, those at risk for development of the disease, and controls with the Bender–Gestalt recall scores and clinical evaluation of the protocols as criterion measures. They found that the mean recall scores significantly discriminated between controls and known cases as well as patients at risk, although clinical evaluation of the protocols did almost as well as the recall score method on hit rate analyses. Neither method was sufficient for individual diagnostic evaluation of persons at risk for Huntington's disease.

Russell (1976) presented a case of a patient with severe left hemispheric damage with clear impairment on the Halstead–Reitan Battery but no clear evidence of impaired neuropsychological functioning on the Bender–Gestalt. He suggested that the Bender–Gestalt is most sensitive to right posterior quadrant cerebral dysfunction (cf. Black & Strub, 1976), and that at least in this case it was insensitive to left hemispheric dysfunction. Limitation of the use of the Bender–Gestalt to the role of a screening test for visual–motor dysfunction rather than to the global category of organic cerebral dysfunction is recommended. Delineation of specific dysfunctional patterns and residual strengths in the individual case requires a detailed battery of specialized tests, but group screening use of the Bender–Gestalt may miss some significantly impaired patients such as the one presented by Russell (1976). Use of the Reitan–Indiana Aphasia Screening Test (see next section of this chapter) will provide a remedy to this problem for screening purposes in many cases.

Bender (1938) also included a mixed group of psychiatric patients in her clinical case series. These included schizophrenics, manic depressives, malingerers, patients with Ganser syndrome, and neurotics. Interest in the use of the Bender–Gestalt in psychiatric settings has continued to produce useful results in the recent literature. Bender–Gestalt errors have been found to be factorially related to "disturbances of affect, mood, judgment, and hallucinations" in acute paranoid schizophrenics. Multiple regression analysis showed that the Bender–Gestalt error score was best predicted by the presence of hallucinations in this patient sample (Nahas, 1976).

An investigation of drawing constriction on Bender–Gestalt protocols of depressed patients found a significant relationship of constriction to depression. The figure constriction sign occurred infrequently (5% incidence) in the group sampled, however, so that its clinical utility in differential diagnosis appeared limited (White, 1976).

Use of a Background Interference Procedure with the Bender–Gestalt has been shown to be an effective way to increase the sensitivity of the test to perceptual–motor deficit (Canter, 1966, 1968, 1971, 1976; see also Golden, 1978, for review). The patient is first given a blank sheet of paper upon which to copy the Bender–Gestalt designs, after which s/he is given another sheet with a complex background matrix that consists of overlapping curved lines that perceptually compete (interfere) with his or her direct perception of the figure reproductions that s/he draws. This procedure was studied with a mixed brain-damaged and schizophrenic population by Holland and Wadsworth (1979). They found that the Background Interference Procedure did not discriminate between groups after correction for intelligence level. Holland and Wadsworth (1979, p. 127) note that, "given the sequence of test administration under consideration, the combination of BIP and recall (i.e., BIP–recall) accentuates the memory difficulties of the brain-damaged group relative to schizophrenics in such a fashion as to increase diagnostic differentiation compared to recall alone." The Background Interference Procedure seems to have value as an interference measure of memory functioning within this diagnostic context.

Dastoor, Klingner, Muller, and Kachanoff (1979) included the Bender–Gestalt in the baseline and three-year follow-up evaluations of a geriatric population with functional and organic disorders. There was a 50% death rate from baseline to follow-up evaluation in this sample. Post-hoc comparison of the survivor versus the deceased subgroups at follow-up showed that the survivors had had significantly higher mean Bender–Gestalt recall scores on a 5-second delayed recall measure.

A useful adjunct to the Bender–Gestalt administration procedure is the multiple choice form of the test produced by Spraings (1966). More recently, a study by Friedman, Wakefield, Sasek, and Schroeder (1977) developed and validated a new scoring system for this multiple choice form. This form allows one to evaluate perceptual dysfunction independent of motor output difficulty, since only matching of the target figure to an array is required. The procedure of Friedman and his associates provided for weighting of alternatives according to their similarity to the correct choice. This provides a score based on degree of similarity to the target stimulus, and it increased the correlation with the Bender–Gestalt overall score.

Critique

The Bender–Gestalt is a relatively brief screening measure of visual–motor functioning. The perceptual component can be studied independently of motor output through the use of the multiple choice paradigm. It is a relatively simple task and it has applicability from age 4 through adulthood. Its low floor level makes it useful as a clinical measure with severely impaired adults as well as normal and disturbed children. Ease of administration fosters motivation in patients who have relatively low energy level such as depressives and in others with marginal motivation for cooperation with lengthy and/or difficult tasks. The patient usually experiences the test as nonstressful unless there is extreme perceptual–motor dysfunction, in which case another type of test would be preferable as an opening task. The Bender–Gestalt is a good opening test for an assessment battery since it usually is experienced by the patient as a success. Speed is not a factor and scoring criteria are not known to the patient.

A disadvantage of the Bender–Gestalt is that it is much more effective with identification of normals than patients with brain dysfunction. For the functional versus organic disorder discrimination, the hit rates have averaged near 70% with the Bender–Gestalt for identification of the organic group, but up to 90% for the functional group (cf. Brilliant & Gynther, 1963; Bruhn & Reid, 1975; Goldberg, 1959, 1974; Golden, 1978; Hain, 1964; Hammeke, Golden, & Purisch, 1978; Levine & Feirstein, 1972; McGuire, 1960; Orme, 1962; Tymchuk, 1974). The Bender–Gestalt is prone to be less sensitive to cerebral dysfunction in patients with mild residual or incipient dysfunction, which is the group that is usually of clinical interest in differential diagnosis. There is no clear overall difference in the errors made by patients with functional versus those with organic disorder, although an errorless score does rule out difficulty with perceptual–motor dysfunction and tends to contraindicate cerebral dysfunction (Golden, 1978).

The Bender–Gestalt compensates for its lack of diagnostic specificity with its general sensitivity, particularly for patients with right hemispheric dysfunction. As such it is a useful screening instrument but it should not be used as the sole or primary measure of perceptual–motor dysfunction or cerebral functioning integrity. The Koppitz developmental scoring criteria have been shown to have value with adult retardate populations, and this application of the developmental scoring system deserves further empirical validation. Research is needed on the effects of normal aging in healthy populations from age 40 through senescence, on a cross-sectional and longitudinal basis. The limits of normal variation may be greater than have been appreciated previously, and such information is useful for accurate clinical identification of relevant performance deficits.

Studies that employ methodology that systematically varies brain lesion locus (cf. Black & Strub, 1976) and employ a comprehensive scoring system such as that of Koppitz (1964) or Pascal and Suttell (1951) would be helpful in the systematic evaluation of deficit performances as they are related to the functional systems of the brain (Luria, 1966, 1973). Ethnic and cultural group differences on the Bender–Gestalt have begun to be investigated (Butler, Coursey, & Gatz, 1976; Gilmore, Chandy, & Anderson, 1975) with mixed results. Gilmore and associates found a significant group effect with poorer scores on the Koppitz developmental system among Mexican–American children after age 7 years. Butler and associates, however, found no consistent group effect for black and white adult brain-damaged patients on Bender–Gestalt protocols scored with the Pascal and Suttell (1951) and Hain (1964) systems. Recent work by Amante, Van Houten,

, and Margules (1977) tends to support the work of Gilmore and ̱s, and suggests that "the prevalence of central nervous system pathology ̱ inversely correlated with socioeconomic status and there appears to be a definite concentration of such cases in the minority group populations." These investigators provide support for their conclusion from the literature of the previous 30 years, which identifies the incidence of disadvantagement of such socioeconomic and ethnic groups in medical, nutritional, social–environmental, and educational areas that combine to produce intellectual and perceptual–motor deficits among members of the lower socioeconomic groups. These results are open to alternative interpretation, and additional controlled studies are necessary to evaluate the merit of the conclusions.

REITAN–INDIANA APHASIA SCREENING TEST

The Reitan–Indiana Aphasia Screening Test (Heimburger & Reitan, 1961) is a modification of the Halstead–Wepman Aphasia Screening Test (Halstead & Wepman, 1949), both of which provide a brief overview of the major syndromes of aphasia, apraxia, and agnosia. Several of the test items involve drawing of simple geometric figures that are similar in complexity and difficulty level to figures on the Bender–Gestalt Test. These are a square, a triangle, an outline Greek cross (similar to an outline drawing of the equal-armed Red Cross symbol), and an old-fashioned skeleton key. The square and triangle are too elementary to discriminate constructional difficulty in any but the most impaired patients without meticulous scoring criteria (cf. Golden, Hammeke, & Purisch, 1980; Golden, Purisch, & Hammeke, 1979). The outline skeleton key is too complex for many neurologically normal subjects (Reitan, 1975).

The Greek cross has proven quite satisfactory as an intermediate difficulty level task. Example criteria for its scoring on a five-point qualitative scale that ranges from normal to severely impaired are provided for adult subjects by Russell, Nueringer, and Goldstein (1970). It is essential that when a subject is asked to copy the Greek cross that s/he not be allowed to lift his or her pencil from the paper during the outline drawing. The perimeter of the figure must be drawn in one continuous line so that the patient is required to cross the perceptual midline during the act of drawing. Important errors to note are omission of one arm of the cross, distortion of half of the figure to one side of the vertical midline, inability to close the figure, and/or drawing the figure far to one side of the page or the other as part of a general strategy across a series of figures. Failure to use half of the page may indicate a problem with a homonymous visual field defect and/or visual neglect. Examples of various errors of these kinds are shown in Figure 2. Testing for those syndromes that suggest perceptual disturbance should follow the recognition of these deficits. Methods for this follow-up testing are presented later in this chapter.

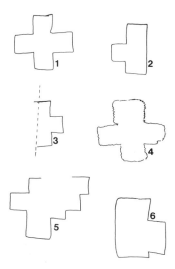

Figure 2. Greek cross reproductions. (1) Essentially normal performance, with minor closure difficulty at vertex and minor dyssymetry on right side of vertical arm; (2) omission of right arm of cross
in patient with left hemispheric stroke and visual field defect; (3) visual neglect with homonymous
visual field defect following right hemispheric stroke (broken midline added); (4) fine hand tremor
with preservation of overall form of cross configuration; (5) constructional difficulty in severe form,
greater in right visual hemifield; (6) omission of left arm and distortion of the overall form of the
cross in a demented patient. Also note simplification of overall design.

The Halstead–Wepman Aphasia Screening Test has continued to be used in
its own right as a clinical tool, with 9.6% of neuropsychological examiners in public psychiatric facilities reporting its clinical use (Craig, 1979). As part of the Halstead–Reitan Neuropsychological Battery the Reitan–Indiana revision of the
instrument has received more general use, with 45.6% of reporting clinicians noting routine use of that battery (Craig, 1979). Thus, over half of the responding
neuropsychological practitioners in representative psychiatric settings are employing one or another form of this instrument. Populations studied have included the
full range of psychiatric disorders and a variety of brain-damaged patients whose
disorders varied widely in location, extent, and etiology. All major diagnostic
groups have been represented (cf. Davis & Reitan, 1966; Doehring & Reitan,
1961; Golden, Osmon, Moses, & Berg, 1981; Reitan, 1954, 1960; Wheeler, 1963;
Wheeler & Reitan, 1962).

Critique

As a brief, easily administered screening measure of language-related functions, the Halstead–Wepman and Reitan–Indiana Aphasia Screening Tests are
quite satisfactory measures. They can be used to predict the presence and laterality

of brain damage effectively by means of a sign approach. Presence of two positive signs identifies 86% of brain-damaged cases, and four positive signs successfully identify 100% of brain-damaged cases (Wheeler & Reitan, 1962). If there is evidence of significant aphasic, apraxic, or agnosic disorder on this screening examination, follow-up testing with a more complete battery of tests for these disorders is advisable (cf. Goodglass & Kaplan, 1972; Schuell, 1965). The Halstead–Wepman and Reitan–Indiana Aphasia Screening Tests were developed as adjunctive measures to more comprehensive batteries of neuropsychological tests, and as such they perform well. As with any other screening measure, negative findings help to rule out serious cerebral dysfunction, but positive findings require more detailed evaluation. These screening tests may be insensitive, however, to mild, residual dysnomia and to subcortical aphasic syndromes of the conduction type. Goodglass and Kaplan (1972) provide a thorough review of these and other major aphasic syndromes in addition to detailed procedures for their diagnostic evaluation.

The Reitan–Indiana Aphasia Screening Test has been studied in regard to its psychometric and clinical attributes. In the context of visual–motor assessment it seems that mild, incipient, or residual constructional difficulty on the square and triangle drawings would be more evident if the criteria developed by Golden, Purisch, and Hammeke (1979) for the Luria–Nebraska Battery were used in the scoring of these items routinely. Further evaluation of the quality of the drawing of the Greek cross in normal populations that vary in age and educational level is needed, for we know much more about clinical poulations than about the range of normal variation on this measure.

MEMORY FOR DESIGNS TEST

Graham and Kendall (1946, 1960; Kendall & Graham, 1948) developed a series of 15 line drawing designs of graded complexity for use in an immediate memory task as a screening measure for brain dysfunction. Their rationale for use of this procedure was the prevailing belief of the time, based on the work of Foster (1920), that inability to perform an immediate memory task with such material was indicative of cerebral dysfunction (see discussion under Bender–Gestalt in this review as well). Graham and Kendall were the first investigators to develop a set of standardized materials and a formal scoring system to test this hypothesis. Bender (1938) already had developed her test as a copying task based on the related hypothesis that cerebral dysfunction would be reflected in visuopractic impairment on a geometric figure line drawing task. The validational success of the Graham and Kendall procedure is reflected in its continued wide use as a neuropsychological screening measure, with 28.9% of practicing clinicians in psychiatric settings reporting its use in a recent survey (Craig, 1979).

The validation and cross-validation samples used with the Graham–Kendall

Memory for Designs Test (MFD) consisted of carefully screened brain-damage cases of a variety of types (see Graham & Kendall, 1960, for details on all samples) and a group of primarily psychiatric patients as controls. Approximately 30% of the original and cross-validation samples were psychotics of various kinds. All of these psychotic patients were tested prior to March, 1952, which insured that there was no antipsychotic drug in use to affect CNS functioning (Graham & Kendall, 1960). Use of the published norms thus provides a particularly relevant screening tool for use of the MFD in a mixed psychiatric and brain-damaged population. This seems to account for the continued popularity of the MFD with clinicians who work in such settings.

Because of its normative data base, the MFD is somewhat more effective than the Bender–Gestalt for differentiation of chronic schizophrenics from brain-damaged, nonpsychotic subjects. There is a large degree of overlap between the Bender–Gestalt as scored by the Hain (1964) system and the MFD, with a correlation of 0.851 between the measures (Quattlebaum, 1968). Hit rates for brain-damaged subjects and controls averaged approximately 75% in the Graham and Kendall validation and cross-validation studies (Graham & Kendall, 1960). Those findings have been upheld by subsequent research (see Golden, 1978, for review), although occasional reports of hit rates up to 90% have been noted (Korman & Blumberg, 1963). Partial listings of the references to the literature on the MFD published and presented without published support are available in two Ammons and Ammons reviews (1978a, 1978b).

Grundvig, Ajax, and Needham (1973) attempted to improve on the sensitivity of the MFD to sensory and perceptual deficits in cerebrally dysfunctional patients with a shorter exposure time, but the standard 5-second exposure yielded greater group differentiation between controls and brain-damaged patients. Birkett and Boltuch (1977) also found evidence for the effectiveness of the MFD as a screening device in differentiation of patients with functional psychiatric disorders as compared with brain-damaged patients (primarily stroke victims). These investigators found that a structured clinical interview (Maudsley Tests of the Sensorium), which consists of tasks that are sensitive to verbal memory and orientation, was as effective as the MFD in making the functional versus organic differentiation.

One study of the MFD as a screening device for identification of patients with penetrating missile wounds of the brain found very low hit rates of 10% or less (Black, 1974). Penetration of the skull and dura mater were proven through neurosurgical treatment. Lesions were recent in this group, injuries were "relatively small," the subjects were young (18–27), and they were well prior to injury. In fact, 62% of the subjects "appeared normal without evidence of medical complications, motor impairment, or cognitive deficits" (Black, 1974, p. 76) at the time of testing. The majority of the focally injured patients also did not have injuries to cortical areas that are associated with either visual perception or constructional

ability, as Black himself notes. These findings suggest that the MFD may be better used as a screening device for visuopractic skills rather than for brain dysfunction or damage in general. It is not surprising, however, that the MFD failed
to demonstrate deficit in patients for whom recovery appeared complete on cognitive and medical measures.

A follow-up study by Klajajic (1976) attempted to expand Black's design to
investigate the utility of the MFD in differentiation of cerebral dysfunction in
patients with a wide variety of neurological disorders from controls. Brain damage
was proven by pneumoencephalography (PEG) and electroencephalography
(EEG), but only 73% of the neurological patients showed abnormalities on neurological examination performed by a neurologist. The "control sample" was
drawn from cases who had been referred (apparently clinically) for PEG, EEG,
neurological examination, brain scan, and/or angiography, but in whom results
of these tests were consistently negative. Subjects in whom brain damage is suspected clinically and in whom no hard signs of neuropathology are demonstrated
by the said tests, however, are not truly control patients. In addition, 20% of the
"control" subjects in this study had abnormal neurological findings. Thus, the
failure to find significant differences between these groups was not surprising, and
the results have no implications for the differential diagnostic validity of the MFD.

A study by Hagberg (1978) found that there was a significant correlation of
regional cerebral blood flow increase in the left cerebral hemisphere temporal and
parietal regions for verbal memory tasks, and in the temporal and inferior frontal
regions for spatial recognition tasks. There was, however, no correlation of MFD
performance to any focal region of the left cerebral hemisphere. In support of these
findings is the data of Kumar (1977), who employed a tactual modification of the
MFD in the examination of commissurotomy patients. In patients with complete
callosal sectioning, marked superiority of the right cerebral hemisphere was demonstrated on the tactual MFD task and on a measure of spatial–configurational
memory.

Kish, Hagen, Woody, and Harvey (1980) found evidence of improvement on
the MFD among other measures during the third week of alcohol abstinence after
a heavy drinking episode. Fine and Steer (1979) found evidence of borderline
range impairment on the MFD in a sample of subjects who had been arrested for
driving while intoxicated. Further evidence of MFD sensitivity to toxic drug
effects is provided by Wecowicz, Fedora, Masons, Radstaak, Bay, and Yonge
(1975), who found that marijuana users in low-dose and high-dose THC groups
showed impaired MFD performance levels. In a study of confabulation estimation, Joslyn, Grundvig, and Chamberlain (1978) found that the MFD Embel-
lishment score significantly distinguished the confabulators in both brain-damaged
and schizophrenic groups. There was no difference between the groups in overall
memory functioning as measured by the Wechsler Memory Scale.

Critique

The MFD is useful primarily as a brief, easily administered, nonstressful screening measure for visuopractic performance and cerebral dysfunction, particularly within a mixed psychiatric and brain-damaged population. It is essentially equivalent to the Bender–Gestalt for this purpose. The MFD is normed in such a conservative manner that few false positives are identified. An easily corrected oversight of the scoring system is the failure to score as an error the omission of a figure due to total recall failure. Such a finding indicates an immediate visual memory problem (Lezak, 1976), which the clinician should investigate further with more detailed techniques.

The cases that the MFD fails to detect as cerebrally dysfunctional appear to be individuals with mild, incipient, or residual cerebral dysfunction. As a result, it is a useful technique with cases that present clear behavioral deficit that is of questionable functional versus organic origin. More sophisticated and comprehensive techniques such as the Luria–Nebraska Neuropsychological Battery (Golden et al., 1980) or the Halstead–Reitan Neuropsychological Battery (Reitan & Davison, 1974; Golden, Osmon, Moses, & Berg, 1981) should be employed in the evaluation of such cases.

Future research could profitably include a measure of figure omissions in the scoring system once the occurrence of such errors in normals and criterion clinical groups has been established. Performances of normals on the MFD has been neglected in the literature, and we have relatively little data on medically ill but neurologically intact controls. It may be that the differentiating power of the MFD has been underestimated by the choice of criterion groups. It would also be useful to study findings in residually brain-dysfunctional subjects such as those who had suffered concussive head injuries several years previously but who now show only mild, residual deficit as compared with medical controls who are neurologically intact. This distinction has direct clinical relevance to the practicing clinician but it remains to be investigated.

BENTON REVISED VISUAL RETENTION TEST

The original Visual Retention Test was introduced by Benton (1945). It and its successor, the Benton Revised Visual Retention Test (BVRT) were designed to be measures of "visual perception, visual memory, and visuoconstructive abilities" (Benton, 1974). The standard form of the revised BVRT is available in three parallel forms of 10 figures each. Benton advocates use of the test as a copying task, an immediate visual memory measure with 5- or 10-second exposure of the stimulus cards before reproduction, and as a delayed memory task. The series of figures on the BVRT present the patient with designs of graded complexity. Illustrative figures of the kind included on the BVRT are presented in Figure 3, but these are not actual items taken from the test. The two initial designs in each series are single figures, which are followed by groups of three figures, two of which are large (major) overlapping or nonoverlapping geometric designs with a smaller peripheral figure to one side of the major figures. Some of the designs are rotated or mirror-image versions of each other (see Figure 3 for illustrative examples). There are deliberate and systematic alterations of the major and peripheral figures throughout the series that are sensitive to effects of perseveration and perceptual distortion such as mirror imaging and rotation. In particular, the examiner who employs the BVRT should be attentive to errors of rotation, left–right misplacement, perseveration, overall distortion, confabulation, and misidentification or omission of internal details. The peripheral figures are considerably smaller than the major figures in order to increase their sensitivity to visual field defects or visual neglect that may be subtle. Benton (1974) provides an elaborate scoring system for the BVRT. The copy and short-term memory administrations have detailed age and intelligence level corrections for adults and children aged 8–14 years, which aid in the clinical interpretation of the test. A special feature is the separate scoring of figures for accuracy (number of designs correct) and for errors. Since a figure may be reproduced incorrectly due to one or multiple reasons, this dual scoring system provides a means of evaluation of the number and variety of errors that are involved.

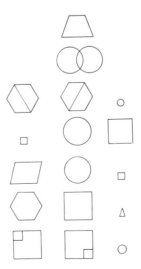

Figure 3. Illustrative design sequence of figures similar to those on the Benton Visual Retention Test. (See text for discussion.)

The usual administration format for the BVRT is to present the figures one at a time for 10 seconds with immediate recall reproduction after the figure has been removed. Poor performance at this phase may be due to an immediate memory problem, a motor output problem, or a perceptual input problem. To clarify the nature of any performance difficulty, the patient is asked to copy the figures on an untimed basis with the figure in plain view during the next portion of the administration. This eliminates the memory component, but poor performance at this stage still may be due to a perceptual problem or a motor problem. The patient may be asked to compare his copied reproductions with the stimulus figures to make any corrections s/he deems necessary with a pencil of another color. This procedure will help to rule out impulsiveness or failure to scan fully for details by providing another opportunity for review of the quality of performance. It clarifies those errors that the patient can identify spontaneously.

To rule out a perceptual problem, it is useful to administer the multiple choice form of the BVRT as the final portion of the administration sequence (Benton, 1950; Benton, Hamsher, & Stone, 1977). This form was developed because many patients were unable to write legibly after a stroke or other neurological disorder had affected voluntary motor control of the dominant hand. Drawing reproduction with the nondominant hand was of questionable significance. A form of the test was developed in which the patient was presented with a stimulus figure and an array of four similar stimuli, one of which is identical to the original stimulus. All figures (stimulus and four alternative choices) are presented simultaneously for all items. The patient is then asked to point to which of the figures in the four-choice array is identical to the original stimulus figure. The differences in the distractor (non-stimulus-match) figures provide a means of objectively assessing what sort of perceptual cues create confusion for the patient. The variation of the errors and distractor cues provides a means of systematically evaluating common perceptual errors in patients with impaired cerebral functioning. A patient who can perceptually match correctly but who makes copying errors is showing a motor output problem. Inability to match the figures correctly shows a perceptual problem.

Recent work with the BVRT has found definite aging effects on error score performance. Arenberg (1978) found small error score increases in men aged less than 50 years, moderate error score increases for those in their 50s and 60s, and "substantial" error score increases for those aged 70 or more. In another study (Arenberg, 1977) he found that verbal cueing increased BVRT performance of male blue-collar workers aged 59–77 years, but not in a comparison group of male high school students with similar educational backgrounds. Verbal cueing about key features of the BVRT geometric designs appeared to have aided verbal mediation for the older group and thus improved recall by providing retrieval cues. There was a ceiling effect with the younger group, so that less score change was notable.

In an interesting study of cerebral laterality, Arena and Gainotti (1978) administered the standard and multiple choice versions of the BVRT to patients with lateralized brain lesions and controls. They found that there were no significant differences between patients with left or right brain damage on measures of visuopractic or visuoperceptual deficit, either for frequency or severity of the deficits. A study by Hagberg (1978), however, showed increased regional cerebral blood flow to the left temporal region only to be associated with performance on the BVRT. Martin-Ramirez, Gadow, and Aksamski (1977) found evidence for impairment of BVRT "apperception capacity and visual retention" in patients with surgically removed cerebral tumors in the frontal or posterior fossa areas, whereas patients with hypophyseal tumors (beneath the cerebral hemispheres proper) did not differ significantly on these measures from controls. Jost (1977) found evidence for diminished BVRT performance in both schizophrenics and brain-damaged patients, with similar deficit performances in these clinical groups as compared to controls.

Critique

The BVRT is a standard psychometric instrument that continues to enjoy a wide application in neuropsychiatric settings where neuropsychological evaluation is done. Craig (1979) reports that 26.3% of the respondents to his survey in settings of this kind make use of the BVRT in their clinical practice. The availability of parallel forms that are psychometrically valid, reliable, and equivalent, as well as a multiple choice form of the test, makes it a highly valuable clinical tool for the assessment of visuopractic and visuoperceptual functioning.

More work is needed to identify patterns of deficit that are characteristic of psychiatric patients with chronic psychotic and serious depressive syndromes as compared to patients with valid cerebral dysfunction only. Benton (1974) gives some clinical guidelines for the evaluation of psychiatric cases, but more systematic work in this area is necessary to clarify the range of clinical variation encountered in neuropsychiatric diagnostic work. Differentiation of such functionally disturbed patients from organically impaired patients is an issue of prime clinical interest in many settings. Because many clinicians continue to use the BVRT as a screening measure for organic cerebral dysfunction with neuropsychiatric patients, more systematic data would help to improve the basis upon which clinical decisions are made from BVRT results.

There also is a need for systematic evaluation of the sensitivity of the BVRT to the differential presentation of focal cerebral lesions. It clearly has merit as a screening device for the identification of cerebral dysfunction in general and perceptuo-motor dysfunction in particular, but studies that systematically vary lesion locus as a function of age and educational level and then evaluate the types of errors made within these groupings would increase our understanding of the clinical interpretation of the BVRT errors. More work with the normal-aged population also is needed. The encouraging results of Arenberg (1977, 1978) suggest that this work also may have implications for amnestic retraining in older persons.

TEST OF VISUAL NEGLECT

Albert (1973) introduced a brief, simply administered measure for evaluation of the syndrome of visual neglect. He defines this syndrome as "a defective and, therefore, a reduced ability to attend to one or more components of the visual world." Classically the syndrome is seen in patients with a right hemispheric lesion that causes a syndrome of hemi-inattention or neglect of the contralateral half of phenomenal space (Weinstein & Friedland, 1977). If the lesion were in the right hemisphere, the patient with this syndrome in full form would act as though all or a large part of the left side of his or her visual field did not exist. The visual neglect syndrome can exist without an associated homonymous visual field defect, and visual field defects may occur without visual neglect (Albert, 1973).

The test material consists of a letter-size piece of unlined paper covered with 40 straight, nonintersecting, 2.5-centimeter lines that are arranged in an obliquely angled fashion all over the page. The long axis of the paper is presented on the patient's left–right axis. The lines are not arranged randomly, although they may appear to be so. Albert's article should be consulted by the potential user of this technique for details of the stimulus figure construction; an illustration of it is provided there. To be sure that the patient has seen all of the lines on the page and that s/he understands the nature of the task, the examiner takes a red pencil and traces over all of the printed black lines on the page while the patient is asked to watch. The subject is then asked to cross out all of the lines by making each of them into an "X" or cross. The examiner demonstrates this by drawing a line through one of the stimulus lines near the center of the array. The patient then is told to cross out all of the other lines on the page in the same manner.

Albert (1973) reports that use of this test for his sample produced a 37% incidence of visual neglect in patients with right hemispheric lesions and a 30% incidence of the syndrome in left hemispheric lesion cases. Albert's neglect criterion was strict so that the amount of visual neglect could have been very mild and still been identified. In clinical practice it is often only the patient who displays the visual neglect syndrome in dramatic form who is diagnosed as showing it. This occurs more frequently with right hemispheric lesioned patients. Severity of visual neglect, when present, was much more pronounced in patients with unilateral right hemispheric damage than in those with left hemispheric damage. Posterior lesion site in either hemisphere was associated with more severe neglect than anterior lesion placement. The occurrence of visual neglect was found in both left and right lesion groups with the *same* pattern: greatest in the left visual hemifield, moderate centrally, and least in the right visual hemifield (Albert, 1973).

These paradoxical findings led Albert to question the concept of visual neglect as a strictly lateralized inattention syndrome and to infer that "the type of visual neglect shown by this test is more a bilateral than a unilateral phenomenon." He speculated that visual perception requires the integrated functioning of both cerebral hemispheres (cf. Luria, 1966, 1973), but that visual sensation is attributable solely to the functioning of the hemisphere opposite to the contralateral visual field. Since the right cerebral hemisphere is dominant for object recognition and visual–spatial integration, the visual neglect syndrome should be more marked after damage to the right cerebral hemisphere. With a brain lesion in either hemisphere, however, there is misperception and failure of proper visual integration of information in the contralateral visual hemifield. This information travels from the damaged cerebral hemisphere via the corpus callosum for integration with information from the normal cerebral hemisphere in a manner that is out of temporal synchrony (due to faulty processing) and spatially distorted. The patient perceives relatively better in the portion of the visual field opposite to the normal hemisphere, but visual input from the damaged hemisphere tends to disrupt the overall integration of visual perception so that some minor errors occur bilaterally, even with a left hemispheric lesion. When the lesion is in the right hemisphere, a similar mixing of normal and disturbed visual input from the two cerebral hemispheres is hypothesized to take place, but here the dominant visual–perceptual integration network is directly disturbed. As a result the syndrome of visual neglect is more pronounced than in left hemispheric lesions, but a bilateral syndrome is seen in the manner noted empirically by Albert.

A subsequent study by Colombo, DeRenzi, and Faglioni (1976) investigated the visual neglect syndrome in patients with left or right hemispheric lesions. They confirmed that patients with right hemispheric damage are nearly unique in displaying visual neglect when they perform "a task that by its very nature demands adequate space exploration." Patients with left hemispheric lesions, by contrast, show the visual neglect syndrome with tasks in which "the exploration is left to the subject's initiative." It appears that Albert's (1973) theory is correct in a measure, but that there is an interaction with task type. Thus his relatively simple visual cancellation task produced a different set of results than the double dissociation of lesion laterality with task type demonstrated by Colombo and associates.

DOUBLE SIMULTANEOUS STIMULATION

A related deficit of simultaneous hemispheric information processing may be demonstrated in the absence of gross sensory deficit, but it may contribute to impaired visual–motor performance. The patient should be tested in the tactile, visual, and auditory modalities with double simultaneous stimulation as is customary in clinical neurological examination (Reitan & Davison, 1974). Only the first two modalities directly concern us in the present context.

To test for tactile suppression, the examiner sits facing the patient, who is blindfolded or is asked to close his or her eyes. The examiner explains to the patient that the testing will involve evaluation of light-touch perception. The backs of the patient's hands are touched as lightly as the patient can recognize and report reliably. A threshold stimulus is desirable and deep pressure should be avoided because cortically mediated light-touch sensation is the modality under investigation. If the right hand is touched, the patient is instructed to say "right." If the left hand is touched, the correct response is "left," and the patient is so instructed. Several unimanual trials are given to be sure that reporting is reliable and that unilateral sensation is intact. Patients should always be questioned about peripheral hand or arm injuries to be sure that these conditions are not associated with sensory deficit, which may be confused with cerebrally related deficit if it is not recognized as a peripheral lesion. Thereafter, random variation of the side of unimanual stimulation continues for several more trials. The stimuli are varied randomly to prevent the patient from developing a set response strategy. Then, without warning, both of the patient's hands are touched *simultaneously,* and s/he is asked to report the stimulus felt. Suppression consists of reporting only one of the hand touches and failing to report (suppressing) the other stimulus. The suppression implies dysfunction of the contralateral parietal lobe, particularly in the maintenance of cortical tone between the brainstem and the cortex by means of the corticoreticular and reticulocortical feedback loops.

Strub and Black (1977) have advanced the theory that suppression under double simultaneous stimulation may be associated with an imbalance in the feedback loop from the ascending reticular activating system of the brainstem and the cerebral cortex that subserves the sensory modality in which suppression occurs (temporal lobe for audition, occipital lobe for vision, parietal lobe for somesthesis). Normally there is an optimal level of "cortical tone" or readiness to respond to stimulation, which is maintained by means of such feedback loops between the reticular system and the cerebral cortex (Luria, 1966). When cortical tone is lowered by a tissue-destructive cortical lesion in one cerebral hemisphere, suppression in the affected modality on the other side of the body tends to occur. Inconsistent suppressions tend to occur after serious head injuries because of the coup and contre-coup effects of closed head injury that produce bilateral cerebral dysfunction. The inconsistency of such findings appears to be due to a concussive mechanism of injury that is less severe in its tissue destructive effects than a stroke or intrinsic brain tumor, which typically are associated with consistent suppression in the affected sensory modality (Reitan, 1959).

One must be very careful to make the bimanual touches to the backs of the hands simultaneously, as even a very brief delay between the two stimuli will allow an impaired patient to process the stimuli independently and the deficit will be missed. It is also important to recognize that suppression can be demonstrated only when unimanual sensation is intact. If the patient evidences sensory loss to unimanual light touch stimulation, the suppression measure is invalidated for that sensory modality.

A similar procedure is used with visual suppression testing. The examiner sits facing the patient at a comfortable distance, usually about three feet, with the examiner's arms extended as far laterally as possible and equidistant between his or her eyes and those of the patient. The smallest visually detectible movement, preferably the wiggling of only one finger at arm's length, serves as the stimulus. Throughout testing, the patient is instructed to stare intently at the examiner's nose and not to look to the sides. The examiner can use his or her own peripheral vision to judge the adequacy of the stimulus presented. Reitan suggests examination of the visual fields above, at, and below eye level to evaluate for quadrantanoptic and hemianoptic suppression and visual field defects, with double simultaneous and unilateral stimuli, respectively. A tangent screen and visual perimetry can be used to supplement evaluation of central and peripheral visual field deficits if any are suspected from unilateral confrontation testing. As with double simultaneous tactile stimulation, unilateral visual stimuli are presented at first and then bilateral stimuli are introduced without prior warning. Failure to report a stimulus in one visual hemifield only during double simultaneous stimulation indicates visual suppression and dysfunction in the contralateral temporo-parietal visual system tracts. Suppression only below eye level implies parietal dysfunction, while suppression only above eye level implies temporal lobe dysfunction of the contralateral hemisphere.

Unilateral testing is done in each sensory modality to insure that basic sensation in that modality is intact. Once this has been demonstrated, one can interpret failure to respond to the bilateral stimuli as evidence of suppression. Inconsistent reporting of suppression phenomena is *not* to be discounted as a random or chance performance. While consistent suppression naturally is more serious, any suppression is significant. Such findings of inconsistent suppression may be residuals of serious neurological disorder such as head trauma, as noted above, and always need to be followed up with additional evaluation. If the examiner is unsure of his or her technique or the reliability of the results, the test should be repeated several times with intervening test material and/or a rest period to insure that the patient does not tire and make fatigue-related errors. In any case, a minimum of four unilateral trials on each side of the body should be given in addition to at least four simultaneous bilateral trials.

TRAIL MAKING TESTS

The Trail Making Tests (TMT) were developed originally by the Adjutant General's Office in the United States Army in 1944 as a subtest of the Army

Individual Test (Reitan, 1958). The tests consist of two parts, A and B. Part A presents the patient with a series of numbered circles that are arranged in an apparently random fashion on the page. The subject's task is to connect the circles in numerical order as quickly as possible. The score for the task is the time in seconds required to make a successful completion of the path or trail through the array. Errors count only in the increased time that the patient requires to correct them. The examiner should watch the patient's performance carefully to point out errors as soon as they occur. Part B is constructed on a similar format, but the ordering of the series is more complex than that in Part A. For Part B the patient is presented with letters and numbers and s/he is instructed to alternate between the alphabetical and numerical series to create an alphanumeric sequence, thusly: 1—A—2—B—3—C . . . and so forth. As with Part A, only time for completion of the task constitutes the formal score for Part B. The time is allowed to run while the examiner briefly identifies the patient's errors as they occur on each part.

This pair of tasks presents the examiner with an excellent opportunity to discriminate visual–perceptual from motor output deficits. The first task, Part A, allows one to assess the patient's spatial orientation and ability to perform sequencing with an overlearned series, the numbers from 1 to 25. Those patients who have difficulty with Part A may have difficulty with visual neglect, as in the case of individuals who fail to search actively on the periphery of the array or in the center of it, and fail to include items in the series as a result. Visual field defects also may be associated with errors of this kind. Other patients reach the circle numbered 9 and become confused about how to proceed. Double-digit numbers create particular difficulty for patients with left posterior parietal lesions since they have lost a grasp of basic number structure (Conley et al., 1980; Luria, 1966). One such patient reached circle 11 and was confused about how to proceed. He explained later that he knew that the next item was the circle with a 1 and a 2 in it, but he did not know whether 12 or 21 was the correct next item in the sequence. Still another patient had no difficulty with visual neglect of number interpretation, but he became lost in attempts to find his way about the page spatially and he had to randomly hunt among the circles for the next item in a trial-and-error fashion. One individual lost his place in the numerical sequence and had to count through the series each time to find what number came next. These patients were able to voice their confusion so that the observant examiner could understand the problem with limited questioning. Understanding of the patient's difficulty intuitively requires additional backup testing to prove the hypothesis correct or incorrect and to eliminate other possibilities for the performance decrement. It is a good general strategy to ask the patient to think out loud while doing the task if this comes naturally, and if not, to have the patient explain his or her strategy after the performance is completed.

Trails B provides an opportunity for the patient to make similar errors, but it adds the need for relatively intact short-term memory to keep two parallel series in intact order. Cognitive flexibility and sequencing skills also are essential to adequate performance on this measure. The brain-damaged patient often will lose track of the task if it is too complex for him or her and will simplify it by reverting to a perseverative attempt at solution by counting, as in the Part A numerical sequence. The series thus changes after the first few alternations and may become: 1—A—2—B—3—4—5— . . . and so forth. Some patients may substitute the alphabetical sequence for the alphanumeric one.

A number of early studies validated and cross-validated the use of the TMT with criterion brain-injured subjects as a screening device (Armitage, 1946; Davids, Goldenberg, & Laufer, 1957; Reitan 1955, 1958). A subsequent study by Reitan and Tarshes (1959) showed significantly poorer mean performance on TMT Part A for the right hemispheric group as compared to the left hemispheric group. Intragroup comparisons, however, showed highly significant differences for the comparison of performances on Parts A and B as a function of lesion laterality. The left cerebral hemisphere lesion group performed at a significantly lower level on Part B as compared to Part A, while the right hemisphere lesion group performed significantly more poorly on Part A as compared to Part B. The TMT is sensitive to the effects of aging, education, and intelligence level, particularly Part B (Davies, 1968; Finlayson, Johnson, & Reitan, 1977; Golden, 1978; Golden, Osmon, Moses, & Berg, 1981; Gordon, 1978).

While the weight of empirical evidence continues to support the validity of the TMT as a psychometric device that produces large intergroup mean differences between criterion groups of brain-damaged patients and controls (cf. Mezzich & Moses, 1980; Sterne, 1973), the value of the TMT as a screening device has been questioned in the recent literature by Norton (1978). Norton found the usual large intergroup TMT differences as described by others. He reported that 21% of the patients who passed the TMT were classified as definitely abnormal by the Wisconsin form of the Halstead–Reitan Battery, and that 33% of the patients who passed the TMT had one or more definitely abnormal neurological studies. These results are reasonably comparable to the findings of Mezzich and Moses (1980) and to the validation study of Reitan (1958), in which approximately 15% false positives and false negatives were found in similar comparisons. Most other screening devices such as the Bender–Gestalt and Graham–Kendall Memory for Designs Tests have similar hit rates for identification of cerebrally dysfunctional patients.

The work of Craig (1979) suggests that clinical neuropsychological screening in many neuropsychiatric settings employ techniques such as the Benton Visual Retention Test and/or the Bender–Gestalt, which have hit rates that are in this approximate range of 75–85%. Rapid screening of large numbers of subjects of this kind is primarily useful for identification of definitely impaired and definitely normal subjects, but patients with clinical evidence of cerebral impairment by examination and/or history that may now be mild deserve more detailed neuropsychological evaluation. This caveat must be kept clearly in mind by the clinician who is not a neuropsychological specialist and who therefore may be limited in his or her options to relatively simple neuropsychological screening devices.

Investigation of psychiatric groups on the TMT have shown that reactively depressed mood does not sufficiently impair performance on the TMT to make the patient appear brain-damaged (Alvarez, 1962). Qualitative evaluation of the performances of schizophrenics on the TMT Part B revealed that they "either complete the task without error, abandon the task, or produce illogical patterns," while the latter two groups of errors were rarely seen in nonpsychotic brain-damaged persons. The brain-damaged patients rather tended to simplify the task by "sequence binding," with return to an alphabetical or numerical sequence without the appropriate alternation of letters and numbers. The other typical strategy employed by the brain-damaged group was to return to an earlier place in the sequence or to begin the task again when difficulty with solution was encountered (Goldstein & Neuringer, 1966).

Sensitivity of the TMT to perceptual motor deficit in alcoholics has been established (Fitzhugh, Fitzhugh, & Reitan, 1960, 1965). More recent studies have shown the sensitivity of the TMT to improvement of cerebral functioning efficiency in ethanol-abstinent alcoholics (Ayers, Templer, Ruff, & Barthlow, 1978; Kish et al., 1980; Page & Schaub, 1977). The sensitivity of TMT performance to the other toxic effects such as paint fume inhalation has been demonstrated as well (Tsushima & Towne, 1977). Sensitivity of TMT scores to cerebral lesions, which reportedly often are undetected by routine clinical medical workup in cases of decompression illness in divers, also has been demonstrated (Peters, Levin, & Kelly, 1977).

Critique

The Trail Making Test still receives fairly wide clinical use among neuropsychiatric hospital practitioners. In Craig's (1979) survey, 10.5% of respondents used the Trail Making Tests singly as a screening device, and 45.6% of the clinicians sampled included the TMT as a standard part of the entire Halstead–Reitan Battery. TMT is an attractive screening device because of its brevity, its sensitivity to a wide variety of clinical disorders of functional and/or organic etiology, and its relative resistance to spurious but common effects such as reactively depessed mood. It can be given quickly by clerical personnel with little formal training. It is inexpensive of staff time and materials. Since the only score is the time in seconds taken to complete the test, there is no difficulty with scoring validity or accuracy. As Goldstein and Neuringer (1966) have shown, however, the observant clinician can gain a good deal of incidental qualitative information about the patient's response strategy, which can be of value in differential diagnosis.

The major disadvantage of the TMT is the issue of false positive and false negative rates, which average approximately 15–20%, depending upon the sample. This is a typical failure rate for neuropsychological screening devices, but considerably improved hit rates can be obtained with an abbreviated form of the Halstead–Reitan Neuropsychological Battery. This measure combines several of the screening measures reviewed in this chapter with other brief measures such as the Stroop Color and Word Test to produce an examination that requires about an hour to administer (Golden, 1976). The choice of a screening measure essentially is a matter of brevity versus accuracy. The clinician who uses the TMT in a repeated measures design also should note that Dye (1979) found a significant practice effect on the TMT with young normals, so that "improvement" in TMT scores over a brief time interval may be due as much to practice effect as to the interposed clinical or experimental treatment.

Future researchers who employ the TMT could profitably increase our knowledge of the effects of normal aging, medication effects in chronic schizophrenia, polydrug abuse, and criterion lateralized or localized lesions on TMT performance. Discriminant function analyses of the differential diagnostic value of the TMT with various clinical groups such as those noted above would be of value to determine the screening power and efficiency of the test with these clinical groups.

WECHSLER ADULT INTELLIGENCE SCALE

The Wechsler Adult Intelligence Scale (WAIS) continues to be widely used among neuropsychological practitioners in neuropsychiatric settings (cf. Goodglass & Kaplan, 1979; Lezak, 1976). Craig (1979) found that in his sample the WAIS was employed by 70.2% of the respondents as a neuropsychological measure, which was a rate second only to the Bender–Gestalt. As a standard intellectual measure with ubiquitous clinical and experimental use, it has excellent validity and reliability (Matarazzo, 1972; Zimmerman & Woo-Sam, 1973). While the entire WAIS subtest array can be used in neuropsychological evaluation (for review see Lezak, 1976), the Block Design and Digit Symbol subtests are particularly useful for qualitative evaluation of perceptual–motor deficits. Each of these subtests will be considered in turn within this context.

WAIS Block Design Subtest

The Block Design subtest from the WAIS is a satisfactory measure of visual–motor coordination and a relatively culture-fair measure of nonverbal reasoning (Zimmerman & Woo-Sam, 1973). The WAIS version of the test presents the patient with blocks that have two of the six sides painted red, two sides painted white, and two sides painted diagonally half-red and half-white. The first two designs are demonstrated by the examiner with a concrete model in the patient's view for the first item that is made from blocks by the examiner while the patient observes. A card design is substituted for the second figure, and the examiner constructs the design in the patient's view. Two trials are allowed if the patient fails on the first attempt at either of the first two items. Thereafter the patient constructs more and more complex designs with four or nine blocks, depending upon the design complexity. The test is sensitive to any locus of brain injury in the cerebral cortex (Lezak, 1976). This is so at least in part because cerebral hemispheres must cooperate to solve the task presented by the Block Design items. This interhemispheric cooperation process is basic to visual perception (Luria, 1973), and it has been graphically demonstrated in a commissurotomized patient by Kaplan (see Geschwind, 1979). Kaplan showed that the outer square configuration or shape of the block designs was maintained but that internal details were confused when the patient attempted to solve the task with the left hand only. This meant that the commissurotomized patient was attempting to solve the task with the right cerebral hemisphere alone. When the same task was attempted with the right hand (left cerebral hemisphere) alone, the configuration was "broken" and the square outline shape was lost. As a result the patient attempted to reproduce the figure piecemeal from an analysis of internal details, and the overall configuration was lost.

Kaplan's results had been anticipated in intuitive form by Goldstein and Scheerer (1941), who noted that some of their patients became perceptually regressed after they had suffered brain injury. These patients subsequently broke the square outer block configurations in an attempt to solve some of the more complex figures that required attention to different parts of the design. For example, a block design might require diagonal block placement with half of the exposed face white and the other half red to contribute to that part of the design on each side of a diagonal stripe pattern. The patients who broke configurations typically could not break up the design into these more discrete units and became perceptually "stimulus bound" or "concrete" in their attempts to solve the task by using solid colored block faces to make rows of blocks with all red or all white elements to make the desired stripe pattern shown in the stimulus figure. Goldstein and Scheerer rightly inferred that the patient who makes such errors "translates his color impressions into that choice or arrangement of blocks which is the simplest for him ... in so doing he need not break up the material into real squares and their subdivisions which would cut through the model or his own pattern." One should thus be aware that the breaking of the square configurational outline on the Block Design Test is a strong clue to impaired right cerebral hemisphere visual–perceptual functioning, while preservation of the square outer configuration with distortion of internal details is typical of left cerebral hemisphere dysfunction.

A systematic study of Block Design errors as an index of constructional difficulty in patients with focal head injuries to one of the four quadrants of the brain was reported by Black and Strub (1976). They found that the highest scaled scores (best performance) on this measure occurred in left anterior lesion cases, and that the poorest performances were found in right posterior lesion patients. There were significantly better performance levels demonstrated on WAIS Block Design in patients with anterior as compared to posterior lesions, and performance level was better in patients with lesions of the left hemisphere than in patients with lesions of the right cerebral hemisphere.

WAIS Digit Symbol Subtest

The Digit Symbol subtest of the WAIS is a measure of visual–motor coordination, dexterity, speed, accuracy, and immediate memory (Zimmerman & Woo-Sam, 1973), particularly in neurologically intact populations. Glosser, Butters, and Kaplan (1977), however, also have noted that in brain-damaged populations there also are relevant "visual processing variables, e.g. visual scanning, contour formation, and organization" that contribute to deficient performance level in such patients on this task. Familarity with the stimulus figures and their perceptual salience for verbal encoding when they are unfamiliar also were noted as significant features that may affect performance.

The Digit Symbol subtest presents the patient with a key in which each of the numbers from 1 through 9 is placed in the top half of a rectangular space with a corresponding symbol underneath it in the bottom half of the space to represent the number. The key has the numbers arranged from left to right in ascending numerical order. Beneath the key is an array of 100 more spaces with the top halves of the spaces containing numbers arranged in random order and the spaces beneath the numbers left blank. The subject's task is to place the correct symbol beneath each number as rapidly as possible. The items must be done in the order that they appear, so that the patient is not allowed to scan the array in an attempt to fill in all of the items that have one symbol at a time, such as all the 2s or all the 8s. Immediate memory and flexibility in alternating between symbols as well as speed of motor output are at a premium for the subject who earns a high score. The examiner completes the first three items for the patient as a model, and the patient then completes the next seven items as a pretest practice series to be sure that s/he has grasped the task. Then 90 seconds are allowed for the patient to complete as many of the following 90 items as s/he is able to do. Rarely do patients complete the entire task in the allotted time limit. Zimmerman and Woo-Sam (1973) suggest that the patient's performance should be noted for fatigue and attentional laxity. The WAIS Digit Span subtest can be used as an index of attentional laxity in addition to clinical observation of the subject's attention to task.

SYMBOL DIGIT MODALITIES TEST

Smith (1968, 1969, 1971, 1972) developed the Symbol Digit Modalities Test (SDMT) as a screening test for organic cerebral dysfunction and as a level of performance measure that was applicable to patients with motor output or speech dysfunction. It has proven successful as a group screening device for children with learning disabilities, mixed brain-damaged patients, mental retardates, and controls. It is thus surprising that Craig (1979) reported its use among only 1.8% of neuropsychiatric facility neuropsychological practitioners.

Smith (1968, 1976) altered Wechsler's technique with the Digit Symbol subtest of the WAIS and reversed the positions of the symbols and digits to create a variant that he called the Symbol Digit Modalities Test. The patient is presented with a key in which the numbers from 1 to 9 are paired with symbols, several of which are variants of each other. In the SDMT the patient is presented with 10 practice items and an array of 110 test items in which the symbols are presented in the upper half of the spaces and the appropriate numbers from the key are to be provided by the patient. Then 90 seconds are allowed for the patient to complete as many test items as possible.

One advantage of the SDMT is that subjects with motor output deficits can be tested by calling out the number of the appropriate symbols, while the examiner records the responses. Testing with the Digit Symbol subtest of the WAIS cannot employ this procedure because there is no convenient and generally accepted way to name the geometric symbols in a brief, easily recognized manner that is conductive to rapid response, as can be done with numbers. Smith (1976) presents evidence that the SDMT has wide cross-cultural applicability because the concept of number has almost universal recognition. Certainly, local norms are necessary when subjects from another culture are tested, but there are encouraging results from cross-cultural research with the SDMT that suggest it is relatively culture-fair with appropriate norms. Smith (1976) also suggests use of the SDMT as a subtle, brain-dysfunction screening measure. It seems particularly well suited to learning and reading disorders in which there are letter and figure reversals because several of the symbols are variants of each other, which should be sensitive to such perceptual errors. Smith suggests comparison of the written and oral forms of the SDMT for clinical interpretation. Deficits in written performance with normal oral performance suggests a difficulty with motor output. The reverse pattern suggests speech output difficulty. Subnormal performance on both the written and oral forms requires further evaluation of the reasons for the deficiency, particularly evaluation of visual acuity. The SDMT can provide a useful, brief, objective means of screening patients singly or in groups for visual–motor problems. If the group administration is chosen, the written form can be done in this fashion, but the oral portion must be done individually.

Critique

The SDMT provides a useful measure for neuropsychological screening, particularly with patients who have dysarthric or aphasic speech difficulty or who have motor output problems. Much more effort is often necessary to separate these effects with other tests, and the SDMT deserves more general clinical use than that reported by Craig (1979) to investigate its clinical utility. It is a relatively new measure, however, and most of the widely used measures are established through long use among clinical examiners. Future research with the SDMT would profitably focus on the performance of broad criterion psychiatric groups such as schizophrenics, reactively depressed medical and psychiatric patients, the normal aged, and sex differences across the age range (Smith, 1976). A successful differential diagnostic combination of the SDMT and the MMPI Depression scale led to higher diagnostic separation of depressive and organic subjects than a variety of other timed tests that have relevance for cerebral functioning (Watson, Davis, & Gasser, 1978). More work in this area is needed to extend the clinical utility and application of the SDMT in neuropsychiatric settings.

REY–OSTERREITH COMPLEX FIGURE TEST

Rey (1941) developed a "complex figure" for the investigation of perceptual dysfunction and visual dysmnesia in brain-damaged patients. Osterreith (1944) standardized the stimulus figure and developed an elaborate scoring system for its component parts with norms for children and adults (for review, see Lezak, 1976). This test is not reported as being in routine use among clinicians in neuropsychiatric settings sampled by Craig (1979), but it appears intermittently in the literature in pilot studies, case studies, and reviews (cf. Goodglass & Kaplan, 1979; Kello & Kovac, 1975; Kosc, 1979; Lezak, 1976; Powell, 1979; Taylor, 1959; Teuber, Milner & Vaughan, 1968).

Goodglass and Kaplan (1979) make perhaps the most cogent argument for the inclusion of this measure in a battery designed to measure visuopractic skills. They present data on a right-hemispheric-damaged patient who showed clear visuopractic deficits on the Rey–Osterreith Complex Figure Test, in which the figure was segmentally drawn, but the spatial arrangement of the individual elements to each other was grossly disorganized. Kaplan (1980) has shown clinically that the same sort of piecemeal internal detail analysis is typical of patients with right hemispheric damage since they attempt to analyze the figure primarily with an intact left hemisphere. Patients with a damaged left hemisphere employ the spared right hemisphere to scan the overall configuration for form and make errors on recall of internal details. This strategy follows directly from the errors noted earlier in patients with lateralized lesions on the WAIS Block Design subtest. See Figure 4 for examples of these drawings.

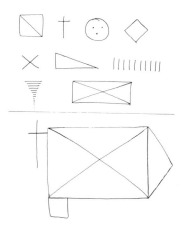

Figure 4. Upper half of figure shows an attempt at recall of the Rey–Osterreith Complex Figure of the type expected from a patient with a severe right hemispheric lesion. Note segmental analysis of internal details. Lower half of figure shows an attempt at recall of the Rey–Osterreith Complex Figure of the type expected from a patient with a severe left hemispheric lesion. Note absence of internal details with preservation of overall form. (See text for discussion.)

Case report data are sufficiently encouraging with the Rey–Osterreith Complex Figure Drawing Test that systematic empirical exploration of the qualitative error scores made by patients with lateralized and focal brain lesions should be performed. The performance of normals on the task to highlight individual differences and the range of normal variation in the elderly on this task have yet to be systematically explored by empirical means.

BOSTON PARIETAL LOBE BATTERY

The Parietal Lobe Battery of the Boston Diagnostic Aphasia Examination (Goodglass & Kaplan, 1972) provides a thorough measure of key apraxic and agnosic disorders that are sensitive to the syndrome of the parietal lobe: constructional difficulty, finger agnosia, acalculia, and right–left confusion. In the context of visual–motor function evaluation we will be concerned only with the first of these skills, constructional difficulty, but the interested reader is referred to the original source for an excellent discussion of the associated testing procedures.

The Parietal Lobe Battery tests two- and three-dimensional constructional praxis by means of line drawings, stick constructions, and block constructions. The six line drawings include a clock face with the numbers and hands indicated, a daisy, an elephant, the Red Cross symbol, a cube in perspective (to show the top and two faces), and a house (to show the roof and two sides). The patient is given a blank half sheet of paper to draw each figure to verbal command. If s/he is unable to do so adequately for any figure, a model is provided and the patient is asked to copy it. Credit is given for the general outline of the figures and for symmetry and accuracy of details. These are not tests of artistic ability *per se*, but measures of how accurately the patient is able to reproduce the essential details of the figures. Ability to do so shows intact perceptual processing that is sufficient to recognize the figures, and a modicum of voluntary motor control that is necessary to reproduce the essential features of the figures. Omission or distortion of details are the sort of subtler errors that are sensitive to residual, higher order, or milder visuopractic deficits.

The stick construction figures are 14 designs of graded complexity that are presented first for reproduction from memory. Each design is assembled before the patient by the examiner as a model for the patient's performance. The patient is told that s/he will have to make the design after s/he has observed the examiner's model. Ten seconds are allowed for the patient to memorize the model, after which it is removed and the patient is asked to construct it from memory. One looks for the same sort of errors that were noted for the drawing tasks mentioned in earlier sections of this chapter. Rotation, simplification, omission, confabulation, mirror imaging, perseveration, and the like may be noted as measures of visual–motor regression, as is the case when they appear as drawing errors. If the patient is unable to make a design from immediate memory, the examiner reconstructs the figure and s/he has the patient copy the design with the examiner's figure as a model in view. If the design is still faulty, one could test the limits by asking the patient if the reproduction is the same as the examiner's model. Inability to recognize errors with the examiner's model in view suggests a perceptual problem, whereas inability to correct the model despite recognition of the error suggests a problem with voluntary praxis.

The three-dimensional block construction task is an extension of the stick construction task principle. The patient is shown a series of 10 photographed, three-dimensional block designs of graduated difficulty, one at a time, and s/he then is asked to reproduce them with square, triangular, and rectangular shaped blocks of various sizes. This task requires analysis of perspective and spatial relationships. It presents the patient with a more challenging problem in perceptual analysis than do the two-dimensional drawing and stick construction tasks. Such a three-dimensional problem may be particularly helpful with the assessment of higher order, subtle, and residual visual–motor functioning deficits.

SYNOPSIS

The tests that have been reviewed as measures of visual–motor skills in this chapter all are easily obtained and relatively inexpensive. Most of them are in common clinical use. They have gained wide acceptance among practicing clinicians because of their reliability, validity, and/or utility in the assessment of clinical neuropsychological syndromes. Clinicians who make use of the standard interpretive principles for these instruments as measures of short-term memory, perceptual–motor integrity, or nonverbal intellectual functioning components, however, often may overlook an opportunity for a careful analysis of the visual–motor, input–output processes that underlie the patient's ability to perform the test tasks. These are essential to a basic understanding of the patient's errors and their significance for adaptive functioning. The analysis necessary for such understanding is relatively simple once it has been operationalized, and it requires little additional work. The busy clinician thereby can gain a good deal more information than would be obtained from an overall evaluation of the results that omits an examination of the patient's information processing strategies and errors.

REFERENCES

Albert, M. A simple test of visual neglect. *Neurology,* 1973, *12,* 659–664.

Alvarez, R. R. Comparison of depressive and brain-injured subjects on the Trail Making Test. *Perceptual and Motor Skills,* 1962, *14,* 91–96.

Amante, D., Van Houten, V. W., Grieve, J. H., Bader, C. A., & Margules, P. H. Neuropsychological deficit, ethnicity, and socioeconomic status. *Journal of Consulting and Clinical Psychology,* 1977, *45,* 524–535.

Ammons, R. B., & Ammons, C. H. Use and evaluation of the Memory for Designs Test: Partial summary through December 1977. I. Published Papers. *Perceptual and Motor Skills,* 1978a, *47,* 795–798.

Ammons, R. B., & Ammons, C. H. Use and evaluation of the Memory for Designs Test: Partial summary through December 1977. II. Reviews, theses, reports at meetings. *Perceptual and Motor Skills,* 1978b, *47,* 809–810.

Andert, J. H. Dinning, W. D., & Hustak, T. L. Koppitz errors on the Bender–Gestalt for adult retardates: Normative data. *Perceptual and Motor Skills,* 1976, *42,* 451–454.

Arena, R., & Gainotti, G. Constructional apraxia and visuoperspective disabilities in relation to laterality of cerebral lesions. *Cortex,* 1978, *14,* 463–473.

Arenberg, D. The effects of auditory augmentation on visual retention for young and old adults. *Journal of Gerontology,* 1977, *32,* 192–195.

Arenberg, D. Differences and changes with age in the Benton Visual Retention Test. *Journal of Gerontology,* 1978, *33,* 534–540.

Armitage, S. G. An analysis of certain psychological tests used for the evaluation of brain injury. *Psychological Monographs,* 1946, *60* (1, Whole No. 277).

Ayers, J. L., Templer, D. I., Ruff, C. F., & Barthlow, V. L. Trail Making Test improvement in abstinent alcoholics. *Journal of Studies on Alcohol,* 1978, *39,* 1627–1629.

Bender, L. A visual motor gestalt test and its clinical use. *American Orthopsychiatric Association Research Monographs,* 1938, No. 3.

Benton, A. L. A visual retention test for clinical use. *Archives of Neurology and Psychiatry,* 1945, *54,* 212–216.

Benton, A. L. A multiple choice form of the Visual Retention Test. *Archives of Neurology and Psychiatry,* 1950, *64,* 699–707.

Benton, A. L. *Revised visual retention test: Clinical and experimental applications* (4th ed.). New York: The Psychological Corporation, 1974.

Benton, A. L., Hamsher, K. de S., & Stone, F. B. *Visual retention test: Multiple choice form I.* Iowa City: Division of Behavioral Neurology, University Hospitals, 1977.

Birkett, D. P., & Boltuch, B. Measuring dementia. *Journal of the American Geriatrics Society,* 1977, *25,* 153–156.

Black, W. F. The utility of the Memory for Designs Test with patients with penetrating missile wounds of the brain. *Journal of Clinical Psychology,* 1974, *30,* 75–77.

Black, W. F., & Strub, R. L. Constructional apraxia in patients with discrete missile wounds of the brain. *Cortex,* 1976, *12,* 212–220.

Brilliant, P. J., & Gynther, M. D. Relationships between the performance on three tests for organicity and selected patient variables. *Journal of Consulting Psychology,* 1963, *27,* 474–480.

Bruhn, A. R., & Reid, M. R. Simulation of brain damage on the Bender–Gestalt Test by college subjects. *Journal of Personality Assessment,* 1975, *39,* 244–248.

Butler, O. T., Coursey, R. D., & Gatz, M. Comparison of the Bender–Gestalt Test for both black and white brain-damaged patients using two scoring systems. *Journal of Consulting and Clinical Psychology,* 1976, *44,* 280–285.

Canter, A. H. A background interference procedure to increase sensitivity of the Bender–Gestalt Test to organic brain disorder. *Journal of Consulting and Clinical Psychology,* 1966, *30.* 91–97.

Canter, A. H. BIP Bender Test for the detection of organic brain disorder: Modified scoring method and replication. *Journal of Consulting and Clinical Psychology,* 1968, *32,* 522–526.

Canter, A. H. A comparison of the background interference procedure effect in schizophrenic, nonschizophrenic and organic patients. *Journal of Clinical Psychology,* 1971, *27,* 473–474.

Canter, A. H. *The Canter background interference procedure for the Bender–Gestalt test.* Nashville, Tennessee: Counselor Recordings, 1976.

Colombo, A., DeRenzi, E., & Faglioni, P. The occurrence of visual neglect in patients with unilateral cerebral disease. *Cortex,* 1976, *12,* 221–231.

Conley, F. K., Moses, J. A., Jr., & Helle, T. L. Deficits of higher cortical functioning caused by posterior parietal arteriovenous malformations: Pre- and postoperative testing with the Luria–Nebraska Neuropsychological Battery. *Neurosurgery,* 1980, *7,* 230–237.

Craig, P. L. Neuropsychological assessment in public psychiatric hospitals: The current state of the practice. *Clinical Neuropsychology,* 1979, *1,* 1–7.

Dastoor, D. P., Klingner, A., Muller, H. F., & Kachanoff, R. A psychogeriatric assessment program. V. Three year follow-up. *Journal of the American Geriatrics Society,* 1979, *27,* 162–169.

Davids, A., Goldenberg, L. & Laufer, M. W. The relation of the Archimedes spiral aftereffect and the Trail Making Test to brain damage in children. *Journal of Consulting Psychology,* 1957, *21,* 429–433.

Davies, A. D. M. The influence of age on Trail Making Test performance. *Journal of Clinical Psychology,* 1968, *24,* 96–98.

Davis, L. J., & Reitan, R. M. Methodological note on the relationship between ability to copy a simple configuration and Wechsler verbal and performance IQs. *Perceptual and Motor Skills,* 1966, *22,* 381–382.

Doehring, D. G., & Reitan, R. M. Language disorders in brain-damaged patients. *AMA Archives of Neurology,* 1961, *5,* 294–299.

Dye, O. A. Effects of practice on Trail Making Test performance. *Perceptual and Motor Skills,* 1979, *48,* 296.

Fine, E. W., & Steer, R. A. Short-term spatial memory deficits in men arrested for driving while intoxicated. *American Journal of Psychiatry,* 1979, *136,* 594–597.

Finlayson, M. A., Johnson, K. A., & Reitan, R. K. Relationship of level of education to neuropsychological measures in brain-damaged and non-brain-damaged adults. *Journal of Consulting and Clinical Psychology,* 1977, *45,* 536–542.

Fitzhugh, L. C., Fitzhugh, K. B., & Reitan, R. M. Adaptive abilities and intellectual functioning in hospitalized alcoholics. *Quarterly Journal of Studies on Alcohol,* 1960, *21,* 414–423.

Fitzhugh, L. C., Fitzhugh, K. B., & Reitan, R. M. Adaptive abilities and intellectual functioning of hospitalized alcoholics: Further considerations. *Quarterly Journal of Studies on Alcohol,* 1965, *26,* 402–411.

Foster, J. C. Significant responses in certain memory tests. *Journal of Applied Psychology,* 1920, *4,* 142–154.

Friedman, A. F., Wakefield, J. A., Sasek, J., & Schroeder, D. A new screening system for the Spraings Multiple Choice Bender–Gestalt Test. *Journal of Clinical Psychology,* 1977, *33,* 205–207.

Geschwind, N. Specializations of the human brain. *Scientific American,* 1979, *241,* 180–182; 186–187; 189–192; 196; 198–199.

Gilmore, G., Chandy, J., & Anderson, T. The Bender–Gestalt and the Mexican–American student: A report. *Psychology in the Schools,* 1975, *12,* 172–175.

Glosser, G., Butters, N., & Kaplan, E. Visuoperceptual processes in brain damaged patients on the Digit Symbol Substitution Test. *International Journal of Neuroscience,* 1977, *7,* 59–66.

Goldberg, L. R. The effectiveness of clinicians' judgments: The diagnosis of organic brain damage from the Bender–Gestalt Test. *Journal of Consulting Psychology,* 1959, *23,* 25–30.

Goldberg, L. R. Objective diagnostic tests and measures. *Annual Review of Psychology,* 1974, *25,* 343–372.

Golden, C. J. The identification of brain damage by an abbreviated form of the Halstead–Reitan Neuropsychological Battery. *Journal of Clinical Psychology,* 1976, *32,* 821–826.

Golden, C. J. *Diagnosis and rehabilitation in clinical neuropsychology.* Springfield, Ill.: Charles C Thomas, 1978.

Golden, C. J., Hammeke, T. A., & Purisch, A. D. *The Luria–Nebraska neuropsychological battery manual.* Los Angeles: Western Psychological Services, 1980.

Golden, C. J., Osmon, D. C., Moses, J. A., Jr., & Berg, R. A. *Interpretation of the Halstead–Reitan Neuropsychological Battery: A casebook approach.* New York: Grune & Stratton, 1981.

Golden, C. J., Purisch, A. D., & Hammeke, T. A. *The Luria–Nebraska Neuropsychological Battery: A manual for clinical and experimental uses.* Lincoln: University of Nebraska Press, 1979.

Goldstein, G., & Neuringer, C. Schizophrenic and organic signs on the Trail Making Test. *Perceptual and Motor Skills,* 1966, *22,* 347–350.

Goldstein, K., & Scheerer, M. Abstract and concrete behavior: An experimental study with special tests. *Psychological Monographs,* 1941, *53,* (2, Whole No. 239).

Goodglass, H., & Kaplan, E. *The assessment of aphasia and related disorders.* Philadelphia: Lea & Febiger, 1972.

Goodglass, H., & Kaplan, E. Assessment of cognitive deficit in the brain-injured patient. In M. S. Gazzaniga (Ed.), *Handbook of behavioral neurobiology* (Vol. 2). New York: Plenum, 1979.

Gordon, N. G. Diagnostic efficiency of the Trail Making Test as a function of cut-off score, diagnosis, and age. *Perceptual and Motor Skills,* 1978, *47,* 191–195.

Graham, F. K., & Kendall, B. S. Performance of brain-damaged cases on a Memory-for Designs Test. *Journal of Abnormal and Social Psychology,* 1946, *41,* 303–314.

Graham, F. K., & Kendall, B. S. Memory-for-Designs Test: Revised general manual. *Perceptual and Motor Skills,* 1960, *11,* 147–188.

Grundvig, J. L., Ajax, E. T., & Needham, W. E. Screening organic brain impairment with the Memory-for-Designs Test: Validation of comparison of different scoring systems and exposure times. *Journal of Clinical Psychology,* 1973, *29,* 350–354.

Hagberg, B. Defects of immediate memory related to the cerebral blood flow distribution. *Brain and Language*, 1978, *5*, 366–377.

Hain, J. D. The Bender–Gestalt Test: A scoring method for identifying brain damage. *Journal of Consulting Psychology*, 1964, *28*, 34–40.

Halstead, W. C., & Wepman, J. M. The Halstead–Wepman Aphasia Screening Test. *Journal of Speech and Hearing Disorders*, 1949, *14*, 9–15.

Hammeke, T. A., Golden, C. J., & Purisch, A. D. A standardized, short, and comprehensive neuropsychological test battery based on the Luria neuropsychological evaluation. *International Journal of Neuroscience*, 1978, *8*, 135–141.

Heimburger, R. F., & Reitan, R. M. Easily administered written test for lateralizing brain lesions. *Journal of Neurosurgery*, 1961, *18*, 301–311.

Holland, T. R., & Wadsworth, H. M. Comparison and combination of recall and background interference procedures for the Bender–Gestalt Test with brain-damaged and schizophrenic patients. *Journal of Personality Assessment*, 1979, *43*, 123–127.

Hustak, T. L., Dinning, W. D., & Andert, J. N. Reliability of the Koppitz scoring system for the Bender–Gestalt Test. *Journal of Clinical Psychology*, 1976, *32*, 468–469.

Hutt, M. *The Hutt adaptation of the Bender–Gestalt Test* (2nd ed.). New York: Grune & Stratton, 1969.

Hutt, M. L., & Briskin, G. J. *The clinical uses of the Revised Bender–Gestalt Test*. New York: Grune & Stratton, 1960.

Joslyn, D., Grundvig, J. L., & Chamberlain, C. J. Predicting confabulation from the Graham–Kendall Memory for Designs Test. *Journal of Consulting and Clinical Psychology*, 1978, *46*, 181–182.

Jost, K. Studies on schizophrenics using the Benton Visual Retention Test. *Diagnostica*, 1977, *23*, 173–178.

Kaplan, E. The right cerebral hemisphere. In E. Kaplan & N. Helm, *Hemispheric specialization: An interdisciplinary approach to the assessment and treatment of acquired neurolinguistic and neuropsychological deficits*. Conference presented at the University of California, University Extension, Berkeley, October 18–19, 1980.

Kello, A., & Kovac, D. A probe into the relationships between emotional lability and memory performance. *Studia Psychologica*, 1975, *17*, 306–308.

Kendall, B. S., & Graham, F. K. Further standardization of the Memory-for-Designs Test on children and adults. *Journal of Consulting Psychology*, 1948, *12*, 349–354.

Kish, G. B., Hagen, J. M., Woody, M. M., & Harvey, H. L. Alcoholics' recovery from cerebral impairment as a function of duration of abstinence. *Journal of Clinical Psychology*, 1980, *36*, 584–589.

Klajajic, I. The MFD and brain pathology. *Journal of Clinical Psychology*, 1976, *32*, 91–93.

Koppitz, E. M. *The Bender–Gestalt test for young children*. New York: Grune & Stratton, 1964.

Koppitz, E. M. *The Bender–Gestalt test for young children* (Vol. 2): *Research and application, 1963–1973*. New York: Grune & Stratton, 1975.

Korman, M., & Blumberg, S. Comparative efficiency of some tests of cerebral damage. *Journal of Consulting Psychology*, 1963, *27*, 303–309.

Kosc, L. To the problems of diagnosing disorders of mathematical functions in children. *Studia Psychologica*, 1979, *21*, 62–67.

Kumar, S. Short-term memory for a nonverbal tactual task after cerebral commissurotomy, *Cortex*. 1977, *13*, 55–61.

Lacks, P. B. The use of the Bender–Gestalt in clinical neuropsychology. *Clinical Neuropsychology*, 1979, *1*, 29–34.

Lacks, P. B., & Newport, K. A comparison of scoring systems and level of scorer experience on the Bender–Gestalt Test. *Journal of Personality Assessment*, 1980, *44*, 351–357.

Levine, J., & Feirstein, A. Differences in test performance between brain damaged, schizophrenic, and medical patients. *Journal of Consulting and Clinical Psychology*, 1972, *39*, 508–512.

Lezak, M. D. *Neuropsychological assessment*. New York: Oxford University Press, 1976.

Luria, A. R. *Higher cortical functions in man*. New York: Basic Books, 1966.

Luria, A. R. *The working brain: An introduction to neuropsychology*. New York: Basic Books, 1973.

Lyle, O., & Quast, W. The Bender–Gestalt: Use of clinical judgement versus recall scores in prediction of Huntington's disease. *Journal of Consulting and Clinical Psychology*, 1976, *44*, 229–232.

Martin-Ramirez, J., Gadow, M., & Aksamski, R. Intellectual efficiency after cerebral tumor surgery. *Archivos de Neurobiologia*, 1977, *40*, 177–196.

Matarazzo, J. D. *Wechsler's measurement and appraisal of adult intelligence* (5th ed.). Baltimore: Williams and Wilkins, 1972.

McGuire, F. L. A comparison of the Bender–Gestalt and Flicker Fusion as indicators of CNS involvement. *Journal of Clinical Psychology*, 1960, *16*, 276–278.

Mezzich, J. E., & Moses, J. A., Jr. Efficient screening for brain dysfunction. *Biological Psychiatry*, 1980, *15*, 333–337.

Nahas, A. D. The prediction of perceptual-motor abnormalities in paranoid schizophrenia. *Research Communications in Psychology, Psychiatry, and Behavior*, 1976, *1*, 167–181.

Norton, J. C. The Trail Making Test and Bender Background Interference Procedure as screening devices. *Journal of Clinical Psychology*, 1978, *34*, 916–922.

Orme, J. E. Bender design recall and brain damage. *Diseases of the Nervous System*, 1962, *23*, 329–335.

Osterreith, P. A. Le test de copie d'une figure complexe. *Archives de Psychologie*, 1944, *30*, 206–356.

Page, R. D., & Schaub, L. H. Intellectual functioning in alcoholics during six months' abstinence. *Journal of Studies on Alcohol*, 1977, *38*, 1240–1246.

Pascal, G. R., & Suttell, B. J. *The Bender–Gestalt Test: Quantification and validity for adults*. New York: Grune & Stratton, 1951.

Pauker, J. D. A quick-scoring system for the Bender–Gestalt: Interrater reliability and scoring validity. *Journal of Clinical Psychology*, 1976, *32*, 86–89.

Peters, B. H., Levin, H. S., & Kelly, P. J. Neurologic and psychologic manifestations of decompression illness in divers. *Neurology*, 1977, *27*, 125–127.

Powell, G. E. The relationship between intelligence and verbal and spatial memory. *Journal of Clinical Psychology*, 1979, *35*, 335–340.

Quattlebaum, L. F. A brief note on the relationship between two psychomotor tests. *Journal of Clinical Psychology*, 1968, *24*, 198–199.

Reitan, R. M. Intelligence and language functions in dysphasic patients. *Diseases of the Nervous System*, 1954, *15*, 131–137.

Reitan, R. M. The relation of the Trail Making Test to organic brain damage. *Journal of Consulting Psychology*, 1955, *19*, 393–394.

Reitan, R. M. Validity of the Trail Making Test as an indicator of organic brain damage. *Perceptual and Motor Skills*, 1958, *8*, 271–276.

Reitan, R. M. *Trail Making Test: Manual for administration, scoring, and interpretation*. Unpublished manuscript, 1958.

Reitan, R. M. *The effects of brain lesions on adaptive abilities in human beings*. Unpublished manuscript, 1959.

Reitan, R. M. The significance of dysphasic for intelligence and adaptive abilities. *The Journal of Psychology*, 1960, *50*, 355–376.

Reitan, R. M. Personal communication, March 19, 1975.

Reitan, R. M., & Davison, L. A. *Clinical neuropsychology: Current status and applications.* New York: Wiley, 1974.

Reitan, R. M., & Tarshes, E. L. Differential effects of lateralized brain lesions on the Trail Making Test. *Journal of Nervous and Mental Disease,* 1959, *129,* 257–262.

Rey, A. L'examen psychologique dans les cas d'encephalopathie traumatique. *Archives de Psychologie,* 1941, *28,* 286–340.

Russell, E. W. The Bender–Gestalt and the Halstead–Reitan Battery: A case study. *Journal of Clinical Psychology,* 1976, *32,* 355–361.

Russell, E. W., Neuringer, C., & Goldstein, G. *Assessment of brain damage: A neuropsychological key approach.* New York:. Wiley-Interscience, 1970.

Schuell, H. *Differential diagnosis of aphasia with the Minnesota Test.* Minneapolis: University of Minnesota Press, 1965.

Small, L. *Neuropsychodiagnosis in psychotherapy.* New York: Brunner/Mazel, 1973.

Smith, A. The Symbol Digit Modalities Test: A neuropsychologic test of learning and other cerebral disorders. In J. Helmuth (Ed.), *Learning disorders.* Seattle: Special Child Publications, 1968.

Smith, A. Nondominant hemispherectomy. *Neurology,* 1969, *19,* 442–445.

Smith, A. Objective indices of severity of chronic aphasia in stroke patients. *Journal of Speech and Hearing Disorders,* 1971, *36,* 167–207.

Smith, A. Dominant and nondominant hemispherectomy. In W. L. Smith (Ed.), *Drugs, development and cerebral function.* Springfield, Ill.: Charles C Thomas, 1972.

Smith, A. *Symbol digit modalities test manual.* Los Angeles: Western Psychological Service, 1976.

Spraings, V. *The Spraings multiple choice Bender–Gestalt test.* Olympia, Wa.: Sherwood Press, 1966.

Sterne, D. M. The Hooper Visual Organization Test and the Trail Making Tests as discriminants of brain injury. *Journal of Clinical Psychology,* 1973, *29,* 212–213.

Strub, R. L., & Black, W. F. *The mental status examination in neurology.* Philadelphia: F. A. Davis Company, 1977.

Taylor, E. M. *Psychological appraisal of children with cerebral defects.* Cambridge, Mass.: Harvard University Press, 1959.

Teuber, H. L., Milner, B., & Vaughan, H. G. Persistent anterograde amnesia after stab wound of the basal brain. *Neuropsychologia,* 1968, *6,* 267–282.

Tsushima, W. T., & Towne, W. S. Effects of paint sniffing on neuropsychological test performance. *Journal of Abnormal Psychology,* 1977, *86,* 402–407.

Tymchuk, A. J. Comparison of the Bender error and time scores from groups of epileptic, retarded, and behavior problem children. *Perceptual and Motor Skills,* 1974, *38,* 71–72.

Van Couvering, N. *A brief outline of clinical neuropsychology.* Unpublished manuscript, 1970.

Watson, C. G., Davis, W. E., & Gasser, B. The separation of organics from depressives with ability- and personality-based tests. *Journal of Clinical Psychology,* 1978, *34,* 393–397.

Wecowicz, T. E., Fedora, D., Masons, J., Radstaak, D., Bay, K. S., & Yonge, K. A. Effects of marijuana on divergent and convergent production cognitive tests. *Journal of Abnormal Psychology,* 1975, *84,* 386–398.

Weinstein, E. A., & Friedland, F. P. (Eds.). *Hemi-inattention and hemisphere specialization. Advances in neurology* (Vol. 18). New York: Raven Press, 1977.

Wertheimer, M. Studies in the theory of gestalt psychology. *Psychologia Forschung,* 1923, *4,* 300.

Wheeler, L. Predictions of brain damage from an aphasia screening test: An application of discriminant functions and a comparison with a non-linear method of analysis. *Perceptual and Motor Skills,* 1963, *17,* 63–80.

Wheeler, L., & Reitan, R. M. Presence and laterality of brain damage predicted from responses to a short aphasia screening test. *Perceptual and Motor Skills,* 1962, *15,* 783–799.

White, R. B. Variations of Bender–Gestalt constriction and depression in adult psychiatric patients. *Perceptual and Motor Skills,* 1976, *42,* 221–222.

Winter, W. D. *Suggested instructions to client for Bender–Gestalt and TAT administration.* Unpublished manuscript, 1969.

Zimmerman, I. L., & Woo-Sam, J. M. *Clinical interpretation of the Wechsler Adult Intelligence Scale.* New York: Grune & Stratton, 1973.

3

Tests of Intellectual Abilities

RICHARD A. BERG

Disturbances of the intellectual functions—those mental activities having to do with the processing of information—figure very prominently in symptom constellations of brain damage. As a result, intellectual functions have received a great deal of attention from neuropsychologists.

Intellectual behavior was originally attributed to a single intellectual function, general intelligence. Early psychological theorists treated the concept of intelligence as if it were a unitary variable that, like physical strength, increased at a regular rate in the course of normal development (Binet, 1908; Terman, 1916) and decreased with the amount of brain tissue lost through accident, disease, or injury (Chapman & Wolff, 1959; Lashley, 1938). As refinements of testing and data handling techniques have afforded greater precision and control over observations of intellectual behavior, it has become evident that behaviors measured by various tests were directly inferable to specific intellectual functions. The concept of intelligence became meaningful as an abstraction from common observations that reflected the tendency for each organism to process all kinds of information at a similar level of efficiency (Lezak, 1976).

For decades, many investigators have worked on the question of the nature and organization of the mental abilities covered by the global concept of intelligence. The statistical methods of factor analysis that were pioneered by Spearman (1927) and Thurstone (1948) have provided a fruitful approach to this problem.

RICHARD A. BERG ● Division of Neurology/Psychology, Saint Jude Children's Research Hospital, Memphis, Tennessee 38101.

Factor analysis is a statistical technique that allows for the reduction of large amounts of data into smaller, more easily used bits of information. Factor analytic techniques enable the user to see whether some underlying pattern of relationships exists such that the data may be "rearranged" or "reduced" to a smaller set of components that may be viewed as source variables, that account for observed interrelations within a given set of data (Kim, 1975). In brief, therefore, factor analysis is a way to summarize large amounts of data.

Factor analytic studies of intellectual behavior have consistently demonstrated a hierarchical organization of mental abilities. At the top of the hierarchy is the general mental ability factor "g" that represents the extent to which all intellectual activities are associated (Spearman, 1927).

Spearman and Jones (1950) noted that a person will perform at much the same level for a variety of different intellectual tasks. This commonly observed tendency gave an operational meaning to the concept of general intelligence (McNemar, 1965). Since this tendency was first documented at the turn of the century, it has regularly been demonstrated in clinical practice (Williams, 1962), in large sample standardization programs (Terman & Merrrill, 1960; Wechsler, 1958), in longitudinal studies (Anastasi, 1965; Garrett, 1946; Jarvik, Eisdorfer, & Blum, 1973), and in studies of individual abilities in which intraindividual correlations between scores on different skills and functions have been investigated (Bennett, Seashore, & Wesman, 1972). Consistency of intellectual performance tends to appear even when uninvited (Lezak, 1976). In other words, even when attempting to evaluate a specific mental function to the exclusion of all other mental functions, a person will tend to perform at roughly the same level on a variety of intellectual tasks. Test makers have typically failed in their efforts to develop test batteries in which the commonality of performance on different kinds of mental tests would be minimal or eliminated altogether (Payne, 1961; Thurstone, 1948). However, "g" does not represent an intellectual function, for it is the one factor that is not defined by its own unique set of operations, nor does it refer to any given activity.

At the next lower level of the mental ability hierarchy are a number of group factors that are common to such broad classes of mental abilities as verbal, computational, or visual organization. The verbal group factor, for example, appears in all factor analyses of tests of verbal skills, whether they be tests of vocabulary, grammar, or verbal abstraction (Lezak, 1976). Within these broad group factors there may be subgroups of factors referable to narrower ranges of abilities. Tests of grammatical skills, for example, would certainly be weighted with the general verbal factor and may also include a further subgrouping related to knowledge and use of grammar. The factors that emerge will, of course, depend on the tests studied.

The performance of most adults on tests of intellectual ability reflects both the tendency for test scores generally to converge at the same level and for some test scores to differ in small, usually insignificant degrees from others (Payne, 1961; Vernon, 1950). In normal adults, specialization of interests and activities and singular experiences contribute to intraindividual differences. A variety of factors, including social limitations, emotional disturbance, physical illness or handicaps, and brain dysfunction, tend to magnify intraindividual test differences to significant proportions.

Intelligence remains a useful concept in intellectual assessment when it refers to the common tendency of the individual to perform many different intellectual tasks at about the same level of proficiency (Lezak, 1976). Spiker and McCandless (1954) have defined *tendency* as the "transitional consistency" of intellectual behavior. This tendency follows naturally from the conditions of normal development during which different parts of the brain are regulated by the same genetic material, receive the same nourishment, are subjected to the same diseases, and share levels of stimulation. Piercy (1964, p. 341) summarizes this view by defining intelligence as "a tendency for cerebral regions subserving different intellectual functions to be proportionately developed in any one individual. According to this notion, people with good verbal ability will tend also to have good non-verbal ability, in much the same way as people with big hands tend to have big feet."

As noted, early psychological theorists treated the notion of intelligence as a unitary capacity. However, test markers have always acknowledged the multidimensionality of intelligence by developing test instruments that measure several facets of what is labeled intelligence. With few exceptions, the most widely used mental ability tests have been what Lezak (1976) terms composite tests comprised of a variety of tasks testing different skills and capacities.

Composite instruments exist in two basic formats. First, there is *the omnibus composite test* (e.g., the Stanford–Binet Intelligence Scale). In this format, the order of task presentation varies so that each test item or subtest differs from the preceding or succeeding item. For example, a mathematics problem may follow a vocabulary item and be followed in turn by a short-term memory or motor control task. Typically, different kinds of tasks reappear at different difficulty levels. This test format (omnibus) provides frequent activity changes to hold the interest of children and mentally impaired individuals of all ages. It also exposes the individual to a variety of tasks in a reasonable amount of administration time. The quick-change format, however, keeps the examiner so busy manipulating test materials and giving new instructions that it may prove more difficult to observe the patient and his test performance.

The other form of composite test is a *test battery* comprised of a number of distinct subtests such as the Wechsler Adult Intelligence Scale. The battery format eliminates the administration problems of the omnibus approach. Fewer shifts from task to task reduce both the amount of necessary instructions and the handling of test materials to more manageable proportions and give the patient sufficient time to perform the task. Subtests with several similar items at varying levels of difficulty permit relatively fine gradation in item-scaling and development of standardized subtest norms for comparing performances on the various subtest tasks. Such features have resulted in the vast majority of tests of intellectual functions being of the battery type.

The remainder of this chapter will cover a variety of intelligence scales currently being used in neuropsychology. Those tests covered here by no means constitute a complete list of intellectual assessment devices available for use currently. Rather, an attempt has been made to limit the discussion to those tests that appear to be most widely in use. Additionally, the chapter will deal with intelligence scales primarily designed for use with adults. With those scales that can be used with children, the discussion will center on use with an adult population. The primary reason for this is because the great majority of neuropsychological research conducted with intelligence tests has been carried out with adults. While diagnosis and evaluation of children has much in common with adult neuropsychology, one must remain aware of the differential effects of brain injury in children as well as the different instuments that must be employed. Such a discussion is beyond the scope of this chapter. (For a discussion of the neuropsychology of children, the reader is referred to Boll & Barth, 1981, and Rourke, 1981.)

THE WECHSLER ADULT INTELLIGENCE SCALE

The Wechsler Adult Intelligence Scale (WAIS) is an individually administered composite test in battery format (Matarazzo, 1972; Wechsler, 1955, 1958). The original version of what became the WAIS (the Wechsler–Bellevue) was developed in 1939 by David Wechsler. The test was developed to serve as an alternative to the Stanford–Binet Intelligence Scale. The original Wechsler–Bellevue scale did away with the concept of mental age, which at the time was prominent in the assessment of intelligence, and introduced the concept of a deviation IQ that measured an individual's relative standing in relation to his or her peer group.

In 1955 the Wechsler–Bellevue was replaced by an extensively revised test, the WAIS. Many of the deficiencies in the original test were corrected by the WAIS and, at the present time, it is the most frequently used adult intellectual test in mental health and educational settings. Since the introduction of the WAIS in 1955, many of the test items have become outdated to some degree. Additionally, questions have been raised as to the current validity of the scale scores and IQ conversions. As a result, the WAIS has recently been revised and restandardized (Psychological Corporation, 1981).

The major purpose of any intelligence examination is to assess an individual's level of inferable intelligence. Initially, such tests were used to identify individuals who were mentally retarded or who possessed very high intelligence, in order to offer them appropriate educational or work placement. The WAIS, however, offers the examiner the possibility of examining scores on different subtests and allows for the identification of particular areas of strength and weakness in the individual. These resulting patterns can be used to provide vocational training or to make diagnostic decisions in a more refined and specific manner than allowed by an overall IQ score. Diagnostic decisions aided by the WAIS include the diagnosis of the type and extent of brain damage (McFie, 1975), the diagnosis of psychiatric disorders (Rapaport, Gill, & Schafer, 1970), and the assessment of such conditions as chronic alcoholism (Gudeman, Craine, Golden, & McLaughlin, 1977). In each of these instances there is more reliance on the pattern of subtest scores rather than the general IQ's generated by the test.

Administration and Scoring of the WAIS

The WAIS consists of 11 subtests, 6 of which are classified as verbal and 5 of which are classified as performance. Each is administered according to detailed instructions offered in the WAIS manual (Wechsler, 1955). The importance of following the instructions exactly as written is emphasized by Wechsler. Therefore, proper administration necessitates extensive familiarity with the test manual and test material.

In the administration of the WAIS, the following should be initially considered: The examiner and examinee should be interpersonally comfortable with one another; general introduction as to the reason for testing, an explanation of the testing and its purpose, and a relaxed, unhurried atmosphere can serve to do this. In the testing situation the examiner should exhibit an unjudgmental attitude toward the subject. No performance attempted by a subject is "wrong," and all performance, whether right or wrong, should be followed by encouragement to motivate the individual to do his or her best. Specific feedback, however, such as saying "good" after only correct answers, should be avoided because it has been demonstrated to increase most test scores (Isenberg & Bass, 1974; Sattler, 1969).

Each subtest is scored according to the rules specified in the manual. After calculating the raw scores, scaled scores are determined. All scale scores are based on the performance of 500 subjects aged 20–34. The mean of this group has been arbitrarily defined as 10 with a standard deviation of 3. All scale scores are based on this group regardless of the subject's age. Raw scores are easily changed into scale scores by using the conversion table available in all WAIS record sheets.

Scaled scores on the six verbal tests are summed up to give a Verbal Weighted Score. Similarly, the five performance tests are summed up to get a Performance Weighted Score. These two scores are then summed up to give a Full Scale Weighted Score. Following this, the three scores are found in the appropriate IQ conversion table for the patient's current age. In conversion tables, the IQ equivalent of each weighted score is given.

The WAIS Subtests

Information

The 29 Information items serve primarily as a measure of an individual's fund of general information. The subtest represents information to which it is expected that the average individual with an average educational background has had access. The items are arranged in order of difficulty from the four simplest, which all but severely retarded or organically impaired persons answer correctly, to the most difficult, which only 1% of the adult population can answer correctly (Matarazzo, 1972). The test measures long-term memory, remote memory, and the ability to assess and use that memory (Golden, 1979). Information scores that are significantly low in an individual who was once graded as normal suggest severe deterioration in intellectual function, which may be related to severe psychosis or degenerative brain disorders (Golden, 1979). The score will also be low in individuals suffering early brain damage of the left hemisphere or damage involving both hemispheres (Golden, 1979).

Comprehension

This subtest attempts to establish the degree to which the individual understands basic social customs and situations. In the more advanced items, ability to interpret proverbs is also included.

This 14-item subtest includes two kinds of open-ended questions: 11 items test common-sense, judgment, and practical reasoning, and the other 3 items ask for the meaning of proverbs. Comprehension evaluates an individual's long-term memory and exerience, the ability to verbalize these factors, the ability to understand common social customs and situations, and the ability of the individual to demonstrate an understanding of what is a "socially" appropriate activity as well as the reasons behind such activities. The subtest also involves the individual's ability to judiciously select from alternative answers and to provide those answers that are most "socially" acceptable and logical (Rapaport et al., 1970).

Poor performance on Comprehension has been associated with early developmental dysfunction such as brain injury or childhood psychosis. Comparatively low scores on comprehension, as with those on Information, will generally be relatively frequent in brain-injured adults. In the estimation of premorbid level of functioning, Comprehension is generally among the highest scores (Golden, 1979).

Arithmetic

This subtest consists of 14 items and provides a basic measure of an individual's ability to work with arithmetic data in logical and daily problems. In addition to basic arithmetic skills, the test also requires verbal comprehension, memory, and concentration.

Frequently, many individuals react quite uncooperatively to arithmetic problems, refusing to even try simple problems. In many instances, these scores must be discounted in determining the individual's intellectual capabilities. If the examiner feels that this was the case with a given patient, she may wish to omit the arithmetic subtest score from the overall scoring and, instead, prorate the patient's IQ score using the technique described in the test manual. Or, the examiner may wish to compute the patient's IQ scores both with the arithmetic score and without this score (by prorating) and then decide qualitatively which of the two resulting IQ scores is the more representative reflection of the individual's capabilities. Arithmetic often is a low score in mentally retarded individuals as well as brain-injured persons (Lezak, 1976). Also, individuals with concentration problems often perform poorly (Golden, 1979). Furthermore, transient high-anxiety states have been found to cause low scores on this test and on Digit Span (Keiser, 1975; Knox & Grippaldi, 1970).

Similarities

The 13 items in this subtest involve identifying similarities between two objects. The format for each question is, "In what way is a (object one) and a (object two) alike?"

Similarities is a measure of an individual's ability to form verbal concepts (specifically, generalizations) when presented with two members of a given verbal class. The test requires both short-term and remote verbal memory, concentration, and the ability to relate the two objects to a common class. These relationships may be done at two levels: concrete ("you eat them") or abstract ("fruit").

The subtest provides a measure of higher cognitive skills. Individuals who attain high scores are often able to work well with verbal abstract ideas and to handle simple reasoning. Similarities varies little from a person's mean score in most diagnostic groups, thus making it a poor diagnostic indicator of premorbid functioning (Zimmerman & Woo-Sam, 1973). However, in individuals who have sustained a brain injury to the left temporal lobe or left parietal lobe, interference with the person's ability to form verbal categories has been noted (Luria, 1966). This skill is generally not affected except by significant organic and/or functional dysfunction (Golden, 1979).

Digit Span

This subtest consists of two sections: Digits Forward and Digits Backward. For Digits Forward, the subject is told that numbers will be spoken and that the subject should repeat them afterwards, exactly as they have been verbalized by the examiner. Digits Backward is administered in a similar manner, but the subject must repeat the numbers given in reverse order rather than exactly as spoken.

Digit Span has been described as a measure of immediate auditory memory. The test requires the ability to attend and concentrate as well as recall. In the Digits Backward section of the test, there is the additional skill of reverse sequencing, which appears to be largely spatial rather than verbal in nature (Golden, 1978). Digit Span is highly sensitive to both anxiety and brain deterioration (Firetto & Davey, 1971; Golden, 1978; Keiser, 1975; McFie, 1975). Both Digits Forward and Digits Backward are affected by left hemisphere brain damage, especially in the temporal lobe, whereas localized right hemisphere injuries, especially in the right frontal lobe, most often affect only Digits Backward (McFie, 1975).

Vocabulary

The subtest consists of 40 words arranged in order of difficulty. Vocabulary measures the individual's ability to learn words and describe their meanings. It is generally recognized as the best single estimate of general (i.e., "g" factor) intelligence (Golden, 1979). In this subtest, it is assumed that each individual has had a sociologically normative experience of education and cultural background. To the extent that these assumptions are valid, it has been found that Vocabulary can correlate up to .9 with full scale intelligence (e.g., Wechsler, 1955). A brain injury will often not affect the individual's level of performance on this subtest (Gonen & Brown, 1968); however, such an injury will affect future learning of Vocabulary related tasks (Parsons, Vega, Burn, 1969). Thus, Vocabulary can be used to estimate premorbid intelligence affected in adulthood and to estimate the age of injury in an individual injured as a child. The exception of this finding is a generally deteriorating disorder such as Alzheimer's disease (Golden, 1979).

Digit Symbol

The Digit Symbol subtest requires the individual to match empty spaces under the numerical symbols 1 to 9 with nonsense symbols exclusively assigned to individual numbers in a table at the top of the work page. The individual has 90 seconds in which to complete 90 items. Wechsler (1955) provides special instructions for left-handed individuals whose writing hand covers the table that gives the association between numbers and symbols. In this situation, a second key is placed before the subject so that the key can be easily seen.

Digit Symbol has been described as measuring a wide variety of skills (Golden, Osmon, Moses, & Berg, 1981). It is the most sensitive WAIS subtest to motor problems in the dominant hand. In addition, the test measures a basic learning skill—the ability to associate a symbol with a number. This requires immediate visual memory, the ability to sustain a flexible yet complex mental set, and the ability to maintain rapid visual–motor activity in a timed test. Thus, the test is sensitive to high levels of anxiety. The test is also useful in detecting brain dysfunction due to its sensitivity to memory and motor deficits. Efficient performance of this task requires an individual to be able to quickly learn the symbol–number associations. If a patient does not or cannot retain the symbol–number associations, performance will be impeded by the constant need to search the key for the correct association. This subtest must be interpreted with caution, however, as a variety of brain lesions can lead to lowered scores (Golden, 1978), although for a different reason in each case. Additionally, the Digit Symbol subtest is sensitive to psychiatric disorders such as schizophrenia, depression, and anxiety neurosis (Heaton & Crowley, 1981; Rapaport *et al.,* 1970).

Picture Completion

This subtest involves the individual viewing a set of pictures included in the WAIS kit, each of which has an important detail missing. The subject must identify the missing detail of each picture.

Picture Completion evaluates the individual's ability to perceive and visually organize a scene, recognize that an essential element of the scene is missing, and communicate the answer to the examiner. During this process the individual must also be able to avoid distractions and nonessential details.

Of all performance subtests of the WAIS, Picture Completion is the least sensitive to focal brain disorders (Lezak, 1976; Woo-Sam, 1971). Thus, in serious left hemisphere injuries that affect the traditional scores that measure premorbid intelligence (Comprehension, Vocabulary, Information), the Picture Completion score becomes the best estimate of that premorbid intelligence (Lezak, 1976).

Block Design

This subtest uses nine blocks, all of which are identical, having all-red sides, all-white sides, and sides half red and half white, divided along the block's diagonal. The task requires the individual to duplicate 10 designs in the Block Design booklet using the blocks.

Block Design is the purest measure of spatial (nonverbal) reasoning in the

WAIS (Golden, 1978; Lezak, 1976; McFie, 1960, 1975). Visual analysis skills and visual–motor coordination are required for this test. The subject is presented with four or nine blocks, depending on the difficulty of the item. The task is to use the blocks to construct three-dimensional replicas of 10 red-and-white designs printed in smaller scale. As the items become more difficult, speed as well as concentration and attention become necessary. The Block Design test also allows for the observation of the method by which an individual solves a problem (i.e., impulsively, with great planning, hit-and-miss, or a combination of these techniques).

This test is frequently affected extensively by brain dysfunction. This is particularly obvious in diffuse injuries as well as injuries involving either parietal lobe (e.g., Mahan, 1976; McFie, 1969, 1975).

Picture Arrangement

This subtest requires the sequential arrangement of pictures so that they will tell a logical, coherent story.

Picture Arrangement enables evaluation of several major skills, including visual perception of individual pictures, organization of a series of pictures, awareness of social sequences, planning skills, ability to form and test hypotheses, flexibility, and general ability to sequence material in a logical order. Brain-injured individuals do not show as great a loss on Picture Arrangement as they do on the other performance subtests, with the exception of Picture Completion (Golden, 1979). Performance of this test can be affected, however, by injuries to the right frontal areas, and may be lower than the other performance tests in certain left hemisphere injuries that disrupt social or verbal skills (McFie, 1969, 1975).

Object Assembly

Object Assembly is the last Wechsler subtest in the standard administration. It consists of four commonly recognizable items that are represented in jigsaw-puzzle fashion. The subject must complete each item within specified time limits. Timing is extremely important on this test as time bonuses are available for each item.

Object Assembly requires visual analysis and visual–motor skills. The individual must recognize what the object is from the pieces presented, or at least their interrelationship. This subtest, therefore, requires little in the way of abstract thinking. The ability to form visual concepts is needed for an adequate performance on this subtest; the ability to form visual concepts quickly is essential for an average or better score (Lezak, 1976).

Poor scores can occur because of left hemisphere injuries resulting in right hand motor impairment, and as a result of verbal and spatial deficits associated with left parietal lobe damage; however, the test is primarily sensitive to right hemisphere disorders (Golden *et al.*, 1981). Right parietal dysfunction as well as temporal and frontal lobe dysfunction can result in poor performance on this subtest (McFie, 1975).

Scoring Issues

There are a number of issues involved in the interpretation of WAIS scores. Of them, the most important with respect to neuropsychology concern IQ scores, sex differences, and the evaluation of the significance of score patterns.

IQ Scores

The interpretation of the meaning of an intelligence quotient has become a highly controversial issue in psychology (Lezak, 1976). Educators have found that the WAIS Full Scale IQ score, which is calculated from the sum of all the subtest scale scores, is a reasonably good predictor of academic achievement (Lezak, 1976). However, neither the IQ scores calculated for the Verbal or Performance subtests nor the Full Scale IQ score are clinically useful in neuropsychological evaluation. That is, IQ scores simply represent averaged estimates of intellectual performance representing such a variety of neuropsychological functions that they become meaningless in the presence of a neuropsychological disorder. An individual may perform exceptionally well on a few subtests and extremely poorly on others. An IQ score acts to average these good and poor performances in such a manner that the individual's overall IQ falls in the normal range. Thus, IQ scores may act to obscure selective deficits in specific subtests (Smith, 1966).

There has been a great deal of research, which has focused on the significance to neuropsychology of differences between the Wechsler Verbal and Performance IQ scores (e.g., Todd, Coolidge, & Satz, 1977; Zimmerman & Woo-Sam, 1973). The underlying assumption of this line of investigation is that differences between these scores would reflect impairment of one or the other major functional system (i.e., verbal vs. nonverbal functions) and, thus, aid significantly in diagnosis (Lezak, 1976). Both Verbal and Performance IQ scores, however, are based on the averages of quite dissimilar functions that bear little neuroanatomical or neuropsychological relationship to one another (Cohen, 1957; Parsons *et al.*, 1969). Differences between Verbal IQ and Performance IQ have been demonstrated to distinguish patients with primarily left hemisphere damage (lower Verbal IQ scores) from those with impairment to the right hemisphere who have lowered Performance scores (Balthazar & Morrison, 1961; Parsons *et al.*, 1969; Reitan, 1955; Reitan & Fitzhugh, 1971; Satz, Richard, & Daniels, 1967; Vega & Parsons, 1969; Zimmerman, Whitmyre, & Fields, 1970). However, there are impaired patients with lateralized impairment who do not produce the expected VIQ-PIQ pattern (Filskov & Leli, 1981). In addition, Small (1973) notes that extreme

VIQ–PIQ differences have much more pathological significance when a patient's IQ is 100 or less than it does when a person has a full scale IQ in the higher range of ability. In clinical practice, a difference of 15 or more points between Verbal and Performance IQ should be further investigated and interpreted with other pertinent data. However, it must be remembered that there are no data to support a magical VIQ–PIQ discrepancy as indicative of brain damage (Filskov & Leli, 1981). Such a finding is simply a pattern of test performance that suggests another hypothesis to be investigated.

Sex Differences

Although men and and women perform differently in some WAIS subtests, the overlap between their scores is too great to allow these differences to enter into interpretations of the scores of an individual case. With few exceptions, studies of the original Wechsler tests found that men regularly obtained slightly higher full scale scores than women (Lezak, 1976). This tendency has persisted in the WAIS (Payne & Lehman, 1966; Wechsler, 1958). The men of the standardization sample for the 1955 WAIS revision of the Wechsler–Bellevue Scales achieved higher scores on Information, Comprehension, Arithmetic, Picture Completion, and Block Design, whereas the women had a very small advantage on Similarities, Vocabulary, and Digit Symbol (Wechsler, 1955).

The years since the WAIS was standardized have seen critical changes in the nature and extent of women's education and vocational pursuits. The changes have not been limited to younger women alone, for the proportion of working older women continues to grow, as does the number of older women returning to school. Hence, without current data, it is not really possible to estimate the presence or pattern of sex differences almost three decades later. It is highly likely that significant differences remain between the sexes in WAIS response patterns, but the nature of these differences as well as how they vary between age groups will be answered only by further study.

Patterns of Scores and Identification of Brain Damage

As it was recognized that differences between Verbal and Performance IQ's were not sufficient for the diagnosis of brain damage, researchers attempted to find alternate ways to identify brain dysfunction using the WAIS. The most widely known of these involves the "hold" and "don't hold" tests. Essentially, the theory behind this approach suggested that some of the WAIS subtests were very sensitive to brain damage; they would be affected every time a brain injury was present. Other subtests were the "hold" tests; performance on these subtests would not be affected by the presence of brain dysfunction. If there was a decrease in the "don't hold" tests, there was brain damage. Numerous combinations of "hold" and "don't hold" tests were suggested (e.g., Bersoff, 1970; Meyer, 1961; Rabin, 1965; Savage, 1970; Wechsler, 1958). All ended with the basic result: They did not discriminate between brain-injured and non-brain-injured patients with any significant degree of reliability (Golden, 1979).

From the recognition that the WAIS is differentially affected by different lesions has come research looking for patterns of WAIS scores that signify different lesions. Using this method, one determines the pattern of impaired test scores for an individual and then matches this pattern against patterns expected in different kinds of brain injury.

A highly ambitious use of the WAIS in this manner was reported by McFie (1975). McFie outlines basic patterns expected in types of localized brain injuries. Left frontal injuries are characterized by a loss in the Verbal IQ. Such injuries will also be accompanied by a deficit in verbal associates learning. Right frontal injuries are characterized by deficits in Picture Arrangement, on memory tasks involving designs, and sometimes in Digits Backwards (Golden, 1978). Left temporal lesions produce losses in Similarities and the Digit Span test (McFie, 1975); right temporal lesions result in a drop in Picture Arrangement and design memory (Luria, 1966, 1973; McFie, 1960). Meier and French (1966) have suggested that a loss in Object Assembly may be seen. Left parietal injuries will cause losses on Arithmetic, Digit Span, Block Design, and sometimes on Similarities (Mahan, 1976). Right parietal lesions will affect memory for Block Design and Picture Arrangement (Golden, 1979; McFie, 1975).

Diffuse injuries will generally lead to loss on most of the tests sensitive to brain injury: Digit Span, Arithmetic, Picture Arrangement, Object Assembly, Block Design, and Digit Symbol (McFie, 1975). Injuries to subcortical areas will generally affect tests with strong motor components: Digit Symbol, Block Design, Object Assembly, Picture Arrangement, in that order (De Wolfe, 1971; McFie, 1975; Woo-Sam, 1971).

Injuries in early childhood, especially before age 2, can lead to deficits that show a considerably different pattern of scores than the patterns seen with later injuries. Generally, the individual will have an IQ below 80 and often in the range of mental retardation. The tests traditionally considered to be "hold" tests (Information, Comprehension, and Vocabulary) will generally be the lowest test scores on the record. It has been speculated that this is due to the inability of the early brain-injured child to fully take advantage of both educational opportunities and daily social learning experiences (Golden, 1979). Often the highest scores for these persons will be on Digit Span, Picture Completion, Arithmetic, and Block Design. Recognition of such a pattern allows for differentiation between relatively early brain damage and brain damage occurring later in life.

The WAIS as a test for organicity is not accurate enough to be used alone. Combined with a test of visual memory, the WAIS can be useful as a screening device for deficits in persons known to be brain injured (Golden, 1979). It is not, however, diagnostically effective enough to be used alone to diagnose brain damage versus no brain damage with confidence (Lezak, 1976). Nonetheless, the WAIS has been shown to be extremely useful when used in conjunction with a more extensive neuropsychological test battery (Golden, 1978; Reitan, undated, 1974; Reitan & Davison, 1974).

THE STANFORD–BINET INTELLIGENCE SCALE

The Stanford–Binet (Terman, 1916) preceded the WAIS as the major measure of child and adult intelligence. (For a review of the historical development of the Stanford–Binet Intelligence Scale, the reader is referred to Matarazzo, 1972, and Sattler, 1974.) The Binet was originally designed as a test of children's intelligence but was later extended to allow the assessment of adult intelligence. The original Binet used the notion of a mental age to assess intelligence. Briefly, this approach attempted to establish the age at which skills possessed by the individual would be considered normal (defined as 50% of an age group having a given skill). When the mental age of the individual was divided by the chronological (true) age and multiplied by 100, the resulting quotient would be an IQ. An IQ over 100 would indicate a brighter than average person while an IQ below 100 would indicate a duller than normal person. Recent editions of the test (Terman & Merrill, 1973), however, have adopted the deviation IQ approach advocated by Wechsler.

Administration of the Stanford–Binet

The Binet tests are arranged in year levels ranging from two years to superior adult. In adminstering the Binet, the examiner must first establish where to begin the test to determine a basal level, a year grouping in which the individual can pass all tests in that section. If the individual does not pass all tests at the level chosen, it is necessary to administer the levels previous to the one chosen until s/he passes all tests at a given level. If the individual only missed one item at the level chosen, it is generally necessary to go back only one level. If the subject misses all or most items at a given level, however, it may be necessary for the examiner to go back more than one level, depending on the examiner's assessment of the individual's abilities. After establishing a basal level, testing is continued until all test items are failed at a given level. Complete instructions for each level are provided in the test manual.

After completing the test, credit is allotted for each test. Full credit for each year up to and including the basal level is given. Thereafter, credit is given for each test passed at each level according to instructions in both the record booklet and test manual. The months' credit earned at each year level is summed to get a total score, which is then located in the appropriate table in the manual to yield an overall IQ score. The resulting Binet IQ can be interpreted much the same as the WAIS Full Scale IQ (Golden, 1978, 1979; Sattler, 1969).

As is the case with the WAIS, a Stanford–Binet IQ of 100 is considered to be average. However, as is true for the WAIS, the resulting IQ score is an averaged estimate of an individual's intellectual capabilities. As such, it tends to obscure deficit areas in an individual's performance. The Stanford–Binet can, however, contribute to a neuropsychological evaluation. It provides a wide enough range of difficulty for testing those individuals who are so seriously impaired that they are unable to correctly perform enough WAIS items to earn subtest scores that differ appreciably from the bottom of the scale. Additionally, many of the individual items of the Binet are good tests of one or more of the functions that are typically evaluated by a neuropsychologist (Lezak, 1976). Stanford–Binet test items may provide information that can help to confirm or reject the presence of a specific kind of intellectual dysfunction. The items can often be used to help clarify the nature of a given dysfunction. Although very few of the items reoccur at enough levels of the test to allow for the discrimination of a deficit at every level, the item-by-item age or ability level grading enables the examiner to evaluate Stanford–Binet subtests separately and also to compare them with performance on tests other than the Binet.

PEABODY PICTURE VOCABULARY TEST (PPVT)

One of the more common brief tests of intelligence is the Peabody Picture Vocabulary Test (Dunn, 1965). The PPVT is easily administered and does not require an oral or written response. The subject responds in a nonverbal manner, most frequently by pointing. The test consists of 150 picture plates, each with four pictures, and a list of 150 words. The examinee is told a word and shown four pictures representing simple words and objects. The subject usually is asked to point to the picture representing the word to be defined. A second, alternate form of the test (Form B, with 150 different words) can be used in the same manner. A basal level is established (six consecutive items correct), and testing is continued until a ceiling is reached (missing six of eight consecutive items). All correct items, including those not administered below the basal level, are summed up to yield a total raw score, which is subsequently converted into an IQ equivalent using the appropriate table in the manual.

The PPVT IQ averages a correlation of about .75 to .80 with WAIS Full Scale and Verbal IQ's (Bonner, 1969; Pool & Brown, 1970; Shaw, 1961). The simplicity of the PPVT pictures makes the test suitable for use with brain-damaged individuals. Such individuals often exhibit much difficulty sorting out the elements in a complex stimulus and frequently are unable to respond to the intended problem. Additionally, the PPVT has been found useful in the evaluation of aphasic patients (Stark, Cohen, & Eisenson, 1968; Zaidel, 1977). Of the three nonverbal vocabulary tests discussed here, the PPVT probably gives the purest measure of recognition vocabulary *per se* and is also the test on which the most seriously impaired patients have the greatest likelihood of success (Lezak, 1976).

AMMONS FULL RANGE PICTURE VOCABULARY TEST

The Ammons Full Range Picture Vocabulary Test (Ammons & Ammons, 1948) consists of pictures representing complex scenes or situations. The individual is given a word and must pick the picture that best represents the word. The test manual covers a wide range of age norms, from age 2 to adult. During testing the subject is presented a stimulus word orally or reads it in written form. Two forms are available, each with a separate set of four pictures. The same pictures are used for all items making administration and scoring simple. The majority of studies available demonstrate correlations of between .7 and .9 when comparing the Ammon's IQ with the WAIS IQ (e.g., Granick, 1971; Sydiaha, 1967; Vellutino & Hogan, 1966). As is the case with the PPVT, this test is useful with brain-injured individuals, particularly those who have difficulty with oral speech (Lezak, 1976).

THE QUICK TEST

A test related to the Full Range Vocabulary Test is the Quick Test (Ammons & Ammons, 1962), which consists of three sets of picture plates, each of which has four pictures depicting a complex scene with 50 words associated with it. The words are presented to the individual either orally or in written form. The subject either points or gives the number of the picture that can best be associated with a given word. All words are given to all subjects, with total administration time of about 50 minutes for all lists of words. As the three sets of words are highly intercorrelated, however, the examiner has the option of administering only one 50 item list in a time of 10–15 minutes. The raw score is the number correct for each list. Tables accompanying the test give the mental age equivalent, percentile, and deviation IQ score for each of the three raw scores separately as well as for each combination of two raw scores and for the summed raw scores for all three lists. Tables provide equivalent IQ's for ages 6 through adult.

The Quick Test is only appropriate for individuals with average or below average IQ, rather than for individuals who cover the full range of IQ scores (Golden, 1979). Quick Test IQ scores correlate with full scale WAIS IQ's from .34 to .88, with the lower correlations occurring in brighter populations for which the test is inappropriate (Ammons & Ammons, 1962). This is primarily because the pictures are sufficiently complex to be useful in making discriminations from age 6 through average adult. However, the test ceiling (i.e., level of difficulty of the most difficult item) is so low that it offers virtually no differentiation between bright and very bright adults (Lezak, 1976). Quick Test scores are reportedly not as sensitive to pathology as are WAIS scores. Thus they will tend to estimate premorbid intelligence rather than reflect impairment in organic groups and other severely pathological groups (Golden, 1979).

RAVEN'S PROGRESSIVE MATRICES

The Raven's Progressive Matrices (Raven, 1960) was intended as a "culture fair" test of intelligence based solely on nonverbal and noncultural items. However, although the test requires neither language nor academic skills for success, educational level has been found to influence performance on the test such that the higher the educational level, the better the performance on the test (Bolin, 1955; Colonna & Faglioni, 1966). Each item in the test consists of a visual design with a piece removed. Given six to eight choices, the individual must select the correct missing piece for the design. The Raven's Matrices require spatial skills, recognition of design, ability to abstract, ability to recognize numerical and spatial relationships, and concentration and attention skills.

The Raven's Progressive Matrices can be easily administered. The instructions are easily explained; for each of the 60 items, the subject simply points to or writes the number of the piece that correctly fills the hole and completes the design. Therefore, it can be self-administered. The test takes approximately 40 to 60 minutes to administer. A shorter, simpler form (The Coloured Progressive Matrices) is available for use with children and also can be used with retarded adults (Lezak, 1976).

Norms are available for ages 8 to 65. Score conversion is to percentiles, with several percentile levels rather than direct conversion to IQ equivalents. For finer scoring, Peck (1970) presents more extensive percentile norms for age groups 25 to 65. These percentiles may be converted to IQ's by converting the percentile to standard z-scores, multiplying the z by 15, and adding the result to 100 (Golden, 1979).

Raven's IQ's have been reported to correlate with WAIS IQ from .43 to .93 in populations including brain-damaged and psychiatric populations. Poor performance on the test is associated with the type of brain injury that tends to cause difficulty on such tests as Block Design. Therefore, scores on the Raven Progressive Matrices Test will tend to be lower than overall WAIS IQ's in individuals with specific losses in these skills who retain verbal and verbal-conceptual skills. Such underestimation may cause the examiner to expect less of the patient. The difficulty in estimating IQ's because of lack of extensive normative data is a major problem when using this test.

CONCLUSIONS

A number of tests of intellectual functioning are widely used in clinical–educational settings. Each of these tests have specific advantages and disadvantages. The WAIS offers an IQ that has been well normed and is the standard instrument against which all other IQ tests are currently measured. Consequently, the use of almost any other test is validated based on its correlation with the WAIS IQ. Therefore, whenever time and other conditions permit, the WAIS is the instrument of choice in clinical settings with adults. The WAIS also offers more than a full scale IQ. It provides subtest scores that can yield a significant amount of information about the functioning of an individual. This can therefore be used to respond to a variety of referral questions. Finally, the WAIS remains the most comprehensively normed adult intelligence scale currently available, with normative data available for numerous psychological service settings, patient populations, and administration conditions.

The WAIS also has its disadvantages. It is not designed for group administrations, causing difficulty in screening large numbers of individuals. There is also the disadvantage of cultural bias. The test is heavily influenced by the cultural and language concepts that reflect the life of the average American but not that of most minority groups. The WAIS is highly susceptible to improvement of scores upon retesting. The "practice effect" (i.e., improvement of scores with retesting) is particularly evident on the WAIS Performance subtests (Karson, Pool, & Freud, 1957; Matarazzo, 1972), as the individual gains more exposure to the testing situation and has further opportunities to manipulate the test materials (Demer, Aborn, & Canter, 1953; Duncan & Barrett, 1961; Griffith & Yamahiro, 1958). As there is no alternate form of the WAIS, the use of the test in situations indicating frequent reevaluations is difficult. Finally, the WAIS tends to overestimate low IQ, a serious drawback (Golden, 1979). Therefore, caution should be exercised in interpreting WAIS IQ's below 80. If documentation is needed for legal cases or other purposes, Golden (1979) suggests the use of the Stanford–Binet (1972 norms) because this will provide the most accurate estimate of a low IQ in an adult.

The alternate tests of intellectual functioning covered in this chapter are often employed in settings where time and personnel requirements make the administration of a WAIS impractical. These briefer tests enable the clinician to identify those individuals who can benefit most from further evaluation with tests such as the WAIS. These tests can also serve as substitutes in testing individuals with speech or physical handicaps that make it impossible for them to adequately perform on the WAIS.

When selecting an alternate test, a number of considerations must be taken into account. The limitations and advantages of each test must be examined carefully by the clinician, analyzing factors such as staff availability, purpose for examination, type of population, and so on. For as Golden (1979, p. 44) has noted, "the use of a procedure or set of procedures that is inadequate for the person being tested is rarely justified, nor is overly extensive testing . . . likely to be of benefit to the patient."

Although the measures of intellectual functioning described in this chapter were not designed for the identification of impaired cerebral functioning, they provide some important descriptions of general aspects of behavior necessary for daily living, in addition to some specific data that might indicate brain dysfunction. Major strengths, as well as deficiencies, can be described that may fit patterns of performance that have been found to be common in brain dysfunction. As such, when used properly, they can offer a first step in an integrated assessment of behavior related to brain functioning. For this reason, it seems safe to assume that the continued use of some measure of intellectual functioning is assured for the forseeable future.

REFERENCES

Ammons, R. B., & Ammons, H. S. *The full-range picture vocabulary test.* Missoula, Mont.: Psychological Test Specialists, 1948.

Ammons, R. B., & Ammons, C. H. *The quick test (QT): Provisional manual. Psychological Reports,* Monograph Supplement, I-VII, 1962.

Anastasi, A. *Differential psychology* (3rd ed.). New York: Wiley, 1965.

Balthazar, E. E., & Morrison, D. H. The use of the Wechsler intelligence scales as diagnostic indicators of predominant left-hand and indeterminant unilateral brain damage. *Journal of Clinical Psychology,* 1961, *17,* 161.

Bennett, G. K., Seashore, H. G., & Wesman, A. G. *Differential aptitude tests manual* (5th ed.). New York: Psychological Corporation, 1972.

Bersoff, D. N. The revised deterioration formula for the WAIS. *Journal of Clinical Psychology,* 1970, *39,* 15.

Binet, A. Le Dévelopment d'intelligence chez les enfants. *L' Année Psychologique,* 1908, *14,* 1.

Bolin, B. J. A comparison of Raven's Progressive Matrices (1938) with the A.C.E. Psychological Examination and the Otis Gamma Mental Ability Test. *Journal of Consulting Psychology,* 1955, *19,* 400.

Boll, T. J., & Barth, J. T. Neuropsychology of brain damage in children. In S. B. Filskov & T. J. Boll (Eds.), *Handbook of clinical neuropsychology.* New York: Wiley, 1981.

Bonner, L. W. Comparative study of the performance of Negro seniors of Oklahoma City high schools on the WAIS and the PPVT. *Dissertation Abstracts,* 1969, *30,* 921A.

Chapman, L. F., & Wolff, H. G. The cerebral hemispheres and the highest integrative functions of man. *Archives of Neurology,* 1959, *1,* 357.

Cohen, J. Factor analytically based rationale for the Wechsler Adult Intelligence Scale. *Journal of Consulting Psychology,* 1957, *21,* 451.

Colonna, A., & Faglioni, P. The performance of hemisphere-damaged patients on spatial intelligence tests. *Cortex,* 1966, *2,* 293.

Demer, G. F., Aborn, M., & Canter, A. H. The reliability of the Wechsler–Bellevue subtests and scales. *Journal of Consulting Psychology,* 1953, *38,* 187.

De Wolfe, A. S. Differentiation of schizophrenia and brain damage with the WAIS. *Journal of Clinical Psychology*, 1971, *27*, 209.

Duncan, D. R., & Barrett, A. M. A longitudinal comparison of intelligence involving the Wechsler–Bellevue I and WAIS. *Journal of Clinical Psychology*, 1961, *17*, 318.

Dunn, L. M. *Expanded manual for the Peabody Picture Vocabulary Test.* Circle Pines, Minn.: American Guidance Service, 1965.

Filskov, S. B., & Leli, D. A. Assessment of the individual in neuropsychological practice. In S. B. Filskov & T. J. Boll (Eds.), *Handbook of clinical neuropsychology.* New York: Wiley, 1981.

Firetto, A. C., & Davey, H. Subjectively reported anxiety as a discriminator of digit span performance. *Psychological Reports,* 1971, *28*, 98.

Garrett, H. E. A developmental theory of intelligence. *American Psychologist,* 1946, *1*, 372.

Golden, C. J. *Diagnosis and rehabilitation in clinical neuropsychology.* Springfield, Ill.: Charles C Thomas, 1978.

Golden, C. J. *Clinical interpretation of objective psychological tests.* New York: Grune & Stratton, 1979.

Golden, C. J., Osmon, D. C., Moses, J. A., Jr., & Berg, R. A. *Interpretation of the Halstead–Reitan Neuropsychological Test Battery: A casebook approach.* New York: Grune & Stratton, 1981.

Gonen, J. Y., & Brown, L. Role of vocabulary in deterioration and restitution of mental functioning. *Proceedings of the 76th Annual Convention of the American Psychological Association*, 1968, *3*, 469.

Granick, S. Brief tests and their interrelationships as intellectual measures of aged subjects. *Proceedings of the American Psychological Association*, 1971, *7*, 599.

Griffith, R. M., & Yamahiro, R. S. Reliability–stability of subtest scatter on the Wechsler–Bellevue intelligence scales. *Journal of Clinical Psychology*, 1958, *14*, 317.

Gudeman, H. E., Craine, J. F., Golden, C. J., & McLaughlin, D. Higher cortical dysfunction associated with long term alcoholism. *International Journal of Neuroscience,* 1977, *8*, 33.

Heaton, R. K., & Crowley, T. J. Effects of psychiatric disorders and their somatic treatments on neuropsychological test results. In S. B. Filskov & T. J. Boll (Eds.), *Handbook of clinical neuropsychology.* New York: Wiley, 1981.

Isenberg, S. J., & Bass, B. A. Effects of verbal and nonverbal reinforcement on the WAIS performance of normal adults. *Journal of Consulting and Clinical Psychology.* 1974, *42*, 467.

Jarvik, L. F., Eisdorfer, C., & Blum, J. E. (Eds.). *Intellectual functioning in adults.* New York: Springer, 1973.

Karson, S., Pool, K. B., & Freud, S. L. The effects of scale and practice on WAIS and W–BI test scores. *Journal of Consulting Psychology,* 1957, *21*, 241.

Keiser, T. W. Schizotype and the Wechsler Digit Span Test. *Journal of Clinical Psychology*, 1975, *31*, 303.

Kim, J-O. Factor analysis. In N. H. Nie, C. Hull, J. G. Jenkins, K. Steinbrenner, and D. H. Bent (Eds.), *Statistical package for the social sciences* (2nd ed.). New York: McGraw-Hill, 1975.

Knox, W. J., & Grippaldi, R. High levels of state or trait anxiety and performance on selected verbal WAIS subtests. *Psychological Reports,* 1970, *27*, 375.

Lashley, K. S. Factors limiting recovery after central nervous lesions. *Journal of Nervous and Mental Disease,* 1938, *88*, 733.

Lezak, M. D. *Neuropsychological assessment.* New York: Oxford University Press, 1976.

Luria, A. R. *Higher cortical functions in man.* New York: Basic Books, 1966.

Luria, A. R. *The working brain.* New York: Basic Books, 1973.

Mahan, H. Sensitivity of WAIS tests to focal lobe damage. Privately mimeographed, 1976.

Matarazzo, J. D. *Wechsler's measurement and appraisal of adult intelligence* (5th ed.). Baltimore: Williams and Wilkins, 1972.

McFie, J. Psychological testing in clinical neurology. *Journal of Nervous and Mental Disease,* 1960, *131*, 383.

McFie, J. The diagnostic significance of disorders of higher nervous activity. Syndromes related to frontal, temporal, parietal, and occipital lesions. In P. J. Vinken & G. W. Bruyn (Eds.), *Handbook of clinical neurology (Vol. 3: Disorders of higher nervous activity)*. New York: Wiley, 1969.

McFie, J. *Assessment of organic intellectual impairment*. New York: Academic Press, 1975.

McNemar, Q. Lost: Our intelligence? Why? *American Psychologist*, 1965, *20*, 871.

Meier, M. J., & French, L. A. Longitudinal assessment of intellectual function following unilateral temporal lobectomy. *Journal of Clinical Psychology*, 1966, *22*, 22.

Meyer, V. Psychological effects of brain damage. In H. J. Eysenck (Ed.), *Handbook of abnormal psychology*. New York: Basic Books, 1961.

Parsons, O. A., Vega, A., Jr., & Burn, J. Different psychological effects of lateralized brain damage. *Journal of Consulting and Clinical Psychology*, 1969, *33*, 551.

Payne, R. W. Cognitive abnormalities. In H. J. Eysenck (Ed.), *Handbook of abnormal psychology*. New York: Basic Books, 1961.

Payne, D. A., & Lehmann, I. J. A brief WAIS analysis. *Journal of Clinical Psychology*, 1966, *22*, 296.

Peck, D. F. The conversion of Progressive Matrices and Mill Hill vocabulary raw scores into deviation IQ's. *Journal of Clinical Psychology*, 1970, *26*, 67.

Piercy, M. The effects of cerebral lesions on intellectual functions: A review of current research trends. *British Journal of Psychiatry*, 1964, *110*, 310.

Pool, D. A., & Brown, R. The PPVT as a measure of general adult intelligence. *Journal of Consulting and Clinical Psychology*, 1970, *34*, 8.

Psychological Corporation: Catalog supplement and price list. New York, 1981.

Rabin, I. A. Diagnostic use of intelligence tests. In B. B. Wolman (Ed.), *Handbook of clinical psychology*. New York: McGraw-Hill, 1965.

Rapaport, D., Gill, M. M., & Schafer, R. *Diagnostic psychological testing*. New York: International Universities Press, 1970.

Raven, J. C. *Guide to the standard progressive matrices*. London: H. K. Lewis, 1960.

Reitan, R. M. Certain differential effects of left and right cerebral lesions in human adults. *Journal of Comparative and Physiological Psychology*, 1955, *48*, 474.

Reitan, R. M. Psychological effects of cerebral lesions in children of early school age. In R. M. Reitan & L. A. Davison (Eds.), *Clinical neuropsychology: Current status and applications*. Washington: Winston, 1974.

Reitan, R. M. *Neuropsychological methods of inferring brain damage in adults and children*. Unpublished manuscript, undated.

Reitan, R. M., & Davison, L. A. *Clinical neuropsychology: Current status and applications*. Washington: Winston, 1974.

Reitan, R. M., & Fitzhugh, K. B. Behavioral deficits in groups with cerebral vascular lesions. *Journal of Consulting and Clinical Psychology*, 1971, *37*, 215.

Rourke, B. P. Neuropsychological assessment of children with learning disabilities. In S. B. Filskov & T. J. Boll (Eds.), *Handbook of clinical neuropsychology*. New York: Wiley, 1981.

Sattler, J. M. Effects of cues and examiner influence on two Wechsler subtests. *Journal of Consulting and Clinical Psychology*, 1969, *33*, 716.

Sattler, J. M. *Assessment of children's intelligence and special abilities*. Boston: Allyn and Bacon, 1974.

Satz, P., Richard, W., & Daniels, A. The alteration of intellectual performance after lateralized brain injury in man. *Psychonomic Science*, 1967, *7*, 369.

Savage, R. B. Intellectual assessment. In P. Mittler (Ed.), *The psychological assessment of mental and physical handicaps*. London: Methuen, 1970.

Shaw, J. H. Comparability of PPVT and WAIS scores with schizophrenics without brain damage. Unpublished study, Nampa State School, Nampa, Iowa, 1961. (Quoted in C. B. Ernhart. The correlation of PPVT and WAIS scores for adult psychiatric patients. *Journal of Clinical Psychology,* 1970, *26,* 470.)

Small, L. A. *Neuropsychodiagnosis in psychotherapy.* New York: Bruner/Mazel, 1973.

Smith, A. Intellectual functions in patients with lateralized frontal tumors. *Journal of Neurology, Neurosurgery, and Psychiatry,* 1966, *29,* 52.

Spearman, C. *The abilities of man: Their nature and measurement.* London: Macmillan, 1927.

Spearman, C., & Jones, L. L. *Human abilities.* London: Macmillan, 1950.

Spiker, C. C., & McCandless, B. R. The concept of intelligence and the philosophy of science. *Psychological Review,* 1954, *61,* 255.

Stark, J., Cohen, S., & Eisenson, J. Performances of aphasics on the PPVT and Auditory Recording Tests. *Journal of Special Education,* 1968, *2,* 435.

Sydiaha, D. Prediction of WAIS IQ for psychiatric patients using the Ammons Full Range Picture Vocabulary and Raven Progressive Matrices. *Psychological Reports,* 1967, *20,* 823.

Terman, L. M. *The measurement of intelligence.* Boston: Houghton Mifflin, 1916.

Terman, L. M. & Merrill, M. A. *Measuring intelligence.* Cambridge, Mass.: Houghton Mifflin, 1960.

Terman, L. M., & Merrill, M. A. *The Stanford–Binet intelligence scale* (1972 norms edition). Boston: Houghton Mifflin, 1973.

Thurstone, L. L. Psychological implications of factor analysis. *American Psychologist,* 1948, *3,* 402.

Todd, J., Coolidge, F., & Satz, P. The Wechsler Adult Intelligence Scale discrepancy index: A neuropsychological evaluation. *Journal of Consulting and Clinical Psychology,* 1977, *45,* 450.

Vega, A., Jr., & Parsons, O. A. Relationships between sensory–motor deficits and WAIS verbal and performance scores in unilateral brain damage. *Cortex,* 1969, *5,* 229.

Vellutino, F. R., & Hogan, T. P. Relationship between the Ammons and WAIS test performances of unselected psychiatric patients. *Journal of Clinical Psychology,* 1966, *22,* 69.

Vernon, P. E. *The structure of human abilities.* New York: Wiley, 1950.

Wechsler, D. *Wechsler adult intelligence scale manual.* New York: Psychological Corporation, 1955.

Wechsler, D. *The measurement and appraisal of adult intelligence* (4th ed.). Baltimore: Williams and Wilkins, 1958.

Williams, H. L. Psychologic testing. In A. B. Baker (Ed.), *Clinical neurology* (2nd ed., Vol. 1). New York: Hoeber-Harper, 1962.

Woo-Sam, J. Lateralized brain damage and differential psychological effects: Parsons, et al., reexamined. *Perceptual and Motor Skills,* 1971, *33,* 259.

Zaidel, E. Unilateral auditory language comprehension on the token test following cerebral commisurotomy and hemispherectomy. *Neuropsychologia,* 1977, *15,* 1.

Zimmerman, I. L., & Woo-Sam, J. M. *Clinical interpretation of the Wechsler adult intelligence scale.* New York: Grune & Stratton, 1973.

Zimmerman, S. F., Whitmyre, J. W., & Fields, F. R. J. Intelligence scales in patients with diffuse and lateralized cerebral dysfunction. *Journal of Clinical Psychology,* 1970, *26,* 462.

4

Assessment of Verbal Abilities for Neuropsychological Purposes

ROBERT L. BRUNNER

Testing of verbal abilities, in common with all neuropsychological evaluation, has two global purposes. The first purpose is in the clinical/diagnostic assessment of functional abilities. This dates from the work of Wernicke, Broca, and other physician–scientists of the nineteenth century who became interested in language disorders resulting from damage to the central nervous system. The clinical techniques administered at bedside have become the basis for a number of systematic language instruments currently available. The second major purpose of language testing is the experimental investigation of "brain-behavioral" relationships.

Keeping in mind these broad purposes, verbal tests used in neuropsychology may be classified into one of the following areas: (1) independent tests of language disorders (aphasia); (2) speech and language examinations that are integrated within more comprehensive neuropsychological test batteries but are not ordinarily administered separately; (3) language portions of standard intelligence tests; (4) tests of educational competency that depend on language abilities; (5) verbal learning and memory tests; and (6) research tests that have a focused aim and more infrequent use. The present chapter will present an overview of tests in each of these categories.

ROBERT L. BRUNNER • Department of Pediatrics, Children's Hospital Medical Center, Cincinnati, Ohio 45229.

ISSUES IN THE ASSESSMENT OF VERBAL ABILITIES

There are specific issues, controversies and hypotheses that have persistently resurfaced in the neuropsychological literature (Benton, 1964). The first of these are the arguments pertaining to utilization of a quantitative–statistical approach versus a qualitative–clinical approach in the understanding of neuropsychological deficit (Mahan, 1980). Today, among those who evaluate verbal ability, some continue to caution against dependence on scores and norms (Schuell, 1973) to the exclusion of "kinds of errors . . . or clinical signs" which may go unnoticed if the only basis for grading is a purely quantitative score (Boller, 1968). However, a dissenting opinion was presented by Benson (1979) in a cogent review describing aphasia testing as "inexact, nonstandardized and constantly changing" (p. 33). This author further noted that while an experienced examiner may obtain a clear view of the patient, because of theoretical biases and differences in clinical expertise, "the need for exact, standardized testing methods is obvious" (Benson, 1979, p. 34).

Another issue has concerned the proposition that certain functions deteriorate rapidly as a result of brain insult ("don't hold") whereas others such as verbal abilities may be less seriously impaired ("hold") (Yates, 1954). Mahan (1980) exactingly described the history of this idea as it related to declines with age, supporting the idea that "verbal ability and particularly vocabulary is the last to show decline as age advances" (Mahan, 1980), and provided a formula to estimate premorbid intelligence (Mahan, 1979). Prior to Mahan's formulators, Lezak (1976) had concluded after reviewing earlier findings that "no one has yet devised a formula based on Wechsler subtest scores that will separate organic patients from control or other patient groups to a clinically satisfactory degree" (Lezak, 1976, p. 195). The question of whether or not verbal test scores are able to represent premorbid status does not appear answerable with a simple "yes" or "no." Instead, there may be conditions under which the "hold/don't hold" distinction is valid. These parameters may be defined by history (education, institutionalization, etc.), location and type of insult, presence and completeness of aphasic symptoms, and age, among others.

The third issue relates to the utilization of a standardized clinical battery approach. This method may, because of its seeming inflexibility or superficiality, find objectors among "experimentalists" who insist on exploring an inferred underlying mechanism, often by increasingly precise, complex, and custom-made methods. Often such methods are not accessible to or practical for the clinician weighed down by a service load.

Fourth, there is the important theoretical question of how to separate, by means of testing, general cognitive disturbances or memory disorders from disorders of verbal behavior. In the same vein is the issue of separating specific deficits in performance on language items (i.e., motor speech from deficits of the integrity of underlying linguistic competence; Hecaen & Albert, 1978). The latter question has generated considerable research and has had a significant effect on verbal test adoption, construction, and interpretation. This problem has been cogently reviewed by Heilman and Valenstein (1979).

BASIC CONCEPTS AND HISTORICAL BACKGROUND

Prior to a discussion of some specific language tests utilized in neuropsychological assessment and research, general views of prominent figures in neuropsychology and their influential writing will be reviewed in order to put this topic in broad perspective.

Luria (1973) described speech processes as a "highly complex chapter of neuropsychology" (p. 322). The basic premise in Luria's thinking is that individuals with lesions in different parts of the brain may suffer damage to various components of speech. In considering the various speech and language problems that Luria described, one might attempt to examine them with evaluative tests available to psychologists, including those tests specifically based on Luria's hypotheses. In Luria's scheme, expressive and impressive (receptive) language include the same components. A coding or decoding process relates a speech scheme to a general idea through the mechanism of internal speech. Luria believed that speech is not only a means of communication because it allows complex categorical thinking and abstraction and it guides one's mental activities. Similarly, memory for an "audioverbal trace" is a simple language process and forms a basis for one of Luria's six categories of language disorder. Speech processes thus vary in level of complexity and stability. The idea of increasing levels of complexity is important in the aim of Luria's testing, namely to associate the damaged components of speech with the anatomical damage. A complex test, such as one of logical–grammatical structuring, assumes that lower level functions like word comprehension and goal-directed activities are at least partially intact. Luria's testing approach has been highly influential and should be encountered first-hand by neuropsychologists in order to appreciate its artfulness (Luria, 1966). Many of the individual items have been reproduced in batteries based on the original writings (Christensen, 1975; Golden, Purisch, & Hammeke, 1979).

Lezak's (1976) review on the topic of verbal tests suggests categorization under the terms aphasia or fluency. Aphasia tests are specifically designated as those that focus on "disorders of symbol formulation and associated problems" (Lezak, 1976, p. 255). These were contrasted with verbal tests that may be affected by more generalized disorders of learning, memory, attention, or intelligence. Lezak (1976) points out that, most commonly, aphasia tests are administered by specially trained speech pathologists. However, the major neuropsychological batteries include a minimum aphasia screening exam, which cannot, according to Lezak (1976), replace careful examination of language functions. So, for example, the Halstead–Wepman Aphasia Screening Test is included in Halstead and Reitan's Test Battery. The emphasis in this instrument is in determining the presence of a particular linguistic disorder but not necessarily with concrete scoring criteria or through comparison with age-related norms. Lezak (1976) presented excellent synopses of five well known aphasia tests that are representative of available instruments. These were Examining for Aphasia, the Porch Index of Communicative Abilities, the Functional Communication Profile, the Minnesota tests for Differential Diagnosis of Aphasia, the Neurosensory Center Comprehensive Examination Test for Aphasia, and the Language Modalities Test for Aphasia.

Brookshire (1973) has also provided a scholarly review and description of major tests aimed at speech and language functioning. He included the Boston Diagnostic Aphasia Examination and the Token Test, as well as those reviewed by Lezak (1976). Furthermore, he has suggested that most aphasia tests are based on a stimulus-processing-response concept. Generally, the stimuli used will be introduced through the modalities of vision, audition, and touch. Responses will be spoken, written, gestured, or selected (e.g., underlined). Brookshire (1973) supports the idea of Lezak (1976), among others, that the test system should be comprehensive for all stimulus and response modalities and that nonlanguage abilities need to be measured in the examination.

Jones and Wepman (1961) had earlier conceptualized language as consisting of a "stimulating situation," a response and an intervening system of central processing. They pointed out that the "stimulating situation" portion may use any of the senses and that the response is likewise modality specific. This seemingly led to their conclusion that the makers of language tests need to be cognizant of this fact and should devise special tests that are both simple for nonaphasic subjects and sensitive to problems of symbol processing. The Language Modalities Test for Aphasia by Wepman and Jones (1961) tests the adequacy of written and spoken responses to visual and spoken stimuli within a linguistic framework.

Goodglass and Kaplan (1976) described the general purpose of aphasia testing as diagnosis and interpretation of types of symptoms (i.e., to assess through test performance the particular problem of linguistic input and output). Level of performance and pattern of strengths and weaknesses are measured in order to plan therapeutic approaches. Goodglass and Kaplan (1976) were in disagreement with Schuell, Jenkins, and Jimenez-Pabon (1964) that various symptoms can be understood as fluctuations of "general language capacity" that cross all language modalities and vary primarily in severity. Nor do they think that a multiplicity of S–R connections solely underlie language, a position they suggest is implicit in Wepman's Language Modalities Test for Aphasia (Wepman, 1961). Instead, they argued that while simple repetition and copying are S–R units, more often there are numerous complex intermediary steps between the stimulus and response.

Assessment of language disorders through formal testing schedules (e.g., Eisenson, 1954; Schuell, 1973) was criticized by McFie (1975) because of his observation that the patient's performance is highly erratic. Instead, a recommendation was made for shorter tests (Oldfield & Wingfield, 1965; Rochford & Williams, 1964) as being useful to detect the precise deficit behind a patient's difficulties (Boller, 1968).

Sarno (1972) suggested that there was no universally accepted aphasia test but that instruments developed by Schuell (1973), Eisenson (1954), and Wepman and Jones (1961) were the most commonly used by diagnosticians. Sarno's (1972) view, however, was that the Token Test, the Functional Communication Profile, and the Neurosensory Center Comprehensive Examination for Aphasia made up the most useful combination of tests available at the moment. On the other hand, Brookshire (1973) concluded that the Boston Diagnostic Aphasia Examination and Minnesota tests were the most comprehensive, but that the PICA (Porch Index of Communicative Ability) may be the most sensitive of the available instruments. He found the Token Test to be useful in clarifying aspects of mild receptive loss but too finely focused to be considered a general comprehension test.

APHASIA TESTS

As recently as 1967, Benton described the field of aphasia test construction as being at a level comparable to intelligence testing prior to the Binet or Wechsler scales, although the first of the modern aphasia batteries was published more than 45 years ago (Weisenberg & McBride, 1935). Benton (1967) argued that the problems of test construction in each field have been (1) conceptual and (2) technical.

In language test construction, the conceptual approach begins with adoption of an underlying theoretical framework to understand language. The models may be broadly conceived of as neurological, behavioral, or linguistic, but most frequently a combination of these. The prominent neurological models have been based either on a localizationist view, represented historically by Broca and Wernicke with updating most notably by Geschwind (1972), or on a holistic notion (Head, 1926; Jackson, 1915), now represented in formal testing by Schuell (1973). Behavioral approaches, such as social imitation (Bandura & Harris, 1966) or associationist views (Skinner, 1957) of language, have not greatly influenced test construction in this field. Neither have the behaviorists prevailed in aphasia classification, an area in which the neurological approach has been most important. This is evidenced by Benson's (1979) comparison of various aphasia classifications.

Linguistic models (Chomsky, 1957; Jakobson, 1964; Osgood & Miron, 1963) have been theoretically a strong force in language studies, and also find their way into diagnosis through the use of terminology such as semantic and syntactic aphasia (Wepman, Bock, Jones, & Van Pelt, 1965). The fundamental idea of the linguistic school has been that an understanding of the linguistic rules governing an individual's language performance was crucial for interpreting the disintegration of language after brain injury. Research on aphasia (Goodglass & Berko, 1960; Goodglass, Berko-Gleason, Sckerman-Bernholtz, & Hyde, 1972) has incorporated a linguistic approach by analyzing performance at semantic, phonemic, and syntactic levels. A neurolinguistic model (Gainotti, Miceli, & Caltagirone, 1977) has been proposed that relies on linguistic distinctions but incorporates clinical observations and psychological findings of disturbances in both verbal and nonverbal tasks. This model also recognizes that extralinguistic disorders (like attention) can affect language performance.

The technical problems in aphasia test construction cited by Benton (1967) involve item selection, normative information, scoring procedures, reliability, and validity. Kertesz (1979a) concurred with Benton (1967) that no single aphasia test has been found universally acceptable. Among the criticisms, in addition to disputing theoretical formulations, are that tests are too long or too specialized. These criticisms plus others related to Benton's technical issues have probably led to the creation of a rather large number of aphasia test procedures.

A review of the literature on aphasia tests suggests several conclusions concerning their use in research. The number of papers citing these tests has more than doubled between the middle and late 1970s. This probably reflects the tremendous growth of neurosciences in general during this period. The Boston Diagnostic Aphasia Examination is easily the most widely reported aphasia instrument in research, with more than 25 citations in 1980 alone. The major use of these instruments has been to establish the presence of aphasia or to classify patients as fitting a particular aphasia classification. All too often, despite having the data, severity of aphasia is ignored and groups are neither homogeneous nor matched for severity of aphasia. This flaw would be considered significant in most psychological research. For example, if two groups of interest are to be compared on a cognitive task, it is expected that intellectual level or mental age will be comparable. Invariably, such disregard for fundamental methodological procedures has frequently occurred in most aphasiologists' research.

Eisenson's Examining for Aphasia Test

This test (Eisenson, 1954) is among the aphasia tests that does not utilize norms and that permits considerable flexibility in administration and scoring. It has, in common with other aphasia tests, a separate evalution of receptive and expressive verbal functions. The test has a 30-minute to 2-hour administration time. The materials include several common objects along with the requisite manual and scoring sheets. Eisenson (1954) made conceptual distinction among subsymbolic behaviors (naming, copying, etc.), low symbolic behaviors (meaning, etc.), and high symbolic behaviors (reading, calculations, etc.) that could be of interest for interpreting loss and recovery following specific injury.

Eisenson's (1954) test, having been primarly devised as a clinical instrument, has not been frequently cited in published research. Eisenson (1964) has published findings concerned with recovery following penetrating wounds (better) compared with tumors/CVA's (poorer). The bulk of Eisenson's theoretical and clinical views on aphasia are presented in his 1973 book.

Minnesota Test for Differential Diagnosis of Aphasia

Schuell's (1973) test is a comprehensive battery that is both descriptive and analytic with the ultimate goal of differential diagnosis. The technical manual that accompanies the test provides the author's view of aphasia classification. Portions of the Minnesota that are most discriminating are listed by aphasia category, as are pathognomic signs and prognostic impressions. Test materials consist of instruction manual, two spiral-bound card pockets, eight special objects, coins, and an individual test booklet that includes a clinical profile sheet. The test is divided into five parts: (1) auditory comprehension/discrimination; (2) visual and reading abilities; (3) speech movements and language capacities; (4) visuo–motor and writing skils; and (5) arithmetic performance. The Minnesota is lengthy (about 2 hours) but may be shortened by estimating a baseline starting point and establishing a ceiling when the subject fails approximately 90% of the items.

The Minnesota has been extensively used to evaluate the presence of aphasia as a prerequisite for participation of subjects in an experimental procedure (eg., Brookshire, 1978; Rosenbeck, Messert, Collins, & Wertz, 1978). In a step beyond a simple screening function, comprehension subtests from the Minnesota (plus parallel subtests from the Boston and PICA) were administered to aphasics and normals (Wilcox, Davis, & Leonard, 1978). The same subjects were also tested for comprehension of videotaped language interactions that included contextual cues. Wilcox *et al.* (1978) found that the standardized aphasia tests tended to underestimate comprehension ability attainable by aphasics in more natural settings.

A portion of the Minnesota (word definition) was used (Rivers & Love, 1980) in comparing left hemisphere lesioned (LH), right hemisphere lesioned (RH), and normal subjects for language performance. Despite blind ratings by judges that the RH group's communication status was "significantly reduced," they performed significantly better than LH patients and not worse than normals on the word definition test. The RH patients were mainly affected on tests that required visual–spatial information processing. They had, for example, difficulty using sentence cues as a basis for finding appropriate word responses or to fully use visual information as a basis for stories. Rivers and Love (1980) concluded that language problems after RH damage were distinct from those known in standard aphasia classifications in the contribution made by visual information processing functions.

Coughlan (1979) used the articulation subtest of the Minnesota as one of several tests to help analyze the basis for verbal memory deficits in LH damaged patients. Only 4 of 29 of the LH patients (all of whom were dysphasic) had below normal articulation scores on the Minnesota subtest. These deficits were mild and thought to be insufficient to explain the LH group's significant verbal memory deficit. Neither were verbal comprehension or intelligence correlated with memory deficits. Coughlan (1979) attributed the memory deficit to a quantitative change in the efficient use of language-based procedures for storage, organization, and retrieval of information in verbal memory. The author's primary conclusion was that study of specific aphasic disorders may reveal corresponding types of verbal memory disorder.

April and Tse (1977) used the Minnesota in both English and Chinese to demonstrate the presence of more severe aphasia in a right-handed bilingual Chinese patient who had suffered a right hemisphere stroke. It was hypothesized that early-childhood learning of Chinese, an ideographic language based on visual spatial percepts, might have been critical for the establishment and maintenance of language dominance in the right hemisphere. The patient's English was left relatively intact, while the Chinese was more severely affected.

A factor analytic study of the Minnesota Differential Diagnosis of Aphasia Test (Schuell, Jenkins, & Carroll, 1962) using 157 aphasic subjects yielded 5 interpretable dimensions. The "language factor," on which all auditory tests loaded heavily, crossed all language modalities but did not include nonlanguage functions. There were a "visual" factor, which involved reading and writing tests, and a motor factor related to the speech apparatus. There were also a visual–spatial factor and one that was described as "stimulus equivalence."

Boston Diagnostic Aphasic Examination

The Boston is a comprehensive battery (Goodglass & Kaplan, 1976) that features three parallel systems for classifying the findings. The Rating Scale Profile is a global severity rating of oral communication on a five-point continuum from "no speech or auditory comprehension" to "minimal discernible speech handicap" that is based on structured clinical interview material. The Rating Scale Profile is used in conjunction with the Rating Scale Profile of Speech Characteristics, which utilizes seven seven-point scales to grade melodic line, phrase length, articulatory ability, grammatical form, paraphasia in running speech, word finding and auditory comprehension. Finally, a z score profile provides a standardized summary of the raw scores for each subtest of the battery. The test materials are 17 stimulus cards and scoring sheets. The tasks for the subject include pointing to named objects, figures of body parts, following instructions to produce motor actions, answering general and specific yes or no questions, answering questions with specific words, speech articulation, mouth movement ability, automatic naming (days of week, etc.), naming visually presented objects or body parts, recitation, singing (the latter two from long-term memory), reproduction of tapping sequences, short-term recall–repetition of single words and sentences, naming animals from memory, reading sentences, matching tasks (words/letters oral/written, etc.), identifying words spelled aloud, and completing fill-in sentences with multiple choice alternatives, writing and spelling from memory and dictation or in response to stimuli. The test requires aproximately 1½ hours to administer.

A wide variety of research has been accomplished with the Boston. Cherlow and Serafetinides (1976) compared individuals after left or right temporal lobe surgery on two subtests (Visual Confrontation Naming and Reading Sentences) from the Boston, finding no significant differences between the groups. Farmer (1977) used the Boston Diagnostic Aphasia Examination to define aphasia subgroups and compare them for self-correction, strategy, and success. Gallagher and Guilford (1977) screened patients for aphasia with the Boston Diagnostic Aphasia Examination, then assessed their ability to answer questions related to 10 pictures of people engaged in activities. They found questions requiring temporal or location responses were more difficult than those requiring subject, object, or adjective responses. Blumstein, Baker and Goodglass (1977) examined the role of phonemic discrimination deficits in various forms of aphasia. Boller, Barturtunski, Mack, and Kim (1977) found no losses on the Token Test or BDAE writing test in a group of hypertensives who showed losses on tests of general functioning, including reaction time and digit span. The BDAE special tests of oral–facial dyspraxia were found to be helpful in understanding patients with developmental verbal dyspraxia (Ferry, Hall, & Hicks, 1975). In this syndrome there is delayed speech, worsening with more complex phonetic combinations, in association with a normal or surprisingly high receptive language level. These patients may often show signs of associated oral dyspraxia. Baker, Berry, Gardner, Zuris, Davis, and Veroff (1975) utilized the BDAE to verify the presence of markedly paraphasic language in patients who could then be taught to receive and transmit information, feelings, and ideas using cards on which arbitrary or ideographic symbols were drawn. This study illustrated that cognitive capacities entailed in natural language may be preserved in the absence of the natural language itself.

Goodglass and Kaplan (1976) presented the results of two factor analytic studies of the Boston Diagnostic Aphasia Examination. In the first, 111 aphasic patients were given the battery plus some received additional tests, and 5 interpretable factors emerged. Factor I, a language factor similar to that found by

Schuell *et al.,* (1962), encompassed preserved naming, auditory comprehension, and reading–writing clusters. This factor was thought to be Broca's aphasia compounded by severity of deficit that allowed maintenance of writing ability ordinarily reduced in Broca's aphasia. Factor II was a cluster of spatial arithmetic and somatographic tasks. Factor III corresponds to Wernicke's aphasia in which there are good fluency and articulation but poor comprehension and repetition. Paraphrasia is present in this factor. Factor IV is equivalent to transcortical sensory aphasia in which the links between speech and cognition are disturbed. In this factor, articulation, fluency, and repetition are satisfactory, but comprehension, naming, matching, and spontaneous speech are not. In Factor V, finger gnosis, right–left discrimination, and academic skills are reduced to a category similar to Gerstmann's syndrome or a general learning disability.

A later study with a larger sample ($n = 189$) factor analysis also resulted in five interpretable factors (Goodglass & Kaplan, 1976). Factor I related to written language tests plus naming of visual stimuli. Factor II included all spatial–quantitative–somatognosic tests but not language subtests. Factor III involved the motor aspects of speech plus naming visual stimuli. Factor IV was determined by scores on auditory comprehension and reading tests. Factor V was a paraphasia factor. The main differences between the two factor analyses were that, in the 1972 analysis, a written language factor emerged and Wernicke's aphasia split into auditory comprehension and paraphasia components.

Western Aphasia Battery

Based on the approach of the Boston workers (Goodglass & Kaplan, 1976), Kertesz and his co-workers (Kertesz & Poole, 1974) have provided this assessment instrument, which was designed for research and clinical applications. The Western Aphasia Battery (WAB) test requires about an hour to administer and allows calculation of an aphasia quotient based on the oral language subtests of spontaneous speech, comprehension (including a brief form of the Token Test), repetition, naming, and information. A separate performance quotient may be computed after administration of reading, writing, praxis, drawing, block design, calculation, and Raven's matrices. Kertesz (1979b) has reviewed the work of his group using the WAB, the bulk of which pertains to recovery of language function. Kertesz and McCabe (1977) found that language recovery was better after head trauma than after stroke. Greatest improvement can be expected in patients initially least severe. Age has an unclear effect on recovery of language function, but Kertesz and McCabe's (1977) evidence favored the fairly widely accepted notion that younger patients profit more with recovery time. The largest proportion of this recovery occurs during the first 6 months after brain injury. Lomas and Kertesz (1978) examined components of language for differential recovery and reported that fluency remained most handicapped whereas comprehension and repetition recovered best.

Neurosensory Center Comprehensive Examination for Aphasia

Spreen and Benton (1969, 1977) began developing the NCCEA in 1962. The examination's underlying conceptualization of language was seemingly along the lines of stimulus–response associations. It is a unique test in two regards: (1) Control tests are included that are aimed at ruling out sensory–perceptual disorders that might cause aphasic symptoms; and (2) children's norms (6–13 years of age) are included. There are 20 subtests in the language battery, including naming, repetition, fluency, reading, writing, sentence construction, and articulation functions. The control tests involve tactile–visual matching, visual–visual matching, and visual–form perception. The test materials include a set of 40 objects plus the abbreviated version of the Token Test of De Renzi and Vignolo (1962) and cards with words printed on them. Profile sheets provide percentile rank conversion of raw scores.

Crockett (1977) used the NCCEA to statistically attack the basic question of aphasia classification schemes. The study identified by statistical means several groups of aphasics whose characteristics could be compared to various theoretical models.

A factor analysis of the Neurosensory Center Comprehensive Examination for Aphasia (Crockett, 1976) resulted in 8 factors: word finding; production of units of expression over time (fluency–dysfluency); semantic, syntactic, and pragmatic expressive skills; attentional factor; reading; syntactic refinement of verbal output; naming; and articulation. The author concluded that this analysis pointed out the importance of including nonpsycholinguistic factors in theorizing about language. Pertinent to the latter point was the observation (Thomsen, 1975) that the presence and degree of concomitant neuropsychological disorders are important for prognosis about aphasia produced by closed head injury.

The Token Test

This test, developed by De Renzi and Vignolo (1962), is a set of colored forms (circles, squares, triangles) placed in front of the subject. A brief version (Spellacy & Spreen, 1969), requiring only about 10 minutes for normal subjects, is often used. The shorter forms are reported to discriminate aphasics from nonaphasics less well (van Harskamp & van Dongen, 1977). The examiner instructs the subject to manipulate the forms in various ways. At the simplest level the subject must touch a form, progressing to more complex responses, in which the subject must touch one form with another form. At a higher level, varying rates of touching speed are demanded, and finally contingencies are arranged such that the subject responds in a particular manner cued by the examiner's manipulation of a form. During the instructions, the forms are hidden or open to the subject's view in order to assess auditory comprehension with or without visual support to assess the effect of delays between instruction and the required performance.

A recent volume (Boller & Dennis, 1979) brought together papers by Vignolo and De Renzi plus contributions by other researchers using this test. The volume examines the relationships of test performance to various anatomical lesions. The overall conclusions in the final chapter of the volume were that right hemisphere (nondominant) integrity is somewhat superfluous for good performance, and that full understanding of how various lesions within the dominant sphere affect Token Test performance remains to be clarified.

Zaidel (1977) used the Token Test as a part of a program of research aimed at understanding right hemisphere contributions to language in commissurotomy and hemispherectomy patients. Normal children of 4 to 5 years were also tested. Both weighted (crediting partially correct responses) and pass–fail scoring methods were used. The isolated right hemisphere performance was markedly poorer than left and was, in fact, poorer than that of the average left-brain-damaged aphasic reported in the literature. In comparison with children, right hemisphere performance approximated that of a 4-year-old child. This was considerably lower than a receptive language score of 11 years, 7 months (Peabody PVT) obtained in a earlier study (Zaidel, 1976). This difference between Peabody and Token performance indicates that there is no single "language age" for the right hemisphere but that there are wide variations depending on the language function being tested.

Zaidel's (1977) explanation involves differential memory requirements for the two tests. The Token Test may rely more on short-term memory, which, because of impairments of subvocalized speech, may be disturbed in storage and decoding aspects. This was supported by Yorkston, Marshall, and Butler (1977), who found that auditory and visual commands together were better than auditory alone, and that extra processing time led to further improvement in this condition. Thus, in a sense, the Token Test may not be restricted to language and in fact may be associated with more generalized neuropsychological processes such as memory (Lesser, 1976). This notion could be critical in understanding the Token Test's sensitivity to all types of aphasia (Boller & Vignolo, 1966; Cohen, Kelter, & Engel, 1976).

Porch Index of Communication Ability

Bruce Porch developed the PICA over a 6-year period. The purpose of this comprehensive test, published in 1967 by Consulting Psychologists Press, was to provide a sensitive, reliable tool with a strong quantitative/statistical foundation. The PICA consists of a test manual, objects, three sets of stimulus cards, and scoring and response sheets. Total time to complete administration of the battery is approximately 1 hour. There are 18 subtests divided into 3 areas: 4 verbal, 8 gestural and 6 graphic. The total number of items is 180. Averages for the three modalities are computed and a profile is drawn. Each response may be elevated along five dimensions: accuracy, responsiveness, completeness, promptness, and efficiency. This seems to represent an advance because Eisenson, Schuell, Wepman, and others have been criticized for not paying attention to an analysis of errors in scoring their test results (Berry, 1976). Actual scores given to a response vary from 1 (no response) to 16 (complex). A score of 16 indicates that the response is accurate, responsive, complex, prompt, and efficient. Porch (1967) provides an informative flowchart to allow the scorer to decide which scoring category is appropriate through a series of questions that one may ask oneself about the patient's response. The author states in his manual that a 40-hour training session plus 10 supervised test administrations is needed for basic competency in PICA administration and scoring.

DiSimoni, Keith, Holt, and Darley (1975) performed step-wise multiple regression analysis on PICA data from 222 aphasic patients to determine the accuracy of prediction of overall score by fewer subtests or items. They found that only four complete subtest scores could predict overall score but, even more surprisingly, that one or two items alone would yield approximatey the same level. DiSimoni *et al.* (1975) concluded that the PICA is highly redundant and that shorter forms should be developed.

Despite the fact that aphasia tests are ordinarily screening measures in studies aimed at aphasic poulations, there are reports of performance in other groups on the PICA. Rada, Porch, Dillingham, Kellner, and Poree (1977) reported improved PICA scores in recovering chronic alcoholics after a 2-week hiatus from drinking, but there was no correlation between PICA scores and variables of alcohol abuse. This suggested a generalized deficit, possibly resulting from nutritional or psychological factors rather than from toxic effects of alcohol. Groher (1977) reported a similar recovery on skills assessed by the PICA after closed head injury with greatest improvement in the first month. Again, as in the case of alcohol, no significant correlation was found between severity (length of coma) and eventual language score.

A recent factor analysis of the PICA (Clark, Crockett, & Klonoff, 1979) showed that three factors accounted for about 83% of the variance. These were verbal competency (fluency), written competency, and a general language disorder. The general language disorder factor correlated with all PICA subtests, but highest correlations were obtained with the simplest subtests. The authors concluded that Porch's assumption that a sum of the subtest scores reflected general communication competency was correct. They did not find support for a separate gestural component postulated by Porch (1967), and suggested additional subtests may be needed to obtain a "clean" gestural factor.

LANGUAGE PORTIONS OF COMPREHENSIVE NEUROPSYCHOLOGICAL BATTERIES

Russell, Neuringer, and Goldstein (1970) pointed out that an aphasia test is part of the traditional neurological examination. Similarly, the two major neuropsychological test batteries include language evaluations. The Halstead–Reitan battery includes a modified Halstead–Wepman Aphasia Screening Test (Halstead & Wepman, 1959), which is a brief examination covering major functions. Research has demonstrated that it is sensitive to lateralized brain damage (Doehring & Reitan, 1962; Heimburger & Reitan, 1961; Wheeler & Reitan, 1963). Russell *et al.* (1970) assigned a numerical score to each item on the test that had to do with language functioning. Errors received one to four points, depending on the item. The Speech Sounds Perception Test is also part of the Halstead–Reitan Battery and involves auditory discrimination ability. No verbal response is required, only underlining from a multiple-choice array. Basic reading competency is needed to complete this test.

The batteries based on Luria's System (Luria, 1951) include those of Christensen (1975), Majovski, Tanquay, Russell, Sigman, Crumley, and Goldenberg (1979), and Golden et al. (1979). The purpose of these tests is to understand impairments in functional systems and brain regions for specific diagnosis. Verbal abilities are comprehensively evaluated in these batteries, perhaps so that when used by an expert, specific aphasic syndromes may be refined from the scores. McKay and Golden (1979) reported associations between clusters of specific items of the Luria–Nebraska and damage to specific brain regions. Verbal performance reductions in the motor, memory, and reasoning areas were related to left frontal damage and the coordination of visual and verbal skills to left sensorimotor damage. Left parietal–occipital damage also affected the integration of verbal and visual skills. Linguistic performance (grammar, phonetic analysis) and verbal memory were related to the left temporal region. McKay and Golden (1979) added that verbal deficits may affect nonverbal performance, whereas the converse seems to be rare.

Receptive Language Tests

Receptive language tests such as the Peabody Picture Vocabulary Test (Dunn, 1965) and the Full-Range Picture Vocabulary Test (Ammons & Huth, 1949; Ammons & Rachiele, 1950; Ammons, Larson, & Shearn, 1950) require that the subject match a spoken word and its pictorial representation. The Peabody is primarily a tool for evaluating children and adolescents, whereas the Full-Range provides adult norms. The receptive language tests may be used to measure comprehension of speech in severely aphasic patients (Smith & Burklund, 1966). Since language rarely consists of a word in isolation from others (Fraser, Bellugi, & Brown, 1963), a task was developed in which a sentence was presented auditorially and was matched with one of two pictures. This procedure allows variation of both syntactic and semantic aspects.

Within the context of a series of subtests, the Illinois Test of Psycholinguistic Abilities (Kirk, McCarthy, & Kirk, 1969) includes a receptive language evaluation. This test, designed for children, is widely used by both psychologists and speech pathologists to ascertain language strengths and weaknesses. The 12 subtests are divided into those termed representational (i.e., symbolic), such as receptive language, and those termed automatic (i.e., nonsymbolic), such as visual closure and digit memory. The test has been primarily used in analyzing and planning remediation of learning disabilities. Test materials include an examiner's manual, stimulus cards and objects, record forms, and profile sheets.

Coupar (1976) obtained correlation coefficients among the Wepman Auditory Discrimination Test, oral sentences from Examining for Aphasia, following directions of the Minnesota Test for Differential Diagnosis of Aphasia, the English Picture Vocabulary Test (Brimer & Dunn, 1968), Raven's Matrices, and the Token Test. Aphasics, right hemisphere damaged, leucotomized, and controls were tested. Except for the Raven, all tests or test portions were considered to assess receptive language. The Wepman and English Picture Vocabulary Test failed to correlate significantly with any other measures or with each other. Interestingly, the Raven scores significantly correlated with all test scores but the Wepman. The Token Test did not correlate significantly with the Picture Vocabulary Test, suggesting again that receptive language has a variety of components.

The Dichotic Listening Test is possibly best classified as a receptive language tool. Originally described by Broadbent (1954) and elaborated in the work of Kimura (1961a), it provides a means of establishing cerebral dominance. As is true for many other functions, auditory signals cross to the hemisphere opposite from the body side receiving the signal due to decussation of afferent fibers. The cerebral hemisphere that is superior (i.e., dominant) for reception of language stimuli can be established by comparing stimuli presented through earphones to each ear separately. The majority of non-brain-damaged individuals show a right ear (left hemisphere) advantage for verbal stimuli (Broadbent, 1954; Kimura, 1961a; Shankweiler & Studdert-Kennedy, 1967). In left temporal lobe injury (Kimura, 1961b), stuttering (Curry & Gregory, 1969), severe aphasia (Johnson, Sommers, & Weidner, 1977), and language-delayed children (Slorach and Noehr, 1973; Sommers & Taylor, 1972), this advantage is reversed or reduced. A shift in cerebral dominance for language may be a causative factor in certain conditions or a compensatory mechanism after injury.

Verbal Learning and Memory Tests

There has been little change since Zangwill (1943) reviewed clinical tests of memory impairment and described digit spans, word lists, memory for facts in stories, and paired associate tasks as in "fairly general use . . . in diagnosis of organic and funtional disorders of memory" (p. 577). Zangwill (1943) was dissatisfied with available methodologies and modified the digit span test by giving repeated trials on the digit span originally failed until the patient learned. The procedure was then repeated with a longer series. Trials to criterion were recorded. The second task involved verbatim repetition of sentences from the Babcock Sentence Repetition Test (Babcock, 1930).

While early research concentrated on discrimination of brain-injured patients from other patients, neuropsychological investigations involving verbal memory tests have more recently investigated styles of cognitive processing in various clinical conditions (Butters, Tarlow, Cermak, & Sax, 1976) and on relating type of deficit to severity of clinical disease (Ellenberg, Rosenbaum, Goldman, & Whitman, 1980). The use of learning and memory tests of words or consonant sequences has continued, but increasing memorization difficulty, either by competing associations (Stark, 1961) or unrelated interfering tasks (Peterson & Peterson, 1959), has improved the applicability of these procedures to disorders having milder consequences. Stimulus words may vary on level of imagery potential (Weingartner, Caine, & Ebert, 1979) or rarity (Rochford & Williams, 1962), reminding may be used (Buschke, 1973; Meudell, Butters, & Montgomery, 1978), or massed practice compared with distributed practice (Butters, Tarlow, Cermak, & Sax, 1976). These techniques permit clarification of specific practices that might or might not be useful in aiding individuals of various diagnostic categories. For example, Weingartner, Cohen, Murphy, Martello, & Gerdt (1981) found that clustering or "chunking" by the experimenter of learned verbal material reduced the difference in recall between controls and depressed patients. In other words, patients were less apt to learn or remember information unless it had been organized for them.

Language disorders are known to be associated with reduced immediate and delayed verbal memory (Butters et al., 1970). Butters et al. (1970) attributed the deficit to verbal processes rather than memory. Flowers (1975) found poorer recall of trigrams in aphasic subjects compared with brain-damaged nonaphasics and controls. Proactive interference seemed to be equally potent among the groups. Primacy and recency effects were observed in the nonaphasic and control subjects, but only primacy effects obtained in the aphasic group. Again, lengthened processing time in the aphasic subjects was implicated in the deficit.

Word Association Tasks

According to Goodglass and Baker (1976), virtually all word association tasks have been modeled after one developed by Kent and Rosanoff in 1910 in which a stimulus word is presented and the subject either emits a word or fails to respond. The task has been used neuropsychologically to describe and differentiate among types of aphasia (Howes, 1967). In general, expressive aphasics gave normal responses after a long delay, but receptive aphasics showed associative disturbances. Lhermitte, Desrouesne, and Lecours (1971), quoted in Boller et al. (1977) found aphasics were impaired in correctly deciding whether words were associated; they made errors of omission or commission. Goodglass and Baker (1976) utilized a procedure in which subjects made a motor response only if they recognized a relationship between individually visually presented target words and orally presented stimulus words. Associative connections were placed in seven categories. Aphasics with severe comprehension deficits had more overall errors and generally longer latencies, except in responding to a stimulus–target combination where both word members were of the same class (e.g., orange–apple). The overall conclusions were that even in the absence of severe comprehension deficits, aphasics can be differentiated from both brain-damaged and normal controls in the pattern and rapidity of semantic associations. The ability to name depends on the integrity of these associations, but type of association does not appear to differentiate among various types of aphasia (Goodglass, Kaplan, Weintraub, & Ackerman, 1976).

Pizzamiglio and Appicciafuoco (1971) varied the ordinary word association task by auditorially presenting a stimulus word to be matched with a picture. One picture was of the stimulus word; the others were of frequent associations made to the stimulus by normal subjects. Patients with comprehension problems did more poorly on this task than did patients with expressive problems.

VERBAL FLUENCY PROBLEMS

Thurstone (1938) first standardized the word fluency test, and Milner (1964) utilized it in an important study showing that frontal lobe injury resulted in poor performance in the absence of other signs of aphasia or memory deficits.

Borkowski, Benton, & Spreen (1967) developed a word fluency test in which subjects were asked to say in 60 seconds all the words they could think of that started with a certain letter. Difficult letters (J and U) were effective in discriminating patients with right and left hemisphere damage in patients with higher intelligence. Easier letters (F, S, P, and T) were better for differentiating brain-damaged and control subjects of lower measured intelligence.

Damasio (1979) notes that word fluency may play a role in the diagnosis of frontal lobe damage. These patients may be spontaneously fluent but unable to produce morphologically or semantically similar words on demand. Butters, Sax, Montgomery, and Tarlow (1978) found that both recent and advanced cases of Huntington's disease generated significantly fewer words than did normals. Fluency has been reported to be a very important factor in differentiating various aphasics (Kertesz & Poole, 1974). The methodology in the latter study involved scoring of spontaneous speech on a 0 to 10 scale using the following criteria: no response or meaningless utterances; recurrent utterances with meaningful intonation; most inappropriate single words; fluent stereotypic utterances or low volume jargon; mostly appropriate single words or prepositional phrases; halting;

telegraphic speech; more complete prepositional sentences; phonemic jargon; fluent circumlocutory speech; mostly complete sentences with some word or word portion finding problems; and normal sentences.

Word fluency deficits have been found to be associated with poor reading in learning disabled individuals (Spellacy & Peter, 1978). The authors further reported that word fluency does not load on a factor including sentence repetition and vocabulary. Word fluency is also considered a measure of frontal lobe functions (Lezak, 1976).

ADDITIONAL LANGUAGE TESTS

Two language tests used chiefly with children deserve mention. The Wepman Auditory Discrimination Test (Wepman, 1958) is used by some neurologists and pediatricians to screen children for language problems. The subject is asked to decide whether 40 pairs of spoken words are the same or different. It is important to know whether the subject comprehends the instructions. This may be a significant problem in aphasia and can preclude the use of this or many other tests with aphasic subjects. The Reynell Developmental Language Scales (Reynell, 1969) have been used by British neuropsychology groups mainly in clinical diagnosis of children under age 5. Bartak, Rutter, & Cox (1977) compared autistic and dysphasic children (on the Reynell) and were able to differentiate the groups as efficiently on the basis of language as on interpersonal/behavioral criteria. They concluded that a cognitive deficit, as yet unspecified, is an essential symptom of autism.

With subjects who are incapable of expressive speech, investigators have asked them to reconstruct sentences that had been written on cards, cut into several pieces, and the elements of each sentence presented in meaningless order (von Stockert, 1972). Similarly, Gazzaniga, LeDoux, and Wilson (1977) had a callosum sectioned subject spell the names of visually presented items by arranging letters. Generally, expressive aphasics have more difficulty than receptive aphasics in sentence construction (Kremin & Goldblum, 1975; von Stockert, 1972). However, simple severity of aphasia does not yet seem to have been adequately ruled out as the critical dimension.

Lansdell (1968) used the Wide Range Vocabulary Test of Atwell and Wells (1937), which involves visual input and word selection as a response, to demonstrate a positive relationship between size of left hemisphere lesion in neurosurgical patients and this verbal measure.

Albert, Yamadori, Gardner, and Howes (1973) developed a verbal concept test known as the "odd word out" to evaluate semantic comprehension in reading disorders. There is a parallel form known as the "odd object out" test (Albert *et al.*, 1973). The "odd word out" test consists of 10 presentations of 5 words each in which 4 of the words belong to the same semantic category. Subjects are asked which word or object is the odd one. Albert, Reches, and Silverberg (1975) used the "odd word out" and "odd object out" test in order to demonstrate the presence of a visual agnosia in the absence of alexia. This finding suggested to the authors that two underlying neuropsychological mechanisms were responsible for the deficit: (1) an interhemisphere visual–verbal disconnection, and (2) a specific categorization deficit for visual, nonverbal, meaningful stimuli.

Gardner and Zurif (1975) tested reading in aphasics by asking them to read simple words; if they failed this, four choices were offered orally by the examiner and the subject chose among them. Order of difficulty for various types of words was similar among aphasic groups, but global aphasics performed most poorly and Wenicke's most proficiently. Non-nouns were more difficult than nouns, and grammatical particles were difficult even for patients who used them in speech. High imagery nouns were easier than abstract nouns, particularly if they had few letters. The conclusions were that semantic processes have a role in the reading ability of aphasics and that reading is not simply matching sounds and graphic patterns.

Many language researchers who have adopted a linguistic approach use a technique in which subjects are asked to group words from a sentence that they think "fit best together" (Kolk, 1978; Zurif, Caramazza, & Myerson, 1972). In nonaphasic subjects, the perceived clusters are consistent with accepted linguistic rules. Expressive aphasics were particularly impaired at this task, failing to organize adjectives or functors (prepositions, articles, pronouns). This was interpreted as a disturbance of representation of sentences at a syntactic level (Kolk, 1978).

As previously described, well learned verbal skills have been thought to remain relatively unaffected or to "hold" during dementing processes. Nelson and McKenna (1975) reported that among verbal tests, word reading showed less decrement in progressive brain damage than did knowledge of word meaning on the WAIS. Nelson and O'Connell (1978) have reported the development of the New Adult Reading Test, which uses words easily subjected to phonetic analysis. Again, it was found that word reading was a relatively well maintained ability among patients with generalized brain atrophy, and that it could be used to predict premorbid intellectual level.

CONCLUSION

It should not be surprising that verbal behavior has historically received the attention it has in the field of human neuropsychology. No other readily recordable behavior has the variations and intricacies observed in verbal behavior. That verbal behavior should be disrupted by disorders of the central nervous system is self-evident. What is remarkable, perhaps, is that in these days of quantification, mathematical models, and so on, the tests of verbal behavior seem so qualitative and traditional. Ironically, with seemingly greater quantitative sophistication, McDonald (1915) made simple frequency counts of the number of different words in the everyday language of ordinary people of various educational backgrounds. He reported the percentage of use of different parts of speech in their language samples and compared them with those of brain-damaged individuals. Brain-damaged patients (generally with expressive aphasia) used a relative overabundance of words in the verb/adverb class with reduction of words in the noun/adjective class. In non-brain-damaged individuals, verb/adverb and noun/adjective classes were used with approximately equal frequency. McDonald concluded that "mere careful attention to a few sentences from the patient may suffice for a diagnosis of brain disease . . ." (p. 560). More recent and sophisticated methodologies such as content analysis (Gottschalk & Gleser, 1969) or scaling of standardized interviews (Crockett, 1976, 1977; Spreen & Wachal, 1973) should be applied to premorbid and current verbal samples of brain-damaged patients as a research or diagnostic tool. The application of such methodologies should greatly enhance the clinical-scientific use of tests of verbal abilities in human neuropsychology.

REFERENCES

Aftanas, M. A., & Royce, J. R. A factor analysis of brain damage tests administered to normal subjects with factor score comparisons across ages. *Multivariate Behavioral Research,* 1969, *4,* 459–481.

Albert, M. L., Yamadori, A., Gardner, H., & Howes, D. Comprehension in alexia. *Brain,* 1973, *96,* 317–328.

Albert, M. L., Reches, A., & Silverberg, R. Associative visual agnosis without alexia. *Neurology,* 1975, *25,* 322–326.

Ammons, R. B., & Huth, R. W. The full-range picture vocabulary test: I. Preliminary scale. *Journal of Psychology,* 1949, *28,* 51–64.

Ammons, R. B., & Rachiele, L. D. The full-range picture vocabulary test: II. Selection of items for final scales. *Educational Psychology Measurement,* 1950, *10,* 307–319.

Ammons, R. B., Larson, W. L., & Shearn, C. R. The full-range vocabulary test: V. Results for an adult population. *Journal of Consulting Psychology,* 1950, *14,* 150–155.

April, R. S., & Tse, P. C. Crossed aphasia in a Chinese Bilingual Dextral. *Archives of Neurology,* 1977, *34,* 766–770.

Atwell, C. R., & Wells, F. L. Wide range multiple-choice vocabulary tests. *Journal of Applied Psychology,* 1937, *21,* 550–555.

Babcock, H. An experiment in the measurement of mental deterioration. *Archives of Psychology (New York),* 1930, No. 117.

Baker, E., Berry, T., Gardner, H., Zuris, E., Davis L., & Veroff, A. Can linguistic competence be dissociated from natural language functions? *Nature,* 1975, *254,* 509–510.

Bandura, A., & Harris, M. B. Modification of syntactic style. *Journal of Experimental Child Psychology,* 1966, *4,* 341–352.

Bartak, L., Rutter, M., & Cox, A. A comparative study of infantile autism and specific developmental receptive language disorders: III. Discriminant function analysis. *Journal of Autism and Childhood Schizophrenia*, 1977, *7*, 383–396.

Benson, D. F. Aphasia. In Heilman, K. M., & Valenstein, E. (Eds.), *Clinical neuropsychology*. New York: Oxford University Press, 1979.

Benton, A. L. Developmental aphasia and brain damage. *Cortex*, 1964, *1*, 40–52.

Benton, A. L. Problems in test construction in the field of aphasia. *Cortex*, 1967, *3*, 32–58.

Berry, P. B. Elicited imitation of language: Some ESNS population characteristics. *Language and Speech*, 1976, *19*, 350–362.

Blumstein, S. E., Baker, E., & Goodglass, H. Phonological factors in auditory comprehension in aphasia. *Neuropsychologia*, 1977, *15*, 19–30.

Boller, F. Latent aphasia: Right and left "non/aphasic" brain/damaged patients compared. *Cortex*, 1968, *4*, 245–256.

Boller, F., & Dennis, M. (Eds.). *Auditory comprehension: Clinical and experimental studies with the Token Test*. New York: Academic Press, 1979.

Boller, F., & Vignolo, L. A. Latent sensory aphasia in hemisphere-damaged patients: An experimental study with the Token Test. *Brain*, 1966, *89*, 815–830.

Boller, F., Barturtunski, P., Mack, J. L., & Kim. Y. Neuropsychological correlates of hypertension. *Archives of Neurology*, 1977, *34*, 701–705.

Borkowski, J. G., Benton, A. L., & Spreen, O. Word fluency and brain damage. *Neuropsychologia*, 1967, *5*, 135–140.

Brimer, M. A., & Dunn, L. M. *English picture vocabulary test 3, 11 to 184*. Bristol: Educational Evaluation Enterprises, 1968.

Broadbent, D. The role of auditory localization in attention and memory span. *Journal of Experimental Psychology*, 1954, *47*, 191–196.

Brookshire, R. H. *An introduction to aphasia*. Minneapolis: BRK Publishers, 1973.

Brookshire, R. H. A Token Test battery for testing auditory comprehension in brain-injured adults. *Brain and Language*, 1978, *6*, 149–157.

Buschke, H. Selective reminding for analysis of memory and learning. *Journal of Verbal Learning and Verbal Behavior*, 1973, *12*, 543–550.

Butters, N., Samuels, I., Goodglass, H., & Brody, B. Short-term visual and auditory memory disorders after parietal and frontal lobe damage. *Cortex*, 1970, *6*, 440–459.

Butters, N., Sax, D., Montgomery, K., & Tarlow, S. Comparison of the neuropsychological deficits associated with early and advanced Huntington's disease. *Archives of Neurology*, 1978, *35*, 585–589.

Butters, N., Tarlow, S., Cermak, L. S., & Sax, D. A comparison of the information processing deficits of patients with Huntington's chorea and Korsakoff's syndrome. *Cortex*, 1976, *12*, 134–144.

Cherlow, D. G., & Serafetinides, E. A. Speech and memory assessment in psychomotor epileptics. *Cortex*, 1976, *12*, 21–26.

Chomsky, N. *Syntactic structure*. Mouton: La Haye, 1957.

Christensen, A. L. *Luria's neuropsychological investigation*. New York: Spectrum Publications, 1975.

Clark, C., Crockett, D. J., & Klonoff, H. Factor analysis of the Porch Index of Communication Ability. *Brain and Language*, 1979, *7*, 1–7.

Cohen, R., Kelter, S., & Engel, D. On the validity of the Token Test. *Nervenarzt*, 1976, *47*, 357–361.

Coughlan, A. K. Effects of localized cerebral lesions and dysphasia on verbal memory. *Journal of Neurology, Neurosurgery and Psychiatry*, 1979, *42*, 914–923.

Coupar, A. M. Detection of mild aphasia: A study using the Token Test. *British Journal of Medical Psychology*, 1976, *49*, 141–144.

Crockett, D. J. Multivariate comparison of Howe's and Weisenburg and McBride's models of aphasia on the Neurosensory Center Comprehensive Examination. *Perceptual and Motor Skills*, 1976, *43*, 795–806.

Crockett, D. J. A comparison of empirically derived groups of aphasic patients on the Neurosensory Center Comprehensive Examination for Aphasia. *Journal of Clinical Psychology*, 1977, *33*, 194–198.

Curry, F., & Gregory, H. The performance of stutterers on dichotic listening tasks thought to reflect cerebral dominance. *Journal of Speech and Hearing Research*, 1969, *12*, 73.

Damasio, A. The frontal lobes. In K. M. Heilman & E. Valenstein, (Eds.), *Clinical neuropsychology*. New York: Oxford University Press, 1979.

De Renzi, E., & Vignolo, L. A. The Token Test: A sensitive test to detect receptive disturbances in aphasics. *Brain*, 1962, *85*, 665–678.

De Reuck, A. V. S. & O'Connor, M. (Eds.). *Disorders of language* (A Ciba Foundation Symposium). London: Churchill, 1964.

DiSimoni, F. G., Keith, R. L., Holt, D. L., & Darley, F. L. Practicality of shortening the Porch Index of Communicative Ability. *Journal of Speech and Hearing Research*, 1975, *18*, 491–497.

Doehring, D. G., & Reitan, R. M. Concept attainment of human adults with lateralized cerebral lesions. *Perceptual and Motor Skills*, 1962, *14*, 27–33.

Dunn, L. M. *Expanded manual for the Peabody picture vocabulary test*. Circle Pines, Minneapolis: American Guidance Service, 1965.

Eisenson, J. *Examining for aphasia. A manual for the examination of aphasia and related disturbances*. New York: Psychological Corporation, 1954.

Eisenson, J. Aphasia: A point of view as to the nature of the disorder and factors that determine prognosis for recovery. *International Journal of Neurology*, 1964, *4*, 287–295.

Eisenson, J. *Adult aphasia: Assessment and treatment*. Englewood Cliffs, N.J.: Prentice-Hall, 1973.

Ellenberg, L., Rosenbaum, G., Goldman, M. S., & Whitman, R. D. Recoverability of psychological functioning following alcohol abuse: Lateralization effects. *Journal of Consulting and Clinical Psychology*, 1980, *48*, 503–510.

Farmer, A. Self-correctional strategies in the conversational speech of aphasia and non-aphasic brain damaged adults. *Cortex*, 1977, *13*, 327–334.

Ferry, P. C., Hall, S. M., & Hicks, J. L. "Dilapidated" speech: Developmental verbal dyspraxia. *Developmental Medicine and Child Neurology*, 1975, *17*, 749–756.

Flowers, C. R. Proactive interference in short-term recall by aphasic, brain damaged non-aphasic and normal subjects. *Neuropsychologia*, 1975, *13*, 59–88.

Fraser, C., Bellugi, U., & Brown, R. Control of grammar in imitation, comprehension, and production. *Journal of Verbal Learning and Verbal Behavior*, 1963, *2*, 121–135.

Gainotti, G., Miceli, G., & Caltagirone, C. A neurolinguistic model for the study of aphasia. *European Neurology*, 1977, *15*, 20–24.

Gallagher, T. M., & Guilford, A. M. Wh-questions: Responses by aphasic patients. *Cortex*, 1977, *13*, 44–54.

Gardner, H., & Zurif, E. Bee but not be: Oral reading of single words in aphasia and alexia. *Neuropsychologia*, 1975, *13*, 181–190.

Gazzaniga, M. S., LeDoux, J. E., & Wilson, D. H. Language, praxis, and the right hemisphere: Clues to some mechanisms of consciousness. *Neurology*, 1977, *27*, 1144–1147.

Geschwind, N. Language and the brain. *Scientific American*, 1972, *226*, 76–83.

Golden, C. J., Purisch, A. D., & Hammeke, T. A. *The Luria–Nebraska neuropsychological battery: A battery for clinical and experimental uses*. Lincoln: University of Nebraska Press, 1979.

Goodglass, H., & Baker, E. Semantic field, naming, and auditory comprehension in aphasia. *Brain and Language*, 1976, *3*, 359–374.

Goodglass, H., & Berko, J. Agrammatism and inflectional morphology in English. *Journal of Speech and Hearing Research*, 1960, *3*, 257–267.

Goodglass, H., & Kaplan, E. *The assessment of aphasia and related disorders.* Philadelphia: Lea and Febiger, 1976.

Goodglass, H., Berko-Gleason, J., Sckerman-Bernholtz, N., and Hyde, M. R. Some linguistic structures in the speech of a Broca's aphasic. *Cortex,* 1972, *8,* 191–212.

Goodglass, H., Gleason, J. B., & Hyde, M. Some dimensions of auditory language comprehension in aphasics. *Journal of Speech and Hearing Research,* 1970, *13,* 595–606.

Goodglass, H., Kaplan, E., Weintraub, S., & Ackerman, N. The "tip of the tongue" phenomenon in aphasia. *Cortex,* 1976, *12,* 145–153.

Gottschalk, L. A., & Gleser, G. C. *Measurement of psychological states through the content analysis of verbal behavior.* Berkeley: University of Californa Press, 1969.

Groher, M. Language and memory disorders following closed head trauma. *Journal of Speech and Hearing Research,* 1977, *20,* 212–223.

Halstead, W. C., & Wepman, J. M. The Halstead–Wepman aphasia screening test. *Journal of Speech and Hearing Disorders,* 1959, *14,* 9–15.

Head, H. *Aphasia and kindred disorders* (2 vols.). London: Cambridge University Press, 1926.

Hecaen, H., & Albert, M. L. *Human neuropsychology.* New York: Wiley, 1978.

Heilman, K. M., & Valenstein, E. *Clinical neuropsychology.* New York: Oxford University Press, 1979.

Heimburger, R. F., & Reitan, R. M. Easily administered written test for lateralizing brain lesions. *Journal of Neurosurgery,* 1961, *18,* 301–312.

Howes, D. Hypotheses concerning the functioning of the language mechanism. Paper presented at the Conference on Verbal Behavior, New York, September 1965.

Howes, D. Some experimental investigations of language in aphasia. In K. Salzinger & S. Salzinger (Eds.), *Research in verbal behavior and some neuropsychological implications.* New York: Academic Press, 1967.

Inglis, J. A. A paired-associate learning test for use with elderly psychiatric patients. *Journal of Mental Science,* 1959, *105,* 440–443.

Jackson, J. H. On the physiology of language. *Brain,* 1915, *38,* 59–64.

Jakobson, R. Towards a linguistic typology of aphasic impairments. In A. V. S. de Reuck and M. O'Connor (Eds.), *Disorders of language* (A Ciba Foundation Symposium). London: Churchill, 1964.

Johnson, J. P., Sommers, R. K., & Weidner, W. E. Dichotic ear preference in aphasia. *Journal of Speech and Hearing Research,* 1977, *20,* 116–129.

Jones, L. V., & Wepman, J. M. Dimensions of language performance in aphasia. *Journal of Speech and Hearing Research,* 1961, *4,* 220–232.

Keenan, J. S., & Brassell, E. G. *Aphasia language performance scales.* Murfreesboro, Tenn.: Pinnacle Press, 1975.

Kent, G. H., & Rosanoff, A. J. A study of association in insanity. *American Journal of Insanity,* 1910, *67,* 27–96.

Kertesz, A. *Aphasia and associated disorders: Taxonomy, localization, and recovery.* New York: Grune & Stratton, 1979a.

Kertesz, A. Recovery and treatment. In K. M. Heilman & E. Valenstein, (Eds.), *Clinical neuropsychology.* New York: Oxford University Press, 1979b.

Kertesz, A., & McCabe, P. Recovery patterns and prognosis in aphasia. *Brain,* 1977, *100,* 1–18.

Kertesz, A., & Poole, E. The aphasia quotient: The taxonomic approach to measurement of aphasic disability. *Le Journal Canadien des Sciences Neurologiques,* 1974, *1,* 7–16.

Kimura, D. Cerebral dominance and the perception of verbal stimuli. *Canadian Journal of Psychology,* 1961a, *15,* 166–171.

Kimura, D. Some effects of temporal lobe damage on auditory perception. *Canadian Journal of Psychology,* 1961b, *15,* 156–165.

Kirk, S. A., McCarthy, J., & Kirk, W. *The Illinois test of psycholinguistic abilities* (rev. ed.). Urbana, Ill.: University Press, 1969.

Kolk, H. H. J. Judgment of sentence structure in Broca's aphasia. *Neuropsychologia,* 1978, *16,* 617–625.

Kremin, H., & Goldblum, M. C. Etude de le comprehension syntaxique chez les aphasiquee. *Linguistics,* 1975, *154,* 31–46.

Lansdell, H. Effect of extent of temporal lobe ablations on two lateralized deficits. *Physiology and Behavior,* 1968, *3,* 271–273.

Lesser, R. Verbal and non-verbal memory components in the Token Test. *Neuropsychologia,* 1976, *14,* 79–85.

Lezak, M. D. *Neuropsychological assessment.* New York: Oxford University Press, 1976.

Lhermitte, F., Desrouesne, J., & Lecours, A. R. Contribution a l'étude des troubles semantiques dans l'aphasie. *Revue Neurologique,* 1971, *125,* 81–101.

Lomas, J., & Kertesz, A. Patterns of spontaneous recovery in aphasic groups: A study of adult stroke patients. *Brain and Language,* 1978, *5,* 388–401.

Luria, A. R. [*Neuropsychological investigation scheme.*] Moscow: Moscow University Press, 1951.

Luria, A. R. *Higher cortical functions in man.* New York: Basic Books, 1966.

Luria, A. R. *The working brain: An introduction to neuropsychology.* New York: Basic Books, 1973.

Mahan, H. C. Measuring intellectual impairment with the WAIS: An improved approach to scoring. *Clinical Neuropsychology,* 1979, *1,* 54–63.

Mahan, H. C. Early quantitative studies of neuropsychological impairment, 1899–1939. *Clinical Neuropsychology.* 1980, *2,* 38–46.

Majovski, L., Tanquay, P., Russell, A., Sigman, M., Crumley, K., & Goldenberg, I. Clinical neuropsychological screening instrument for assessment of higher cortical deficits in adolescents. *Clinical Neuropsychology,* 1979, *1,* 3–8.

McDonald, W. Mental disease and language. *Journal of Nervous and Mental Diseases,* 1915, *42,* 482–491, 540–563.

McFie, J. *Assessment of organic intellectual impairment.* London: Academic Press, 1975.

McKay, S., & Golden, C. J. Empirical derivation of experimental scales for localizing brain lesions using the Luria–Nebraska Neuropsychological Battery. *Clinical Neuropsychology,* 1979, *1,* 19–23.

Meudell, P., Butters, N., & Montgomery, L. The role of rehearsal in the short-term memory performance of patients with Korsakoff's and Huntington's disease. *Neuropsychologia,* 1978, *16,* 507–510.

Milner, B. Some effects of frontal lobectomy in man. In J. M. Warren & K. Akert (Eds.), *The frontal granular cortex and behavior.* New York: McGraw-Hill, 1964.

Nelson, H. E., & McKenna, P. The use of current reading ability in the assessment of dementia. *British Journal of Social and Clinical Psychology,* 1975, *14,* 259–267.

Nelson, H. E., & O'Connell, A. Dementia: The estimation of premorbid intelligence levels using the New Adult Reading Test. *Cortex,* 1978, *14,* 234–244.

Oldfield, R. C., & Wingfield, A. *A series of pictures for use in object naming.* M.R.C. Psycholinguistic Research Unit Special Report No. PLU/65/19, 1965.

Osgood, C. E., & Miron, M. S. *Approaches to the study of aphasia.* Urbana: University of Illinois Press, 1963.

Porch, B. *Porch index of communicative ability.* Palo Alto: Consulting Psychologist Press, 1967.

Peterson, L. R., & Peterson, M. J. Short-term retention of individual verbal items. *Journal of Experimental Psychology,* 1959, *58,* 193–198.

Pizzamiglio, L., & Appicciafuoco, A. Semantic comprehension in aphasia. *Journal of Comparative Diseases,* 1971, *3,* 280–288.

Rada, R. T., Porch, B. E., Dillingham, C., Kellner, R., & Poree, J. B. Alcoholism and language function. *Alcoholism: Clinical and Experimental Research*, 1977, *1*, 199–205.

Reynell, J. *Reynell developmental language scales*. London: NFER Publishing, 1969.

Rivers, D. L., & Love, R. J. Language performance on visual processing tasks in right hemisphere lesion cases. *Brain and Language*, 1980, *10*, 348–366.

Rochford, G., & Williams, M. Studies in the development and breakdown of the use of names: Experimental production of naming disorders in normal people. *Journal of Neurology, Neurosurgery and Psychiatry*, 1962, *25*, 228–233.

Rochford, G., & Williams, M. The measurement of language disorders. *Speech Pathology and Therapeutics*, 1964, *7*, 3–11.

Rosenbeck, J., Messert, B., Collins, M., & Wertz, R. T. Stuttering following brain damage *Brain and Language*, 1978, *6*, 82–96.

Royce, J. R., Yeudall, L. T. & Bock, C. Factor analytic studies of human brain damage: I. First and second-order factors and their brain correlates. *Multivariate Behavioral Research*, 1976, *10*, 381–418.

Russell, E. W., Neuringer, C., & Goldstein, G. *Assessment of brain damage. A neuropsychological key approach*. New York: Wiley-Interscience, 1970.

Sarno, M. T. (Ed.). *Aphasia: Selected readings*. New York: Appleton-Century-Crofts, 1972.

Schuell, H. *Differential diagnosis of aphasia with the Minnesota Test*, (2nd ed.). Minnesota: University of Minneapolis Press, 1973.

Schuell, H., Jenkins, J. J., & Carroll, J. B. A factor analysis of the Minnesota Test for differential diagnosis of aphasia. *Journal of Speech and Hearing Research*, 1962, *5*, 350–369.

Schuell, H., Jenkins, J., & Jimenez-Pabon, E. *Aphasia in adults—Diagnosis, prognosis, and treatment*. New York: Harper & Row, 1964.

Shankweiler, D., & Studdert-Kennedy, M. Identification of consonants and vowels presented to left and right ears. *Quarterly Journal of Experimental Psychology*, 1967, *19*, 59–63.

Skinner, B. F. *Verbal behavior*. New York: Appleton-Century-Crofts, 1957.

Slorach, N., & Noehr, B. Dichotic listening in stuttering and dyslalic children. *Cortex*, 1973, *9*, 295–300.

Smith, A., & Burklund, C. W. Dominant hemispherectomy: Preliminary report on neuropsychological sequelae. *Science*, 1966, *153*, 1280–1282.

Smith, M. D. On the understanding of some relational words in aphasia. *Neuropsychologia*, 1974, *12*, 377–384.

Sommers, R., & Taylor, M. Cerebral speech dominance in language disordered and normal children. *Cortex*, 1972, *8*, 224–232.

Spellacy, F., & Peter, B. Dyscalculia and elements of the developmental Gerstmann syndrome in school children. *Cortex*, 1978, *14*, 197–206.

Spellacy, F. J., & Spreen, O. A short form of the Token Test. *Cortex*, 1969, *5*, 390–397.

Spreen, O., & Benton, A. L. *Neurosensory Center comprehensive examination for aphasia*. Victoria, B.C., Canada: Department of Psychology, University of Victoria, 1969. (Rev. ed., 1977.)

Spreen, O., & Wachal, R. P. Psycholinguistic analysis of aphasic language: Theoretical formulations and procedures. *Language and Speech*, 1973, *16*, 130–146.

Stark, R. An investigation of unilateral cerebral pathology with equated verbal and visual-spatial tasks. *Journal of Abnormal and Social Psychology*, 1961, *62*, 282–287.

Swiercinsky, D. *Manual for the adult neuropsychological evaluation*. Springfield, Ill.: Charles C Thomas, 1978.

Thomsen, I. V. Evaluation and outcome of aphasia in patients with severe closed head trauma. *Journal of Neurology, Neurosurgery and Psychiatry*, 1975, *38*, 713–718.

Thurstone, L. L. *Primary mental abilities*. Chicago: University of Chicago Press, 1938.

van Harskamp, F., & van Dongen, H. R. Construction and validation of different short forms of the Token Test. *Neuropsychologia,* 1977, *15,* 467–470.

von Stockert, T. R. Recognition of syntactic structure in aphasic patients. *Cortex,* 1972, *8,* 323–334.

Walton, D., & Black, D. A. The validity of a psychological test of brain damage. *British Journal of Medical Psychology,* 1957, *30,* 270–279.

Walton, D., White, J. G., Black, D. A., & Young, A. J. The modified word-learning test: A cross-validation study. *British Journal of Medical Psychology,* 1959, *32,* 213–220.

Warnock, J. K., & Mintz, S. I. Investigation of models of brain functioning through a factor analytic procedure of neuropsychological data. *Clinical Neuropsychology,* 1979, *1,* 43–48.

Weingartner, H., Caine, E. D., & Ebert, M. H. Imagery, encoding and retrieval of information from memory: Some specific encoding–retrieval changes in Huntington's disease. *Journal of Abnormal Psychology,* 1979, *88,* 52–58.

Weingartner, H., Cohen, R., Murphy, D. L., Martello, J., & Gerdt, C. Cognitive processes in depression. *Archives of General Psychiatry,* 1981, *38,* 42–47.

Weingartner, H., Gold, P., Ballenger, J. C., Smallberg, S. A., Summers, R., Rubinow, D. R., Post, R. M., & Goodwin, F. K. Effects of Vasopressin on human memory functions. *Science,* 1981, *211,* 601–603.

Weisenberg, T., & McBride, K. *Aphasia, a clinical and psychological study.* New York: Commonwealth Fund, 1935.

Wepman, J. M., *Auditory discrimination test.* Chicago: Language Research Associates, 1958.

Wepman, J. M., *Language modalities test for aphasia.* Chicago: Education Industry Service, 1961.

Wepman, J. M., & Jones, L. V. *Studies in aphasia: An approach to testing.* Chicago: University of Chicago Education–Industry Service. 1961.

Wepman, J. M., & Jones, L. V. Five aphasias: A commentary on aphasia as a regressive linguistic phenomenon. In Rioch, D., and Weinstein, E. (Eds.), *Disorders of communication.* Baltimore: Williams and Wilkins, 1964.

Wepman, J. M., Bock, R. D. Jones, L. V., & Van Pelt, D. Psycholinguistic study of aphasia: A revision of the concept of anomia. *Journal of Speech Disorders,* 1965, *21,* 468–477.

Wheeler, L., & Reitan, R. M. The presence and laterality of brain damage predicted from responses to a short aphasia screening test. *Perceptual and Motor Skills,* 1962, *15,* 783–799.

Wheeler, L., & Reitan, R. M. Discriminant functions applied to the problem of predicting cerebral damage from behavioral testing: A cross validation study. *Perceptual and Motor Skills,* 1963, *16,* 681–701.

Wilcox, M. J., Davis, G. A., & Leonard, L. B. Aphasics comprehension of contextually conveyed meaning. *Brain and Language,* 1978, *6,* 362–377.

Yates, A. The validity of some psychological tests of brain damage. *Psychological Bulletin,* 1954, *51,* 359–380.

Yorkston, K. M., Marshall, R. C., & Butler, M. R. Imposed delay of response effects on aphasic's auditory comprehension of visually and non-visually cued material. *Perceptual and Motor Skills,* 1977, *44,* 647–655.

Zaidel, E. Auditory vocabulary in the right hemisphere following brain bisection and hemidecortication. *Cortex,* 1976, *12,* 191–211.

Zaidel, E. Unilateral auditory language comprehension on the Token Test following cerebral commissurotomy and hemispherectomy. *Neuropsychologia,* 1977, *15,* 1–18.

Zangwill, O. L. Clinical tests of memory impairment. *Proceedings of the Royal Society of Medicine,* 1943, *36,* 576–580.

Zurif, E. B., Caramazza, A., & Myerson, R. Grammatical judgements of agrammatic aphasics. *Neuropsychologia,* 1972, *10,* 405–417.

5

The Use of Test Batteries in Clinical Neuropsychology

DAVID C. OSMON

INTRODUCTION AND OVERVIEW

For purposes of studying the development of test batteries in neuropsychology, it is instructive to look at the progression of two dimensions through four eras in the evolution of brain function evaluation methodologies. The first dimension concerns the use of standardized versus unstandardized methods of assessment; while the second dimension involves qualitative versus quantitative techniques of evaluation.

The four eras are represented by the neurological exam, the use of single psychometric tests, the use of empirically derived, atheoretical test batteries, and the use of theoretical test batteries. The development of the two dimensions through these four eras and the assessment techniques associated with each era provide a useful heuristic device with which to view the current state-of-the-art of neuropsychological assessment.

The neurological exam represents the combination of an unstandardized method of assessment combined with a powerful qualitative method of diagnosis. While the medical profession continues to use this methodology today, psychologists brought their own brand of techniques to bear, in the form of single psychometric instruments. This kind of standardized and quantitative method of assessing brain damage quickly was found to lack the power of the more qualitative neurological exam. The test battery approach grew out of the first attempt to

DAVID C. OSMON ● Department of Psychology, University of Wisconsin-Milwaukee, Milwaukee, Wisconsin 53201.

regain the power of previous methods while retaining the consistency of standardized, quantifiable psychometric techniques.

Finally, our understanding of brain function began to catch up with the practice of neuropsychology, and the power of qualitative analysis of brain function was combined with standardized and quantifiable techniques of assessment. This last and most current era of brain function evaluation methodologies is represented by theoretical test batteries. Unlike previous test batteries, a test item is included based upon its theoretical relationship with a specific brain area and the function associated with that area. All items are interrelated according to the assumptions of the theory of brain function used to construct the battery. However, before looking more closely at the four eras in the evaluation of brain function, it is important to review briefly two dimensions of neuropsychological assessment.

STANDARDIZED VERSUS UNSTANDARDIZED METHODS

For purposes of this chapter, the definition of standardized method is broadened beyond its traditional meaning. Three different issues are included under the term. The first is the issue of "uniformity of procedure" as defined by Anastasi in *Psychological Testing* (1954). The second issue concerns the establishment of comparison or reference norms, referred to as "standardization" of a test by Cronbach in *Essentials of Psychological Testing* (1949). The final aspect of standardized method refers to the use of a rigid versus a flexible battery of tests.

Uniform Procedure of Administration

Since testing in America first began around the start of the twentieth century, standard administration procedure has been recognized as a necessary part of psychometric assessment in this country. This approach has not been the only method of assessment practiced. What Cronbach (1949) calls "impressionistic testing" is often an unstandardized or nonuniform method of assessment. This type of testing is especially prevalent in evaluating complex behavior such as in the assessment of personality or brain function. Here a task may be administered in one of several different ways, depending upon the idiosyncratic conditions presented by the individual tested. This approach to testing emphasizes the necessity of interpreting test results in light of the unique characteristics of each person being examined.

An example of an unstandardized neuropsychological technique may involve a subject in which a spatial deficit is being evaluated. The task may be to determine whether the deficit is due to poor perception of the visual stimulus, to an inability to judge spatial relations such as slope and directionality of line, or to a difficulty in the spatial problem-solving strategy where the subject does not actively investigate the problem situation before deciding upon a plan of solution.

In an unstandardized examination using, for example, the WAIS Block Design subtest, the task could be administered in three different ways depending upon which aspect of spatial function was to be evaluated.

If misperception of the stimulus figure is suspected, then the administration may emphasize that the subject describe the stimulus pattern before actually setting about to execute the task. This procedure is followed in order to determine if visual agnosia (the inability to perceive properly a visual stimulus) is present. Likewise, a different emphasis of interpretation would be obtained with a patient suspected of faulty judgement of spatial relations. In this case, the subject's performance would be inspected for errors which indicate a poor ability to judge directionality or slope. For example, a subject may rotate or reverse the visual configuration, indicating poor spatial perception as opposed to visual agnosia as represented in the first example where the subject is unable to "see" the stimulus figure. In the last case, the object of the examination might be to investigate the subject's problem-solving strategy so that whether or not the right answer was obtained is of little consequence. Instead, the manner in which the subject solves the task is the objective of assessment.

In summary, the standardized method of assessment is seen predominantly as a way of reliably identifying whether or not a deficit exists, while the unstandardized method can, albeit in a less objective way, identify not only that a deficit exists but also the reason for the deficit. For now, standardized and nonstandardized techniques will be considered as independent and mutually exclusive assessment procedures. Later in the chapter, however, a type of technique that possibly combines the advantages of both a standardized and a nonstandardized method will be examined.

Reference Norms

One of the major purposes of creating a standardized test situation is for the purpose of developing comparison levels. Reference norms tell us how to interpret a patient's performance and are dependent upon creating a replicable measurement process in which the skills are measured in the same manner and under the same conditions with each subject. Therefore, reference norms are impossible to obtain with a nonstandardized instrument. Instead, pathognomonic signs must be assessed by nonstandardized techniques.

A pathognomonic sign is a type of performance that by its very presence indicates the existence of the condition being tested for. The example of the visual agnosia used above is a pathognomonic sign. Brain damage is immediately indicated by the presence of visual agnosia because a non-brain-damaged person would not evidence this deficit.

In the case where pathognomonic signs are not present, the usual way of determining whether the performance is indicative of a brain dysfunction is by comparing the level of performance attained with the appropriate reference sample. This method, however, cannot be utilized efficaciously without a reliable, standardized instrument for which reference norms can be established.

Rigid versus Flexible Battery

While most neuropsychologists use a battery of tests rather than a single instrument, there are two basic schools of thought as to how to use the battery of tests. The flexible battery approach is predicated upon the notion that the complexity of brain function makes every patient a unique assessment challenge. This challenge necessitates a step-by-step process where the findings of the preceding step provide information that is used to decide how the assessment should progress.

Again using the spatial deficit example, a flexible battery approach might start with a general test of spatial skills such as the WAIS Block Design subtest. The performance on this task would then tell the examiner how to proceed. Say, for example, that the subject looked confused throughout the entire task and was unable to complete even the simplest design. In this case, the examiner might decide that visual agnosia may be present, and tests designed specifically to assess for this deficit would then be administered.

This example is exaggerated and perhaps oversimplified, but one which, nevertheless, illustrates the logic of a flexible battery approach in the evaluation of brain function. A neuropsychological examination is seen as a complex process whereby adequate testing depends upon decisions that are made during the assessment process. How, then, can a rigid battery of tests provide useful information?

Instead of deciding what functions to evaluate based upon the subject's performance, an examination that evaluates many major aspects of brain function can be put together. Using this battery, many neuropsychological functions are evaluated, and no decision-making process during the examination is necessary. In a flexible battery approach, however, where the examiner decides what tests to give based upon what deficits emerge during the examination, not all of the major neurological functions are evaluated and some deficits may go unnoticed.

The disadvantage of some rigid batteries lies in their poor ability to account for the reasons for the manifest deficits. For example, is a spatial deficit due to an inability to perceive a visual stimulus, to poor spatial relations judgement, or to defective problem-solving skills? In a situation such as is the case with the flexible battery approach, hypotheses about why a deficit occurred are made and tested during the examination. This procedure adds power to the assessment, which is more difficut to attain with a rigid battery approach where task performance is quantitatively evaluated without regard for the qualitative aspects of performance.

Because there are advantages to both approaches, most neuropsychologists utilize a combination of the rigid and the flexible battery approach. The rigid battery gives the examiner the assurance that most brain functions are evaluated.

Therefore, most examiners administer a comprehensive set of tests from which performance can be evaluated. This initial testing provides information that may point out areas that the examiner may then wish to evaluate further. Additional testing can focus more specifically upon a few identified deficits, and qualitative evaluation of the reason for the deficit can be obtained.

QUALITATIVE VERSUS QUANTITATIVE EVALUATION

Qualitative and quantitative types of evaluation refer not to the kinds of tests used (e.g., standardized or rigid battery), rather to the way in which the abilities are assessed. A quantitative method stresses measuring each skill in a manner that allows quantification of the level of skill attainment. The objective of a quantitative measurement is to determine if a task can be correctly completed, and if so, then to what extent. For example, time to finish the task, number of trials necessary before correct performance is attained, and frequency of correct responses are all examples of objective, quantified measurement.

A qualitative evaluation, however, is directed at determining why a particular skill is deficient. This type of evaluation assumes that each skill tested is composed of several underlying, basic brain functions. These basic functions combine to make up all complex psychological abilities. Conducting an assessment of this type, then, becomes a process of evaluating how a task is completed or solved in order to determine which underlying functions are disrupted. Again referring to the test of spatial ability, there could be three basic skills to be evaluated: visual perception of the stimulus, spatial analysis, and spatial problem solving. If a deficit were present, then a qualitative examination would try to assess which of these three basic functions were contributing to the deficient performance.

By contrast, a quantitative assessment would simply identify the deficit by scoring the accuracy of the response, the speed of the response, the frequency of correct responses, or some other objective measurement of performance. No attempt would be made to assess why the deficit occurred because the underlying functions cannot be readily quantified in isolation of each other. Brain-damaged performance on a given task, then, is determined by whether or not the score is above or below some specified cut-off level. The cut-off score is derived by finding the optimal separation between a known brain-damaged group and a known non-brain-damaged group (see "Reference Norms" earlier in this chapter).

Traditionally, the quantitative method (e.g., Halstead–Reitan test battery) relies strictly upon tested empirical relationships that demonstrate the level of performance associated with a brain-injured population. Such a method is atheoretical in concept and lacks an appreciation of how the brain combines its basic functions, such as visual perception, sense of directionality, and nonverbal reasoning, into complex abilities such as the Block Design task. However, the qualitative assessment technique (e.g., Christensen's adaptation of Luria's techniques; Christensen, 1975) is often based upon a theory of brain function that delineates the basic brain functions that combine to make up the complex neuropsychological abilities that are tested.

While it may be unfashionable to speak of a theoretical construct that underlies some observable event, students of the qualitative school of assessment speak of the necessity of such an approach in neuropsychology, where the same test deficit can occur for widely different reasons. For example, a reading deficit can occur as a result of a posterior left parietal lesion that disrupts the ability to understand complex logical–grammatical relationships. A lesion in the occipital–parietal area can occur that interferes with visual perception so that a reading deficit results because the subject cannot maintain his place from line to line in the text or is unable visually to decode the letters. A left temporal lobe lesion may also interfere with reading ability because the discrimination of phonemes is disrupted. This deficit results in an inability to read correctly words that contain similar sounds.

Other lesions can also adversely affect such a complex ability as reading but, again, causing the deficit for widely disparate reasons. The understanding of the basis for a single neuropsychological deficit is, then, very important in deciding upon lesion location and the appropriate rehabilitation techniques. If the reading deficit occurs after an occipital–parietal lesion, the basis for the deficit (visual perception) and the remediation of that deficit are vastly different than if the reading problem occurs subsequent to a temporal lobe lesion.

Quantitative approaches have been devised to minimize the need for unstandardized administration procedures. Such nonuniform procedures are common in qualitative techniques that are designed to arrive at the basic brain function underlying a neuropsychological deficit. New techniques (e.g., the Luria–Nebraska test battery) seek to combine a quantitative measure of performance with a qualitative interpretation of the results. This is accomplished by determining basic brain functions so that each may be assessed independently from one another. Rather than testing reading ability, for example, each of the basic functions underlying the skill is isolated and assessed individually. This process is not completely successful because basic functions such as speech sound perception cannot be assessed completely independent of all other functions. However, with knowledge of the way in which the brain puts together a complex ability such as reading, neuropsychological deficits can be analyzed in a more comprehensive and systematic fashion.

The advantages of both a quantitative and a qualitative method of assessment are combined in such a technique. The quantitative aspects of the method allow reference norms to be established that are used to identify brain-damaged performance. The qualitative nature of the approach, however, allows more detailed analysis of the deficits to determine the basic brain functions and hence the area(s) of the brain that are disrupted (see "Theoretical Test Batteries" later in this chapter).

FOUR ERAS IN THE EVALUATION OF BRAIN FUNCTION

Having delineated two important dimensions of techniques that measure brain function (quantitative versus qualitative evaluation and standardized versus nonstandardized tests), the development of test batteries in neuropsychology can be better examined. Methodologies for the evaluation of brain function can be seen as passing through four generations that can be characterized by: neurological exam; single psychometric tests; empirical test batteries; and theoretical test batteries. Within this "bare-bones" outline are the progressions of the two dimensions of brain function evaluation that are reviewed above and that eventually lead to the creation of a test battery. This historical overview is not meant to be an exhaustive survey of neuropsychological assessment techniques. Rather, its purpose is as a heuristic device to be used as a guide to the important issues in examining brain function. The reader is urged to study the progression of the two dimensions and their eventual merger in the last phase.

Neurological Exam

The neurological exam is essentially a "physical examination" of the central nervous system. Just as the physician pokes, probes, looks, listens, and otherwise examines the external manifestations of the body's workings, so does the neurologist examine the manifest functions of the brain. An exhaustive treatment of the neurologic exam is beyond the scope of this chapter; however, a general overview is provided so that a basic understanding of the exam can be gleaned and its relationship to the development of neuropsychological test batteries can be demonstrated.

The complete neurological exam is divided into six different sections (after Chusid, 1976). The first part is a mental examination and is analogous to a psychiatric mental status exam. General appearance, mood, level of awareness, and cognitive functions are evaluated. The neurologist clinically and qualitatively assesses for unconventional modes of deportment and unusual affect or alertness that could be indicative of organic deterioration. Extensive aspects of intellectual functioning are examined, although there are no uniform procedures to follow, and the content and exact form of the exam vary widely from physician to physician.

Coordination, gait, and equilibrium; sensation; reflexes; and the motor system are the next four sections of the neurological exam. These sections are designed to evaluate many functions, most of which relate to the motor–sensory system. This evaluation is largely directed at centrally controlled functions, although peripheral functions are also examined. Performance in this part of the exam is again evaluated in a rather unstandardized, intuitive manner consistent with the notion that a flexible method of evaluation is necessary to evaluate adequately such a complex, multifaceted system as the brain. The neurologist uses his knowledge of how the brain controls movement to interpret the specific deficits of performance that the patient exhibits. For example, a patient presents with deficits on each of the six different sections of the neurological examination. Mental status reveals slowness and inaccuracy in naming objects and slight difficulty in delayed recall, while reading and arithmetic abilities remain intact. Motor and sensory dysfunction is seen on the right body side with the lower extremity more severely affected than the upper extremity. Simple and complex sensory disturbances are noted, including inability to locate tactile stimulation, increased reflexes, a Babinski response, misperception of simultaneous stimulation, and misidentification of numbers and letters drawn on the skin. Paresis of the right side is present with the leg more noticeably impaired than the arm. Also noted is a slight right central facial weakness.

From this profile of deficits and strengths, the neurologist makes a diagnosis by hypothesizing from his knowledge of brain function a brain lesion that will account for this pattern of performance. The unilateral motor and sensory deficits indicate a unilateral brain lesion. Further, the left motor/sensory strip is indicated by the arm and leg paresis and the simple sensory deficits (increased reflexes, etc.) A more anterior parietal lobe lesion is indicated by the naming deficit in the absence of calculation and reading difficulties on the mental status portion of the exam. Furthermore, the more impaired dysfunction of the leg when compared to the arm and face tells the neurologist that more damage occurs higher on the parietal lobe because this is where the leg is represented on the cortical surface.

The cranial nerve examination, the sixth and final section of the neurological examination, is an exhaustive evaluation of the 12 cranial nerves. This portion of the exam acts as a thorough evaluation of the subcortical structures of the brain and is represented in the above example in the facial weakness.

It can be seen from this brief description of the neurological exam that brain function is evaluated in an unstandardized and qualitative manner. There are no strict norms by which to interpret much of the performance on the exam. For example, general mood and appearance, and even the cognitive portions of the exam, are not interpreted in light of standardized scores. Rather, the neurologist makes an intuitive evaluation of the performance that is based upon his/her years of experience with brain-damaged patients.

Other parts of the exam, for example, the Babinski reflex, are qualitatively assessed and are conducted according to whether the patient manifests a pathognomonic sign. On testing the Babinski reflex, the examiner looks for a performance that by its very nature indicates brain damage (a pathognomonic sign). If a Babinski response is present—that is, if the toes are upward going when the sole of the foot is stroked—then brain damage is highly likely. Knee-jerk and other deep tendon reflexes are evaluated according to a three point rating scale that on the surface looks like a quantitative scoring method. A rating of one indicates diminished reflexive reaction while a rating of three suggests hyperactive reflexes, with a two rating being normal reflexive action. While a rating assigns a quantitative score, the method of assigning that score is qualitative. The assignment is not objective in the sense that an answer on a multiple choice question is objective (either right or wrong). This rating is given by the neurologist based upon a subjective opinion on whether or not the reflex is normal. Everyone differs on the intensity of reflexive action so that an objective quantitative scoring is impractical if not impossible. Thus, the neurologist must judge whether or not for this particular person the reflex is normal.

Since there are no reference norms on which to interpret performance, the exam is based upon a theory of brain function that allows interpretation of the results of the neurological exam. In the example above, the results of the exam indicate the localization of a brain lesion because it is known that certain performances correspond to lesions in certain areas of the brain. For example, the motor/sensory strip is known to control motor and sensory output in a point-by-point fashion. That is, a certain point of the cortical surface represents a certain point of the body surface. Thus, when the leg is more impaired than the arm in motor and sensory functions, then it is known that the area that controls function for the leg is more damaged than the area for the arm. The theory that explains the deficits and successfully predicts the location of a brain lesion based upon an analysis of the manifest performance on the neurological exam is then necessary where unstandardized and qualitative techniques are used.

Single Tests

Rather than begin from a theory of brain function and develop assessment techniques out of this theory, those who utilized single tests to evaluate brain-damaged patients did so from an empirical basis. That is, the "unitary construct" of organicity prevailed (Reitan & Davison, 1974) and a theory of brain function was therefore necessary. It was assumed that all forms of brain damage are alike and lead to the same kinds of performance problems. Therefore, it was thought possible to develop a single test in which all forms of brain damage could be identified. The only requirements were to find a technique that reliably differentiated a brain-damaged group from a non-brain-damaged group.

The single test approach utilized standardized and quantitative methods of assessment in developing a test for organicity. This approach grew out of the American psychometric tradition and is best represented by the use of tests like the Bender–Gestalt and Memory-for-Designs. Utilizing these tests in a standardized and quantitative manner is a method that is diametrically opposed to the manner of evaluation seen in the last section on the neurological exam. Both tests involve drawing various types of geometric figures. The Bender–Gestalt requires copying the figures from visual stimuli while the Memory-for-Designs test requires drawing from memory (Bender, 1938; Graham & Kendall, 1960).

In utilizing single tests, this approach often makes use of drawing techniques because these tasks are among the most complex to execute for the brain-damaged subject. The task is complex in the sense that widely different areas of the brain are involved in its execution. For example, in drawing a geometric figure such as is required in the Memory-for-Designs test, both the right and left hemisphere play a significant role in the successful completion of the task. The task requires the left hemisphere to control motor execution (for right-handed subjects) of the drawing. Conversely, the spatial analysis and synthesis is executed largely in the right hemisphere.

Because both hemispheres are significantly utilized in the task, most brain lesions adversely affect the execution of the test. In fact, hit rates as high as 90% have been reported in some populations (Golden, 1978). Such hit rates are misleading, however, because the detection of a brain-damaged subject relies heavily upon the occurrence of either a motor or spatial deficit. Brain-injured subjects who show no motor or spatial problems would not necessarily be detected by these instruments, especially where the results are not qualitatively interpreted. Even in those subjects where deficits are detected, little more than the information that the person is brain damaged is learned. The localization of the damage or the extent and exact nature of the neuropsychological dysfunction remains unknown.

Nevertheless, some deficiencies of the neurological exam approach to evaluating brain dysfunction are partially addressed by the single test method. The lack of uniform procedure with which to reliably assess the subject's performance for brain-damaged signs is corrected for by the standardized techniques lent by the traditional psychometric approach. In gaining quantitative measures of performance, the actual level of skill attainment can be gleaned. This information is necessary to determine if the subject's performance is characteristic of brain dysfunction. In the neurological exam, this distinction is made strictly on a qualitative basis taken from the theory of brain function that underlies the exam. The criticism of qualitative interpretation is the uncertainty in the process afforded by the examiner's clinical skill. With the standardized administration and the quantitative scoring of the psychometric approach, this uncertainty is largely eliminated. Empirical investigation establishes the performance level that is characteristic of brain dysfunction, and clinical skills are not necessary to interpret whether or not a deficit in performance exists.

Despite correcting some of the deficits of the neurological exam, the single test approach loses much of the diagnostic power that is inherent in the neurological exam. In those cases where empirical interpretation fails because the brain-damaged subject does not perform in the brain-damaged range of performance, a more qualitative interpretation of the test performance may be of use. In fact, those who use the Bender–Gestalt often resort to such methods to increase the accuracy of the test. For example, qualitatively recognizable pathognomonic signs such as unilateral spatial inattention and differentiation of "frontal" construction dyspraxia from "parietal" construction dyspraxia (Benton, 1968) can be used to detect subtle brain dysfunction that is missed by the global statistical/empirical techniques that characterize the single test method.

The use of qualitative methods of interpretation require a theoretical understanding of how the brain works and how complex psychological functions are derived by the brain. Ideally, the tests used to detect brain dysfunction would be constructed from this theoretical basis so that qualitative interpretation as well as quantitative measurement would follow logically from the test format. More will be said about this notion at the end of the next section.

As the understanding of the brain and its workings began to grow, neuropsychologists recognized that psychological functions were far too complex to be adequately evaluated by a single test. It became apparent that single instruments could not identify all forms of neuropsychological deficit. To do so, it was necessary to develop an evaluation that surveyed an entire range of neuropsychological abilities. Hence, the test battery approach to neuropsychological diagnosis was born.

Empirically Derived Test Batteries

The development of a single comprehensive battery of tests to evaluate brain function began with the realization that brain function is too complex to evaluate with a single test. Batteries were developed for specific purposes. For example, the Columbia–Greystone battery was developed for the specific purpose of evaluating the effects of psychosurgery (Landis, 1952). Specific areas of the brain were singled out and batteries were developed to assess their functions independently (e.g., Halstead, 1947, and Benton, 1968, developed frontal lobe batteries). With the proliferation of specific-purpose batteries, it was not long before the field of neuropsychology produced comprehensive general-purpose batteries.

Arthur Benton has long been a leading pillar in the edifice that is empirical neuropsychology. While he does not advocate any one particular rigid battery, he regularly uses a core set of tests, many of his own devising, that survey all manner of apraxic, agnostic, and aphasic symptoms. Table 1 shows the extensive list of some instruments utilized in the Benton battery.

Perhaps more than any other, Benton's approach characterizes the empirically derived test battery. Each test is standardized with quantifiable scoring procedures and represents an instrument that by itself is highly accurate in identifying brain-damaged subjects.

Aaron Smith also advocates an empirical test battery approach. Smith (1975) utilizes the Wechsler IQ test, the Visual Organization test, the Raven's Progressive Matrices test, Form A and C of the Benton Visual Retention test, the Purdue

Table 1
Representative Sample of Tests in Benton's Flexible Battery

Orientation and Memory	Language
Wechsler Memory Scale	Neurosensory Center Comprehensive Examination for
Orientation—Temporal, Person,	Aphasia
Place	Boston Diagnostic Aphasia Test
Recall of Recent Presidents	Multilingual Aphasia Examination
Line Cancellation Test	
Reaction Time	
Trail Making Test	
Perceptual Functions	
	General Intelligence and Achievement
Right–Left Discriminations	
Finger Localization	Shipley–Hartford Scale
Dichotic Listening for Words	WAIS
Facial Recognition Test	WRAT
Color Perception	Digit Sequence Learning
Benton Visual Retention Test	Verbal Paired Associate Learning Test
Pantomime Recognition	

Pegboard, the Symbol Digits Modalities test, the PPVT, and several other unpublished tests of verbal, memory, and sensory functions. Used as a rigid battery, a fairly comprehensive yet portable and short examination can be completed.

Lezak (1976) presents her own set of tests, which also may be characterized as an empirically derived battery. Included are the WAIS (excepting the Vocabulary and Digit Symbol subtests), the Symbol Digits Modality test, the Rey-Auditory-Verbal Learning test, the Subtracting Serial Sevens test, Draw-a-Bicycle, administrations A and D of the Benton Visual Retention test, the Purdue Pegboard, the Trail Making test, the Rorschach, and the Bender–Gestalt test. On the whole, this collection of measures represent standardized and quantitative techniques. Lezak (1976) does not, however, advocate that a rigid battery of tests be routinely administered.

The Montreal Neurological Institute Battery devised by Milner, Taylor, and associates (see Kolb & Whishaw, 1980) is also an empirically derived battery. Its 27 measures taken from various and separate tests represent a carefully selected battery that can evaluate 10 different neuropsychological functions. The 10 functions include: determining the lateralization of speech, intelligence, visual perception, memory, spatial perception, somatosensory function, language, hippocampal function, frontal lobe function, and motor function. Theoretical underpinnings are perhaps the most evident in this empirical battery; however, the individual components of the battery are not theoretically related by design. Each test was constructed separately so that the battery does not yet represent a unified theoretical structure. Instead, the battery is a collection of single techniques, each measuring some discrete neuropsychological function.

The above-mentioned techniques are all part of the empirically derived battery approach that characterizes the first generation of neuropsychological assessment batteries. The Halstead–Reitan battery (Reitan, 1955, 1959, 1964, 1966) is the prototype of the first generation of techniques and is currently the most widely acclaimed instrument of neuropsychological assessment. The Halstead–Reitan possesses the broadest research base and, as a rigid battery, is the most tangible subject for discussing the empirically derived batteries.

Halstead–Reitan Battery

As an empirical test battery, the Halstead–Reitan represents an outgrowth of the single test approach. The battery consists of nine standardized and quantitative subtests: Category, Rhythm, Speech Sounds Perception, Finger-tapping, Tactual Performance test, Trail Making test (A & B), Sensory–Perceptual Examination, and Aphasia Exam. Despite the lack of a unifying theoretical structure underlying the test battery as a whole, each of the individual subtests is theoretically related to certain brain functions. These relationships will be discussed for each of the subtests. For a more complete description of the apparatus and the administration and scoring procedures, refer either to Golden, Osmon, Moses and Berg (1981) or the test manual published privately by Reitan (1959).

The Category Test. This procedure is designed to test concept formation and, as such, represents the best instrument in the battery for evaluating frontal lobe function (Golden, 1978). The subject is presented with a visual stimulus with four alternatives and must select the appropriate alternative according to some abstract principle that underlies the group of items. There are seven groups of items, and the subject must determine the underlying principle in each of the seven groups. Thus, the task requires the ability to generate hypotheses (i.e., form concepts), validate these hypotheses against experience, and change flexibly from one hypothesis to another when the available evidence conflicts with the currently held hypothesis.

In addition to concept formation, other abilities play a prominent role in the successful completion of the task. For example, many of the visual stimuli are complex geometric configurations and thus require well developed perceptual and spatial reasoning skills. The last group of items on the test are a compilation of items that are governed by the principles underlying the previous six groups of items and, therefore, require adequate memory skills. Attention, concentration, and simple counting skills are also a necessary component of the test.

The Rhythm Test. This test is basically a measure of nonverbal auditory perception. The subject hears two rhythms, each composed of five to seven beats, and must decide whether the two are the same or different. This task is particularly sensitive to right temporal lobe lesions; however, it is often poorly performed by subjects with left temporal lobe lesions. The test is also generally sensitive to brain damage, for by its nature the task requires good attention and concentration (Reitan, 1959).

The Speech–Sounds Perception Test. This test is the verbal counterpart to the Rhythm test. This task requires the subject to discriminate single- and double-letter sounds by matching a visual representation to the sound heard on a tape recorder. The test is particularly sensitive to left temporal lobe disorder where phonemic discrimination takes place (Luria, 1966). Golden *et al.* (1981) note that right hemisphere lesions, particularly in the temporal lobe, may also yield deficits on this test.

The Finger-Tapping Test. The tapping test is a measure of simple motor speed derived from the subject's performance on the finger oscillation machine (Reitan, 1959). Cortical deficit on this measure represents dysfunction of the motor/sensory strip, although brain-damaged performance can be associated with other lesions. Subcortical dysfunction as well as middle to anterior parietal lobe lesions may also result in deficient tapping scores.

The Tactual Performance Test (TPT). The TPT examines the subject's ability, while blindfolded, to place variously shaped wooden blocks into their appropriate holes on a modified Sequin–Goddard form board. This task represents a complex neuropsychological ability that involves various brain functions. Spatial and tactual perceptual abilities are the prominent components of the task. As such, dysfunction on this test oftentimes represents parietal lobe damage. Frontal lobe damage may also result in a poor TPT performance because the subject is unable to generate an appropriate problem-solving strategy. Qualitative evaluation of the subject's TPT performance is necessary to differentiate between an anterior lesion and a posterior lesion.

The Trail Making Test. Two parts are included. In both parts the task consists of connecting circles according to a principle. In Part A the circles are numbered from 1 to 25 and the task is a measure of visual-scanning, motor, and sequencing skills. Part B, however, is more complex and involves alternately connecting numbers and letters in their proper order. The addition of a second principle makes the task a measure of cognitive flexibility and the ability to direct behavior according to a complex verbal plan. Part A is generally considered most representative of right hemisphere function, while Part B represents left hemisphere function. Neither test has precise localizing value, although Part B does reflect left frontal lobe involvement under some circumstances. When a large difference exists between Parts A and B, with Part B being severely impaired (over 275–300 seconds), left frontal lobe involvement may be present if other indicators such as poor Category Test performance also occur.

The Sensory–Perceptual Examination. This compilation of tasks resembles those used by a neurologist in the neurological exam. The tasks involve basic sensory function of both sides of the body in the tactile, auditory, and visual modalities. More complex tactile functions are also tested, including finger gnosis, stereognosis, and tactile form recognition. The examination is intended to identify lateralized dysfunction of basic and complex perceptual functions. The test often provides precise localizing information to identify posterior cortical lesions. The test is also sensitive to subcortical and peripheral injuries.

The Aphasia Exam. Designed as a screening test of all major forms of speech and language deficits, this test includes items to examine for the inability to: name objects (dysnomia); read (dyslexia); write (dysgraphia); recognize numbers and letters (visual letter and number dysgnosia); calculate (dyscalculia); spell (spelling dyspraxia); and discriminate right and left without confusion (right–left confusion). In addition to left hemisphere speech and language deficits, this exam also tests for various right hemisphere difficulties. Drawing tasks are used to evaluate for spatial deficits that show up as construction dyspraxia. Unilateral spatial neglect or inattention also shows up quite clearly on the drawing tasks.

In addition to these 9 subtests, the Halstead–Reitan Neuropsychological Test Battery also includes the Weschler Adult Intelligence Scale (WAIS), the Wide Range Achievement Test (WRAT), and the Minnesota Multiphasic Personality Inventory (MMPI). Two other tests in the original battery (Time Sense Test and Critical Flicker Frequency Test) are generally disregarded in current forms of the battery. The WAIS plays a significant role in the diagnosis of brain damage with the test battery and often has considerable localizing value. The MMPI and WRAT are useful in determining the patient's psychiatric status and premorbid level of functioning.

Advantages and Disadvantages of an Empirical Battery

As an outgrowth of the single test approach, the Halstead–Reitan battery is a quantitative and standardized instrument. A few measures of neuropsychological function (repeatedly represented in the 9 Halstead–Reitan subtests plus the WAIS subtests) are sampled by means of a uniform procedure of administration. These subtests also yield quantitative measures of performance for which reference norms are available to determine the level of performance.

These few neuropsychological measures represent a relatively comprehensive evaluation of brain function. Benton (1975) identifies several major neuropsychological functions to be evaluated: attention, concentration, speed of response, orientation, memory, perceptual functions, perceptual–motor functions, flexibility, language, reasoning, and general intelligence. While the Halstead–Reitan does not have a systematic theory of brain function underlying its construction, it nevertheless appears to evaluate most if not all of these neuropsychological abilities. Attention, concentration, and orientation are repeatedly evaluated by the numerous tests, such as the Rhythm and Speech-Sounds Perception tests, that require focused as well as sustained performance. The speed of response is well tested on the Rhythm and Speech–Sounds tests, where a continuous flow of stimuli bring to light any inability to orient and respond in a paced and expeditious manner.

The Halstead–Reitan lacks a systematic investigation of memory functions, although various types of verbal and nonverbal memory are assessed at various points during the examination. The Digit Span WAIS subtest, the Rhythm test, and the Speech–Sounds test assess immediate auditory memory, verbal and nonverbal. Recent visual memory assessment occurs on the last subtest of the Category test. Incidental tactual perceptual memory is evaluated on the Tactual Performance test. The interference effects of interpolated activities between presentation and recall are not evaluated.

The sensory and motor tasks on the Sensory–Perceptual Exam and Finger-Tapping Test evaluate perceptual and perceptual–motor functions. The TPT tests higher order perceptual–motor functions. Language is evaluated predominantly from the WAIS and the Aphasia Exam.

The Category Test, in addition to several other functions, also provides a measure of higher cognitive abilities. Flexibility is tested by the manner in which the subject is able to discard old hypotheses and generate new ones in the face of the available evidence. Reasoning and general intelligence are also a large part of this process. The results of the Category test, in combination with some subtests of the WAIS and the overall IQ scores, provide a means of evaluating these different functions.

Such a test battery marks an advance over the single test approach in that more neuropsychological abilities are tested. If the main purposes of the battery are neuropsychological assessment and the delineation of the cognitive and personality deficits that arise from brain damage, then the more neuropsychological functions that are evaluated, the better. The empirical battery is made up of various tests that have demonstrated relationships to brain damage and appear conceptually related to various neuropsychological functions. These functions represent different areas of the brain so that making a topographical diagnosis of brain damage is possible. By comparing various tests, the localization of the brain damage is inferred. Taking a simple comparison, tactile perceptual functions on the Sensory–Perceptual test are deficient in the absence of deficits on the Finger-tapping test. Such a test comparison reveals the likelihood that a posterior lesion (behind the central sulcus) exists, since tactile perceptual deficits are associated with parietal lobe injury and the absence of motor speed loss indicates that the motor areas of the posterior frontal lobe are intact.

Utilizing the Halstead–Reitan battery in the manner described above goes somewhat beyond the empirical battery approach. Research has demonstrated some empirical rules to utilize in interpreting the neuropsychological profile. These few rules, however, fall far short of accomplishing the task faced by most clinical neuropsychologists. Making a topographical diagnosis of brain damage from the Halstead–Reitan battery in the manner demonstrated above requires the utilization of a theory of brain function with which to interpret performance on the various tests.

The tests included in the Halstead–Reitan battery are not systematically related to one another, however, because no unifying theory of brain function guided the construction of the battery. Consequently, conceptual gaps plague the neuropsychologist when attempting to understand the relationships between various tests on the battery. If the Rhythm test represents the right temporal lobe, and the Speech–Sounds Perception test corresponds to the left temporal lobe, why does this patient show deficits on both tests when he is known to have a left temporal lobe lesion? This disadvantage argues for a second-generation test battery (see "Theoretical Test Batteries" in this chapter), where deficits are systematically related to one another because the battery has a unified theoretical structure.

Another significant disadvantage of the empirical battery is the amount of time and cost of such an extensive examination. The Halstead–Reitan may require up to 8 hours or more of testing time. If the patient is severely impaired, the entire battery may take several sessions and well over 8 hours. Since a brain-damaged population often fatigues easily, this is a severe drawback leading to inadequate measurement and appraisal of the person's strengths and weaknesses.

One way out of this dilemma is the flexible battery approach. The Halstead–Reitan is designed to be a rigid battery (see "Rigid versus Flexible Battery" earlier in this chapter). However, in an effort to save time, many clinicians administer only those portions of the battery that seem pertinent. Based upon the referral question and the patient's presentation, tests are selected that will adapt the battery to the unique assessment situation of the individual patient. Obviously, the skills of the clinician determine in large measure the success of the assessment procedure using this type of approach. Independent of the clinician's skill, however, there is the added disadvantage that some deficits will be missed altogether. In not administering the entire battery, certain neuropsychological functions are not evaluated and some effects of the lesion may go unnoticed.

Consistent with the information presented in the first section of this chapter, it is believed that a specified set of tests or a rigid battery provides the best base for a neuropsychological evaluation. The advantage of a systematically constructed test battery derived from a unified theory of brain function was also recognized. This was the historical sequence that led to the second generation of neuropsychological test batteries, the theoretical test batteries.

Theoretical Test Batteries

The development of a test battery that is constructed according to a theory of brain function was the next logical step in the evolution of brain function evaluation. The empirically derived test battery approach added many tests so that a comprehensive neuropsychological evaluation could be obtained. It still did not, however, explain the relationships between the various measures of brain function. Research demonstrated that relationships existed but did not say why. For example, the relationship between Trail Making Part A and Part B often indicated lateralized brain dysfunction. When Part B was poorly performed relative to Part A, then the left hemisphere was more impaired than the right hemisphere. Why this relationship existed was explained by a theory of brain function that hypothesizes that verbal functions are associated with the left hemisphere, and the Trails B test requires more complex verbal skills with the addition of the second set of symbols (alphabet) to be sequenced in alternation with the first set of symbols (numbers).

Qualitative analysis of the deficits is often necessary to understand otherwise conflicting relationships between the various tests. For example, it is not uncommon on the Halstead–Reitan to find one test relationship that indicates left hemisphere dysfunction and another relationship that suggests right hemisphere dysfunction for the same patient. One common example of such a contradiction is Trails B more poorly performed than Trails A (left hemisphere indicator), while the WAIS Performance IQ is lower than the WAIS verbal IQ (right hemisphere indicator). It is not until qualitative analysis reveals, however, that the Trails B performance deficit results from cognitive inflexibility and the PIQ deficit reflects disruption of immediate adaptive abilities that the apparent paradox is understood.

By qualitatively analyzing the Trails B deficit, it becomes clear that cognitive inflexibility is the aspect of the task that is deficient, not the more complex verbal skills also required to complete the test. Therefore, the empirical relationship linking the test with the left hemisphere function is somewhat misleading. In fact, the present deficit on Trails B reflects left prefrontal lobe damage. Likewise, the PIQ–VIQ differential does not reflect the verbal–spatial difference that makes PIQ deficits more often indicative of right hemisphere damage. Qualitative analysis instead reveals that left prefrontal damage is responsible for loss of immediate adaptive abilities, which are better represented on the performance scales.

Qualitative analysis with the Halstead–Reitan is a difficult process that necessitates taking several steps away from the data in order to postulate what underlies the manifest test relationships. The test battery is not designed for qualitative analysis of test performance because the combination of tasks was based upon which tests demonstrated the strongest empirical relationships to a general brain-damaged population.

In order to design a theoretical test battery that is amenable to qualitative analysis, a different approach to determining which tasks to include is necessary. Rather than including only those tests that individually identify a general brain-damaged sample with a high level of accuracy, tasks that discriminate only a certain type of brain dysfunction with a high level of accuracy are included. Each task, then, is designed to detect only a certain type of brain-related deficit rather than detecting all types of brain dysfunction.

For example, the Halstead–Reitan includes a single general test for motor functions, the tapping test. This test evaluates overall motor skill and does so in such a way as to maximize discrimination of brain-damaged from non-brain-damaged subjects. However, the theoretical test battery (e.g., Luria–Nebraska) includes several different types of motor ability tasks. Each task is included not because it maximally discriminates brain-damaged from non-brain-damaged subjects, but because it tests for one specific theoretical component of motor function. The theoretical battery attempts to assess independently the various motor components involved in such diverse motor tasks as the Halstead–Reitan tapping test, TPT, Aphasia Examination drawing items, and Aphasia Examination motor reproduction items. The theoretical battery includes separate measures of the various motor tasks including, for example, simple motor movement, optic–spatial motor reproduction, lateral coordination, oral movement, speech-regulation of movement, kinesthetically based movement, and the selectivity of motor function. Each of these functions is an important theoretical component of motor ability and should be assessed individually.

The theoretical test battery also differs in the sampling procedure of various brain functions. Rather than repeatedly sampling a relatively few number of brain functions, such as occurs on the Halstead–Reitan battery, a small sampling of numerous different abilities is made. For example, where the Halstead–Reitan has 30 items to test pitch and rhythm skills (Rhythm subtest), the Luria–Nebraska has 12 (Rhythm scale). Furthermore, the only difference between the 30 Halstead–Reitan items is the graded level of difficulty. The Luria–Nebraska sampling of pitch and rhythm skills, however, evaluates four different aspects of the function. The ability is broken down into its component parts according to the way in which the brain theoretically carries out the function (see the *"Rhythmic Function"* later in this chapter).

In order to design a quantitative technique allowing qualitative analysis, it is necessary to break down each neuropsychological function into its component parts. For pitch and rhythm skills, the four parts that Luria (1966) delineated included: perception of pitch relationships; reproduction of pitch relationships; perception of acoustic signals; and motor performance of acoustic signals. By evaluating each of these aspects of the function, it becomes clear why the ability is disrupted.

For example, according to Luria's theory of brain function, four different areas of the brain can be disrupted, causing a rhythm deficit. Damage to the primary and secondary areas of either temporal lobe can result in an auditory perceptual deficit that will cause poor performance on the perception of pitch relationships and perhaps the perception of acoustic signals tasks. Motor and sensory strip dysfunction may cause deficits on the reproduction of pitch relationships and the motor performance of acoustic signals tasks. Finally, damage to the premotor areas of the dominant hemisphere may result in deficits on those tasks included in the motor performance of acoustic signals section.

In the preceding example with the Halstead–Reitan, it was necessary to guess which aspect of the Trails B test was deficient. Several components are included in the task, any one of which could be responsible for the deficit. The more complex verbal skills, the counting skill, the conceptual ability involved in the strategy, the cognitive flexibility required to execute the strategy, and the sustained attention are all aspects of the task that combine to allow successful completion of the test. Sorting through these various skills is a difficult process because the Halstead–Reitan is not designed to test each component separately. The underlying deficit is, therefore, difficult to determine.

The theoretical breakdown of each neuropsychological function into its component parts on the theoretical battery allows a qualitative analysis of the basic deficit underlying the dysfunction. For example, a rhythm and a receptive speech deficit manifests itself on the Halstead–Reitan as poor performance on the Rhythm and Speech–Sounds Perception tests. Such a deficit combination is a contradiction of the established empirical relationships on the Halstead–Reitan because the Rhythm test is generally associated with the right hemisphere and the Speech test is associated with the left hemisphere. If a lateralized deficit is apparent, the contradiction is resolved on these two Halstead–Reitan tests by lateralizing the deficit to the side indicated by the test which is more severely dysfunctional.

On the Luria–Nebraska, however, the two deficits are qualitatively analyzed in order to determine the basic underlying deficits. In the present case, it might be that the rhythm deficit results from a poor perception of acoustic signals, and the receptive speech deficit occurs as a result of a poor discrimination between similar sounding phonemes. Such a qualitative analysis reveals, then, that both the rhythm and the receptive speech deficits stem from an auditory perceptual problem that arises secondary to a left temporal lobe lesion. What appear to be two very different deficits on the empirical test battery become a single basic deficit under the scrutiny of a qualitative analysis of the theoretical test battery results. If the results on the rest of the battery agreed, a left temporal lobe lesion would be postulated that explained the auditory perceptual deficit underlying the rhythm and receptive speech dysfunction.

Luria–Nebraska Battery

For a full understanding of how a standardized theoretical test battery is used, it is useful to examine the construction of the Luria–Nebraska. The battery consists of 269 theoretically related items, each requiring only very short, limited responses. This construction differs from the Halstead–Reitan, where each task is composed of several items and the entire performance requires sustained concentration over several minutes. The Luria–Nebraska can be interrupted after any one item without disrupting the flow of the test battery. The 269 items are divided into 11 sections. Each section represents a complex psychological function, and these 11 functions include: Motor, Rhythm, Tactile, Visual, Receptive Speech, Expressive Speech, Writing, Reading, Arithmetic, Memory, and Intelligence. A discussion of each of these 11 sections and the theoretical structure of each of the 11 neuropsychological functions follows.

Motor Function. Luria (1966) divided the motor section of his test battery into three main divisions: the motor functions of the hands, oral praxis, and the speech regulation of the motor act. Motor function, then, is one of the most complex sections on the Luria–Nebraska. The investigation of motor function of both the hands and the mouth is divided into several subsections, including simple movement, kinesthetic basis of movement, dynamic organization of movement, and complex forms of praxis. Three other subsections include optic–spatial organization of hand movement, selectivity of motor function, and speech regulation of motor acts. These 11 subsections reduce to 7 factors on factor analysis (Golden, Osmon, Sweet, Graber, Purisch, & Hammeke, 1980a), which agree in essence with Luria's formulations. It appears that when evaluating motor abilities, several components of the function should be kept in mind. The tactile and visual perceptual basis of the movement must be separately evaluated along with bilaterally coordinated movement. Oral movement is also a separate function and must be evaluated separately, as is the ability to draw simple geometric figures. These functions all represent basic neuropsychological abilities and must be separately assessed in any comprehensive neuropsychological evaluation.

Rhythmic Function. Luria (1966) divides rhythmic function into two basic components. The first component actually includes two different functions, which involve the perception and the motoric reproduction of pitch relationships. The subject is asked to distinguish between variously pitched sounds as well as to reproduce these pitch relationships. The second component involves the perception and motoric reproduction of complex rhythmic structures. In these tasks the subject must auditorily distinguish and motorically mimic rhythmic patterns. For example, the subject is asked to count the number of beats in a group or to tap out a group of beats played over a tape recorder.

Tactile Function. The tactile functions are composed, Luria (1966) postulates, of simple cutaneous and deep tactile sensation and of more complex higher order tactile functions that are termed stereognostic ability. Simple tactile sensation is investigated on the Luria–Nebraska by testing the subject's ability to localize a tactile stimulus, determine tactile stimulus intensity, detect tactile stimulus directionality, and kinesthetically recognize limb position. Stereognostic abilities are tested by having the subject try to recognize common objects by the sense of touch alone. The factor structure of this section of the test suggests that two factors are important: simple tactile sensation and stereognostic ability (Golden *et al.*, 1980a).

Visual Function. Luria (1966) notes three different aspects of visual functions, which are represented as visual perception, spatial orientation, and intellectual operations in space on the Luria–Nebraska. Deficits may arise as a result of poor integration of the visual information where the basic perception of the test stimuli is faulty (visual agnosia). Orientation in space or the ability to discriminate directionality with respect to a system of spatial coordinates is a separate function that must be independently assessed (spatial orientation). Spatial problem solving (intellectual operations in space) is the higher order cognitive function that utilizes the two basic perceptual functions (visual gnostic ability and spatial orientation) and may be independently defective. A complete neuropsychological examination must, then, separately evaluate all three visual functions.

Receptive Speech Function. Language is a complex neuropsychological function composed of several basic brain abilities. As such, the receptive speech section of the Luria–Nebraska test is composed of several basic components. Luria (1966) identifies four basic divisions that are used in the battery to evaluate receptive speech ability: phonemic hearing, word comprehension, simple sentence comprehension, and comprehension of complex sentences that have difficult logical–grammatical constructions. Factor analysis identifies two factors that correspond to phonemic hearing and complex sentence comprehension (Golden, Purisch, Sweet, Graber, Osmon, & Hammeke, 1980b). The other two components of this scale, word comprehension and simple sentence comprehension, are apparently not completely independent of the other two factors. Nevertheless, they represent important clinical divisions of brain abilities that can be disrupted and, for this reason, warrant separate evaluation.

Expressive Speech Function. This scale is also a complicated one consisting of many subdivisions organized around four main divisions. These four divisions include articulation, nominative functions, narrative speech, and grammatical expressions. Factor analysis bears out these divisions (Golden, *et al.*, 1980b).

Articulation is a complex ability and apparently consists of three important components. Articulating from two different stimulus modalities apparently represents two different abilities. The ability to express a sound, word, phrase, or sentence when presented with a visual stimulus is, according to Luria (1966), a parietal–occipital function, while the ability to repeat the material when given an auditory stimulus is a parietal–temporal function. Another aspect of articulation is important to consider and involves the analysis and synthesis of the phonetic structure of complex verbal material. Some words are simple and are automatically articulated. Multisyllabic words or unfamiliar words often require the person to sound out the individual syllables and combine them before the word can be properly pronounced. The ability to analyze and synthesize the component parts of complex words is a separate brain function from the ability to pronounce simple and familiar words, and must be evaluated along with the other two expressive aspects of articulation.

Two other expressive speech functions include verbal production, which corresponds to narrative speech function, and verbal organization, which corresponds to grammatical expression. Complex forms of verbal expression include the ability to understand the rules of grammar as well as the ability to narrate or spontaneously generate meaningful sentences. For example, in writing this paragraph, I first decide on the idea to be conveyed (the two expressive speech functions to be evaluated); then, using the rules of grammar to organize the expression, I produce sentences that express the idea. While these two abilities (verbal organization and production) are intimately related, Luria (1966) concludes that they are indeed separate brain functions composed of different functional systems in the brain.

Writing Function. Luria (1966) notes two basic components to writing, which fit the derived factors of the factor analysis study (Golden, Sweet, Hammeke, Purisch, Graber, & Osmon, 1980c). The first component involves the phonetic analysis of the verbal material. Writing deficits can result simply from an inability to decipher the phonetic structure of the verbal material. The second component to be evaluated involves the motor aspect of the act of writing. Can the person translate the verbal material into motor acts? On the test battery the second component is divided into simple and complex functions. Simple function involves the ability to copy letters and elementary words from visual stimuli. The more complex motoric aspects of writing include the ability to generate letters, words, and phrases from dictation as well as the ability to write an extemporaneous composition. In deciphering a deficit in writing function, then, it is important to distinguish between temporal lobe dysfunction, which is represented by the deficits in phonetic analysis and synthesis, and deficits in the parietally controlled motoric function of writing as well as the intellectual aspects of writing represented by the ability to write an extemporaneous composition.

Reading Function. Luria's (1966) divisions of the reading section, which are used on the Luria–Nebraska, are not supported in the factor analysis study. There are two factors found in the Reading section that do, however, fit well with Luria's theory of brain function. The first factor is called automatic reading and is composed of tasks involving reading simple words and individual letters. This factor appears to represent temporal lobe function in which the basic brain ability is one of phonemic analysis and synthesis. The second factor includes tasks that require reading more complex words. The ability most closely aligned with this factor seems to be the ability to sound out complicated words. This ability represents parietal lobe function where kinesthetic feedback from the vocal apparatus is important in pronouncing the words.

The qualitative analysis of reading function appears to be a matter of evaluating two different basic abilities. The ability to hear and distinguish similar sounding phonemes is one important basic ability in reading and is evaluated from the items that make up the first factor. The ability to pronounce complex words that have to be sounded out or internally rehearsed is important and is evaluated as the second factor.

Arithmetic Function. Luria (1966) notes two basic abilities that combine to make up arithmetic function. The first ability is labeled arithmetic operations and involves the ability to calculate. The second ability represents the comprehension of the structure of number and is often conceived of as a spatial function. This deficit manifests itself as a poor ability to write a four-digit number. For example, "one thousand twenty-three" is written "100023" because the person has lost the ability to understand the representational notion of the columns in such a number.

The test battery divides arithmetic functions along the lines of these two basic abilities. Comprehension of the categorical structure of number is broken down into two subcategories: writing and recognizing numbers, and numerical differences. Writing numbers from dictation and identifying numbers from visual stimulus, and identifying which of a pair of numbers is larger make up the tasks in these two subsections. Arithmetic operations is broken down into four subdivisions: simple operations, complex operations, arithmetic signs, and serial addition. These subdivisions allow evaluation of the level of performance of the person with a deficit in arithmetic operations. Also, arithmetic reasoning is evaluated in the task by requiring the subject to decide which sign is appropriate for an equation such as $10 \_ 2 = 20$.

Memory Function. The evaluation of memory function is a complex and poorly understood area because the localization of "memory" appears to be an outdated concept. Luria (1966) does note three important clinical aspects of memory function, however. The learning process is intimately related to memory function, and Luria advocates evaluating this process by means of determining the number of trials necessary to repeat seven words correctly twice in a row after presentation.

A second major aspect of memory function, according to Luria (1966), is retention and retrieval. Luria advocates evaluating the ability to retain and retrieve information from visual, tactile, and auditory modalities. Memory for verbal material is further divided into two sections: the retention and retrieval of words under both heterogeneous and homogeneous interference, and retention and retrieval of sentences and paragraphs.

A third aspect of memory function is what Luria calls logical memorization. This function is evaluated by means of a paired associate task in which a word is coupled with a picture that can be easily associated with the word. For example, a picture of the ocean is associated with the word energy. The subject sees seven of these word–picture pairs, then must repeat the word on the second presentation of the seven pictures.

Factor analysis does not agree with Luria's division of memory function. Only two factors derive from the factor analysis, and they do not correspond with any of the three major divisions that Luria notes. The first factor involves items requiring rote repetition of the stimulus material immediately after presentation. This factor appears, then, to be related to temporal–limbic function in that the items represent immediate memory and test the strength of the memory trace impression.

The second factor is composed of items for which the response is more complex than simple rote repetition of the presented material. A cognitive factor is added to the memory task so that before the material is repeated it must be intellectually transformed in some manner. For example, a short story is presented to the subject and the task is to repeat as many of the ideas in the story as possible. This much information cannot be repeated in a rote fashion by most people. The preferred method of performing the task is to listen for content so that a conceptual organization is imposed upon the information that thereby enhances recall.

Luria's divisions of memory function appear to assume a cortical locus and seem to represent useful clinical components of the memory process. The factors in the factor analysis study, however, appear to define a broader theoretical interpretation of memory function. The first factor identifies the more basic process of trace impression strength while the second factor represents the higher cortical aspects of the memory process. It would appear that Luria's components of memory function should always be interpreted in light of two factors found in the factor analysis study.

Intellectual Function. The intellectual section is designed as an assessment of general neuropsychological competence and, as such, provides an estimate of IQ. Perhaps the major strength of this section, however, is as a test of frontal lobe function. Three divisions of this section are derived from Luria's theoretical formulation of frontal lobe function. The first division involves the interpretation of thematic pictures.

Luria (1966) notes a deficit in preliminary synthesis as an indication of frontal lobe dysfunction. The subject is unable to interpret a thematic picture because the interpretation is built upon one or two salient features of the picture. The "preliminary synthesis" of the problem-solving strategy is incomplete.

The remaining two divisions include concept-formation and problem-solving skills, which are also frontal lobe abilities. Luria (1966) identifies the role the frontal lobe plays in organizing complex voluntary behavior. The frontal lobe generates a behavioral plan, executes the plan, and evaluates the results of the plan so that concept formation and problem-solving abilities are necessary skills of this area of the brain.

Advantages and Disadvantages of the Luria–Nebraska Battery

The major advantage of the Luria–Nebraska battery is the systematic investigation of brain-behavior relationships afforded by the particular construction of the test. All basic brain abilities are assessed in relation to their participation in the functional systems of the 11 major neuropsychological abilities represented by the Luria–Nebraska scales. Although quantitative measures of performance are obtained, however, a qualitative analysis of brain–behavior relationships is not precluded. In fact, qualitative evaluations are encouraged by the construction of the battery so that the basic brain abilities that underlie deficits in complex neuropsychological function can be easily identified.

The Luria–Nebraska also overcomes the extreme costs in time and expense that have continually plagued those clinicians who have attempted to do a comprehensive neuropsychological investigation. The Luria–Nebraska provides a comprehensive evaluation in 2 to 2½ hours. The test is also more amenable to rest breaks because each item is independent and no single task lasts more than 2 minutes. The test is also easily administered at bedside because the battery is completely portable and can be carried in an attache case.

The most significant disadvantage of the Luria–Nebraska battery is the newness of the test and the relatively sparse research literature in comparison with that of the Halstead–Reitan battery. Clinically, the test has proven to be a powerful diagnostic instrument, and the research literature to date has shown the instrument to be capable of identification, lateralization, and localization of all manner of forms of brain damage (see Golden, Hammeke, & Purisch, 1980). Vicente and associates (Vicente, Kennelly, Golden, Kane, Sweet, Moses, Cardelline, Templeton, & Graber, 1980) have shown the Luria–Nebraska to be highly correlated with the Halstead–Reitan and to have more test–retest reliability; convergent validity research is still needed, however. Further modifications of the battery may prove necessary as well. For example, as the Visual section now stands, it is sometimes difficult to differentiate right hemisphere spatial deficits from left hemisphere spatial deficits. The addition of a more spatially complex construction praxia item such as a Greek cross may eventually prove to be a valuable addition to the battery. More extensive investigation of memory disorders is also needed.

Test Battery Characteristics

Lezak (1976) has noted three general principles with which to evaluate the efficacy of neuropsychological test batteries. The *suitability* of a battery refers to how well the examination is suited to the patients' needs. A *practicable* battery is one that fits the limitations of the assessment situation. A *useful* battery, on the other hand, provides the information necessary to handle the clinical problem presented to the neuropsychologist. These clinical and theoretical considerations lead to 10 specific points on which all batteries should be evaluated. The 10 points are derived from various sources (Golden, 1978; Kolb & Whishaw, 1980; Lezak, 1976), including the author's own clinical experience.

Portability. Given the limitations of a brain-damaged population where patient immobility is commonplace, a test battery must be mobile. It is preferable that a battery be able to be transported by the examiner alone and set up at bedside by the examiner with a minimum of effort and inconvenience.

Cost. Cost, in terms of initial investment for equipment and price of the examination for the patient, are important considerations in interfacing neuropsychology with the medical profession. Inexpensive examinations allow the neuropsychologist diagnostic access that might not otherwise be available.

Administrative Ease. An easy-to-administer and brief test battery affords two advantages. Concise and uncomplicated administration procedures allow the use of psychometric technicians that in turn cut down the cost of doctoral level examiners. A brief exam is almost a necessity when testing brain-damaged patients who tire easily.

Adaptable. The test battery must be capable of adapting to physical handicaps such as paresis or diminished sensory capabilities in one or more modalities. In such cases, items may have to be administered in a manner that circumvents the physical handicaps.

Accessibility. For a test battery to gain empirical support and acceptance, it must be available to clinicians and researchers.

Comprehensive. To provide an accurate neuropsychological assessment that will yield clinically useful predictions, a comprehensive examination of most cortical functions is necessary.

Systematic Exam. Redundancy is often encountered (Kolb & Whishaw, 1980) in test batteries compiled of already existing instruments. Batteries constructed according to a theory of brain function dictating theoretically related items that measure basic brain functions provide for more efficient inclusion of items. The interrelationships among the items are clear, which provides for a more systematic interpretation of existing deficits.

Qualitative Interpretation Potential. Quantitative scores are summaries or generalizations of the processes being measured. Hence, information is lost that is recovered through qualitative interpretation of why the deficit occurred. Batteries that provide easily for the qualitative interpretation of deficits are at an advantage.

Rehabilitation Potential. Tests that by design suggest the patient's rehabilitation potential provide an advantage to the clinician.

Research Base. Tests that lend themselves easily to empirical study by construction, accessibility, and comprehensive, systematic examination of cortical functions are a necessity if neuropsychology is to progress as a scientific and clinical discipline.

FUTURE PROSPECTS

With the third generation of neuropsychological techniques not yet in sight, the current task of the field of neuropsychology seems to lie in further developing current forms of test batteries. Test batteries must be modified as our knowledge of brain-behavior relationships increase, and as research data indicate the need for change. The remediation of brain-related deficits is a capability that is fully within the purview of the field as envisioned from Luria's theoretical perspective (Golden, in press).

The area of rehabilitation and remediation is only beginning to receive the attention it deserves. The clinical utility of neuropsychological techniques ultimately rests with the ability to make statements about treatment implications. The ability to localize brain lesions is primarily of academic interest in the search for an understanding of brain function. Of perhaps more immediate and practical importance is the ability to provide neuropsychological information concerning the clinical course and day-to-day functioning of the brain-injured person. It is this capability that provides the field of neuropsychology with an interface with the medical branch of the neurosciences. The task that now awaits us is to develop the theoretical test batteries and to explore their potential for aiding the rehabilitation of the brain-injured client.

REFERENCES

Anastasi, A. *Psychological testing*. New York: Macmillan, 1954.

Bender, L. *A visual motor gestalt test and its clinical use*. New York: American Orthopsychiatry, 1938.

Benton, A. L. Differential behavior effects in frontal lobe disease. *Neuropsychologia*, 1968, *6*, 53–60.

Benton, A. L. Psychological tests for brain damage. In H. L. Freedman, H. Kaplan, & B. J. Sadock (Eds.), *Comprehensive textbook of psychiatry/II*. Baltimore: Williams & Wilkins, 1975.

Christensen, A. L. *Luria's neuropsychological investigation*. New York: Spectrum, 1975.

Chusid, J. G. *Correlative neuroanatomy and functional neurology*. Los Altos, Calif.: Lange, 1976.

Cronbach, L. J. *Essentials of psychological testing*. New York: Harper & Row, 1949.

Golden, C. J. *Diagnosis and rehabilitation in clinical neuropsychology*. Springfield, Ill.: Charles C Thomas, 1978.

Golden, C. J. Rehabilitation and the Luria–Nebraska Neuropsychological Battery: Introduction to theory and practice. In B. Edelstein & E. Couture (Eds.), *Behavioral assessment and rehabilitation of the traumatically brain damage*. New York: Plenum Press, in press.

Golden, C. J., Hammeke, T. A., & Purisch, A. *The Luria–Nebraska neuropsychological battery: A manual for clinical and experimental uses*. Lincoln, Nebr.: University of Nebraska Press, 1980.

Golden, C. J., Osmon, D. C., Moses, J. A., & Berg, R. *Interpretation of the Halstead–Reitan Neuropsychological Test Battery: A casebook approach*. New York: Grune & Stratton, 1981.

Golden, C. J., Osmon, D. C., Sweet, J., Graber, B., Purisch, A., & Hammeke, T. Factor analysis of the Luria–Nebraska Neuropsychological Battery: III. Writing, arithmetic, memory, left and right scales. *International Journal of Neuroscience*, 1980, *11*, 309–315. (a)

Golden, C. J., Purisch, A., Sweet, J., Graber, B., Osmon, D. C., & Hammeke, T. Factor analysis of the Luria–Nebraska Neuropsychological Battery: II. Visual, receptive, expressive and reading scales. *International Journal of Neuroscience*, 1980, *11*, 227–236. (b)

Golden, C. J., Sweet, J., Hammeke, T., Purisch, A., Graber, B., & Osmon, D. C. Factor analysis of the Luria–Nebraska Neuropsychological Battery: I. Motor, rhythm, tactile, scales. *International Journal of Neuroscience*, 1980, *11*, 91–99. (c)

Graham, F. R., & Kendall, B. S. Memory-for-designs test: Revised general manual. *Perceptual and Motor Skills*, 1960, *11*, 147.

Halstead, W. C. *Brain and intelligence.* Chicago: University of Chicago Press, 1947.

Kolb, B., & Whishaw, I. Q. *Fundamentals of human neuropsychology.* San Francisco: W. H. Freeman, 1980.

Landis, C. Remarks on psychological findings attendant on psychosurgery. In Milbank Memorial Fund, *The biology of mental health and disease.* New York: Hoeber, 1952.

Lezak, M. D. *Neuropsychological assessment.* New York: Oxford University Press, 1976.

Luria, A. R. *Higher cortical functions in man.* New York: Basic, 1966.

Reitan, R. M. An investigation of the validity of Halstead's measure of biological intelligence. *Archives of Neurology and Psychiatry*, 1955, *73*, 28–35.

Reitan, R. M. *Manual for administration of neuropsychological test batteries for adults and children.* Privately published, 1959. (Available from: Neuropsychology Lab, 1338 East Edison Street, Tucson, Arizona 85719.)

Reitan, R. M. Psychological deficits resulting from cerebral lesions in man. In J. M. Warren & K. Akert (Eds.), *The frontal granular cortex and behavior.* New York: McGraw-Hill, 1964.

Reitan, R. M. Problems and prospects in studying the psychological correlates of brain lesions. *Cortex*, 1966, *2*, 127–154.

Reitan, R. M., & Davison, L. A. *Clinical neuropsychology: Current status and applications.* New York: Wiley, 1974.

Smith, A. Neuropsychological testing in neurological disorders. In W. J. Friedlander (Ed.), *Advances in Neurology* (Vol. 7). New York: Raven Press, 1975.

Vicente, P., Kennelly, D., Golden, C. J., Kane, R., Sweet, J., Moses, J. A., Jr., Cardelline, J. P., Templeton, R., & Graber, B. The relationship of the Halstead-Reitan Neuropsychological Battery to the Luria–Nebraska Neuropsychological Battery: Preliminary report. *Clinical Neuropsychology*, 1980, *2*, 140–141.

6

Diagnosis of Central Nervous System Disorders with Projective Techniques

HENRY LELAND

CENTRAL NERVOUS SYSTEM—ORGANIC DISORDERS

When discussing the problem of the relationship between central nervous system disorders and projective techniques, one needs to simultaneously present the theoretical considerations relating to brain damage (or CNS disorders) with the theoretical considerations regarding projective techniques. Because this is not possible, it is necessary to present these pieces individually and then to try to weave them together. For these purposes this chapter will be divided into two major parts. The first will discuss some theoretical considerations relating to CNS disorders, projective techniques, and some general commentary on the question of diagnosis. The second part will illustrate some of these concepts as they relate to specific projective instruments and processes and cite some of the available research.

Brain Damage

From a strictly physiological point of view, one would define brain injury or brain damage in terms that include the nonfunctioning or malfunctioning of the brain. It would simplify things if that were the psychological definition, but daily experience brings us to the realization that we have to think of a CNS disorder as relating primarily to a brain that is not functioning in a *predictable* manner

HENRY LELAND ● Psychological Services, Nisonger Center for Mental Retardation, Ohio State University, Columbus, Ohio 43210.

(Luria, 1980). We think of a normal brain as having all the expected parts, which are the appropriate size, have the appropriate shape, and maintain the appropriate relationship to each other (Bykov, 1957). The disordered or abnormal brain is one where there are errors in this original construct or in the related physiology (Ross, 1968), producing functions that are different than those one expects from the normal brain.

These "different" functions refer to all abnormal behaviors, whether they are due to genius or mental retardation. The problems of genius potentially represent as much psychological difficulty as do the problems of mental retardation, although they are of a different nature and society views them in a different manner (Hirsch, 1896; Hock, 1960; Moreau, 1859).

Severe mental retardation is easily ascertainable, and does not require psychodiagnostic tests or complicated analysis to illustrate the relationship to errors of daily functioning. It has been found that even with "untestable" retarded persons, through play activity (Deutsch, 1978) and other types of activities, there is a great deal of performance that clearly differentiates brain dysfunction in the behaviors of these children and adults (Wagner, Klein, & Walter, 1978).

From a developmental frame of reference, there are behaviors that are associated with childhood stages of development. One may see on a Bender–Gestalt Test (Bender, 1946) that certain types of drawing are developmental and are only considered errors or construed as being due to a CNS disorder in an older person. That is, one has to raise the question of why an adolescent or an adult is drawing a figure the way a young child would draw it. It may be that some of these developmental errors remain too long and lead us to speak of "developmental delay," indicating that the behaviors have not improved at a sufficient rate. As this child moves into adolescence and adulthood without remediation, the lack of use of the brain capabilities increases the malfunction. We then have maladaptive behavior and related social maladjustment, based on the early or cogenital dysfunction.

The well structured brain is able to appropriately compartmentalize various daily activities (Lewin, 1935), and emerges with an organized personality, and with adaptive processes for dealing with the daily demands of the environment. The more labile or rigid personality emerging from a dysfunctional brain organization cannot cope appropriately with the day-to-day demands of the environment. The well ordered brain responds in the anticipated manner, both to the demands of the environment and to projective instruments. The disordered brain either develops internal responses that are essentially chaotic or, in an attempt to deal with chaos, the structures become so rigid that the necessary flexibility for appropriate coping is lacking.

This situation has led to many attempts to define "organic" responses in psychological terms. For example, Strauss and Werner (1943) established five areas: forced responsiveness to stimuli; fixation and perseveration; instability or fluctuations of reactions; meticulosity and pedantry; and substitute activity. Later, Reitan

(1955) described a group of behaviors related to specific parts of the brain and concluded, "affective disturbances, primarily of a neurotic-like nature, are the rule rather than the exception in brain-damaged patients." During this same period, Doll (1953) identified 18 patterns of "organic" behavior associated with a psychological examination.

The major point we want to make is that we have a whole range of brains that come under the broad heading of developmentally disordered or dysfunctional. These are abnormal brains that may not have a clear-cut anatomical identity and are often defined mainly in psychological terms. There is an implication that psychopathological phenomena may arise from neurological causes (Small, 1980).

When we talk about the diagnosis of CNS disorders by projective techniques, we are seeking to pick out the type of processing errors that typically would be related to the disorder (Barclay, 1968). These processing errors relate to personality development and maturation, the manner in which decisions are made, the manner in which new learning occurs, and the relationship between any form of psychological testing and personality growth and behavior. Solving a test problem is not important; how the problem is solved is important. This process reflects the clinical aspects of intelligence, including sensory–motor development, the rate of learning, the development of cognition (which for our purposes is divided into reception, perception, and apperception), the questions of adaptive behavior and social awareness (Leland & Smith, 1974). Projective instruments look primarily at apperception, that is, the aspect of cognition representing a highly individualized and personal construct of the material that has been received from the environment. Obviously, if the sensorium is not functioning appropriately or if motoric development is not permitting typical physical interactions with the external world, the result is an individual who, in relationship to his own inner promptings, apperceives elements in a manner different than persons who have a normal sensorium or whose physical contact with the external world is more consistent with expected development. Sensory–motor development, cognition, rate of learning, adaptive behavior, and social awareness all grow out of the peculiarly human physical formation, and if there are errors in that formation, the experiences the individual will have will vary from the expected norm. Personality growth patterns will be different and responses to projective instruments will be different. The existence of a handicapping condition by definition produces intellectual and personality variations (Mayman & Gardner, 1960).

Projective Theory

Theories of projective techniques basically assume that everything that the individual does, or is, is a projection of the personality of that individual. The difficulty is to sufficiently organize observations of these behaviors so as to be able to "read" the information being shared. This does not mean that every aspect has a complex explanation, nor does it necessarily mean that each detail of the personality is contained within a specific activity. For example, if a male individual decides to sport a beard, this may be done for a variety of reasons. The surface one typically is considered to be a mode of dress within a particular group of individuals with whom the person wishes to identify. At another level, it may also be a way of indicating that he does not wish to identify with another group of individuals. Also, it is a visible expression of a personality variable, and the question is why the individual feels that he wants to be visible, including the presumed penalty for not being visible. Further, the way the beard is worn may relate to other variables such as social conformity and individuality. The carefully combed, manicured beard demonstrates a different personality than the beard that obviously has been allowed to grow without attention. The combination of the beard and the rest of the items being worn give additional information. In some instances the beard may be a conformist item (e.g., the director of the enterprise also wears a beard). In others, it may reflect nonconformity. These variations make up the elements from which one would draw personality conclusions if the only data one had were the beard and some of the supporting items of clothing.

In developing any kind of test, one has to introduce a sufficient level of structure to assure that everybody is looking at the same key response elements to insure that the information derived from observing those elements has a certain degree of consistency (Masling & Lewis, 1966). Projective diagnosis is often drawn from the absence of this constancy in areas where it is typically expected. Thus, on the Rorschach there are a certain number of responses that are considered "popular." The individual who is unable to produce popular responses is noteworthy because such an individual is giving unusual responses. There is no implication at this point that they are pathological responses, but there is always the possibility that unusual responses may reflect pathology. Obviously no one would give a diagnosis based purely on the absence of popular responses. But this is a "red flag" that must be observed and understood on the road to diagnosis (Anzieu, 1973; Piotrowski, 1950).

The use of environmental cues provides a basis for a perceptual response that, theoretically, all persons of similar orientation will gain from observing the same specific stimulus. It is anticipated that most individuals who are raised with similar environments and have had an opportunity to be in contact with similar experiences either directly or indirectly (e.g., television or movies) will accommodate information along very similar lines. Nothing is seen exactly the same, but an individual who radically fails to perceive in an expected manner is immediately considered to have a condition that is actively, functionally interfering with the process of perception itself.

At the next level the individual internalizes these data and assimilates the material. Assimilation is not as consistent among persons because it is dependent on what the external data means to the individual. Thus, one may look at a chocolate sundae and feel that it is a good thing for dessert, or one may look at it and feel that it is a thousand extra calories. These are different assimilations of the same environmental cue. There is no right or wrong. The process of assimilation is one of utilizing the data to meet the personal needs of the individual within the requirements of coping with the demands of the environment.

These elements are described as two aspects of perception that, coming together, are absolutely necessary to create an appropriate adaptive balance between the person as an individual and the person as a member of a social unit (Piaget, 1952). Beyond this, there is the level of cognition that has been described as apperception. One can make the analogy of peeling away the layers of an onion, moving further and further from the dry exterior skin and getting closer to a central core. These apperceptive layers are the basis from which the assimilative process was derived.

There are presumed functional reasons why the individual chooses to assimilate external data in a specific manner. Referring again to the example of a chocolate sundae, obviously the person who saw it as a thousand extra calories had some concern about weight, about the social image that the weight was creating, or possibly about the relationship between this social image and their love life or their job situation. The apperceptive process is the manner in which individuals deal with their inner promptings and with the demands of society as filtered through other aspects of their inner promptings. It becomes a very circular kind of process, and the end product, the behavior or response, is based on this circularity. Generally, in terms of activities of daily living, as separate from highly specialized cognitive activities, these apperceptive responses dominate the response patterns.

What is the relationship between control and coping mechanisms as demonstrated by apperceptive responses? Some people may look at other people and feel that they want to hit them, but they do not do so because of their ability to maintain social inhibitions. In fact, they not only do not hit, but they may smile in a friendly manner and say "Good Morning. How are you?" The "how are you" may be followed by an unspoken statement such as "I hope you are dropping dead," but it is typically not verbalized and the two individuals pass each other without any visible animosity. The individual who cannot or will not exercise these controls simply is considered maladaptive. One of the purposes of projective testing is to determine whether the individual possesses sufficient apperceptive control mechanisms to permit functioning on a day-to-day basis in a socially acceptable manner. We must first make sure that the individual's daily behavior, as reflected through a case history, is consistent with the test results, or at least does not contradict them. Social acceptability does not follow a consistent pattern, and the adaptive individual, the individual who copes successfully, has to work through the differences in various "social realities" in order to stay within societal limits even though there may be very obvious contradictions within the range.

There are times when the alternative behavior is the better behavior. Individuals seek a certain amount of social visibility by deliberately exceeding limits, particularly if the social reality is intolerable. Thus the marches in the southern states against "Jim Crow" laws certainly violated the social reality in those states. There is in each instance a price paid for this latter type of behavior. Those who are not capable of paying that type of psychological price need to be aware of this and regulate their behavior accordingly.

As we look into the question of exercising control, we come to the mechanisms of decision making, behavioral response, evaluation of cost, and so forth. The individual who is able to do this successfully and consciously is considered in one light; the individual who cannot do this successfully or does not take responsibility for his or her own behavior is considered in another light. It is these kinds of considerations that lead us to diagnosis of organicity or other potential causal factors when we observe maladaptive or uncontrolled behavior.

Diagnosis

No single "sign" can be used to diagnose central nervous system disorders and cues may be misread because of sociocultural differences. They may also be misread because of social inference errors. These latter are caused by the individual's inability to understand clearly "the social price of admission" or the specific rules in the home, school, or community (Edmonson, Leland, & Leach, 1970). This lack of understanding, for example, may lead to talking in school or church, or ignoring a red light in traffic. These behaviors may be due to a misreading of the cues, to sociocultural differences, or to a CNS disorder, and we need some way of differentiating these three possibilities. Therefore, instead of making a diagnosis of brain dysfunction solely on the basis of misread cues, we are on much firmer ground if we say that misreading of these cues leads to abnormal responses and that a person who consistently responds abnormally in such situations would also respond abnormally in other situations with the same or similar demands. We need a diagnostic process that will help us differentiate between the possible sources for these behaviors. We must recognize that in general the basic reason for giving a test is that the individual is already behaving sufficiently different to have become abnormally visible (Leland, 1968).

This leads us to questions of differential diagnosis. We will not discuss differential diagnosis in as much detail as others (Bialer, 1970; Klopfer & Spiegelman, 1956), but we do need to consider some basic issues. In this conceptualization, diagnosis must not be considered simply a way to gain a "label" that potentially may contain a treatment or "cure" (Ross, 1968); rather, diagnosis should emphasize the way in which an individual processes information from the world.

Diagnosis requires assessment first through structured observations and tests, second through comparisons with the previous history of the individual, third through field observations of ongoing functioning, and fourth through comparisons with behavior generally expected of persons of similar age, social origin, geographical area, and other relevant factors. The third element is particularly important, both to validate the test results and to determine if the behavior is related to special areas of activity that may differ from the more generalized responses that the individual expresses. Thus, a person may have major difficulties in a job situation because of various types of interpersonal relationships or skill problems, but not necessarily present the same difficulties in a living situation. However, it is not always possible to follow our clients around on a systematic basis over a broad period of time to derive this information. Since field observations often are not available, this puts a great demand on the examiner. It means that while tests give useful information, the utility of that information is restricted by the limits of knowledge and experience of the examiner, and the ability to interpret various types of responses into the cultural frame of the client. This is not always easy and has been a major source of error in clinical psychological procedures. However, to the extent that this can be accomplshed, it is possible to utilize tests for the kind of differential diagnosis demanded within the situation. Fortunately, the client who produces a more "organic" type of protocol is often easier to "read" because this client has a tendency to be able to deal only with less complex ideational systems and is consequently more "open."

PROJECTIVE TESTS AND "ORGANIC" DIAGNOSES

Rorschach Inkblot Test

The Rorschach Psychodiagnostic (Rorschach, 1942) or "ink-blot" test consists of 10 symmetrical ink-blot designs, centered on white paper and mounted on stiff cardboard. Five of the cards (I, IV, V, VI, VII) are gray and five (II, III, VIII, IX, X) have bright colors. The cards are always presented in exactly the same order.

When discussing the use of projective instruments in the diagnosis of brain damage, the Rorschach is the one most commonly mentioned (Anderson & Anderson, 1951; Murstein, 1965; Small, 1980). The literature carries a large amount of material citing the Rorschach with varying results, and it is interesting to note that the thorough discussion presented by Baker (1956) covered much of the ground that would still be covered today (Schwartz & Lazar, 1979). This is not to say that nothing has developed in the intervening years; rather, there has been a pattern of reiteration of findings with a fairly solid core of concepts developed that have stood up over this period (Anzieu, 1973; Small, 1980).

As stressed earlier, no single "sign" can be considered a sole indicator of organicity, but it is helpful to discuss why "signs" have emerged and what aspects of personality are being tapped, although many "signs" of organicity have been proposed. The most cited list of "signs" is that developed by Piotrowski (1950), and his work is used as a basic outline for this discussion. While others have presented additional or different signs (Anzieu, 1973; Small 1980), Piotrowski's list is overall the most useful outline for our approach to both the Rorschach and other major projective techniques. They illustrate well the type of information on projective tests that can be used to detect organic conditions.

1. *The total number of responses (R) will be less than fifteen.* This is not a "strong" sign of organicity and the quality of the response is certainly as important as the number. However, the number of responses relates to several factors that are possibly related to organic problems such as feelings of personal insecurity, disturbances in memory, evidence of direct anxiety, limitations in creative thinking, avoidance, and elements related to perplexity, impotence, and perseveration (signs number 6, 8, and 9). It should also be noted that many highly intelligent individuals also give a limited number of responses. The variations are differentiated by the more intelligent individual's giving more complex and intricate types of organizations but still resulting in one response per card. In terms of our discussion on genius, this may also be an indicator of abnormal brain function. It is certainly a clear response difference from the individual with "normal" intelligence.

2. *Less than 70% good form* would be considered a "strong" sign, except that it does not clearly differentiate between "organic" and psychotic persons who also give a high percentage of poor form. A response is judged as having good form if normal individuals frequently perceive the shape in the same way. Poor form is related to many of the personality variables mentioned above plus an indication of possible visual–motor perception problems. Since the concept of "good form" is related to how well the response concept fits the actual form of the ink blot, there is a possibility that psychotic individuals who give a high percentage of poor form may themselves have brain dysfunctions. The question of differential diagnosis between "organics" and psychotics is a difficult question because there is debate on the question of whether psychosis is in fact an organic condition, and on whether the difference in style is due to time of onset.

3. *Less than two "human movement" (M)* responses is generally considered a "strong" sign. "Human movement" is scored when the patient sees humans engaged in activities on the card. Lack of "human movement" reflects difficulty with self-image, self-identification, and maturation.

4. *Less than 25% popular (P) responses* is not a "strong" sign, but as we have already discussed, if an individual is unable to see what other people typically see, there is possible evidence of perceptual distortion or other pathology.

5. *Color naming (Cn)* is a very "strong" sign and is thought by some to be pathognomic for organicity. The concept is that subjects are completely overwhelmed by the impact of the color, thus creating a sort of perceptual chaos. They respond by doing the one thing they are sure of, which is naming the color of the

ink on the card. Thus, there is a relationship between the confusion that the stimulus produces and the mental insecurity that the individual feels. Color naming should not be confused with color description. In color naming the individual simply names the color. In color description there is a preoccupation with color tones, and this tends to indicate an effort to gain control of a disoriented process and is thus more related to neurosis and psychosis.

6. *Perseveration* (or repetitious responses) is a very "strong" sign; this occurs when the concept does not match the blot area used and there is no effort to reconcile the concept with the shape of the blot. Repetition may occur under normal circumstances, but in those instances the concept matches the blot area. Perseveration is related to contamination in that the subject may use the stimulus on one card as the basis for a response to the next. Under those circumstances the response is often repeated exactly or with only minor variation.

7. *Total test time (T) (to describe cards initially) greater than an average of 1 minute per card.* This is not a "strong" sign and, in fact, in those instances where perseveration occurs, the average response on the card may be very rapid. It is one of the signs that gives a representation of "organicity" when it is present, but its absence cannot be used to rule out anything. It represents efforts by brain-damaged patients to be cooperative and to find something in the blots that they feel secure in stating. This takes them more time, which may increase the feeling of helplessness and frustration, which further increases the time. Efforts to be cooperative are typical of those brain damaged patients whose feelings of helplessness have not yet produced a major emotional disturbance.

8. *Impotence* involves giving a response in spite of recognition of its inadequacy, and is usually associated with an inability to either withdraw the response or to improve it. This sign typically emerges in response to questions about the patients' answers. Large numbers of "inadequate" patients may give impotent responses in the main examination, but they are usually able to improve or modify them when questioned later. The "organic" clients, whether or not they realize the inadequacy of the response, seem completely frozen and unable to deal with it beyond what they have already stated, and this becomes a very "strong" sign.

9. *Perplexity* is marked by clients' distrust of their own ability, which produces tremendous difficulty in responding to the card at all. They may reject the card or go through many struggles (in which they often incorporate the examiner) in trying to find an appropriate response. The perplex response may be marked by verbal blocking or it may be marked by a tremendous outflow of words unrelated to the stimulus material. The confusion and lack of self-concept coupled with the emotional state of the client all combine to block the production of an adequate response. This is a very "strong" sign.

10. *Automatic or "pet" phrases (AP)* is primarily a time-buying device. The clients, in their effort to be cooperative, feel that they should be saying something, but they cannot find a response so they make a remark and continue to make that

same or a very similar remark through a majority of the cards. They use that verbal device to postpone the moment when they have to give the response. This type of behavior occurs under a wide variety of circumstances and is by itself a relatively "weak" sign, though in conjunction with other signs it gives supportive evidence.

In addition to Piotrowski's signs, there has also been an indication that responses based solely on the location of the portion of the blot area used also emerge particularly with epileptic subjects (Delay, Pichot, Lemperiere, & Perse, 1955). The position response is somewhat similar to color naming in that individuals, not knowing what to say, indicate that the blots mean something because of where they are located in relationship to some other arrangement of blots with which these individuals feel a little more secure. This may produce a very bizarre combination, which they may recognize but nevertheless defend on the basis of location on the card.

Certainly if all of the "signs" are present, the probability of brain damage is very high, but there is also the probability that such an individual does not need a Rorschach to be diagnosed. The combination of major "signs" (poor form, less than two "human movement," perseveration, impotence, and perplexity) can be very strong indicators, particularly if these are associated with color naming. However, any combination of five signs is considered a possible indicator. It must also be remembered that the examiner has the diagnostic responsibility to explain the absence of the other signs, for the overall pattern of results is more important than any single sign.

Thematic Apperception Test (TAT)

The second major instrument is the *Thematic Apperception Test or TAT* (Murray, 1938). The TAT or "picture" test consists of 20 pictures selected from classical and magazine art, around which stories could be constructed. The pictures were selected on the basis of "Themas" (10 general, 7 male or female, 2 age–sex, and 1 blank) for the purpose of arousing imaginative apperceptive responses to classical human situations. While this is a major projective instrument, it is not typically utilized in the measurement of brain damage. Some researchers have used the TAT effectively in conjunction with specific groups (Foote & Kahn, 1979; Touliatos & Lindholm, 1975), but generally speaking, the TAT is not considered a useful instrument in this area (Small, 1980).

It still should be recognized that an emotionl status of the individual, as measured by the TAT, which shows an overemphasis on denial, the use of magic to produce results, signs of depression, feelings of neglect, the need for help, or memory difficulties (Small, 1980), is indicative of the same kinds of confusions, insecurities, and perplexities that are noted on the Rorschach. Further, because the TAT requires story telling, among "organics" there is generally more blocking, more use of time-buying phrases, poverty stricken language development, and other indications of difficulty (Bachrach, 1971, discusses some of these verbal problems).

The TAT is a useful projective instrument to spotlight and/or verify areas that may emerge in other projective tests, but is not by itself an instrument that can give "readable" information for the diagnosis of brain damage.

Human Figure Drawings

Human figure drawings are projective instruments that have become a part of the average clinical battery. The most common is a version of the Draw-A-Person Test or DAP (Machover, 1949, 1953). This test requires only a pencil and three sheets of paper. The client is handed a sheet and asked to "draw a person." When the client has completed the first drawing, the sex of the person drawn is ascertained, and the client is given another sheet of paper and asked to draw a person of the opposite sex. When that drawing is complete, a third sheet is given and a "self" drawing is requested. Each drawing is accompanied by a short interview. This technique has a large literature behind it, particularly in the area of intelligence (Goodenough, 1954; Hartlage, 1966; Small, 1980). Because intelligence is often affected by brain injury, the DAP is useful for screening possible brain-damaged subjects.

This was primarily a children's test, and various age-related developmental patterns, which may lead to poor figure drawing, have to be taken into consideration. However, when the DAP is administered to adolescents or adults, we again ask, "Why would an adolescent or adult draw like a young child?" It is relatively easy to differentiate between difficulties of CNS origin and those that relate more to affect disorders. There are few problems with drawings from individuals who draw human figures in a very crude, unrecognizable manner, similar to the drawings associated with severe or profoundly retarded persons. As we have indicated, such drawings are extremely revealing and usually serve the primary purpose of verifying personal observations concerning the behaviors of the client. When the same types of drawings emerge from a client whose general behavior does not suggest such extremes (that the produced images do not have recognizable human characteristics), the test becomes a good indicator of potential brain dysfunctions. It is also a very useful quick test because it can also reveal information concerning self-concept, social interaction, identification, mental state, and other important areas.

Adult individuals of presumed normal intelligence have a tendency to distort the drawings of those parts of their body that are causing them problems. When such an individual draws a distorted head, it becomes a clue that the client feels the head is not working. This may be an early indicator of deeper problems, worthy of referral for a neurological examination. Because this information centers around an estimate of a distorted part, based on the rest of the figure being drawn within normal limits, this estimation may not be reliable with individuals who, for other reasons, cannot produce a "normal" figure.

There are four categories of patients with whom one can utilize the DAP as a CNS screening device. The first category is children to the age of 14. The major indication relates to drawings that are not consistent with those expected for children their age. Questions emerge concerning distortions, difficulty in controlling lines, impairment of organization, balance problems, major details missing, and cephalopodic or unrecognizable figures (as well as the drawing errors usually associated with the Bender Test). As a child grows older, these drawing errors become more significant, and their presence tends to indicate possible mental retardation or developmental delay in a child who probably also has brain damage.

The second category of those for whom the DAP provides a CNS screening device is older children of presumably normal intelligence who draw in the manner described above. There are additional considerations concerning the interrelationships of learning disability and emotional disturbance with the types of drawing errors, particularly the crudity of the drawing, that generally reveal these difficulties.

The third category is adults who draw human figures in a manner similar to first-category individuals. There is suspicion here of schizophrenia or brain damage or both. Some of the drawing patterns seem to be more typically related to schizophrenia; examples are fragmentation of parts, very choppy lines, robotlike drawings, or very "fantastic" drawings that do not relate to the common conceptualization of a human figure. Many adolescents also draw the "fantastic" types as an indication of their "revolt," but the inquiry will reveal whether the individual is drawing in this manner because of smart-aleck feelings or because there is an intense emotional investment leading to the bizarre drawing. "Organic" drawings tend to show recognizable distortion, difficulty in handling the pencil or controlling the lines, or bilateral asymmetry (one side of the figure distinctly different from the other). Both "organics" and psychotics may give very catastrophic types of reactions, flatly refusing to draw, but there is a tendency for the "organic" individual to cooperate eventually, while the psychotic individual often will not.

The fourth category is adults of normal or superior intelligence who have intellectual control of their organicity and produce drawings that are very intricate in detail, obsessively drafted, but which lack organizational qualities, symmetry, or a sense of balance, and present general indications of poor motor control. These adults tend to conceal their behaviors with "artistic" creations, and many of their drawings are very good, yet these adults find instructions to execute a simple drawing almost impossible to follow. Emotional components also play a major role.

While the DAP would seem to be the ideal tool for measuring brain dysfunction, and it is often used that way in specific areas (e.g., reading; Stavrianos,

1970, 1971) or learning disability (Black 1976), the drawing pattern in everyone is extremely variable from one session to the next. The individuals are easily influenced by everything in their environment, and their drawings reflect that influence. Indeed, if the drawings remain stable despite environmental modification, this in itself is a sign of noninteraction between client and environment.

We can summarize by saying that such factors as size (Black, 1976), expansiveness (Persinger & Holmes, 1978), distortion and general drawing difficulties, lack of control, poor planning, peculiar placement, and so forth, all indicate possible "organicity" (Crannell & Plaut, 1955; Hartlage, 1966; McLachlan & Head, 1974; Small, 1980). These characteristics vary with different social and environmental relationships. While the material may be highly diagnostic, it is quite difficult to interpret and thus serves mainly as a screening device to alert the clinician to problems in these areas.

Bender Visual–Motor Gestalt Test

One of the most common psychological tests for brain damage is the Bender–Gestalt Test (Bender, 1938, 1946; Hartlage, 1966). The test was designed for this purpose and has proven its effectiveness. The test involves copying a series of increasingly complex designs. Although it was originally normed on children, it is in some respects less effective with children than adults because of a much greater variability in children. A large number of factors may produce developmental delay in young children and create a category of individuals who are not drawing the figures appropriately but who are also not brain damaged. These alternative factors include such things as cultural patterns, sensory deprivation, various other environmental factors, nutritional and health factors, and so on, and we find essentially three groups of children: (1) those who draw within the normative range; (2) those who do not draw within that range because of brain damage; and (3) those who do not draw within that range because of an "at risk" status, which is especially common in younger children. The latter two groups are not always easily distinguishable, and the test loses some of its effectiveness in younger groups, although it clearly distinguishes individuals who are potential problems. The greatest area of confusion lies in distinguishing between those who represent brain dysfunction and those who, although drawing in the same manner, represent environmental or cultural differences (Welcher, Wessel, Mellits, & Hardy, 1974).

Further, Bender (1974) indicates that the instrument is "not a projective test," meaning that while various personality variables affect the way the drawings are performed, there is nothing that discriminates different types of personality. Thus, some schizophrenic persons demonstrate certain drawing patterns that are different from some "organics." These differences center primarily around the ability to draw the designs properly, making changes in the original design without making major modifications in the "gestalts" (overall patterns). Brain-damaged clients lose this basic integrity of design. The test is generally most useful with older children, adolescents, and adults (Cooper, Dwarshuis, & Blechman, 1967; Parsons, McLeroy, & Wright, 1971; Wachs, 1966).

With those reservations in mind, the general errors one observes include tracing designs with fingers, use of excessive time, rotating either the cards, the drawings, or the paper (here it is noted that individuals who do rotate emerge as "organic," but there are many "organics" who do not rotate; Sandberg, 1977), uncertainty about the number of dots (even after they are counted), no effort to correct errors, substitution of circles for dots, failure to join tangent parts, overlap or penetration of parts, collisions between different designs, disproportion of parts within the figures, substitution of curves or lines for angles or dots (noting the age of the subject and the developmental level), and a number of other similar types of drawing errors also associated with the DAP (Small, 1980).

An effective scoring system should be an aid to diagnosis. Because we are dealing primarily with the presence or absence of certain drawing errors, the only effective scoring system would be one that might help us decide the basis of the errors that were present. There is currently no scoring system that will accomplish this. Another limitation, noted by Russell (1976), is that because the Bender is a visual–motor test, it is related to right hemisphere processes, and if the damage is primarily left hemisphere, the Bender may miss it. This comment underlines the extreme importance of utilizing combined information from a variety of projective tests rather than trying to rely on single scores within a specific test.

If the Bender is administered twice, with a copying performance and a memory performance (the client is asked to draw the figures without reference to the cards) immediately afterwards, it increases its value as a discriminator of "organicity" because loss of immediate memory is a major indicator throughout all projective instruments. The failure of the client to remember at least five of the nine forms is often a clarifying indicator as to whether the performance errors are due to "organicity" or other factors, for brain-injured patients may show more memory problems than patients with other disorders.

The Wechsler Tests of Intelligence

As we have indicated, intelligence affects performance on projective instruments, and the emotional state of the individual or the presence of a CNS disoder affects performance on intelligence tests. The best examples of this are the Wechsler tests (*Wechsler Adult Intelligence Scales* and *Wechsler Intelligence Scales for Children*, both recently revised; Wechsler, 1974, 1980) if they are regarded as criterion measurements rather than IQ tests. We will not discuss their use as IQ tests because they are discussed as such elsewhere in this volume; rather, we will focus on projective uses.

If one starts with a conceptual relationship between learning and test performance, judging what in the learning continuum each of the subtests is attempting to test, there emerge patterns that are indicators of possible CNS disorder. The Wechsler tests allow for identification of this type of information in individuals with otherwise normal or superior intelligence. Recognizing that an extremely high scale score on a singe subtest is just as noteworthy as an extremely low scale score, and that it represents an equally accurate measure of the patient's intelligence, the examiner must account for both sets of scores. Utilizing this approach, it is possible to draw a great deal of information from the test of psychodiagnostic value. However, because the tests are primarily measures of a previous rate of learning within the individual (Leland & Smith, 1974), it is not always a reliable indicator of current difficulties. Thus, if an individual did not, for example, do well in school, there is no indication that learning problems are still present, even though the low scores are. One could immediately assume, however, that this individual was having self-concept difficulties, was not interacting well in the intellectual world, and was reacting accordingly. If the current behavior is consistent with the expected pattern from a criterion analysis of the Wechsler, and if we have reason to believe that the test was taken conscientiously, there are many useful indicators that can help us, as they relate to social interaction, adaptive behavior, emotional maturity, and the day-to-day performance of the individual.

The elements that need to be analyzed are the major differences between the subtests, bearing in mind that all aspects of the performance have apperceptive implications. The various possible distributions can and do indicate a wide variety of problems. A peculiar profile distribution with unusual highs and lows within the criterion analysis is representative of a problem area such as CNS disorder (Dean 1978; Kunce, Regan, & Eckelman, 1976), but it is not possible to determine if it is specifically a CNS disorder.

If the Verbal Scale (VS) is higher than the Performance Scale (PS), the rationale is that the individual is preoccupied with intellectual and egocentric factors, and therefore there is a possibility of psychogenic involvement. This cannot be determined specifically, but this difference between scale scores can give certain indications that must later be supported. Certain items, however, such as Comprehension falling below either Information or Vocabulary, are often supporting indicators.

If the VS is lower than the PS, the factors may be related to cultural or academic deprivation, and these must be ruled out before any other diagnostic interpretation of the high PS (to be discussed shortly) can be utilized. A low VS, in other words, is not necessarily the result of a high level of social manipulation, but may exist because of factors related to functional retardation in relationship to community opportunity or deprivation.

A PS that is higher than the VS may indicate a psychogenic pattern because it requires anxiety-free social manipulative ability over and above verbal ability.

Thus, the individual who is spending his psychic energy in manipulating life and people, has very little of it left with which to learn the type of material required on the VS, but has enough inherent intelligence to do fairly well on the PS.

A low PS may indicate a high level of anxiety for, because the tests are timed, the patient finding himself having to "beat the clock" may break down and be unable to function. This supports the contention that a high VS may be a psychogenic indicator. In this case the high VS would be due primarily to the inability of the patient to perform on the PS because of anxiety. However, it should be stressed that patients with orthopedic difficulties, and certain types of brain damage, will also do very poorly on the PS because of their "organicity" and not because of psychogenic factors.

The test can indicate that there is a serious problem that needs to be analyzed with the use of other tests. One exception is a comparison between Wechsler administrations. If there is a major change in the subtests, one may ascertain evidence of deterioration. This is particularly true if we find consistently declining scores in a geriatric population. It is probable that Wechsler test analysis will be most valuable in picking up the organic problems in aging populations by analysing where this deterioration has occured within the test (Blusewicz, Schenkenberg, Dustman, & Beck, 1977; Overall & Gorham, 1972; Overall, Hoffman, & Levin, 1978; Temmer, 1965).

CONCLUSION

We have discussed, in this very brief overview of major projective instruments, some of the possible diagnostic indicators of central nervous system disorders. If tests designed primarily to indicate the existence of emotional disturbance, personality aberrations, and general overall mental status can at the same time give indications of "organic" problems, we have very valuable instruments that provide the major information we require, with a high level of efficiency because of the general convenience in the administration of projective type tests. We have indicated that this is possible through the utilization of projective batteries even though no one test can give this information. The instruments do not give an indication of basic etiology, nor were they intended to, and they do not always differentiate between "organic" and psychotic behavior; but utilizing them as a battery usually provides enough information, through both the testing situation and the nature of the responses, so that the examiner can gain solid clues as to where the treatment priorities should lie. This information is vital to the planning of appropriate treatment programs, to the decision of whether to maintain individuals in the community or to hospitalize them, and to various other relevant decisions concerning their eventual rehabilitation. We would thus say that projective instruments used as a battery are essential in any diagnostic procedure.

REFERENCES

Anderson, H. H., & Anderson, G. L. *Introduction to projective techniques.* Englewood Cliffs, N.J.: Prentice-Hall, 1951.

Anzieu, D. *Les methodes projectives.* Paris: Presses Universitaires de France, 1973.

Bachrach, H. Studies in the expanded Word Association Test: I. Effect of cerebral dysfunction. *Journal of Personality Assessment,* 1971, *35,* 148–58.

Baker, G. Diagnosis of organic brain damage in the adult. In B. Kloper (Ed.), *Developments in the Rorschach techniques* (Vol. 2). Yonkers-on-Hudson, N.Y.: World Book Co., 1956.

Barclay, A. The discriminate validity of psychological tests as indices of brain damage in the retarded. In J. L. Khanna (Ed.), *Brain damage and mental retardation.* Springfield, Ill.: Charles C. Thomas, 1968.

Bender, L. A visual–motor test and its clinical use. *American Journal of Orthopsychiatry,* 1938, Monograph #3.

Bender L. *Instruction for the use of the Visual–Motor Gestalt Test.* New York: American Orthopsychiatry Association, 1946.

Bender, L. *Symposium with Lauretta Bender.* Videotapes No. M-1084A & M-1084B. Columbus, Ohio: Nisonger Center, Ohio State University, 1974.

Bialer, I. Relationship of mental retardation to emotional disturbance and physical disability. In H. C. Haywood (Ed.), *Social–cultural aspects of mental retardation.* New York: Appleton-Century-Crofts, 1970.

Black, F. W. The size of human figure drawings of learning disabled children. *Journal of Clinical Psychology,* 1976, *32,* 736–741.

Blusewicz, M. D., Schenkenberg, T., Dustman, R. E., & Beck, E. C. WAIS performance in young normal, young alcoholic, and elderly indices. *Journal of Clinical Psychology,* 1977, *33,* 1149–1153.

Bykov, K. M., *The cerebral cortex and the internal organs.* (W.H. Gantt, Ed. and trans.). New York: Chemical Publishing Co., 1957. (Originally published in Moscow, 1954.)

Cooper, J. R., Dwarshuis, L., & Blechman, G. Techniques for measuring reproductions of visual stimuli: III. Bender–Gestalt and severity of neurological deficit. *Perceptual and Motor Skills,* 1967, *25,* 506–508.

Crannell, C. W., & Plaut, E. Drawings of a three-dimensional object by mental patients: A preliminary report. *Journal of Psychology,* 1955, *39,* 351–354.

Dean, R. S. Distinguishing learning disabled and emotionally disturbed children on the WISC-R. *Journal of Consulting and Clinical Psychology,* 1978, *46,* 381–382.

Delay, J., Pichot, P., Lemperiere, T., & Perse, J. *Le Test de Rorschach et le personnalité épileptique.* Paris: Presses Universitaires de France, 1955.

Deutsch, M. *The development of a diagnostic play procedure for developmentally disabled children.* Unpublished doctoral dissertation, The Ohio State University, 1978.

Doll, E. A. *Behavior syndromes of CNS impairment.* Devon, Penn.: Devereux Schools, 1953.

Edmonson, B., Leland, H., & Leach, E. M. Social Inference training of retarded adolescents. *Education and Training of the Mentally Retarded,* 1970, *5,* 169–176.

Foote, J., & Kahn, M. W. Discriminative effectiveness of the Senior Apperception Test with impaired and nonimpaired elderly persons. *Journal of Personality Assessment,* 1979, *43,* 360–364.

Goodenough, F. L. *Measurement of intelligence by drawings.* Yonkers-on-Hudson, N.Y.: World Book, 1954.

Hartlage, L. Common psychological tests applied to the assessment of brain damaged. *Journal of Projective Techniques and Personality Assessment,* 1966, *30,* 319–338.

Hirsch, W. *Genius and degeneration.* New York: D. Appleton, 1896.

Hock, A. *Reason and genius.* New York: The Philosophical Library, 1960.

Klopfer, B., & Spiegelman, M. Differential diagnosis. In B. Klopfer (Ed.), *Developments in the Rorschach technique: Fields of application* (Vol. 2). Yonkers-on-Hudson, N.Y.: World Book, 1956.

Kunce, J. T., Regan, J. J., & Eckelman, C. C. Violent behavior and differential WAIS characteristics. *Journal of Counsulting and Clinical Psychology,* 1976, *44,* 42–45.

Leland, H. *An overview of the problem of the psychological evaluation in mental retardation.* Springfield, Ill.: Charles C Thomas, 1968.

Leland, H., & Smith, D. E. *Mental retardation: Present and future perspectives.* Worthington, Ohio: Charles A. Jones Publishing, 1974.

Lewin, K. *A dynamic theory of personality.* Boston: McGraw-Hill, 1935.

Luria, A. R. *Highly cortical functions in man* (2nd ed.). New York: Basic Books, 1980.

Machover, K. *Personality projection in the drawing of the human figure.* Springfield, Ill.: Charles C Thomas, 1949.

Machover, K. Human figure drawings of children. *Journal of Projective Techniques,* 1953, *17,* 85–91.

Masling, J., & Lewis, P. The social psychology of the use of psychological tests to predict brain damage. *Journal of Projective Techniques and Personality Assessment,* 1966, *30,* 415–417.

Mayman, M., & Gardner, R. W. The characteristic psychological disturbance in some cases of brain damage with mild deficit. *Bulletin of Menninger Clinic,* 1960, *24,* 26–36.

McLachlan, J. F. C., & Head, V. B. An impairment rating scale for human figure drawings. *Journal of Clinical Psychology,* 1974, *30,* 405–407.

Moreau, J. (de Tours). *La psychologie morbide.* Paris: Librairie Victor Masson, 1859.

Murray, H. A. *Explorations in personality.* New York: Oxford University Press, 1938.

Murstein, I. (Ed.). *Handbook of projective techniques.* New York: Basic Books, 1965.

Overall, J. E., & Gorham, D. R. Organicity versus old age in objective and projective test performance. *Journal of Consulting and Clinical Psychology,* 1972, *39,* 98–105.

Overall, J. E., Hoffman, N. G., & Levin, H. Effects of aging, organicity, alcoholism, and functional psychopathology in WAIS subtest profiles. *Journal of Consulting and Clinical Psychology,* 1978, *46,* 1315–1322.

Parsons, L. B., McLeroy, N., & Wright, L. Validity of Koppitz's developmental score as a measure of organicity. *Perceptual and Motor Skills,* 1971, *33,* 1013–1014.

Persinger, B. D., Jr., & Holmes, C. B. Closure difficulty, figure-size expansion and figure-size construction on 240 Graham–Kendall, Memory-for-Design records. *Perceptual and Motor Skills,* 1978, *47,* 343–347.

Piaget, J. *The origins of intelligence in children.* New York: International Universities Press, 1952.

Piotrowski, Z. A. A Rorschach Compendium. In J. A. Brussel, K. S. Hitch, & Z. A. Piotrowski. *A Rorschach training manual.* Utica, N.Y.: State Hospitals Press, 1950.

Reitan, R. M. Affective disturbances in brain-damaged patients. *AMA Archives of Neurology and Psychiatry,* 1955, *73,* 530–532.

Rorschach, H. *Psychodiagnostics* (2nd ed.). New York: Brune & Stratton, 1942.

Ross, A. A. Conceptual issues in the evaluation of brain damage. In J. L. Khanna (Ed.), *Brain damage and mental retardation.* Springfield, Ill.: Charles C Thomas, 1968.

Russell, E. W. The Bender–Gestalt and the Halstead–Reitan battery: A case study. *Journal of Clinical Psychology,* 1976, *32,* 355–361.

Sandberg, B. Rotation tendency and cerebral dysfunction in children. *Perceptual and Motor Skills,* 1977, *44,* 343–356.

Schwartz, F., & Lazar, Z. The scientific status of the Rorschach. *Journal of Personality Assessment,* 1979, *43,* 3–11.

Small, L. *Neuropsychodiagnosis in psychotherapy.* New York: Brunner/Mazel, 1980.

Stavrianos, B. K. Emotional and organic characteristics in drawings of deficient readers. *Journal of Learning Disabilities,* 1970, *3,* 488–495.

Stavrianos, B. K. Can projective test measures aid in the detection and differential diagnosis of reading deficit? *Journal of Personality Assessment,* 1971, *35,* 80–92.

Strauss, A. A., & Werner, H. Comparative psychopathology of the brain-injured child and the traumatic brain-injured adult. *American Journal of Psychiatry,* 1943, *99,* 835–838.

Temmer, H. W. Wechsler intelligence scores and Bender–Gestalt performance in adult male mental defectives. *American Journal of Mental Deficiency,* 1965, *70,* 142–147.

Touliatos, J., & Lindholm, B. W. TAT need achievement and need affiliation in minimally brain injured and normal children and their parents. *Journal of Psychology,* 1975, *89,* 49–54.

Wachs, T. D. Personality testing of the handicapped: A review. *Journal of Projective Techniques and Personality Assessment,* 1966, *30,* 339–355.

Wagner, E. E., Klein, I., & Walter, T. Differentiation of brain damage among low I.Q. subjects with three projective techniques. *Journal of Personality Assessment,* 1978, *42,* 49–55.

Wechsler, D. *Wechsler intelligence scale for chidren.* New York: The Psychological Corporation, 1974.

Wechsler, D. *Wechsler adult intelligence scale.* New York: The Psychological Corporation, 1980.

Welcher, D. W., Wessel, K. W., Mellits, E. D., & Hardy, J. B. The Bender–Gestalt Test as an indicator of neurological impairment in young inner-city children. *Perceptual and Motor Skills,* 1974, *38,* 899–910.

7

The Neuropsychologist in Neurological and Psychiatric Populations

CHARLES J. GOLDEN

The majority of neuropsychologists currently in practice works with either psychiatric or neurological populations. This is done in a wide variety of settings: private practice, university-based medical centers, psychiatric hospitals, general community hospitals, mental health centers, university psychology departments, prisons, and many other similar settings. This is of course not surprising: neuropsychology has generally developed within neurological settings, and its major use in the United States for many years was answering the question of whether psychiatric patients were suffering from "organic" or "functional" (emotional) disorders. Recently, neuropsychologists have become more involved in specifying the nature of brain-related disorders and applying this information to rehabilitation and education.

In general, the psychologist employed in these settings has at present several major responsibilities. The first falls in the broadly defined area of diagnosis. This area includes several subareas: (1) identifying the presence of a brain injury or related disorder, including differentiating between disorders caused by emotional problems and those caused by injury to the function of the brain; (2) specifying the nature of the deficit caused by brain damage, including localizing the injury to specific areas of the brain; and (3) identifying or helping to identify the cause of the brain injury (the underlying process).

The second broad area of responsibility involves assessing the effects of treat-

CHARLES J. GOLDEN ● Department of Psychiatry, University of Nebraska Medical Center, Omaha, Nebraska 68106

ment. This usually involves the evaluation of patients before or after a given treatment (or lack of treatment), which allows one to chart the course of symptoms shown by a patient. This allows inference as to how successful a given surgery or drug treatment may have been, as well as to chart the course of a given disease process.

The final, and newest, responsibility of the neuropsychologist is the design of rehabilitation programs. While fewer neuropsychologists are involved in rehabilitation, it is becoming increasingly important and will come to represent a much more significant responsibility in the future. This responsibility, however, will not be discussed here as it is discussed more completely in Chapter 8 by Lynch in this volume.

The remainder of this chapter will discuss the role of the neuropsychologist and the activities done in the first two areas described above.

DIAGNOSIS

As noted above, the broad area of diagnosis falls into three major subcategories. These subcategories comprise the majority of the work for many neuropsychologists involved with neurological and psychiatric patients. We shall cover each of these general areas individually.

Brain Damage versus Normal

Neurologists have long been involved in attempting to discriminate between brain-damaged and normal individuals (for example, see reviews by Lezak, 1976, and Golden, 1981). In earlier times, the exclusive focus on this was justified on the equipotential assumption (see Chapter 1) that all brain injuries are essentially alike in terms of the cognitive deficits exhibited, although they may differ in terms of severity. Under this assumption, it was only necessary to evaluate a patient for the presence of brain damage and its general severity in order to fully understand the problems that the patient was having. Thereby, decisions could be made for vocational training, statements about prognosis, and so on.

This belief led to a plethora of tests whose major aim was not to describe specific deficits but to define whether an individual was or was not organic. Some of these tests have been discussed in the previous chapters dealing with various types of test approaches. Tests like the Bender–Gestalt were very popular for these purposes and are still in wide use at the present time by psychologists (as well as others) to screen for the presence of brain damage.

As neuropsychology became more sophisticated, it became recognized that such approaches are based on highly questionable assumptions. Studies of individual cases of brain-injured people have revealed that such people are highly different from one another, and that any assumption that all brain-injured patients are alike is both oversimplified and incorrect (Luria, 1966). Thus, a given individual test may or may not pick up brain damage in a patient, depending upon such factors as the location and severity of the injury. This is not a problem in severely injured patients, where many skills are likely to be lost due to involvement of numerous brain areas. It is, however, a problem in more subtle and specific cases of brain injury. Because the latter rather than the former cases are those that present diagnostic problems, this is a serious flaw in the approach.

Because of these observations, many neuropsychologists turned toward test batteries that were chosen to measure a wide range of skills. Two primary approaches are used in the selection of test batteries. First, the flexible approach indicates the test battery to be chosen on the basis of the symptoms shown by the patient. On the positive side, this results in the focusing of the battery on problems suffered by the patient and ignores areas of normality, potentially making the examination more efficient. On the negative side, ignoring areas of supposed normality may make the clinician miss areas of dysfunction that are not immediately obvious, or can lead to incorrect assumptions about how pervasive a disorder may be in affecting different areas of behavior.

The alternate approach in the selection of test batteries has focused on the use of standardized test batteries (described in a prior chapter). In these cases, the same tests are given to all patients regardless of diagnosis. On the positive side, these batteries present a more or less comprehensive evaluation of the major areas of possible dysfunction as defined by the designers of the battery. This approach prevents the clinician from missing areas of dysfunction. It also allows the clinician to compare patterns of test results for one patient with those of other patients who may have the same disorder. This allows the clinician to put together objective rules of classification that can be tested and employed in assessment of future patients. It also allows clinicians in different settings to give similar examinations and thus to compare the results across clinicians and settings. Finally, test result patterns can be empirically identified to predict a wide range of behaviors, including behaviors that were not directly measured by the test.

On the negative side, such a battery cannot cover every possible deficit that a patient may show without taking an excessive amount of time. (In some settings, to eliminate this possibility, test batteries may last three or more days, an investment of time not possible in all settings.) Thus, important areas of dysfunction may be missed in a specific patient, causing an incorrect finding. In addition, areas may be covered unnecessarily, causing excessive time to be used with an individual patient. In these cases there is often a trade-off between how much time one wishes to spend in an area with an impaired patient and how much time one wishes to invest in a nonimpaired patient.

As can be seen, both approaches have limitations and advantages. As a result of this, there have been attempts to modify and combine these approaches. These combination approaches have generally become most dominant, even with those individuals who use the Halstead–Reitan or the Luria–Nebraska as their primary instrument (Golden, 1981). These approaches usually combine some sort of standard battery, which is given initially, and then add tests as seen necessary either for clinical reasons or because of ideas formed from the results of the standard test battery. Individual clinicians differ greatly in the length of the standard test battery they use. Test batteries may consist of a well standardized battery such as the Halstead–Reitan or may alternately consist of tests used because they are liked by the particular clinician for theoretical reasons, or as a result of habit and training.

Similarly, the number of additional tests added to the "standard" battery may vary quite considerably. In some cases, such testing may amount to a relatively short time on the average, while in others a day or more additional testing may be done. In each case, this is the decision of the individual clinician who is conducting the assessment. It is also related in many situations to the practical reality of the work setting in which the neuropsychologist is practicing.

Additional Sources of Information

Although less commonly discussed in books about neuropsychology, the neuropsychologist also uses information gathered from sources other than psychological tests. The foremost of these is getting an accurate history from the patient or someone close to the patient. The history is quite important because many neurological disorders have predictable and identifiable patterns of onset that, when recognized, can aid immensely both in identifying the likelihood of the presence of brain damage as well as in specifying its location and cause. Indeed, many of the questions that cannot be answered with testing alone can be answered by a well evaluated history.

The evaluation of a neuropsychological history, especially in subtle cases, can be difficult and demands a great deal of knowledge from the neuropsychologist, who must be aware of the patterns of onset characteristic of different neurological and psychiatric disorders, as well as what effects medical disorders in other parts of the body may have on the brain. For example, patients with chronic lung diseases, connective tissue diseases, and other disease states may have resultant neuropsychological problems (see Chapter 11 on medical disorders by Ariel and Strider in this volume).

The neuropsychologist must also be aware of the potential effects of various drugs on the brain, including illegal drugs the patient may be taking as well as prescribed drugs. Side effects, reflected in poor brain function, are common for many of the major classes of drugs, including a large number that are not aimed specifically at brain function.

Another set of information that needs to be analyzed by the neuropsychologist deals with the results of a wide variety of neurological techniques that attempt to measure the activity or structure of the brain. Computed tomography (most commonly called the "CT scan") is an x-ray technique that yields data on the structure of the brain by determining differences in density across different brain areas. The CT scan is especially effective in disorders in which there is a large foreign object in the brain (such as a tumor) and in disorders where the structure of the brain is radically altered (such as when the ventricles enlarge due to blockage in the movement of cerebrospinal fluid). The CT scan is weak in disorders where changes are at a more microscopic rather than macroscopic level, and when the disorder does not cause changes in density in any area of the brain. For example, a tumor may not show up if it has the same density as the surrounding brain tissue.

The electroencephalogram (EEG) measures changes in electrical activity at the outer (cortical) surface of the brain. It is most useful in epileptic disorders where the electrical activity of the brain is severely disrupted, but it can miss these disorders if the electrical disorder is transient and does not occur while the testing is going on. While other disorders may be identified by the EEG, it is generally not considered an effective test in most nonepileptic disorders. As is generally the case in all of these techniques, absence of findings does not necessarily indicate normality, only that nothing was found. A common error is the assumption that a normal CT scan, EEG, or neuropsychological evaluation indicates that a problem is not present. This, unfortunately, is not necessarily borne out by scientific studies.

A newer approach in the EEG area is the determination of evoked responses. Essentially these techniques involve looking at the type and the speed of the response of an individual to a stimulus. The most commonly used stimuli are auditory or visual signals. While these techniques are not as common as the standard EEG techniques, they have proven valuable in such disorders as multiple sclerosis and are being investigated in a wide number of disorders.

Although EEG and CT scan techniques are those most likely to be seen in most settings, other techniques are gaining prominence as measures of brain function as well. Positron emission tomography (PET) enables the neuroradiologist to trace the density of radioactive substances in the brain in a very precise manner. As a result, radioactive glucose ("blood sugar") may be introduced into the brain, and the areas that use the glucose can be identified. In this way, those areas of the brain that are metabolically active (using glucose the most) can be measured. This is a significant advance over the CT scan because it allows the detection of areas that may be structurally intact on a gross level but that are not working on a more subtle level. Nuclear magnetic resonance works by discriminating differences in magnetic resonance yielded by atoms or molecules in different chemical combinations, allowing the identification of the distribution of specific substances. Both the positron emission tomography and the nuclear magnetic resonance techniques are experimental at the time of this writing and available for only relatively few patients.

Regional cerebral blood flow (RCBF) is a technique that measures the rate of blood flow to specific areas of the brain. This is done by introducing a mildly radioactive form of xenon into the bloodstream, either through inhaling the gas or through injection. Because blood flow to a particular area is related to oxygen consumption, which in turn represents level of metabolism, this measure also yields a measure of cerebral metabolism. However, this technique as it is commonly used is less precise than the techniques already discussed, but it has the advantage of being more available and at present less costly. More precise versions of these techniques are currently being studied.

A related technique is the angiogram, in which an x-ray opaque dye is introduced into the cerebrovascular system. A subsequent x-ray can then show the course and size of the cerebral vessels, allowing the physician to identify a variety of vascular abnormalities, including aneurysms and complete or partial blockage of blood flow.

Each of these techniques is characterized by being relatively noninvasive, except in some cases for the injection of a substance into an artery. Another class of techniques is more invasive and therefore inherently more dangerous to the patient. Briefly, these techniques include lumbar puncture, in which a needle is introduced into the spinal canal to determine pressure and to get a sample of cerebrospinal fluid (CSF). Analysis of CSF can be useful in the diagnosis of a variety of infectious diseases as well as disorders of the vascular system. In the pneumoencephalogram, air is introduced into the ventricular system, allowing the ventricles to be identified by standard x-rays. This can help identify disorders where the ventricles are enlarged or pushed over by space occupying lesions. However, the pneumoencephalogram has largely been supplanted by the CT scan.

The most invasive technique of all is to open up the brain itself, either to get a sample of brain tissue or to explore a given disorder that other techniques have failed to properly diagnose. The latter is rare, given the many instruments such as the CT scan that have become available within the last 10 years. However, brain biopsy, the taking of specific tissue, can be useful in the specific diagnoses of many diseases.

All of the results from such tests, along with the history and the observations of the patient, must be integrated with the psychological test data in order to determine the likelihood of brain damage. The data may then be analyzed, as discussed in further sections, to determine the localization of a disorder as well as the probable cause of the patient's problems. Such decisions often need to be made in collaboration with specialists in various other areas of medicine due to the potential complexity of such cases.

Brain Damage versus Psychiatric Disorders

One of the major questions facing neuropsychologists in many settings is the differentiation of brain damage from the major psychiatric disorders. Often, the typical referral question is, "Is this patient schizophrenic or brain damaged?" or the equivalent, "Is the illness functional or organic?" There are some basic problems with these questions, which have been recognized due to the increasing sophistication of neuropsychologists working in this area.

The first and most obvious problem is that being schizophrenic (or depressed) does not protect one from becoming brain damaged A schizophrenic is just as likely to suffer head trauma, drug abuse, infections, vascular problems, and the like as anyone else of a similar age and socioeconomic level. Indeed, it can be argued that because schizophrenics and other psychiatric patients are apt to be less effective in self-care skills and more deficient in judgement, they are more likely to suffer from some of these disorders. Thus, the attempt to discriminate schizophrenic or other psychiatric patients from neurological patients as if they were mutually exclusive groups, is clearly inappropriate.

The second difficulty lies in the question of whether schizophrenia and severe depression are in themselves neurological disorders. Recent research, especially in the area of schizophrenia but involving other chronic psychiatric disorders as well, has strongly suggested that there is at least a subgroup of psychiatric patients with brain damage. For example, Weinberger, Torrey, Neophytides, and Wyatt (1979) found enlarged cerebral ventricles (implying some atrophy of the brain) in the CT scans of schizophrenia. Golden, Graber, Coffman, Berg, Newlin, and Bloch (1981) found that these changes in the CT scan related roughly to changes in neuropsychological testing. Golden et al. (1981) found changes in the density of schizophrenic brains when compared to normal brains.

Other studies have found deficits in cerebral metabolism. In the earliest of these studies in schizophrenics, Ingvar and Franzen (1974) found reduced cerebral blood flow in older schizophrenics, a finding replicated by Franzen and Ingvar (1975). This study was recently cross-validated by Ariel, Golden, Berg, Quaife, Dirksen, Forsell, Wilson, and Graber (1983), who found results similar to those reported by Ingvar and Franzen. Studies with newer techniques (such as positron emission tomography and nuclear magnetic resonance) are coming up with similar findings. The implication of these data is not only that schizophrenics can sustain brain injury just as anyone else can, but that schizophrenia itself may also be caused by brain damage. Theories have been postulated that other psychiatric conditions may also be the result of brain damage, although the research on these disorders is not as far along, nor is it at present as conclusive.

Given these problems, it should be clear that brain damage and schizophrenia are not mutually exclusive disorders, and that the diagnostic questions may be answered with a statement that the person has both schizophrenia and brain damage, with a history in which one may have preceded the other.

Can it then be assumed that schizophrenics who test out as brain damaged are indeed brain damaged? Unfortunately, this assumption presents problems as well, primarily because of the reliability of testing with schizophrenics. Because schizophrenics vary in their degree of motivation and cooperation far more than do normal patients, it is possible to get poor test results in schizophrenics who are neurologically intact. In addition, drugs and other somatic treatments given to the schizophrenic or depressed patient may interfere with cognitive efficacy. These and similar problems represent conditions that affect both the reliability (ability to repeat the same results a second time) and the validity (accuracy) of the testing. It is the responsibility of the diagnostician to evaluate these factors and appraise the way in which they may have affected the test results. Thus, diagnosticians must be careful not to rely solely on test results without taking into account these related factors.

Localization

One of the major advantages of the test battery approach, as opposed to single tests, is the ability of the neuropsychologist to go beyond the simple question of the presence or absence of brain damage and to address the more important question of the deficits caused by that brain damage. This may only take the form of describing the patient's deficits, or it may take the form of attempting to fit the deficits seen into a prediction about where in the brain a given deficit is located.

The idea of brain localization has caused a great deal of controversy within clinical neuropsychology. Some significant problems arise in this task. First, individuals with the same injury may have a very wide range of symptoms and psychological test performance. This range appears to be related to a wide variety of factors that include (but are not limited to) age at time of injury, current age, cause of the injury, speed of onset of the injury, pattern of injuries, treatments received, the patient's emotional reaction to the problem, the patient's education, and similar factors. Thus, without attempting to define the direct and interactive effects of these variables, it can be seen that there will be wide differences among patients with similarly located injuries.

This makes localization to specific areas of the brain a difficult task at best. To further complicate matters, as data have become available on finer and finer levels of the structure and function of the brain, it has become increasingly clear that the simplistic conceptions of brain function found both in the popular press and in many textbooks are inadequate to describe the real behavior of the brain. As such, one-to-one correlations between deficits and injuries are rare at best, especially when one deals with higher cognitive and intellectual functions (Luria, 1966). Further, the experts in the area disagree with one another about how the brain is organized. It is probably safe to assert that no one at present has come up with a model that explains all aspects of brain function, although different theories vary in their utility as a model for understanding psychological test results.

With this state of affairs, most clinicians have become somewhat more wary about precise localization and usually attempt only to specify the hemisphere of an injury, although even this simpler task is potentially fraught with difficulty.

Of more importance to the patient is not a precise physiological localization of the injury, but a "neuropsychological" localization that describes the injury in terms of the behavioral deficits and patterns of deficits shown by the patient. This is useful in that much of our knowledge on rehabilitation techniques (for example, see Luria, 1963) is based on assumptions regarding the basic deficits underlying a patient's overall condition. As an example, a patient may have difficulty reading and understanding what is said to him or her. The basic deficit in this case may be an inability to understand or analyze phonemes and to relate them to visual material (words and letters). In this case, our rehabilitation techniques might focus on techniques to help strengthen this basic area or, alternately, to find ways for the patient to perform a task like reading that does not depend as strongly on phonemic analysis, such as sight reading or reading for the meaning of a sentence rather than its specific words.

By specifying the basic deficits involved, we can increase our understanding of the patient's ability to cope in the real world. In the above case, any task requiring strong phonemic analysis skills might be impaired, while other behaviors may be relatively intact. This information can be quite helpful in counseling both the patient and the patient's family.

The material here should not be interpreted to suggest that localization of lesions by psychological means is impossible, rather that such an undertaking can be difficult. Accuracy in difficult cases usually comes only after extensive training and experience. In the following sections, this chapter will briefly describe some of the major ideas about specific functions of cortical areas in the brain.

Functional Systems

An important concept in understanding localization within the brain is the notion of functional systems. Functional systems refer to the fact that no brain area is specifically responsible by itself for any behavior that can be observed by the psychologist. In essence, all overt and covert observable behavior is the product of numerous areas of the brain. The pattern in which areas of the brain interact is described as the functional system for that behavior. In general, many behaviors can be accomplished by more than one functional system. Thus, going back to the example used previously, reading may be accomplished in several different ways, each of which constitute an alternate functional system for reading. With a brain injury, it is possible to injure one functional system for reading, but not another. In such cases, the individual with multiple systems available will continue to read, while the person with only one functional system available might cease reading completely with the same identical lesion.

In general, functional systems are believed to be taught. Our experience has generally been that persons develop alternate functional systems for tasks they perform more frequently. In addition, more intelligent people tend to have more alternate functional systems available to them.

Thus, when we talk about a given skill being "localized" to a particular area of the brain, we are not saying that the skill involved would continue even if the rest of the brain were injured. Rather, when the area is intact, that skill is available for inclusion into functional systems. When an area is injured, or loses its connections to other areas of the brain, that skill is no longer available for inclusion into functional systems. It should be noted that an area of the brain can lose its connections to one or more areas of the brain without the area itself being injured. As a result, although a given localized area is intact, it cannot be included in functional systems.

Major Units of the Brain

Luria (1966, 1973) divides the brain into three major behavioral units that are useful to understand the gross localization of functions within the brain. These units can be called: Unit 1—responsible for arousal, activation, emotion, and other basic responses; Unit 2—responsible for the input, analysis, and integration of sensory information, most educationally related skills, as well as basic abstractive abilities; and Unit 3—responsible for motor output, planning skills, evaluation skills, sequencing, and higher abstractive abilities. Unit 3 is also related to higher cortical control of the basic functions within Unit 1.

Unit 1 is located within the subcortical areas of the brain (see the Appendix to this volume for very brief discussions of neuroanatomy terms) and is responsible for maintaining the arousal level or tone of the brain. This area is necessary for an individual to stay awake. Maintenance of an optimal level of arousal is necessary for optimal functioning of the brain as a whole. Changes in levels of arousal will result in general inefficiency in performing behaviors, with those behaviors requiring the greatest attention and concentration being the most heavily affected.

The subcortical areas of the brain also act to transmit information from the sensory organs to the cortex (the second unit) and to transmit motor commands from the third unit to the muscles of the body. The corpus callosum is responsible for communication between the right and left hemispheres, while other "white matter" tracts (so called because of their actual color) act to communicate information between different areas within and between the three units of the brain. Interruption of these connections can lead to disconnection syndromes in which functional systems cannot interact because the various parts of the system cannot be integrated with one another.

The second unit of the brain, located within the posterior half of the cortex, can be divided into three types of subareas. The primary areas are involved with sensory input from the visual, auditory, and somatosensory modalities. There is a primary area for each modality within each hemisphere, with each hemisphere generally responsible for the activities of the opposite side of the body. The primary areas are responsible for the input and very basic organization of the sensory information they receive.

Adjacent to each of the primary areas is a secondary area. Each secondary area is concerned with the analysis of the information received by the adjacent primary area. Thus, the secondary area adjacent to the primary area that receives auditory information, is charged with the analysis of the acoustic characteristics of that information. This would include such dimensions as analysis of speech, analysis of rhythm and pitch, and so on. The secondary areas within the left hemisphere also specialize in the analysis of verbal information, such as the recognition of speech sounds or the recognition of letters. The secondary areas within the right hemisphere specialize in nonverbal material in most people, such as the analysis of the spatial location of an object or the tone of voice in which something is said. The right hemisphere also appears to play a major role in the analysis of a new or unusual stimulus, while the left hemisphere will be relatively more important in the analysis of overlearned stimuli. Thus, drawing is normally a right hemisphere task in most people, but could become a left hemisphere task in individuals, such as a professional artist, in which all or some of the aspects of drawing become overlearned.

The final subarea within the second unit is comprised of the tertiary areas. There is one tertiary area within the second unit in each hemisphere; this tertiary area lies adjacent to the three secondary areas. The tertiary areas are responsible for integration of the material analyzed in the secondary areas and are thus responsible for cross-modality integration. The left hemisphere tertiary area is responsible for such tasks as location of the body in space, reading skills, arithmetic, and syntax. The right hemisphere tertiary area is responsible for visual–spatial analysis and integrative analysis of new cross-modality inputs.

The third unit of the brain located in the front (anterior) half of the cortex in both hemispheres, can also be subdivided into primary, secondary, and tertiary areas. There is one third-unit primary area located in each hemisphere. These areas are responsible for sending signals (via the subcortical areas and the spinal cord) to the muscles of the body, thereby directing the carrying out of voluntary motor movements. There are also two secondary areas, adjacent to each of the primary areas, which are responsible for the complex organization of motor impulses. These areas program the sequence of impulses needed to carry out even the simplest motor movements. This information is then transferred piece by piece to the primary units, which relay the information to the body. The left secondary area is specifically responsible for the organization of speech production. The subarea involved in speech production is often referred to as "Broca's area."

There is one tertiary third-unit area in each hemisphere, located above the eyes and behind the forehead. This area represents the highest and most complex brain area, and is only found to a significant degree in humans (at least on this planet). The tertiary third-unit areas, also known as the prefrontal areas, are responsible for most of the behaviors associated with adults. Thus the ability to control emotions, to plan ahead for the future, to evaluate one's own behavior, to hold an effective ethical and moral philosophy, and to make complex decisions involving the consideration of many variables are all tasks demanding significant prefrontal activity. Complex, higher order visual–spatial skills in three dimensions, as well as the ability to change and alter sequences of objects or information, are prefrontal skills that appear relatively specialized to the right prefrontal area.

The left prefrontal area, according to Luria (1973), acts as an "executive" system that helps coordinate all activities of the brain and is responsible for many decisions made by the individual and the way in which one tries to carry out those decisions. Luria believed that this control is located here because of the use by the left prefrontal lobe of verbal symbols and concepts to analyze, plan, and carry out behavior.

As may be gathered from even this brief description of the activities of the brain, behavior clearly can involve numerous areas of the brain. As behavior becomes more complex, more and more of the brain will become involved. Indeed, even relatively simple behaviors may involve most of the brain when one recognizes all the individual steps that make up the behavior. It is for this reason that localization of deficits is difficult unless detailed analysis of the patterns of a patient's behavior is made, because a behavior may be disrupted for any of a number of reasons. For example, following a simple verbal command requires arousal and tone, the reception of the oral command, the analysis of the command, the interpretation of the command, the formation of an intent to follow the command, the organization of the motor impulses involved, and the sending of those motor impulses in the proper sequence to the body muscles that are involved. As a consequence, errors of localization can be easily made in the absence of detailed examination of the patient.

Identification of Process

The identification of process is a difficult area that requires both a detailed and extensive neuropsychological examination as well as detailed knowledge of neurological and medical diseases and their effects on the brain and the nervous system as a whole. In general, a history is also necessary to make distinctions among these disorders, although a given pattern may be frequently associated with a given disorder. Knowledge also of the likelihood of each of the diseases involved in different age, sex, and ethnic groups is also useful, as is a history of diseases in the individual's family. The following sections will discuss some of the more common neurological disorders and some of their neuropsychological characteristics. In general, the information repetitive of the previous localization information will be avoided (since all disorders are obviously located in one or both of the hemispheres of the brain), and discussion will instead concentrate on historical details and deficit patterns associated with each of the disorders.

Tumors

Tumors come in a variety of forms that can be divided into two major categories: infiltrative tumors, which take over and destroy brain tissue, and noninfiltrative tumors, which cause brain tissue displacement by occupying space within the skull, causing the brain to be compressed. These types will be addressed separately.

The most common of the infiltrative tumors are the gliomas. These are tumors of the glial cells, which normally serve as the supportive or structural cells of the brain. Of the gliomas, the most common and most destructive is glioblastoma multiforme, a tumor that most often arises in middle age and that grows very rapidly, sometimes significantly expanding in a matter of weeks. If the tumor is removed by surgery, care must be taken to get the entire tumor or it may grow again.

Neuropsychological signs of this disorder are both clear-cut and severe. There is always a strong focal area of dysfunction where psychological processes (functional systems) related to this area are nearly completely destroyed. There is also a general decline across the board, even in skills in areas relatively removed due to the disruptive effects of these tumors on the vascular and ventricular system of the brain.

Astrocytomas are infiltrative tumors arising from the astrocytes, a specific type of glial cell. They are generally slower growing than glioblastoma, although their rate of growth may vary quite considerably from relatively rapid to extremely slow. Astrocytomas, as well as other gliomas, can be classified by grade. The grade of a tumor is determined largely by its speed of growth, with grades ranging from 1 (slowest) to 4 (fastest).

The neuropsychological effects of these tumors are also determined by grade. A slow growing tumor may cause a small area of focal impairment, but will have relatively little overall effect on brain function. A grade 4 tumor will have effects identical to that of glioblastoma. Grades 2 and 3 represent intermediate levels of neuropsychological deficit with similar characteristics. In general, the length of time the symptoms have existed for a tumor before identification is inversely related to the rate of growth. Indeed, some patients have died without anyone suspecting the presence of a slow growing tumor (without the tumor being the cause of death), while other tumors have only been identified because of an epileptic seizure (see later section on epilepsy).

The most common of the noninfiltrative tumors are meningiomas, which represent 15% of all tumors (Robbins, 1974). These tumors generally arise within the meninges (the protective covering of the brain). The neuropsychological effects of these disorders are generally less focal and severe because they cause deficit not by destruction of brain tissue but by pressure. There is an area of relatively more deficit that will be surrounded by an area of decreasing deficit as distance from the meningiomas increase with few clear lines of demarcation between impaired and unimpaired areas.

It should be noted that noninfiltrative tumors may not actually cause deficits where they are located but elsewhere. In these cases, rather than compressing the brain, the meningioma "shoves" the brain out of the way, causing an area opposite the direction of the shove to be compressed against the skull. As a result, the deficit is in this compressed area, which may be substantially removed from the location of the tumor.

Metastatic tumors arise secondarily to cancers that may have begun in the lungs, breasts, adrenals, or lymphatic system. They are usually multiple and account for a large percentage of tumors in the elderly and in patients with a history of cancer. While noninfiltrative, these tumors are considerably faster growing than meningiomas. They may grow either inside or outside the brain (Robbins, 1974).

These tumors generally show multiple foci within the brain, with the size of the foci varying considerably. This will cause alternating patterns of intact and injured brain areas. In later stages, the pattern may seem one of general impairment throughout the brain.

Acoustic neuromas arise at the origin of the cranial nerve that runs from the brain to the auditory system. The initial symptoms are ringing in the ears followed by partial deafness. The patient may show signs of increasing intracranial pressure (see below) and have difficulty in processing auditory inputs. Other cognitive functions are relatively umimpaired unless intracranial pressure is substantially increased.

Increased Intracranial Pressure

In addition to the focal effects of tumors, there will also be effects to the brain caused by elevated intracranial pressure. Intracranial pressure changes may be caused by many neurological disorders, with acute disorders most likely to result in increased intracranial pressure. These pressure changes may result from adding mass to the brain or through disruption of the ability of the brain to reabsorb fluid. Blockages of the ventricles or raised pressure within the ventricles may raise pressure by causing expansion of the ventricular system. In some cases, enlargement of the ventricles may be caused by normal pressure levels within the ventricles when the brain is not able to resist the pressure. This condition is known as normal pressure hydrocephalus.

The effects of this increased pressure may include headaches, vomiting, or papilloedema of the eyes. Papilloedema causes impairment of the peripheral vision, which may extend to more general losses of vision in later stages. When hydrocephalus is present, motor symptoms and disturbances of arousal levels are possible. If not treated, such disorders can lead to long-term impairment of higher cognitive skills.

Infections

A large variety of infectious disorders can cause relatively diffuse impairment to brain processes, although more complex cognitive skills may be more sensitive to the disruption of these disorders. Meningitis is due to an infection of the meninges, and results in fever, vomiting, drowsiness, headache, and impairment of consciousness. If not treated effectively, death may result. Children with this disease are more likely to show long-term deficits.

Encephalitis is due to an infection of the brain caused by a virus or other disease agent. There are several different forms of encephalitis, including forms secondary to other systemic infections. Patients may later develop symptoms similar to Parkinson's disease (see later section on Parkinsonism). Encephalitis presents with symptoms similar to those of meningitis.

Infections of the brain itself, as well as other infections in the body, can result in the formation of an abscess. Abscesses begin as an area of generalized inflammation and progress to a walled off, localized pocket of pus within the brain. The abscess presents symptoms similar to those seen in a tumor, along with the more general effects of any infection that may be present. As the abscess develops, it may initially look like a slow growing tumor that appears to become a fast growing tumor. There is usually a history of infection, although an abscess may develop so slowly that the infection appears to have been treated successfully several months earlier. The abscess destroys brain tissue and can leave permanent focal deficits even when successfully treated.

Head Trauma

The effects of head trauma vary considerably, depending on the strength of the trauma, the physiological resilience of the head, and the relative movements of the injured head and the injuring object. Head traumas may produce no lasting deficits at all or may produce profound and permanent impairment. Head traumas can be classified into several subgroups listed below.

Concussions occur when an individual loses consciousness due to a head trauma. If the trauma is limited to a concussion, there may be no permanent injury or an injury limited to only a small part of the brain. The significance of such an injury, of course, depends on the relative importance of the skills lost to the patient. These deficits are generally limited to the focus of the injury and the exact opposite side of the brain (along the angle of the blow), which is called a contrecoup injury. Contrecoup injuries result from a thrusting of the brain against the irregularities of the skull.

The effects of a concussion are generally focal at the site of the injury and relatively more diffuse in the area of the contrecoup. The severity of the injury is roughly related to the length of unconsciousness (Klonoff & Paris, 1974); however, relatively severe impairments have been found with short periods of unconsciousness, while some individuals with unconsciousness lasting more than a month have recovered with few deficits. The length of unconsciousness is probably related more to the severity of the injury at the subcortical brain stem level rather than to the effects on the cortex itself. It is not surprising, however, that these effects should be relatively correlated.

The focal deficit rarely takes on the highly specific and highly destructive character of tumors. Immediately after the patient regains consciousness, there may be generalized deficits in cognitive skills (Becker, 1975) and in memory functions (Brooks, 1976). The focal symptomatology is likely to appear only as consciousness fully reappears and the patient is able to display normal attention and concentration skills. Early testing when attention and concentration have become stable may serve as a baseline for later recovery. In many instances, the deficits that are worst at this time eventually are the patient's worst problems, although they are likely to improve considerably for a period of 12 to 24 months.

A second form of head trauma is contusion. Two general types of contusion have been identified (Robbins, 1974). A small object striking the head may cause a contusion or bleeding in the brain at the site of the injury. Similarly, a large object may hit the skull, causing the skull to move away from the object at a faster rate than the brain itself moves. This results in a separation between the skull and brain at a point opposite the injury. In this circumstance, blood vessels interconnecting the brain and the meninges may tear, causing a contusion at the opposite side of the brain.

The neuropsychological effects of contusions are generally more severe and focal then those seen in concussions because of the focal bleeding. Generally there is a less focal deficit at the opposite side of the brain from the contusion. The amount of injury is directly related to the size of the contusion. These deficits are more likely to involve higher cognitive functions than more basic sensory and motor functions, as is the general case in most head traumas (Reitan & Fitzhugh, 1971).

The third form of head trauma is called laceration. Laceration occurs when there is a disruption of the continuity of the brain tissue alone. These can arise in severe contrecoup injuries where the brain is ripped by the strength of the deviation between the skull and the brain, or they can be caused by penetrating head injuries where an object actually enters into the brain after passing through the skull and the meninges. This latter case is called an open head trauma, as opposed to other forms of head trauma in which the skull is not penetrated, which are called closed head traumas.

The neuropsychological deficit caused by laceration is generally more severe than seen in contusion or concussion and is related to the amount of injury. It is not unusual for there to be secondary injuries opposite the laceration. Lacerations may show up as very precisely limited injuries (after the more general effects of head trauma have disappeared). If the laceration involves a major artery, there can be extensive bleeding characteristic of a hemorrhage (see the next section on vascular disorders).

All head traumas leave the patient at risk for epilepsy, especially in the first 5 years after the accident. It is theorized that the epilepsy is related to scarring on the brain as a result of bleeding in lacerations and contusions. Head trauma may also result in hematomas. Hematomas are the result of disruptions of arteries in the brain. These hematomas may be subdural hematomas, which occur from bleeding or tearing of the meninges within the meninges that allow blood and cerebrospinal fluid to accumulate in a pocket.

When these disorders occur at the time of the accident, prompt treatment can usually avoid any long-term effects. However, a second form of hematoma may arise after the accident. These chronic hematomas are caused by the rupture of small blood vessels at the site of the injury or the contrecoup. These vessels slowly leak blood into the subdural space, accumulating over time into a significant encapsulated mass. This mass acts to compress the brain much as is seen in a meningioma. Such hematomas may take many months to form, sometimes long after a patient has decided that he or she has recovered. The symptoms of the hematoma may lead one to misdiagnose it initially as a tumor if a history of the head trauma is not properly elicited. In older people, where the arteries may be relatively weak, hematomas may develop after very mild head traumas.

Vascular Disorders

Vascular disorders represent a major cause of brain injury. Because of the complexity of the vascular system and its necessary involvement with all areas of the brain, vascular disorders may potentially affect any psychological skill, although some disorders are more common than others.

Disruptions of the major arteries of the brain cause characteristic problems consistent with the areas of the brain served by that artery. The middlecerebral artery generally causes the most blatant symptoms since this artery serves the major motor and sensory areas of the brain as well as, in the left hemisphere, those areas concerned with the production and analysis of speech, and in the right hemisphere, those areas concerned with visual–spatial analysis. The symptoms of left middle cerebral artery disruption include paralysis and loss of sensory skills on the right side of the body along with disruption of speech (aphasia). The specific kind of aphasia found is dependent on which part of the middle cerebral artery is disrupted.

Symptoms of right middle cerebral artery disruption include paralysis and loss of sensory skills on the left side of the body along with problems in drawing and general construction tasks, spatial skills, rhythmic analysis, and related non-verbal analytic skills.

Disorders related to the anterior cerebral artery may include motor and sensory symptoms involving the leg opposite the side of the disruption and mental symptoms consistent with impairment of the frontal lobes (the third functional unit tertiary areas). Disorders of the posterior cerebral artery are generally infrequent and are characterized by losses in the visual fields of the patient and, in some cases, loss of sensory input through interruption of subcortical pathways. Memory disorders may also be seen. Disorders of the basilar artery may cause extensive subcortical impairment as well as symptoms characteristic of the posterior cerebral artery since this artery acts as the major blood supply for the posterior arteries. Disruption of the internal carotid artery generally looks like a middle cerebral artery function since that artery serves as the blood supply for the middle cerebral. The internal carotid also serves as the major blood supply for the anterior cerebral artery. However, the anterior cerebral artery may also receive blood from the basilar artery system. As a result, anterior cerebral artery symptoms are much less likely to be seen.

Disruption of the arteris may occur through several processes. In infarction, an area of the brain is deprived of proper oxygenation. This can be due to a general failure of the vascular system, such as in a heart attack, or through an occlusion. An occlusion is most often caused by a clot lodging in a vessel and blocking bloodflow through the artery at that point. The middle cerebral artery is the most common site of such a disorder. It should be noted that gradual as opposed to sudden occlusion may not cause serious problems. As an occlusion develops slowly, the brain can reorganize the ways in which a given area receives its blood supply so that when the blockage is complete no area is deprived of blood flow. In addition, gradual partial blockage may result in no problems as an increased rate of flow of blood can compensate for decreased size of the artery.

Hemorrhage results from the disruption of a blood vessel causing the spilling of blood into the cerebral tissue. Because of the destruction of tissue by the blood spilling into the tissue, the hemorrhage results in severe impairment, often over a very wide area. The prognosis of such conditions is generally poor. Hemorrhages may also be massive and cause death.

Aneurysms represent weak areas in the walls of an artery that cause the artery to balloon, causing a space-occupying disorder similar to a slow growing tumor in its effects. Such disorders generally show highly localized findings with little general disruption of brain tissue. Aneurysms may hemorrhage, with the bleeding being massive and causing death, or they may show minor bleeding and cause severe but still somewhat limited neuropsychological deficits. Most aneurysms occur in the distribution of the middle cerebral artery.

When symptoms of an aneurysm occur in children or young adults, this may be the result of a congenital vascular anomaly. These represent defects in the vascular walls present from birth. These disorders may remain undetected throughout life, or may begin to cause symptoms, due to such factors as high blood pressure, that in turn cause the anomaly to expand.

Epilepsy

At the present time, epilepsy cannot be diagnosed through neuropsychological tests alone. Epilepsy is a disorder of the function of the brain that may be secondary to some other disorder (such as a tumor or head trauma), or it may be a primary disorder not known to be related to any other cause. Epilepsy is characterized by abnormal fluctuations in the electrical activity of the brain, which in turn reflects abnormal metabolic processes within the brain. When secondary to other disorders, epilepsy may be caused by the irritative nature of the primary disorder (such as a scar on the brain after a contusion). In cases where no known cause is recognized, the disorder is called idiopathic. Depending on the etiology of the epilepsy, the patient may have few neuropsychological symptoms in between the epileptic seizures (which are generally time limited) or may show extensive permanent neuropsychological damage.

There are a number of major forms of epilepsy. Temporal lobe epilepsy is associated with disturbances of consciousness in which the person may perform highly organized acts, such as making a bed (Hansotia & Wadia, 1971). Such disorders may also be associated with changes in the emotional status of the patient. This disorder is most commonly associated with disorders of the anterior half of the brain.

Petit mal epilepsy is accompanied by a loss of consciousness. The patient does not fall, but may pause and stare. Afterwards, the patient may continue previous behavior with no awareness of the intervening period. Grand mal epilepsy often has an aura—a sensory phenomenon of some sort, such as seeing a given visual stimuli or feeling a given tactile sensation—that precedes the actual seizure. The patient then becomes unconscious, falls to the ground, and often has a general convulsion. The patient may stop breathing and may show foaming at the mouth or biting of the tongue. Generally the neuropsychological deficits associated with this disorder are quite severe (Matthews & Klove, 1967).

Other forms of epilepsy may be set off by specific sensory events in the environment (such as a flashing light) or may show convulsions that radiate from one small part of the body to the entire body in a progressive sequence.

At present, no neuropsychological signs have been identified that either predict which injured patients will get epilepsy (although generally the worse the injury the higher the probability) or whether a given individual has epileptic seizures, although research is going on in this area.

Alcoholism

Chronic alcoholics with a drinking history of more than 10 years have been reported to show significant neuropsychological deficits (Page & Linden, 1974). These deficits appear to fall into three major categories: deficits of frontal lobe functions. such as planning and evaluation; deficits of emotional stability and memory; and deficits of spatial (nonverbal) integration and execution (e.g., Cermak, Butters, & Goodglass, 1971; Chandler, Vega, & Parsons, 1973; Tarter, 1972). The deficits appear roughly related to the duration and amount of the drinking, but there are apparently considerable individual differences in a patient's long-term reaction to alcoholism. This may be related to the patient's diet and general physical condition, but the relationship of the factors is unclear.

Similar types of problems may be found in patients with chronic usage of other drugs as well as in a variety of generalized metabolic disorders. Most of these conditions have not been adequately investigated at present, however.

Alzheimer's Disease

This is the major example of a large group of disorders commonly diagnosed as senile dementias. Alzheimer's disease is marked by a gradual loss of memory and disturbances in speech and spatial orientation in its early stage. This is followed by disorientation of time and place in later stages. In the final stages, there is a total degeneration of personality and intellectual skills. In general, more complex and less used skills are impaired before more basic and overlearned abilities.

Another cause of senile dementias, Pick's disease, is characterized by relatively specific losses of skills in the anterior areas of the brain as opposed to the more generalized problems seen in Alzheimer's disease. As with Alzheimer's disease, the early symptoms revolve around memory and higher intellectual functions. There may be lapses in social behavior characterized by either hyperactivity or extreme apathy. In later forms, the patient is often mute with behavior limited to stereotyped actions. The mutism is more characteristic of Pick's disease than it is of Alzheimer's disease. It can, however, be difficult to discriminate the diseases on the basis of neuropsychological deficits alone. Final diagnosis may not be confirmed until an autopsy is done or unless a brain biopsy is completed.

A third major cause of senile dementia is related to problems with the vascular system. Vascular problems include generalized arteriosclerosis, in which there is inadequate oxygen delivered to the brain, as well as a succession of small strokes. In the latter case, the deterioration is stepwise (marking the occurrences of the strokes) rather than a slow, continuous deterioration. (See Chapter 10 by Goldstein on normal aging and dementia.)

Parkinson's Disease

There are currently seven different etiologies recognized for Parkinson's disease. All are characterized by a disturbance of the extrapyramidal system and result in changes in the metabolic balance of the brain. The primary form of the disease is idiopathic, a form that has no known etiology. Other forms are known to follow encephalitis, certain antipsychotic medications, liver disease in children and adolescents, or injury through trauma, stroke, or other neurological problems to the midbrain or the basal nuclei (in the subcortical areas of the brain).

The course of Parkinson's disease reflects five major stages. Initially, symptoms are mild and unilateral. There is often a tremor in the affected limbs at rest. In the second stage, the patient's overall pattern of movement is slow. The patient walks stooped over. The third stage includes a pronounced gait disturbance and generalized disability. In the fourth stage, the disabilities become more severe and general; in the last stage, disability is complete.

In neuropsychological testing, the patient's drawings are often small in an attempt to correct for the tremor. A similar problem, called micrographia, is seen in the patient's writing. While basic verbal skills are intact, higher abstractive tests and tests requiring significant attention and concentration may be impaired. In later stages, more basic functions become progressively involved.

Multiple Sclerosis

Multiple sclerosis (MS) is a degeneration of the myelin sheath covering the white matter (nerve axons) of the brain. These are the tracts of the brain responsible for intercommunications among the neurons of the brain. Myelin allows these "connectors" to transmit signals in the most efficient and effective manner. It is also the myelin sheath that is responsible for the white colored appearance of these axons. The disease primarily attacks the subcortical areas, but will affect cognitive integrity as the disease progresses.

The early symptoms are primarily sensory and motor rather than cognitive. The symptoms are inconsistent, varying over time with the patient showing periods of exacerbation and remission. The disease may be exacerbated by both emotional and physical stressors. In later stages, higher cognitive skills are affected. The degree to which cognitive skills are affected differs widely in individual cases, but can progress to an MS dementia in some cases. Visual deficits are common, and evoked potentials involving visual stimuli may be one of the earliest behavioral signs of the disease. Because of the inconsistent nature of the symptoms, MS patients can be misdiagnosed as psychiatric rather than neurological patients.

Final Comments on Process

Although the above is certainly not a full account of all the possible neurological problems, nor even a full account of the problems mentioned, it should be clear that neuropsychological problems can be caused by a very wide range of disorders causing overlapping and identical symptoms. As a consequence, identification of process is difficult and requires a good history as well as extensive testing, especially in subtle cases where the cause is undetermined. Skill in this area generally comes only after extensive years of experience.

ASSESSING TREATMENT EFFECTS

Often cases seen by neuropsychologists do not need a diagnostic work-up covering most of the issues discussed in the previous sections. In these cases, the cause of the patient's deficits is obvious, and the general nature of the deficits as well as their implications are also reasonably clear. Neuropsychological testing may therefore be used basically to document the exact extent of the patient's problems in an objective manner. This may be done in some cases for legal purposes because of a lawsuit pending in the case, or simply because the patient, family, or physician is interested in knowing the information. The process of doing this is much the same as in determining the questions of localization and process.

In an increasing number of instances, however, the purpose of referring such patients is to analyze the effects of treatment procedures used with patients. As the field has become more sophisticated, the need to document the effects and value of treatment has become important. Documentation aids in determining what approaches are successful as well as what programs or approaches deserve funding from limited rehabilitation resources.

The basic pattern of such work is simple: the patient is tested both before and after the treatment has occurred, and differences in the patient's performance (positive and negative) are discovered. There are of course difficulties with such an approach. First, if the patient improves, one does not know if the treatment given to the patient was reponsible for the improvement or whether the improvement was due to some other factor. For example, patients with recent injuries may improve on their own (due to the recovery of the brain) for 12 to 24 months. In research, such problems are handled by comparing patients to a no-treatment group that had similar problems. This, however, cannot be easily done in the individual clinical case. As a consequence, the clinician must be aware of this factor and attempt to relate changes in the patient to all the factors in the patient's life that may have played a role. This awareness is necessary if the clinician is interested in understanding the role of a specific treatment in a given case.

A second problem in this area is the fact that performance on some tests improves when taken for a second time within a given time period. Thus, it is important for the clinician to know what is called the test–retest reliability of the test in untreated cases. If an untreated patient will automatically improve 10 points on a test over 3 months, then the treated patient must show considerably more improvement for the treatment to be worthwhile. Unfortunately, information on the effects of retesting is relatively difficult to find for many tests. This factor limits the conclusions one can reach.

A third question in many cases revolves around the question of what the purpose of treatment is. Traditionally, we think of treatment as curing a disorder. In neuropsychology and with chronically brain-injured patients, this is not an appropriate goal. In these cases, the patient is not expected to recover in the sense of regaining an intact brain, but can be taught ways to get around his or her deficits and can thus lead a more effective and pleasant life. In doing this, however, more impact takes place on patients' day-to-day lives rather than on their psychological test performance. Thus, measures of the patient's adaption to their environment must be included, in addition to the more traditional measures discussed in the last several chapters.

The opposite problem arises when treatment is concentrated on teaching people to do psychological tests. This can result in improved test performance but may make no impression on the person's day-to-day life. This of course is of little value to the patient.

Finally, there are questions as to the type of testing appropriate to an assessment of the treatment. Some clinicians advocate using tests specific to the area in which improvement is expected. This has the advantage of giving detailed information in the area being explored. On the other hand, by ignoring other areas, one may miss areas of improvement and may also miss areas where treatment makes the patient worse, an equally important consideration. For example, if a patient slated for surgery is tested in only the areas in which he or she is having problems, the fact may be missed that the procedure led to increased difficulty in a formerly normal area.

The alternative, using a more comprehensive battery with an extra emphasis on those areas that are most of interest, appears more reasonable in designing such evaluations. This approach has the defect of the time such a test battery would take, but avoids the limitations of the first approach.

Treatment Types

The types of treatments evaluated using these approaches can be divided into several major categories. The first is the evaluation of surgical approaches. In these cases, there is an evaluation preceding and following the surgical procedure, and a reevaluation at least several months later because brain surgery may cause acute disruption of brain processes that later recover. Another common area is the assessment of drug effects. In these cases, one is frequently evaluating whether the drug made the patient worse rather than better in terms of neuropsychological functioning. A good example of such treatment is the use of chemotherapy or radiation for various forms of cancer. Although the drugs used in these treatments may cure the cancer, they may also have the side effect of interfering with brain function. Major tranquilizers may calm a schizophrenic patient, but may also interfere with cognition. Drugs for hyperactivity in children can be assessed to see if the child's neuropsychological performance is better or worse.

The third and final area is behavioral treatments. These can be aimed at teaching the patient specific tasks, teaching methods of approaching problems or remembering material, or providing practice in an area of weakness for the patient. It is with this type of treatment that the error of mistaking the learning of a psychological test for real improvement is likely to take place. Some of these techniques are discussed in the chapter by Lynch.

CONCLUSIONS

As can be seen, the neuropsychologist in these populations has a wide range of potential questions and involvement. Specialization in these areas requires an extensive knowledge of neurology, neurological diseases, medical diseases, psychiatry, psychiatric disorders, and such related areas as anatomy, neuropathology, and neuroradiology. The neuropsychologist is involved in diagnostic questions, in determining the extent of a patient's disorder, and in evaluating the effectiveness of treatment in addition to those areas to be discussed in later chapters. The neuropsychologist is involved with patients in all age groups and with a wide variety of disorders, potentially offering a role in almost all major areas of traditional clinical practice.

REFERENCES

Ariel, R. N., Golden, C. J., Berg, R. A., Quaife, M. A., Dirksen, J. W., Forsell, T., Wilson, J., & Graber, B. Regional cerebral blood flow in schizophrenics with 133-xenon inhalation method. *Archives of General Psychiatry*, 1983, *40*, 258–263.

Becker, B. Intellectual changes after closed head injury. *Journal of Clinical Psychology*, 1975, *31*, 307.

Brooks, D. N. Wechsler Memory Scale performance and its relationship to brain damage after severe closed head injury. *Journal of Neurology, Neurosurgery, and Psychiatry*, 1976, *39*, 593.

Cermak, L. S., Butters, N., & Goodglass, A. The extent of memory loss in Korsakoff patients. *Neuropsychologia*, 1971, *9*, 307.

Chandler, B. C., Vega, A., & Parsons, O. A. Dichotic listening in alcoholics with a history of possible brain damage. *Quarterly Journal of Studies on Alcohol*, 1973, *34*, 1099.

Franzen, G., & Ingvar, D. Abnormal distribution of cerebral activity in chronic schizophrenia. *Journal of Psychiatric Research*, 1975, *12*, 199.

Golden, C. J. *Diagnosis and rehabilitation in clinical neuropsychology* (2nd ed.). Springfield, Ill.: Charles C Thomas, 1981.

Golden, C. J., Graber, B., Coffman, J., Berg, R. A., Newlin, D. B., & Bloch, S. Structural brain deficits in schizophrenia as identified by CT scan density parameters. *Archives of General Psychiatry*, 1981, *38*, 1014.

Hansotia, P., & Wadia, N. H. Temporal lobe epilepsy with absenses. *Diseases of the Nervous System*, 1971, *32*, 316.

Ingvar, D., & Franzen, G. Abnormalities of cerebral blood flow in patients with chronic schizophrenia. *Acta Psychiatrica Scandanavica*, 1974, *10*, 425.

Klonoff, H., & Paris, R. Immediate, short term and residual effects of acute head injuries in children: Neuropsychological and neurological correlates. In R. M. Reitan & L. A. Davison (Eds.), *Clinical neuropsychology: Current status and applications.* Washington, D.C.: Winston, 1974.

Lezak, M. D. *Neuropsychological assessment.* New York: Oxford University Press, 1976.

Luria, A. R. *Restoration of function after brain injury.* New York: Macmillan, 1963.

Luria, A. R. *Higher cortical functions in man.* New York: Basic Books, 1966.

Luria, A. R. *The working brain.* New York: Basic Books, 1973.

Matthews, C. G., & Klove, H. Differential psychological performances in major motor, psychomotor, and mixed classifications of known and unknown etiology. *Epilepsia,* 1967, *8,* 117.

Page, R. D., & Linden, J. D. "Reversible" organic brain syndrome in alcoholics. *Quarterly Journal of Studies on Alcohol,* 1974, *35,* 98.

Reitan, R. M., & Fitzhugh, K. B. Behavioral deficits in groups with cerebral vascular lesions. *Journal of Consulting and Clinical Psychology,* 1971, *37,* 215.

Robbins, S. L. *Pathologic basis of disease.* Philadelphia: Saunders, 1974.

Tarter, R. E. Brain damage associated with chronic alcoholism. *Diseases of the Nervous System,* 1972, *33,* 759.

Weinberger, D. P., Torrey, E. F., Neophytides, A. N., & Wyatt, R. J. Lateral cerebral ventricular enlargement in chronic schizophrenia. *Archives of General Psychiatry,* 1979, *36,* 735.

8

Neuropsychological Assessment and Rehabilitation

WILLIAM J. LYNCH

The role of clinical neuropsychological assessment in rehabilitation settings is not a novel concept. The post World War I and World War II eras were characterized by a focusing of interest upon rehabilitation of traumatically injured military personnel. Goldstein (Goldstein & Scheerer, 1941) and later Luria (1963) were the most prominent of the early investigators who concerned themselves with the identification of the location and effects of penetrating missile wounds of the head. As the various brain-imaging techniques (pneumoencephalography, angiography, electroencephalography, and isotope brain scans) became increasingly available and accepted, the need to identify or localize brain lesions became less prominent. With the introduction of computerized tomographic (CT) and position emission transaxial tomographic (PETT) scans in the middle 1970s, the need for localization of brain lesions with neuropsychologic techniques virtually ceased to be an issue.

However, characterization of patterns of neuropsychologic deficit, as well as identification of spared functions, remained as unique contributions of neuropsychological assessment. As Luria (1963) points out, a thorough evaluation of cognitive, sensory, and motor abilities is necessary in any rehabilitation effort. In order to devise an effective treatment strategy, the clinician must be aware of both assets and liabilities in the patient with brain dysfunction.

An additional application of neuropsychological assessment is that of quan-

WILLIAM J. LYNCH • Brain Injury Rehabilitation Unit, Palo Alto Veterans Administration Medical Center, Palo Alto, California 94304.

tifying change over time. This could involve serial evaluation or simply pre–post assessment. The former refers to a design whereby a patient is thoroughly evaluated prior to commencement of treatment (base-line evaluation), and is then reevaluated at periods during treatment (follow-up evaluations). By utilizing quantified measures, a comparison can be made between the patient's condition at the beginning and at various points during treatment. The data provide the staff and the patient with objective evidence of change (or lack of it) so that effectiveness of treatment can be continually monitored.

Pre–post testing can be helpful in situations in which a specific treatment (such as endarterectomy or ventricular shunting) is carried out. Particularly when the anticipated neuropsychological changes are apt to be subtle, a careful assessment of higher cortical functions is indispensable.

ASSESSMENT TECHNIQUES RELEVANT TO REHABILITATION

Neuropsychological Batteries

A thorough discussion of neuropsychological test batteries is provided elsewhere in this volume (Chapter 5). For this reason, I will only describe them briefly. Perhaps it would be more accurate to replace the term "battery" with the word "system," since many clinicians do not utilize precisely the same tests in precisely the same physical form in all settings.

There are two principal systems of neuropsychological assessment in the United States today. A third system has evolved from one of these (although paternity has at times been vigorously denied).

The first system began with the work of Halstead (1947) and has been carried on by Reitan (1955). The resulting set of assessment techniques has formed the basis for the Halstead–Reitan Battery (and its variants for children and adolescents), as well as the test batteries used by groups in Michigan (Smith, 1971), Wisconsin (Beardsley; Matthews, Cleeland, & Harley, 1972), and Canada (Knights & Watson, 1968). There are differences in the tests included in each system, and there are a number of variations in the manner in which certain tests are administered. What remains constant, however, is the fact that a number of tests that have proven validity are gathered together, presented in a standard fashion, and evaluated by comparing the raw scores to an established "cut-off" score, which discriminates impaired from nonimpaired performances. Occasionally, scores are converted to standard scores (usually T-scores) prior to interpretation. The tests included in these batteries contain measures of intellectual functions, cortical sensory functions, simple and complex motor functions, language functions, and memory functions. Frequently, a measure of personality status is included. In most instances, a summary score or index is calculated as a way of concisely representing the patient's general level of performance. These indices include the Impairment Index (Reitan, 1955), Deficit Index (Knights & Watson, 1968), or Average T-score (Kiernan & Matthews, 1976).

The second major neuropsychological assessment system derives from the work of Luria (1966). He made his position quite clear in an article a short time before his death, in which he stated that he did not feel that the "test battery" concept, which typified the mainstream of American clinical neuropsychology, was the best approach to analyzing higher cortical functions (Luria & Majovski, 1977).

Christensen (1975) published a set of materials, a manual, and text under the title *Luria's Neuropsychological Investigation*. This represented an attempt to standardize the clinical evaluation techniques employed and developed by Luria over a 30-year period. It did *not* represent an attempt to create a Luria version of a neuropsychological battery. The procedures outlined in the test manual are aimed at evaluating the integrity of specific cortical zones, as well as of the primary cerebral functional systems (arousal, sensory, and motor).

Golden, Purisch, and Hammeke (1979) have developed a highly standardized battery (now known as Luria–Nebraska Neuropsychological Battery), which draws heavily from Christensen's rendition of Luria's techniques. The procedure consists of 269 items organized into 14 separate scales. The reader is referred to Chapter 5 for a more detailed description of the derivation and interpretation of these scales.

The Halstead–Reitan and Luria–Nebraska systems provide a thorough analysis of perceptual–motor, sensory, and cognitive functions. As Golden and his colleagues have shown (Golden, Hammeke, & Purisch, 1978), the two systems are roughly equivalent in their ability to detect the presence and location of brain dysfunction. Certain patterns of performance have been found to provide information regarding the extent, lateralization, and lobular location of the lesion(s) present. Two major shortcomings of both systems are their inadequate assessment of memory and language functions. Since these functions are vital to any rehabilitation effort, it is necessary to obtain detailed information regarding the integrity of the patient's memory and language systems.

Evaluating Memory Functions

Impaired memory is the most frequent cognitive complaint of brain-injured patients. It is therefore necessary to carefully and thoroughly evaluate memory prior to establishing a program for rehabilitation.

Measures of Auditory Memory

Patients usually are first aware of having difficulty recalling what they have heard in the immediate or recent past. This problem is especially troublesome because patients miss appointments, fail to carry out directions, or repeat what they have recently said without recalling the previous incident.

Auditory memory may involve memory for content, sequence, or recognition. Evaluating memory for content involves presenting the patient with a list of words or a brief story which he/she must repeat in any order. Memory for auditory sequences could involve simple measures such as Digit Span, or more complex stimuli such as words or phrases. The principal difference between content and sequence memory lies in the additional requirement that the stimuli be recalled in a precise order in sequence memory.

Patients possessing adequate content memories but impaired sequence memories are able to remember most of the isolated elements of a task to be performed but are unable to organize these elements into a proper sequence. They may recall most of the steps in a five-step command, but they lose track of the order in which the steps were to be carried out.

Recognition memory is evaluated by presenting auditory stimuli (sounds, patterns of tones, words, phrases, sentences) in a series that features periodic repetitions of previous items in the series. The patient is required to recognize stimuli that have already occurred as well as those that are occurring for the first time. Patients with faulty recognition memory fail to experience a sense of recognition when they begin to say something that they have already said. A related problem occurs when others (family, friends, co-workers) repeat a request or suggestion that the patient has evidently forgotten. The patient sincerely feels as if he is hearing the request for the first time, and may become offended when others point out that he had, indeed, heard the request before.

The assessment devices that are useful in evaluating auditory memory include the logical memory and associate learning subtests of the Wechsler Memory Scale (Wechsler, 1945), the Rey Auditory–Verbal Learning Test (Rey, 1964), Buschke selective reminding procedure (Buschke & Fuld, 1974), and the Goldman, Fristoe, and Woodcock (1974) Auditory Memory Tests. Both the Rey and the Goldman, Fristoe, and Woodcock (GFW) tests contain a recognition memory component. Sequence memory can be assessed by digit span, by unrelated word lists, or by presenting word sequences that the patient must recapitulate using pictures of the words that were presented. The latter technique is employed on the GFW, and is especially helpful in patients who may have expressive language problems.

Measures of Visual Memory

Recall for what one has seen is frequently disrupted by brain injury. The deficit is rarely a purely visual one, in the sense that the patient typically has difficulty with spatial concepts as well. In a sense, the patient may have problems recalling visual content as well as spatial placement of the content. Thus, a patient may be able to describe five objects that were shown to him, but may be unable to recall their correct spatial placements. Deficits such as these may result in problems learning the layout of a room, ward, or building.

Patients may attend fairly well to large, familiar, or centrally located visual stimuli while failing to attend to more subtle, unfamiliar, or peripheral features of a visual array. The memory disorder may be relatively greater for verbal than for nonverbal (such as faces or designs) stimuli, depending upon the location of the brain lesion. Here, as in auditory memory, the clinician can measure both recall and recognition by varying the assessment strategy. Recall can be measured by presenting the stimuli (letters, words, sentences, objects, designs, or photographic scenes) for a prescribed period of time (varying from milleseconds up to several minutes), after which the patient is required to demonstrate recall by naming, copying, or picking out the stimulus from among several possible choices. For patients with speaking and/or writing difficulties, a multiple choice format is desirable. Here the patient simply points or indicates his choice in some fashion as the examiner points to each possibility.

Useful tests for evaluating visual memory include the Visual Recognition Subtest from the Wechsler Memory Scale (Wechsler, 1945), Benton Visual Retention Test (Benton, 1974), The Benton Visual Retention Test—Multiple Choice (Benton, Hamsher, & Stone, 1977), as well as a number of procedures such as recall of nonverbal patterns as devised by Warrington and James (1967), which we have developed at our clinic as visual analogues to the GFW Auditory Memory—Recognition Memory subtest. Other tests that may be found useful are the Graham–Kendall Memory for Designs Test (1960) and the Bender–Gestalt Test recall procedure (Tolor, 1958).

Certain other forms of memory may be impaired by brain disorders. For example, "incidental memory" (i.e., the ability to recall information from previous experience without prior instruction or forewarning) is often impaired to a greater extent than performance on standard memory tests. Incidental memory may be assessed first by presenting an address or list of three words to the patient for immediate repetition; then by suddenly asking the patient to recall the same information 30 to 60 minutes later. In addition, on the Halstead–Reitan Battery, the Tactual Performance Test (TPT), Memory and Localization components measure incidental tactile (recall of shapes) and spatial (recall of their exact locations on the board) incidental memories, respectively.

Because it has been shown (Russell, 1975) that significant delays between learning and recall, especially with heterogeneous interpolated activity, can identify subtle memory deficits, the clinician is well advised to consider including some sort of delay procedure in whatever memory measure he/she employs. It should be borne in mind that measures such as Digit Span or Arithmetic have little to do with memory, save in the very broad sense of the term. Practical or effective memory must deal with delays and distractions, and thus our clinical assessment should strive to be more lifelike and less concerned with procedural quickness or experimental elegance.

Evaluating Language Functions

A thorough evaluation of the patient's ability to comprehend and express linguistic information is essential in a rehabilitation program. Testing is best carried out by a Speech Pathologist or by a neuropsychologist trained in speech pathology.

Once we have determined that a patient's auditory and vocal systems are intact, the patient is referred for a formal speech evaluation that typically consists of a clinical interview along with one or more of the following measures (in whole or in part): The Aphasia Language Performance Scales—or ALPS (Keenan & Brassell, 1975), Boston Diagnostic Aphasia Examination (Goodglass & Kaplan, 1972), Porch Index of Communicative Ability—or PICA (Porch, 1967), or the Minnesota Test for the Differential Diagnosis of Aphasia (Schuell, 1965).

These measures are of extreme importance in that they allow us to understand the nature and extent of any language disorder present. In addition, they provide information concerning the patient's linguistic *abilities,* specifically the ways in which he/she communicates most frequently and efficiently. Such detailed information is valuable in our interpretation of test performances throughout the assessment. For example, it has been suggested recently (Crosson & Warren, 1982) that the clinician must exercise great caution in interpreting test performances of aphasic patients on nonlanguage tasks that contain complex instructions or verbal output requirements.

Evaluating Personality Functions

Alterations in personality are a common source of concern in the brain-injured patient. Families consistently report that changes in the patient's personality were the most troublesome of all the changes with which they had to deal (Lezak, 1978). Aside from traditional interview techniques, certain psychological tests can be used to assess the presence, type, and extent of personality disturbance.

Probably the most common instrument in use today is the Minnesota Multiphasic Personality Inventory or MMPI (Hathaway & McKinley, 1943). The clinician working with brain-injured persons consider using some of the available modifications of the standard MMPI. The need for modification is dictated by the fact that patients are often impaired in one or more sensory or motor functions, and thus may not be able to concentrate, read, or mark responses properly. Shortened versions such as the 373-item format or the MMPI-168 (Overall & Gomez-Mont, 1974) are useful alternatives to the full 566-item version. The MMPI-168 is probably the easiest of the very short versions to use since the clinician needs only to administer the standard, group form of the MMPI, stopping after item 168. In addition, one can use a tape-recorded presentation as well as a recent orally presented form that features a rewording of the items so that they can be responded to by "yes" or "no" (Sbordone & Caldwell, 1979).

Other questionnaires or inventories that are useful are the California Personality Inventory or CPI (Gough, 1956) and the Personality Research Form or PRF (Jackson, 1974). The CPI and PRF tend to be less intimidating than the MMPI due to the content of their items. The CPI and PRF permit a more direct identification of variations in "normal" personality traits without relying upon the more pathology-oriented MMPI scales. The task of identifying those in need of assertion training, for example, is best carried out by the CPI, PRF, or other similar instruments.

Certain briefer inventories or questionnaires are available for specific purposes. For example, current distress, along with a number of dimensions, can be evaluated by the Symptom Checklist or SCL-90 (Derogatis, Lipman, & Covi, 1973). While not intended to measure "personality," the SCL-90 (or its revised form, the SCL-90-R) is quite helpful in identifying particular areas of distress that warrant therapeutic investigation and perhaps intervention. An additional benefit of the SCL-90 is the fact that it may be given fairly frequently—as often as once a week. This is not true of such instruments as the MMPI, CPI, or PRF, which are too lengthy and complex for such frequent administration.

Other specific scales are concerned with level of depression. While both the MMPI and SCL-90 can provide information regarding level of dysphoria, the clinician may wish to employ a measure that is specifically designed for that purpose. Two of the most commonly used depression scales are Zung's Self-Rating Depression Scale (Zung, 1965) and Beck's Depression Inventory (Beck & Beck, 1972). Zung's scale consists of 20 statements to which the patient responds by circling one of four possible choices varying from "none or a little of the time" to "most or all of the time." Beck's inventory consists of 13 categories of depressive symptoms and complaints, each of which has 4 statements describing varying degrees of intensity of that symptom. The patient circles the statement(s) that best describe his/her current status.

Evaluating Independence in Daily Living

The major goal of rehabilitation, regardless of the system employed, is to return the patient to a point at or near his/her former level of independence. The evaluation of activities of daily living (ADL) has been an integral part of the initial assessment of brain-injured patients. There are numerous checklists or guides that have been developed locally by clinicians who desired to obtain structured ADL information. The Veterans Administration has compiled a "Self-Care Functional Evaluation" form (VA Form 10-2617, published in 1953), which evaluates activities such as Eating, Communication, Hygiene, Dressing, Locomotion, and Household.

The Vineland Social Maturity Scale (Doll, 1965) can be used as a measure of ADL skills, and since it yields a Social Age and Social Quotient, it provides numerical summary scores that can be readily manipulated statistically.

Many clinicians have adopted the American Association on Mental Deficiency's Adaptive Behavior Scale—or ABS (Nihira, Foster, Shellhaas, & Leland, 1975) for use as a technique for quantifying ADL. The ABS is divided into two parts: part one consists of 10 "domains" relating to independence such as Language Development, Numbers and Time, and Vocational Activity. Part two contains 14 behavioral domains such as Violent and Destructive Behavior, Withdrawal, and Hyperactive Tendencies. While it is comprehensive and objective, the ABS norms are for mentally retarded persons in institutions, and thus the clinician must use caution in inferring normality or nonnormality from the percentile profiles provided.

Some other available ADL measures include Assessing Basic Competence (Guyett, 1975), The Barthel Index (Mahoney & Barthel, 1965), and the Burke Stroke Time-Oriented Profile or BUSTOP (Feigenson, Polkow, Meikle, & Ferguson, 1979). Some briefer methods have recently appeared in the literature, and these are quite useful for quick screening where time does not permit a more thorough assessment (Meissner, 1980a, 1980b).

At the Brain Injury Rehabilitation Unit, we have adopted an experimental ADL form developed by Porch and Collins (1974). The measure is entitled the Rating of Patient's Independence (ROPI), and it consists of three major categories: Self-Care, Socialization, and Communication. Each major category is subdivided into five separte areas.

Each of the areas consists of five standard behaviors or observations that constitute that functional area. What is unique about the ROPI is its reliance upon a complex multidimensional scoring system ranging from 1 to 15. The scores are assigned according to a series of binary choices, beginning with the determination of whether the task is carried out independently. Additional dimensions include: Versatility (i.e., does the patient do all or only some of the task); Consistency (does the patient carry out the task consistently or inconsistently); and Ability (does the patient carry out the task with normal or premorbid ability or with reduced ability).

The numerical results of the ROPI consist of three area averages, along with a global "Overall Average," in addition to 15 subarea scores. All of these measures are plotted on a profile sheet for quick reference and for comparison with previous and/or future evaluations. The multidimensional scoring system allows for subtle differentiations among levels of performance that may be obscured by broader scale methods such as "plus–minus," "yes–no," or even 4- or 5-point rating scales.

Clinicians should choose an ADL measure that suits their needs, both with regard to time of administration and specificity of the information obtained. It would seem that a fairly thorough appraisal of ADL skills would be a requisite for any active treatment program, and that objective and quantified measures are to be preferred over those that are subjective or impressionistic. A recent national survey (Walton, Schwab, Cassatt-Dunn, & Wright, 1980), for example, showed that while respondents gave high ratings to techniques and concepts of ADL evaluation, they indicated a significantly low level of *use* of these concepts and techniques. Clearly, there is need for more intensive research and utilization in the area of ADL skills assessment.

Additional Consultations and Evaluations

There are a number of other consultations that should be considered before admitting a patient for treatment. Aside from the traditional consultations with rehabilitation medicine (physical, occupational, and corrective therapies), referrals should also be made to neurology, psychiatry, audiology, opthalmology, and radiology.

A referral for a clinical neurologic examination should be a routine admission procedure, and should be ordered at once in the event of sudden deterioration in the patient's condition. Information regarding the integrity of the central nervous system is essential in establishing an accurate diagnosis and treatment plan. The neurologist is also able to assess the need to begin or continue antiseizure medication, or to determine the need for additional studies, such as an electroencephalogram (EEG) or cortical evoked potentials.

The psychiatrist can make an independent evaluation of mental status and the presence of mental or personality disorders. Neuropsychologists can assess these observations in the light of their own determinations from the history, interview, and test data. By carefully reviewing past and current medication history, the psychiatrist is then able to recommend dosage changes, discontinuing current medications, or initiating a new medication.

The audiologic examination should be a part of every workup in a rehabilitation setting. The modern techniques of audiometry go far beyond the simple mapping of frequency/intensity thresholds. Some of the newer techniques include completing sentences, speech sounds reception, dichotic listening, and detection of nonorganic hearing losses. Clearly, the clinician must establish the integrity of the auditory system before assessing organic language disorders involving auditory input.

In a similar fashion, the visual system must be determined to be intact prior to evaluating visually dependent functions such as reading, writing, and perceptual–motor skills. The ophthalmologist should be consulted if there is any question of reduced visual acuity and certainly if there are indications of restricted visual fields on clinical testing. Psychological evaluations alone should *never* be accepted as proof of the presence or extent of a visual field loss unless confirmed by careful ophthalmologic testing.

The radiologist should be consulted for the purpose of obtaining a computed tomographic (CT) scan of the head. This procedure will yield a detailed representation of the skull and brain substance that can often be helpful in establishing a treatment plan and prognostic estimate. While serial or repeated CT scans are usually not indicated, pre–post treatment scans are often helpful in attempting to correlate brain anatomical changes with changes in clinical status. Since the CT scans are noninvasive, and are vitually without mortality or morbidity risk (although iodine based contrast media may result in allergic reactions in some patients), patients tolerate the procedure well, as they can remain dressed in their pajamas or street clothes; and the entire process takes less than 20 minutes to complete.

The CT scan will provide objective evidence of the site and extent of many common brain lesions. In addition, the location, size, and content of the ventricles are easily determined with this procedure. Unfortunately, the CT scan provides a "snapshot" that is a static view of brain structure, and not a "motion picture" that is a dynamic view of ongoing brain function. Some newer procedures that provide a more dynamic picture of the brain "in action" are being developed and applied to human brain disorders.

ANALYSIS AND SUMMARIZATION OF NEUROPSYCHOLOGICAL DATA

Use of Profiles

One of the major advantages of standardized neuropsychological assessment is that the clinician may gather normative data on a number of different populations, calculate group means and standard deviations, and finally generate standard scores in the form of T-scores (mean = 50; standard deviation = 10). The test data from a given patient or group of patients can be transformed to T-scores, and then transcribed onto profile forms. Figure 1 illustrates the type of T-score profile form used at the Brain Injury Rehabilitation Unit of the Veterans Administration Medical Center, Palo Alto, California. There are numerous variations in the complexity and structure of these T-score profiles (see, for example, Golden *et al.,* 1979, or Knights & Watson, 1968), but the principle remains the same: to represent neuropsychological test data in a concise, easy-to-read format that does not require intimate knowledge of the meaning of every subtest raw score.

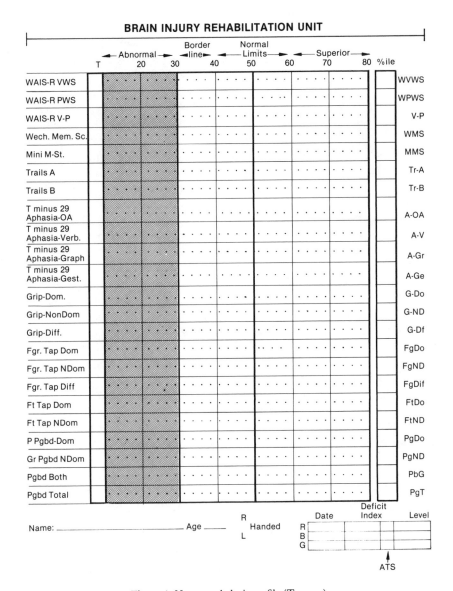

Figure 1. Neuropsychologic profile (T-scores).

Appropriate Norms

However elegant the T-score profiles employed may be, they are apt to be misinterpreted if the reference groups upon which they are based are not relevant to the patient being examined. For example, among normals, there is a definite age factor to be considered on any motor skills measure. According to the WAIS-R manual (Wechsler, 1981) a Digit Symbol raw score of 57–60 is "average" for a 16- to 17-year-old; yet at age 75 a raw score of only 29–33 is considered average. In fact, on virtually every neuropsychological measure, there is a meaningful age effect, especially when one goes beyond age 50 or 60. To compensate for this fact, it is highly advisable to employ "age-weighted" norms whenever possible.

To be maximally useful, normative data should be appropriate to the population under study. For example, if the person is a veteran or a psychiatric patient, the clinician should attempt to utilize norms for those groups. Various authors have presented norms for use with nonhospitalized adults (Pauker, 1977) and children (Knights, 1966), as well as for psychiatric veterans (Swiercinsky, 1978).

It should be noted that not all clinicians support the use of norms in evaluating neuropsychological information. Some prefer to proceed deductively by searching for syndromes or pathognomonic signs. This approach is utilized by those who employ Luria's Neuropsychological Investigation, for example. However, those who use the Luria–Nebraska or Halstead–Reitan methods are using, directly or indirectly, norms that determine the level of cut-off scores. The use of T-scores derived from these norms has the advantage of specifying just how normal or deviant a test performance happens to be. A great deal of useful data is lost when we restrict ourselves to simplistic concepts such as "above" or "below" a given cut-off point. Knowing *how far* above or below can be useful both from the standpoint of identifying problems for treatment and for the determination of prognosis.

NEUROPSYCHOLOGICAL DATA IN THE DETERMINATION OF PROBLEMS, TREATMENTS, AND OUTCOMES

Determining the Problems to be Treated

Once the prospective patient's workup has been completed, the next step in the process involves the generation of the problem list. This process may be carried out in a loose, informal fashion, or it may involve use of a standard problem list. There are a number of such lists in existence (e.g., Meldman, McFarland, & Johnson, 1976), but we have developed a list specifically designed for brain-injured patients (Lynch & Mauss, 1981). Table 1 illustrates a portion of this list.

Table 1

Brain Injury Rehabilitation Unit's Standard
Problems List (Parts I and II)

I. Cognitive problems

A. Memory difficulty
   1. Auditory
   2. Visual
   3. Spatial
   4. Temporal disorientation
B. Impaired receptive language in:
   1. Reading comprehension
   2. Word recognition
   3. Auditory comprehension
C. Impaired expressive language in:
   1. Writing
   2. Word finding
   3. Fluency
   4. Spelling
D. Math difficulty

II. Sensory motor problems

A. Impaired sensory analysis
   1. Visual
      a. Field cuts
      b. Suppression/inattention
      c. Low acuity
   2. Impaired hearing
   3. Impaired body awareness
B. Impaired motor function
   1. Constructional apraxia
   2. Impaired fine-motor coordination
   3. Impaired gross-motor coordination
   4. Extremity weakness
   5. Impaired physical conditioning
   6. Impaired flexibility
   7. Impaired ambulation
   8. Difficulty swallowing
   9. Dysarthria

By carefully reviewing each problem on the list for each patient, it is possible to arrive at a comprehensive problem list that encompasses all potential areas of dysfunction. A thorough neuropsychological assessment is indispensable in identifying and quantifying problem areas. While such a procedure may result in rather lengthy problem lists, it does allow the clinician to then decide which problems are more critical and in need of immediate attention. Frequently, problems may be identified but not treated, or they may be deferred for some specified time.

Table 2

Standard Treatments and Outcome Measures to Accompany Problem List

Problem	Treatment	Outcome measure
IV. Emotional		
A. Depression/anxiety	A. Rap group Psychotherapy Relaxation training Swimming Medication Patient education	A. Depression or Anxiety Scale (Zung, Beck, SCL-90-R, or MMPI)
B. Low self-esteem	B. Assertion training Rap group Language group Social skills group Physical conditioning	B. MMPI (ES and D scales)
C. Nonassertion	C. Assertion training Rap group Social skills group	C. Assertion Index (From PRF)
D. Aggressive behavior	D. Assertion training Behavior modification Anger control class	D. Individualized behavioral measure
E. Family discord	E. Marital counseling Family counseling Family support group Individual therapy	E. Taylor–Johnson Temperament Analysis
V. Social		
A. Impaired self-care (e.g., dressing, grooming, toileting)	A. Occupational therapy Specific retraining Adaptive devices	A. ROPI—Self-care Scales A–E
B. Impaired interpersonal skills	B. Social skills and communication group Assertive training Rap group	B. ROPI— Socialization B
C. Impaired independent living		
1. Clothing	1. Teaching machines (TMs) Consumer "clothing"	1. ROPI—Self- care, A-1 Socialization, E-1
2. Finances	2. TMs—Various financial/ money management programs	2. ROPI— Socialization E
3. Food	3. TMs—Consumer "food"	3. Able to buy and prepare food
4. Housing	4. TMs—Consumer shelter Social work referral Counseling Staff assistance	4. Independent living (if appropriate)
D. Impaired use of transportation	D. Teaching machine (Consumer affairs— transportation)	D. ROPI— Socialization C

(continued)

Table 2. (*Cont.*)

Problem	Treatment	Outcome measure
	V. Social	
E. Job impairment	Transportation class (Foothill Community House) Supervised experience Driver education E. Teaching machines (Full-time employment) Vocational rehabilitation Volunteer work Vets workshop Strong–Campbell II	E. ROPI— Socialization D

The mere process of identifying problems serves the purpose of bringing a focus to the rehabilitative effort. Staff and patient are made aware of what is (and what is not) to be treated, and this provides a coherence to the treatment process. It is important to share the original problem list with the patient and his/her family, both at the onset and throughout treatment.

Determining Appropriate Treatments

The problem list is only a means to an end. The purpose of generating a list of problems is to develop a treatment approach that will be maximally effective. There are excellent guides for treating general and specific neurological dysfunction in a long-term rehabilitative setting (see, for example, Craine & Gudeman, 1981; Golden, 1978; Institute of Rehabilitative Medicine, 1979). We have borrowed from these authors and developed a tentative list of "standard treatments" to accompany our standard problem list (Lynch & Mauss, 1981). Table 2 illustrates a portion of this list, showing both the problem name and recommended treatment.

Luria (1963) as well as Golden (1978) has described the process of analyzing neuropsychological deficits and strengths as a first step in developing a treatment approach. Essentially, the clinician is advised to seek to utilize spared functional systems or parts of systems to assist in retraining those that are dysfunctional. This simple but elegant prescription is all too often ignored in many treatment approaches, which seem to view impaired higher cortical functions as being somehow "weak" and in need of strengthening through more practice.

The specific treatment approaches to be employed cannot be considered universal across patients or programs. Indeed, it is often advisable to prescribe several *different* (although related) techniques, in order to provide variety and maintain patient interest. The clinician should attempt to select treatments that are both effective and tolerated well by the patient.

It is important, also, to vary the level of difficulty of the treatment tasks within and between sessions. For example, it is often possible to divide tasks into varying levels of difficulty, such as easy, somewhat difficult. very difficult, and impossible to perform. Generally, easy and impossible tasks are not useful to practice. The former do not require practice, while the latter can be frustrating and humiliating. Retraining sessions should focus upon abilities that are within the patient's repertoire—however difficult they may be.

Some clinicians have developed highly structured approaches that skillfully blend easy tasks with more difficult ones (La Pointe, 1978; Porch, 1967). The former serve as "warm-up" tasks as well as "exit" tasks, which reinforce feelings of success during each treatment session.

In summary, the most appropriate treatments are those that directly attack the problem in question but do so in an interesting, comprehensible, and quantifiable fashion.

Determining Outcome

There is a need to define treatment outcome in such a way that it can be measured readily. Generally, if thorough assessment has been carried out initially, and the patient's problems have been carefully articulated, the choice of outcome measures is not difficult. The outcome measure should bear directly upon the particular treatment being employed. A common technique consists of readministering the test that was used to identify the problem initially, thus providing a measure of change (presumably) due to treatment. The question of *significance* of difference between pre- and posttreatment is a difficult one to resolve, however.

Certainly, such factors as task difficulty, level of motivation, and time-since-injury will contribute significantly to the occurrence and magnitude of test–retest differences in a rehabilitation setting. Tests that have a known standard error of measurement (such as the Wechsler Intelligence Scales) are helpful, in that one can assume that differences exceeding this range can be considered significant. Unfortunately, most neuropsychological tests do not have published standard errors of measurement. The clinician should bear in mind, however, that the critical objective in rehabilitation is not to demonstrate changes in test scores, but to bring about observable and consistent changes in ADL, affective state, level of communication, memory, or ambulation.

One of the most direct methods for determining treatment outcome is to compare posttreatment status in a given area with pretreatment predictions for that area. Using a technique such as Goal Attainment Scaling (Kiresuk & Sherman, 1968), each problem that is identified upon admission is given a realistic, probable target level to be accomplished after a reasonable treatment period. Other levels of possible outcome may then be expressed: much less than expected; less than expected; greater than expected; or much greater than expected. A specific measurement is prescribed in advance, along with the approximate date for the follow-up evaluation. Thus at the end of 6 months, the patient is reevaluated to determine whether the predicted targets have been reached. In this fashion, effects of a specific treatment, as well as the success of treatment as a whole, can be quickly determined by inspection.

The particular outcome measures to be chosen should be psychometric tests that yield specific numeric scores. When this is not possible, more observational or impressionistic assessment techniques may be suitable. This is especially true of such problems as "aggressive behavior," "inappropriate passivity," or "impaired interpersonal skills," which do not lend themselves easily to precise measurement.

For determining more general levels of outcome, there are several useful scales available. These include the Glasgow Outcome Scale (Jennett, Teasdale, & Knill-Jones, 1975) or the scales described by Roberts (1979) for assessing central neural disability (CND) and mental disability (MD).

The Glasgow Outcome Scale (GOS) consists of five levels of outcome ranging from Death to Good Recovery. The GOS has attained some popularity both in Europe and in the United States. The Roberts scales are more complex and include numerical weights ranging from no disability (a score of 0) to decerebrate dementia (a score of 5).

Each grade on the Roberts scales has specific criteria to assist the evaluator. The clinician will find these scales useful as means of specifying the patient's general status at various points in the rehabilitative process. The numeric values also permit certain prognostic generalizations based upon a large scale research study (Roberts, 1979).

BRIEF OVERVIEW OF FACTORS DETERMINING PROGNOSIS

There are a number of variables that contribute to prognosis when dealing with brain-impaired patients. Some of these will be outlined below, although a thorough discussion of each would extend beyond the scope of this chapter.

Age at Onset

It is generally agreed that the older a patient is at onset of disability, the more profound the initial deficit seems to be, and the more permanent the impairment becomes (Roberts, 1979). This is perhaps best illustrated by the fact that patients who sustain extensive dominant hemisphere brain damage at or shortly after birth

Table 3
Relationship between Age at Injury and
Percentage of Death (D) and Persistently
Vegetative State (PVS)[a]

Age at injury	Percentage D or PVS
0–19	37
20–59	53
60 or older	88

[a]Adapted from Jennet (1976).

are often able to acquire normal language abilities while a similar lesion in an adult results in profound aphasia. A related factor is that older patients often contract more illnesses and are subject to "normal" brain changes due to aging. As a result, they may not be able to participate with full intensity in a rehabilitation progam (Golden, 1978).

Jennett (1976) showed that there was a relationship between age at injury and the percentage of patients who either died or attained only a persistently vegetative state. (See Table 3.) Bakay and Glasauer (1980) point out that age is an important factor in survivors of head injuries, such that in younger patients only 5% to 15% suffer permanent serious sequelae such as aphasia or debilitating motor deficits. Therefore, from the above data, it is clear that age is an important determining factor in the short and long-term effects of head injury.

Location and Type of Injury

Head inuuries that affect the lower brain center (brain-stem) tend to create more profound and lasting neurological deficits. As Bakay and Glasauer (1980) pointed out, severe midbrain damage (characterized by deep coma, fixed, dilated pupils, or decerebrate posturing) is associated with a poor prognosis. Jennett (1976) noted that when eye movements remain normal, 31% of head-injured patients either die or remain vegetative; yet when eye movements are *impaired*, the rate rises to 64%, and when eye movements are *absent*, to 95%. He also observed that 83% of patients evidencing an abnormal (i.e., extensor or flaccid) response to pain have an outcome of either death or vegetative state.

Roberts (1979) states that in his series some children who were decerebrate for 2½ *weeks* recovered almost completely; yet, *no* patients who were decerebrate for more than 3 months recovered to beyond the vegetative state.

The side of the brain that sustains the initial impact has been shown to be a significant factor in outcome. Roberts (1979) concludes that in uncomplicated injuries (i.e., nonpenetrating injuries that are not surgically decompressed), right head impact results in aphasia over twice as often as left head impact. Complicated injuries (penetrating injuries or surgically treated injuries) showed no right–left head impact difference with regard to the occurrence of aphasia. Of the 85 patients in Roberts' series who became aphasic, 52 had right head impact and 33 had left.

The phenomenon of "contre-coup" is critical in understanding the Roberts (1979) data. Contre-coup refers to the common occurrence of cerebral injury at a point diametrically opposite the site of impact. The fact that the brain is surrounded by cerebrospinal fluid and therefore "floating," results in considerable movement of the brain within the skull upon sudden acceleration or deceleration. Often the injury is greater distal to the site of impact because the brain is suddenly driven into the inner surface of the skull at a point opposite the point of initial impact. Additional injury occurs when the inferior surface of the brain is scraped across the uneven basal surface of the skull.

With regard to the type of injury, it appears that direction of the impact is an important variable. Linear impact is less damaging than rotational impact of equal force . Linear impact is that which is directly front-to-back or back-to-front, or left-to-right or right-to-left in relation to the head's central axis. Rotational impact is anything other than straight front–back or side–side, and which therefore produces greater movement of both cortical and subcortical structures. Closed head injuries carry a more favorable prognosis than penetrating injuries or injuries that require surgical decompression (Roberts, 1979).

Sudden deceleration (as in an automobile accident) appears to be more damaging than sudden acceleration (as when one is struck on the head by a blunt object) where the head is free to move (Bakay & Glasauer, 1980).

Duration of Coma

Duration of coma has long been considered a key determinant of outcome from head injury. In one study of the significance of posttraumatic coma in 320 patients (Carlsson, von Essen, & Löfgren, 1968) it was concluded that ultimate recovery or "restitution" (return to work or return to self-care) was independent of coma duration in patients of 20 years and younger.

In the 21–50 age group, all patients who were in coma for 1 day or less reached the level of restitution. When coma persisted for a period of up to a week, the percentage who recovered fell to 50%, and if coma extended beyond 12 days, recovery was not observed. In patients 51 and older, about 50% recovered if coma did not exceed 5 days.

Heiskanen and Sipponen (1970) defined the limits of coma, which were compatible with subsequent return to work for four age groups. In the under-20 group, 4 weeks was found to be the maximum duration of coma for those who returned to work; for ages 20–40, the allowable duration fell to 3 weeks; for the 40–60 group, 1 week; and for the over-60 group, 24 hours.

Roberts (1979) noted that while decerebration following head injury sustained over the age of 35 is highly predictive of severe cognitive disability, those who were merely confused (and not comatose) and with a posttraumatic amnesia of less than 2 weeks, fare much better. He found that 36 of 43 such patients were back at work within 3 months.

Overall, while certainly an important variable in assessing the severity of brain trauma, coma is only one factor and its exact contribution is not completely understood (Bricolo, Turazzi, & Feriotti, 1980).

Duration of Posttraumatic Amnesia

Posttraumatic amnesia or PTA is defined as the period between a head injury and the return of normal memory functions. Recently, more objective criteria for determining the existence of PTA have been suggested (Artiola, Fortuny, Briggs, Newcombe, Ratcliff, & Thomas, 1980; Levin, O'Donnell, & Grossman, 1979). Jennett (1976) found that if PTA lasts less than 1 week, 91% of his series had a good recovery (GR). However if PTA lasted more than 2 weeks, only 53% had a GR, and with a PTA greater than 4 weeks, the percentage of GRs fell to 11%.

Roberts (1979) reported that in his series, those who were decerebrate and had a PTA exceeding 5 weeks were severely disabled or worse both cognitively and neurologically.

It seems clear from the available evidence that PTA reflects the severity of the head injury, and this is inversely related to the potential for general cognitive recovery after craniocerebral trauma.

Neuropsychological Test Patterns and Prognosis

There are certain test factors that contribute to prognosis after brain trauma. The first of these is overall level of performance. Briefly, the better a patient performs initially, the better he will perform at the completion of treatment. Thus, an insignificant Impairment Index (Reitan, 1955), an average T-score of 40 or more (Kiernan & Matthews, 1976), or a Deficit Index of less than .20 (Knights & Watson, 1968) on a battery of neuropsychological tests should be considered a favorable indicator on initial testing. Such a finding would argue against the presence of severe cognitive or perceptual–motor dysfunction.

A second factor is that of the distribution of deficit. Focal, circumscribed deficit is felt to be more favorable than bilateral, generalized, or diffuse impairment. Theoretically, the more brain that remains functional, the less chance that significant functional systems will be compromised (Luria, 1964). In addition, a focal lesion is not likely to stem from severe brain trauma (which usually results in both coup and contrecoup injury, edema, and possible space-occupying accumulations of blood).

With regard to patterns of test scores, variability is generally considered to be indicative of a potential for change. The greater the variability, the more opportunity for improvement. The implication is that if there are spared, as well as impaired, functions, the former will facilitate recovery of the latter.

Certain tests in the neuropsychological battery are quite sensitive to general cortical efficiency. The Category Test, Tactual Performance Test location score, and Part B of the Trail Making Test are examples of such tests (Reitan, 1966). High scores on any of the three are suggestive of some intact higher cortical functions, which can be exploited in treatment in spite of coexisting memory or motor deficits.

The absence of a severe language disorder on aphasia testing is a favorable indicator (Richardson, 1973). In general, patients with receptive or sensory language disorders fare less well than those with expressive or motor language dysfunction (with adequate comprehension).

Finally, it is known that patients who evidence marked behavioral changes featuring disinhibition, concreteness, depression, or irritability are less likely to respond to a typical program of rehabilitation unless their emotional difficulties are dealt with simultaneously (Richardson, 1973).

CONCLUSION

Recent Trends in the Field

In the past 10 years, a number of developments have taken place that have exerted a significant influence upon the field of rehabilitation neuropsychology. For example, the development of cortical evoked potentials as a diagnostic as well as a research tool has led to an expansion of our knowledge of brain functions (see, for example, Greenberg, Becker, Miller, & Mayer, 1977; Greenberg, Mayer, Becker, & Miller, 1977; John, 1977; or Starr, 1978).

In the middle 1970s, computed tomography (CT) began to take its place of prominence as a neurodiagnostic tool. Oldendorf (1978) reviewed the development of the CT scanning process in a recent article, which also describes the other principal brain-imaging techniques such as angiography and radionuclide brain scanning. The current status of CT scanning has not eliminated the need for neuropsychological assessment. Rather, it has necessitated a shift in emphasis from that of "lesion hunting" to that of describing patterns of neuropsychological deficits and strengths for both diagnostic and prognostic purposes. In my view, this development represents a long overdue refocusing upon a unique contribution of clinical neuropsychology.

The measurement of regional cerebral blood flow has become more refined in recent years (Ingvar & Ciria, 1975; Raichle, 1975). This technique has permitted a view of the brain that is more dynamic and concerned with describing functional, rather than structural, properties of normal and abnormal brains.

In recent months, new attention has been directed upon a procedure termed positron emission tomography (PET). PET is a technique whereby a radioactive substance with a brief half-life is injected into the bloodstream in order that a series of detectors situated around the head can detect the emission of positive electrons (positrons) that are released within the skull (Buschbaum *et al.*, 1982; Ter-Pogossian, Raichle, & Sobel, 1980).

Positron emission tomography can be used to detect blood flow, as well as oxygen or glucose metabolism, within the cerebral hemispheres. Here, again, a dynamic view of the brain "in action" is made possible by this technological development. Ingvar and Ciria (1975) and others have shown that presenting stimuli (auditory, tactile, or visual) to the patients or requesting that they speak or move results in appropriate regional increases in blood flow. The information on regional blood flow or metabolism of oxygen or glucose can be helpful in understanding the energy requirement levels and patterns in both normal and impaired brains. Such data are valuable in comprehending the specific effects of brain lesions, as well as the optimum type and timing of neuropsychological rehabilitation.

New Developments and Future Trends

Neuropsychological assessment in rehabilitation promises to be a rapidly growing subspecialty within the field of clinical neuropsychology. Some likely new developments would include increased use of automated techniques to present, analyze, and interpret neuropsychological test data. This trend is made necessary by the increase in available normative data, which require translation of raw scores into appropriate standard scores (typically, T-scores). Without an automated system of analysis, the clinician is forced to refer to numerous sets of normative data, depending upon whether his/her patient is a child or adult, veteran or nonveteran, or psychiatrically healthy or impaired. An original attempt at a scoring and interpretive program was published by Russell, Neuringer, and Goldstein (1970). Other automated approaches have been developed for both children (Knights, 1973; Knights & Watson, 1968) and adults (Adams, Rennick, & Rosenbaum, 1975).

However, further work needs to be carried out, preferably in a collaborative effort among several centers, so that data from a sufficient sample of patients of varying ages, lesion types, and chronicity of lesion can be obtained. The need to develop more rigorous methods for gathering and analyzing neuropsychological data is evident from several recent papers dealing with factorial patterns inherent in neuropsychological batteries (see, for example, Swiercinsky, 1979). Such studies should lead to a reorganization of the current neuropsychological test batteries and even to the total elimination of certain subtests that are redundant or noncontributory.

A further development in neuropsychological assessment in rehabilitation will be the generation of predictive formulas that will permit early prognostic statements. Such work has already begun in the fields of brain trauma (Jennett, Teasdale, Braakman, Minderhood, & Knill-Jones, 1976; Roberts, 1979; Stablein, Miller, Choi, & Becker, 1980) and stroke rehabilitation (Porch, Collins, Wertz, & Friden, 1980). These investigators have attempted to develop predictive rules based upon what is known about the effects of such factors as age at onset, type of lesion, or duration of coma and PTA. It has been demonstrated, not surprisingly, that accuracy of prediction increases with time, that is, the further beyond the onset one makes the prediction, the more correct the prediction is apt to be. Also, the more general the prediction (e.g., live or not live), the more accurate it will be.

There is every reason to anticipate that neuropsychologists will develop decision rules or regression equations similar to those of the investigations noted above. In so doing, they will greatly increase the value of their assessments in rehabilitation settings.

REFERENCES

Adams, K., Rennick, P., & Rosenbaum, G. *Automated clinical interpretation of the neuropsychological battery.* Paper presented at annual meeting of International Neuropsychology Society, Tampa, Florida, 1975.

Artiola, L., Fortuny, I., Briggs, M., Newcombe, F., Ratcliff, G., & Thomas, C. Measuring the duration of posttraumetic amnesia. *Journal of Neurology, Neurosurgery, and Psychiatry,* 1980, *43,* 377–379.

Bakay, L., & Glasauer, F. *Head injury.* Boston: Little, Brown, 1980.

Beardsley, J., Matthews, C., Cleeland, C., & Harley, J. Neuropsychological test battery: Adults 15 and older. Unpublished mimeograph, University of Wisconsin at Madison, 1972.

Beck, A., & Beck, R. Screening depressed patients in family practice. *Postgraduate Medicine,* 1972, *52,* 81–85.

Benton, A. *Revised visual retention test* (4th ed.). New York: Psychological Corporation, 1974.

Benton, A., Hamsher, K., & Stone, F. *Visual retention test: Multiple choice I.* Iowa City: Division of Behavioral Neurology, 1977.

Bricolo, A., Turazzi, S., & Feriotti, G. Prolonged posttraumatic unconsciousness—Therapeutic assets and liabilities. *Journal of Neurosurgery,* 1980, *52,* 625–634.

Buschbaum, M., Ingvar, D., Kessler, R., Waters, R., Cappelletti, J., van Kammen, D., King, A. C., Johnson, J., Manning, R., Flynn, R., Mann, L., Bunney, W., & Sokoloff, L. Cerebral glucography with positron tomography. *Archives of General Psychiatry,* 1982, *39,* 251–259.

Buschke, H., & Fuld, P. Evaluating storate, retention, and retrieval in disordered memory and learning. *Neurology,* 1974, *24,* 1019–1025.

Carlsson, C. A., von Essen, C., & Löfgren, J. Factors affecting the clinical course of patients with severe head injuries. Part I: Influence of biological factors. Part II: Significance of posttraumatic coma. *Journal of Neurosurgery,* 1968, *29,* 242–251.

Christensen, A. L. *Luria's neuropsychological investigation.* New York: Spectrum Publications, 1975.

Craine, J., & Gudeman, H. (Eds.). *The rehabilitation of brain functions: Principles, procedures, and techniques of neurotraining.* Springfield, Ill.: Charles C Thomas, 1981.

Crosson, B., & Warren, R. Use of the Luria–Nebraska neuropsychological battery in aphasia: A conceptual critique. *Journal of Consulting and Clinical Psychology,* 1982, *50,* 22–31.

Derogatis, L., Lipman, R., & Covi, L. SCL-90: An outpatient psychiatric rating scale—Preliminary report. *Psychopharmacology Bulletin,* 1973, *9,* 13–28.

Doll, E. *Vineland social maturity scale condensed manual of directions.* Circle Pines, Minn.: American Guidance Service, 1965.

Feigenson, J., Polkow, L., Meikle, R., & Ferguson, W. Burke stroke time-oriented profile (BUS-TOP): An overview of patient function. *Archives of Physical Medicine and Rehabilitation,* 1979, *60,* 508–511.

Golden, C. *Diagnosis and rehabilitation in clinical neuropsychology.* Springfield, Ill.: Charles C Thomas, 1978.

Golden, C., Hammeke, T., & Purisch, A. Diagnostic validity of a standardized neuropsychological battery derived from Luria's neuropsychological tests. *Journal of Consulting and Clinical Psychology,* 1978, *46,* 1258–1265.

Golden, C., Purisch, A., & Hammeke, T. *The Luria–Nebraska neuropsychological battery.* Lincoln: University of Nebraska Press, 1979.

Goldman, R., Fristoe, M., & Woodcock, R. *G-F-W auditory memory tests.* Circle Pines, Minn.: American Guidance Service, 1974.

Goldstein, K., & Scheerer, M. Abstract and concrete behavior. *Psychological Monographs,* 1941, *53* (Whole no. 239).

Goodglass, H., & Kaplan, E. *The assessment of aphasia and related disorders.* Philadelphia: Lea & Febiger, 1972.

Gough, H. *The California psychological inventory.* Palo Alto, Ca.: Consulting Psychologists Press, 1956.

Graham, F., & Kendall, B. Memory-for-designs-test: Revised general manual *Perceptual and Motor Skills,* 1960, *11,* 147–188.

Greenberg, R., Becker, D., Miller, J., & Mayer, D. Evaluation of brain function in sevre human head trauma with multimodality evoked potentials: Part II. *Journal of Neurosurgery,* 1977, *47,* 163–177.

Greenberg, R., Mayer, D., Becker, D., & Miller, J. Evaluation of brain function in severe human head trauma with multimodality evoked potentials: Part I. *Journal of Neurosurgery,* 1977, *47,* 150–162.

Guyett, I. P. *Assessing basic competence.* Pittsburgh: Institute for Human Services, 1975.

Halstead, W. *Brain and intelligence: A quantative study of the frontal lobes.* Chicago: University of Chicago Press, 1947.

Hathaway, S., & McKinley, J. *The Minnesota multiphasic personality inventory.* New York: The Psychological Corporation, 1943.

Heiskanen, O., & Sipponen, P. Prognosis of severe brain injury. *Acta Neurologica Scandinavia,* 1970, *46,* 343–348.

Ingvar, D., & Ciria, M. Assessment of severe damage to the brain by multiregional measurements of cerebral blood flow. In CIBA Foundation Symposium 34: *Outcome of severe damage to the central nervous system.* New York: American Elsevier, 1975, pp. 97–117.

Institute of Rehabilitation Medicine. *Working approaches to remediation of cognitive deficits in brain damaged.* New York: IRM, 1979.

Jackson, D. *Personality research form manual.* Goshen, N.Y.: Research Psychologists Press, 1974.

Jennett, B. Assessment of the severity of head injury. *Journal of Neurosurgery and Psychiatry,* 1976, *39,* 647–655.

Jennett, B., Teasdale, G., Braakman, R., Minderhood, J., & Knill-Jones, R. Predicting outcome in individual patients after severe head injury. *Lancet,* 1976, *1,* 1031–1034

Jennett, B., Teasdale, G., & Knill-Jones, R. Prognosis after severe head injury. CIBA Foundation Symposium 34: *Outcome of severe damage to the central nervous system.* New York: American Elsevier, 1975, pp. 309–324.

John, E. *Neurometrics: Clinical applications of quantitative electrophysioogy.* Hillsdale, N.J.: Lawrence Erlbaum Associates, 1977.

Keenan, J., & Brassell, E. *Aphasia language performace scales.* Murfresboro, Ind: Pinnacle Press, 1975.

Kiernan, R., & Matthews, C. Impairment Index versus T-score averaging in neuropsychological assessment. *Journal of Consulting and Clinical Psychology,* 1976, *44,* 951–957.

Kiresuk, T., & Sherman, R. Goal attainment scaling: A general method for evaluating comprehensive community mental health programs. *Community Mental Health Journal,* 1968, *4,* 443–453.

Knights, R. *Normative data on tests for evaluating brain damage in children from 5 to 14 years of age.* London, Ont.: Department of Psychology, University of Western Ontario (Research Bulletin No. 20), 1966.

Knights, R. Problems of criteria in diagnosis: A profile similarity approach. *Annals of the New York Academy of Sciences,* 1973, *205,* 124–131.

Knights, R., & Watson, P. The use of computerized test profiles in neuropsychological assessment. *Journal of Learning Disabilities,* 1968, *1,* 696–709.

La Pointe, L. Aphasia therapy: Some principles and strategies for treatment. In Donnell F. Johns (Ed.), *Clinical management of neurogenic communicative disorders.* Boston: Little, Brown, 1978.

Levin, H. S., O'Donnell, V. M., & Grossman, R. G. The Galveston Orientation and Amnesia Test: A practical scale to assess cognition after head injury. *Journal of Nervous and Mental Disease,* 1979, *167,* 675–684.

Lezak, M. Living with the characterologically altered brain injured patient. *Journal of Clinical Psychiatry,* 1978, *39,* 592–598.

Luria, . R. *Restoration of function after brain injury.* New York: Macmillan, 1963.

Luria, A. Neuropsychology in the local diagnosis of brain damage. *Cortex,* 1964, *1,* 3–18.

Luria, A. *Higher cortical functions in man.* New York: Basic Science Books, 1966.

Luria, A., & Majovski, L. Basic approaches used in American and Soviet clinical neuropsychology. *American Psychologist,* 1977, *32,* 959–968.

Lynch, W., & Mauss, N. Brain injury rehabilitation: Standard problem lists. *Archives of Physical Medicine and Rehabilitation,* 1981, *62,* 223–227.

Mahoney, F., & Barthel, D. Functional evaluation: Barthel index. *Maryland State Medical Journal,* 1965, *14,* 61–65.

Meissner, J. Assessing a geriatric patient's need for institutional care. *Nursing '80,* 1980, *10* (March) (a), 86–87.

Meissner, J. Evaluate your patient's level of independence. *Nursing '80,* 1980, *10* (September) (b), 72–73.

Meldman, M., McFarland, G., & Johnson, E. *The problem-oriented psychiatric index and treatment plans.* St. Louis: C. V. Mosby, 1976.

Nihira, K., Foster, R., Shellhaas, M.. & Leland, H. *AAMD adaptive behavior scale.* Washington, D.C.: AAMD, 1975.

Oldendorf, W. The quest for an image of the brain: A brief historical and technical review of brain imaging techniques. *Neurology,* 1978, *28,* 517–533.

Overall, J., & Gomez-Mont, F. The MMPI-168 for psychiatric screening. *Educational and Psychological Measurement,* 1974, *34,* 315–319.

Pauker, J. Adult norms for the Halstead–Reitan neuropsychological test battery: Preliminary data. Unpublished paper presented at Annual Meeting of International Neuropsychological Society, February 1977.

Porch, B. *The Porch index of communicative ability.* (Vol. 1). Palo Alto, Calif.: Consulting Psychologists Press, 1967.

Porch, B., & Collins, M. *The rating of patients' independence (ROPI)*. Albuquerque: VA Medical Center, 1974. (Mimeograph)

Porch, B., Collins, M., Wertz, R., & Friden, T. Statistical prediction of change in aphasia. *Journal of Speech and Hearing Research,* 1980, *23,* 312–321.

Raichle, M. Cerebral blood flow and metabolism. In CIBA Foundation Symposium 34: *Outcome of severe damage to the central nervous system.* New York: American Elsevier, 1975.

Reitan, R. An investigation of the validity of Halstead's measures of biological intelligence. *Archives of Neurology and Psychiatry,* 1955, *73,* 28–35.

Reitan, R. A research program on the psychological effects of brain lesions in human beings. In Norman R. Ellis (Ed.), *International review of research in mental retardation* (Vol. 1). New York: Academic Press, 1966.

Rey, A. L'examen clinique en psychologie. Paris: Presses Universitaires de France, 1964. Cited in M. Lezak, *Neuropsychological assessment.* New York: Oxford, 1976.

Richardson, A. Rehabilitation following central nervous system lesions. In J. Youmans (Ed.), *Neurological sugery (Vol. 3).* Philadelphia: Saunders, 1973.

Roberts, A. *Severe accidental head injury.* New York: Macmillan, 1979.

Russell, E. A multiple scoring method for the assessment of complex memory functions. *Journal of Consulting and Clinical Psychology,* 1975, *43,* 800–809.

Russell, E. Neuringer, C., & Goldstein, G. *Assessment of brain damage: A neuropsychological key approach.* New York: Wiley, 1970.

Sbordone, R., & Caldwell, A. The "OBD-168": Assessing the emotional adjustment to cognitive impairment and organic brain damage. *Clinical Neuropsychology,* 1979, *1,* 36–41.

Schuell, H. *The Minnesota test for the differential diagnosis of aphasia.* Minneapolis: University of Minnesota, 1965.

Smith, A. Objective indices of severity of chronic aphasia in stroke patients. *Journal of Speech and Hearing Disorders,* 1971, *36,* 167–207.

Stablein, D., Miller, J., Choi, S., & Becker, D. Statistical methods for determining prognosis in severe head injury. *Neurosurgery,* 1980, *6,* 243–248.

Starr, A. Sensory evoked potentials in clinical disorders of the nervous system. *Annual Review of Neuroscience,* 1978, *1,* 103–127.

Swiercinsky, D. *Manual for adult neuropsychological evaluation.* Springfield, Ill.: Charles C Thomas, 1978.

Swiercinsky, D. A factorial pattern description and comparison of functional abilities in neuropsychological assessment. *Perceptual and Motor Skills,* 1979, *48,* 231–242.

Taylor, R. *Taylor–Johnson temperment analysis manual.* Los Angeles: Psychological Publication, 1968.

Ter-Pogossian, M., Raichle, M., & Sobel, B. Positron emission tomography. *Scientific American,* 1980, *243,* 170–181.

Tolor, A. A comparison of the Bender–gestalt test and the digit span as measures of recall. *Journal of Clinical Psychology,* 1958, *14,* 14–18.

Veterans Administration. *Self-care activities—Functional evaluation* (VA form No. 10-2617). Washington, D.C.: Government Printing Office, 1953.

Walton, K., Schwab, L., Cassatt-Dunn, M. & Wright, V. Independent living: Perceptions by professionals in rehabilitation. *Journal of Rehabilitation,* 1980, *46,* 57–63.

Warrington, E., & James, M. Disorders of visual perception in patients with localized cerebral lesions. *Neuropsychologia,* 1967, *5,* 253–266.

Wechsler, D. A standardized memory scale for clinical use. *Journal of Psychology,* 1945, *19,* 87–95.

Wechsler, D. *WAIS-R manual: Wechsler Adult Intelligence Scale—Revised.* New York: Psychological Corp., 1981.

Zung, W. A self-rating depression scale. *Archives of General Psychiatry,* 1965, *12,* 63–70.

9

The Neuropsychological Examination of Alcohol and Drug Abuse Patients

OSCAR A. PARSONS and RUSSELL L. ADAMS

The neuropsychological examination has been developed to identify, measure, and describe behavioral changes associated with brain dysfunction. As noted in other chapters in this book, in the neuropsychological examination particular attention is paid to altered higher cortical functions such as abstracting, memory, information processing, problem solving, perceptual spatial analysis, construction, calculating ability, language skills, and sensory–perceptual and sensory–motor functioning. Acute doses of alcohol and other psychoactive drugs may produce temporary and reversible impairment in one or more of these functions. The neuropsychological examination may be used to determine which functions are affected by acute doses of a given drug, but such studies are more in the nature of clinical research with groups of subjects rather than clinical assessment of individuals. In contrast, the chronic use of alcohol and certain other drugs can result in a relatively enduring (at least not easily reversible) impairment in selected higher cortical functions. For persons suffering from such conditions, the individual clinical neuropsychological examination provides information of relevance to diagnosis, treatment, outcome, and rehabilitation. Considering that in the United States there are some 9 to 10 million problem drinkers (Seltzer, 1980; Stinnett, 1977), that depressant drugs are among those most commonly prescribed (Jaffe, 1975),

OSCAR A. PARSONS and RUSSELL L. ADAMS ● Center for Alcohol and Drug Related Studies, Department of Psychiatry and Behavioral Sciences, University of Oklahoma Health Sciences Center, Oklahoma City, Oklahoma 73104. The writing of this chapter was facilitated, in part, by NIAAA Grants AA03032 and AA01464 to Oscar A. Parsons.

that marijuana smoking is rampant in younger people, and that other mind-alter-
ing drugs such as "acid," cocaine, or heroin are used by tens of thousands (Freedman, 1980; Grinspoon & Bakalar, 1980; Ramsey, 1977), the contributions of the
neuropsychologist to what appear to be continuing problems in our culture will
be in demand for decades ahead.

What kinds of questions are posed to clinical neuropsychologists, that is,
what specific contributions may they make to the many problems posed by chronic
alcohol and drug abusers? A sampling of the kinds of cases referred to our neuropsychology laboratory will exemplify the range of such questions.

TYPICAL CASE REFERRALS

Case 1. A 42-year-old man, with a history of drinking a fifth a day for over
15 years, was confused, disoriented, distractable, irritable, and had visual hallucinations for 1 week following admission to the alcohol treatment program. Symptoms worsened in the evening. By the second week these symptoms had disappeared, but at 2 months he had short-term memory disturbances, could not find
his way around the hospital, had calculation difficulties, and was very confused.
Personal grooming was poor and he was depressed. Referral questions: Is there
evidence for dementia, and if so, how severe is it? What potential is there for
rehabilitation?

Case 2. A 55-year-old white male had a history of numerous hospitalizations
for alcoholism. Finally he was admitted for a severe neurological condition with
ataxia of gait, opthalmoplegia, nystagmus, and confusion. Vitamin therapy (B1–
Thiamine) resulted in reduction of symptoms. However, he then developed short-
and long-term memory deficits and confabulation (filling in memory gaps with
incorrect or fanciful presentations). Referral questions: He appears to have an
amnestic syndrome. How pervasive is the memory loss? What rehabilitation procedures would be helpful in compensating for memory loss?

Case 3. A 45-year-old white woman had become addicted to Valium, originally prescribed to "quiet her nerves." Following medical advice, she stopped taking Valium. In several days she became restless and irritable, couldn't sleep, and
paced the floor. She had a seizure, although she had no previous history of epilepsy. At 1 month she is better but complains of insomnia and difficulties in concentration and attention. There is some suspicion that she takes an occasional Valium tablet, although she denies this. Referral question: Prolonged withdrawal
syndrome is suspected. Is there evidence for an acute brain syndrome?

Case 4. An 18-year-old white female had taken several hundred acid (LSD)
trips and had gradually become more strange in her behavior. On the afternoon
of her admission, she had a "bad trip" characterized by anxiety, fears of going
crazy, thoughts that everything was unreal, and continuing visual hallucinations.

Her behavior was so striking that her friends grew concerned and brought her to the emergency room. After several days of hospitalization, the symptoms subsided but she continued to have "flash back" hallucinations over the next several weeks, even though no LSD was taken. Fears that she might be crazy persisted. Referral question: Given this patient's history, is there evidence for a residual dementia?

Case 5. A 22-year-old white woman was brought to the emergency service of the hospital by the police. She had dilated pupils, tachycardia, and nausea. She was very talkative and skipped from topic to topic. She had been at a party and had physically attacked several other young women, claiming they didn't like her and were trying to split up her relationship with her boyfriend. Treated by the hospital's psychiatry service, after a week she lost most of the symptoms but had disturbed sleep and remained convinced that the young women she had attacked were trying to split up her relationship, although her boyfriend reported that this was not the case. The patient had been a regular user of amphetamines for 4 years. Referral questions: Is there evidence for presence of an organic brain syndrome? Prognosis for recovery?

Case 6. A 35-year-old white female tried to commit suicide twice by overdose of phenobarbitol. Each time she had to have resuscitation by an emergency squad, and in one instance she was unconscious for at least several hours. She was distractible, suffered memory loss, and had poor concentration. She was also quite depressed. Currently she complains only of memory loss and depression. Referral question: Is the memory disturbance associated with the continuing depression, or is there mild dementia present?

Case 7. A 24-year-old white male had two successive automobile accidents. He became addicted to barbiturates given for painful residual from the accidents but stopped taking them. Drug screening tests corroborate his contention. However, his personality has changed considerably. Previously outgoing and active, he is now apathetic and dull. Mentation appears slowed but patient denies depression. Referral request: Please evaluate with respect to possible residual organic brain syndrome.

Case 8. A 16-year-old white male had been sniffing paint for several hours a day for the last year. Two weeks ago he had an acute organic brain syndrome. The symptoms have subsided and he seems back to his "normal self" according to the family. Referral questions: Please evaluate intellectual capabilities. Are there any signs of residual organic dementia? Will he be able to finish high school? Prognosis for recovery of function?

Case 9. A 20-year-old white male had a serious head injury (one month in a coma). After recovering sufficiently, he went to vocational rehabilitation for advice and help. According to the vocational counselor, the patient states that he does not drink but he smokes a "joint" every day. Referral questions: Evaluate present level of functioning. What is the potential effect of marijuana smoking in an impaired individual? What strengths does he have for potential training?

Case 10. A 22-year-old white male veteran had a severe psychotic episode after taking a particularly large dose of "angel dust" or PCP (phencyclidine). He had had repeated experiences previously with PCP but none resulting in such a profound reaction. He has recovered and is no longer psychotic, but he is confused, withdrawn, and unable to hold a job. Referral request: Please evaluate for cortical dysfunction and indicate prognosis for recovery.

What information or background must the neuropsychologist have to answer these qestions? First, knowledge of the general type of organic brain syndromes and their characteristics is necessary. Second, background knowledge of the classification of drugs and basic pharmacological concepts would be helpful. Third, a perspective on the natural history of drug abuse as it relates to brain impairment is useful. Fourth, awareness of the effects of certain critical variables on neuropsychological testing is needed. Fifth, the empirical findings from drug and alcohol neuropsychological studies are basic information needed for adequate interpretation, especially as these findings relate to levels of impairment, patterns of impaired and intact abilities, treatment, outcome, and rehabilitation. Sixth, it is necessary to have a familiarity with the basic principles of neuropsychological examination, that is, knowledge of methods of measurement of higher cortical functions and their relationships to presence and type of brain dysfunction in the drug and alcohol abuser. Finally, how are the clinical findings organized and reported? In the subsequent sections of this chapter we will discuss these topics.

ORGANIC BRAIN SYNDROMES AND ORGANIC MENTAL DISORDERS

In 1980, the Third Edition of the Diagnostic and Statistical Manual of Mental Disorders (DSM-III) of the Committee on Nomenclature of the American Psychiatric Association was published (APA, 1980). In the section on Organic Mental Disorders (e.g., those behavioral states in which a temporary or relatively permanent brain dysfunction is present) two classifications are distinguished. "Organic brain syndromes" refer to "a constellation of psychological or behavioral signs and symptoms without reference to etiology (e.g., Delirium, Dementia); organic mental disorder designates a particular brain syndrome in which the etiology is known or presumed (e.g., Alcoholic Withdrawal Delirium, Multi-infarct Dementia)." Thus the Organic Brain Syndromes are the fundamental classification system. Ten syndromes are identified, of which five are particularly important to the clinical neuropsychologist because they all involve changes in higher cortical functions. These five syndromes are Dementia, Amnestic, Delirium, Intoxication, and Withdrawal. Dementia (Case 1 of the Vignettes) and the Amnestic Syndrome (Case 2) both are characterized by loss of intellectual abilities, particularly memory. Dementia, however, involves a more widespread cognitive loss of sufficient magnitude that social and occupational functions usually are diminished. This syndrome is one of the more common accompaniments of organic brain diseases. The Amnestic Syndrome is much more specific (e.g., impairment in short- and long-term memory but otherwise relatively intact intellectual functioning). It is an infrequent disorder and is seen mainly in Korsakoff patients. Both syndromes are considered to be chronic states or disturbances and are diagnosed in the absence of Delirium, Intoxication and Withdrawal.

The Delirium, Intoxication, and Withdrawal syndromes are more temporary and acute states. In the Delirium Syndrome (initial symptoms in Case 1), there is a reduced awareness of the environment, disturbed attention, disorientation, and memory impairment. Perceptual disturbances are frequent. The symptoms may fluctuate over the day. Intoxication and Withdrawal both involve specific substances. Ingestion of these substances (e.g., alcohol, amphetamines, marijuana, LSD) results in symptoms that vary with the substance (e.g., Case 4, initial symptoms). The Withdrawal Syndrome (Case 3) is a specific constellation of behaviors that appear when use of an abused substance is discontinued (e.g., the alcohol and barbiturate withdrawal syndromes).

The remaining Organic Brain syndromes are diagnosed in the absence of delirium and dementia. In the Organic Delusional Syndrome, delusions (beliefs not based on reality) are the major symptoms (Case 5) with no prominent hallucinations (false perceptions); in the Organic Hallucinosis Syndrome, the reverse is the case (Case 4, residual symptoms). In the Organic Affective Syndrome, there is either pronounced depression or mania (euphoric "high") and the absence of delusions and hallucinations (Case 6). For the Organic Personality Syndrome the distinguishing characteristic is a marked personality change, that is, from normal to continual belligerence or apathy (Case 7) and of course the absence of the features of the preceding syndromes. For changed behaviors, in response to a known etiological brain dysfunctional agent, that do not meet any of the above criteria, there is the Atypical or Mixed Organic Brain Syndrome (Cases, 8, 9, and 10).

DRUG CLASSIFICATION AND PHARMACOLOGICAL CONCEPTS

There are many ways of classifying drugs, but for our purposes the classification by Kissin (1977) is the most satisfactory. On the basis of the effects of the drugs on the central nervous system and behavior, Kissin grouped the drugs under three major categories: depressants, stimulants, and hallucinogens. In Table 1, the commonly used and abused drugs and, where appropriate, their trade names, are listed within each of the major classifications. Note that the "depressant" category is by far the largest and is composed of three subcategories: the alcohol group, the barbiturate–sedatives, and morphine and its derivatives. The mode of central ner-

Table 1

Common Psychoactive Drugs[a]

Depressants			Stimulants	Hallucinogens
Alcohol group	Barbiturate–sedatives	Morphine and derivatives		

Alcohol group	Barbiturate–sedatives	Morphine and derivatives	Stimulants	Hallucinogens
Ethanol (alcohol)	**Barbiturates**	Morphine	Cocaine	d-Lysergic acid
Chloral hydrate	Pentobarbital (Nembutal)	Diacetylmorphine	Amphetamine	diethylamide (LSD)
Paraldehyde	Secobarbital (Seconal)	(Heroin)	(Benzedrine)	Psilocybin
Ethchlorvynol (Placidyl)	Amobarbital (Amytal)	Dihydromorphinone	Dextroamphetamine	Bufotenin
Ethinamate (Valmid)	Butabarbital (Butisol)	(Dilaudid)	(Dexedrine)	Dimethyltryptamine (DMT)
Carbromal	Phenobarbital (Luminal)	Codeine	Methamphetamine	Mescaline (peyote)
	Barbital (Veronal)	Camphorated opium tincture	(Desoxyn)	Phencyclidine
	Glutethimide (Doriden)	(Paregoric)	Phenmetrazine	Yohimbine
	Methyprylon (Noludar)	Meperidine (Demerol)	(Preludin)	Δ-Tetrahydrocannabinol
	Methaqualone (Quaalude)	Methadone	Chlorphentermine	Marijuana
	Meprobamate (Miltown;	Pentazocine (Talwin)	(Presate)	Myristicin (nutmeg)
	Equanil)	Dextropropoxyphene	Diethylpropion	
	Benzodiazepines	(Darvon)	(Tenuate; Tepanil)	
	Chlordizepoxide (Librium)			
	Diazepam (Valium)			
	Oxazepam (Serax)			
	Hydroxyzine (Atarax;			
	Vistaril)			

[a]Adapted from Kissin, B., Alcoholism and drug dependence. In R. C. Simons and H. Pardes (Eds.), *Understanding Human Behavior in Health and Illness*. Baltimore: Williams & Wilkins, 1977.

vous system action differs for each major category. Depressants are thought to reduce central nervous system neural excitability with a consequent slowing of behavior and mentation. Stimulant drugs, on the other hand, result in increased neural excitability and a corresponding increase in mental and physical activity. The hallucinogens disrupt normal nervous system activity and result in disturbances in concentration and perception and, with higher doses, hallucinations.

In addition to the classification in Table 1, there is another group of abused drugs that is receiving increasing attention: inhalants. These drugs are so diverse (glue, paint, hydrocarbons) in their behavioral and pharmacological effects that a summarizing description of their central nervous system action is not possible.

Drug abuse is hard to define. However, there are some guidelines that help. First, there is the concept of drug dependence. Does the individual have a psychological need for repeated use of alcohol or other drugs? Does the individual manifest tolerance, that is, taking increasingly larger or more frequent doses to achieve the same effect? Has physical dependence occurred? Physical dependence is the condition where an altered physiological state exists in response to continued use of a drug so that when the drug is discontinued a withdrawal syndrome occurs. Is the person "addicted"? Addiction is defined differently by different authors. For Kissin (1977) addiction is drug dependence involving tolerance and physical dependence and probably only applicable to the depressant drugs and the amphetamines. For Jaffe (1975) addiction refers to a behavioral pattern of compulsive drug use that does not necessarily involve physical dependence. Regardless of which definition is employed, "addicted" individuals are likely to be drug abusers (i.e., using drugs to an extent that interferes with their life adjustment in one or more areas such as health or occupational, familial, or community functioning). Thus, drug abuse usually involves three components: (1) a pattern of pathological use (e.g., inability to control use, need for use to be able to function adequately, use despite health contraindications); (2) impairment in social or occupational functioning; and (3) duration of drug use sufficiently long such that a repetitive pattern can be established (in DSM-III, the minimal time period to establish drug abuse is one month).

The "withdrawal syndrome" is of particular importance for the neuropsychological examiner. When an individual terminates or reduces dosage of a drug that he or she has previously taken to the point of intoxication, a temporary central nervous system reaction may occur. This reaction may differ for different abused drugs, but common symptoms are anxiety, restlessness, irritability, insomnia, and impaired attention (APA, 1980). Abused depressant drugs such as alcohol, the barbiturates, and opiates almost always lead to a withdrawal syndrome. In its mild form, the withdrawal symptoms can be no more severe than those seen with a mild influenza, but extreme withdrawal can result in severe symptoms such as seizures and, in the case of delirium tremens, death. Stimulants such as amphetamines and cocaine give rise to a milder withdrawal reaction characterized by prolonged sleep, low energy levels, easy fatigability, and depressive mood (Jaffe, 1975). Hallucinogens (such as marijuana) and the various inhalants apparently do not lead to withdrawal syndromes (APA, 1980; Kissin, 1977). The time course for the withdrawal syndrome is varied, depending upon drug, dosage, age, and so forth. Most reactions appear to have subsided after 1 week, at least in their overt clinical manifestations. However, areas of disturbed functioning may persist; for example, Begleiter and Porjesz (1979) have recently reported withdrawal changes in brain waves (Event Related Potential) that lasted up to a month! The major point here is that the study of disturbed neurophysiology accompanying withdrawal is in its infancy and that the time course with respect to such subtle changes is unknown for most drugs.

It should be emphasized that the withdrawal syndrome is not confined to instances where drug taking has been totally stopped; it can also occur with *reduction* in amount of drug abused. Thus the syndrome could be maintained by occasional use of the abused drug to relieve the more severe symptoms. The occurrence of even a mild withdrawal syndrome could lead to a quite misleading and pessimistic interpretation of the results of the neuropsychological examination, if the examiner is unaware of its presence and believes the patient is both drug and withdrawal free. The same holds true for presence of mild intoxication from alcohol and other drugs. It is therefore extremely important that the drug abuser be carefully questioned as to current drug or substitute drug usage. Preferably each patient should be given a biomedical screening for drugs by urine or blood tests and, in the case of alcoholics, a breath analysis. The importance of such procedures is underscored by the findings of Grant, Adams, Carlin, Rennick, Judd, Schoof, & Reed (1978), who studied neuropsychological functioning in polydrug abusers. Fifteen percent of 68 polydrug abusers had measurable amounts of drugs in their blood despite the fact that clinical and behavioral self-report scales failed to pick up any signs of intoxication or withdrawal.

NATURAL HISTORY OF ALCOHOL AND DRUG-RELATED DISORDERS

In a recent article, Grant, Reed, and Adams (1980) have contributed a valuable perspective for the neuropsychologist who is examining drug and alcohol abusers for behavioral evidence of brain impairment. Their main points as to time course of neurotoxic effects are summarized in Figure 1. Assuming that a person is born with a healthy brain and the latter remains healthy until point $A(X)$, where the first exposure occurs to a particular neurotoxic substance (e.g., alcohol) that if abused is known to lead to brain dysfunction such as dementia. From $A(X)$ to $A(Y)$, when the first irreversible neuronal changes begin, is termed the latent

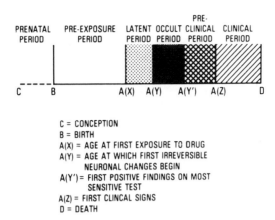

Figure 1. Model for the natural history of neurotoxin-induced dementia (from Grant, Reed, & Adams, 1980, with permission).

period, and no impairment will be found. In the period of $A(Y)$ up to $A(Y')$, however, the first positive findings on testing are observed. From here to $A(Z)$ is the preclinical period in which the prodromal signs are increasing (e.g., in alcoholism, neuropsychological tests of memory or abstracting may show deficits, but a frank organic syndrome is not yet in evidence). At $A(Z)$ the disorder has reached full clinical expression and a definable organic brain syndrome is present. With continued drug abuse and without treatment, the final stage of death (D) occurs.

Using their results and the work of others, Grant *et al.* (1980) estimate that if X is defined as the onset of heavy drinking of alcohol, and if $A(X)$ is 25 years, the latent and occult periods last about a dozen years to age 37, and the preclinical period another dozen to age 49. So the period of time from onset of heavy drinking to the emergence of a clinically diagnosable organic brain syndrome could be about 24 years, although sensitive tests may pick up deficits in patients in their mid-30s. Depending upon the strength of the neurotoxic agent, the amount taken, and the frequency of use, this period could be shortened or lengthened considerably.

One note of caution is that this model assumes that the effects of the neurotoxin are permanent (i.e., once a point such as Y' is reached, deficits will be present from that time on, regardless of cessation of drug taking). Grant *et al.* (1980) point out that this model is oversimplified in that many alcoholics and drug abusers recover at least partially from their deficits if they become abstinent. This has led workers in the field to postulate the presence of an "intermediate stage" of brain damage (Smith, 1977) in alcoholics and polydrug users (Judd & Grant, 1978). Unfortunately, Grant *et al.* (1980) do not alter their model to incorporate this observation. It is extremely important that the neuropsychological examiner recognize that the presence of deficits in the drug abuser in the first several months of abstinence need not indicate a permanent loss of ability.

The attempt by Grant *et al.* to provide a model of the natural history of drug abuse in relation to brain impairment is a good orientation for the neuropsychological examiner. Especially pertinent are the implications that: (a) the neuropsychological examination may be among the first biobehavioral tests to reveal impairment; (b) the absence of behavioral deficits does not mean that brain impairment has not occured; and (c) the finding of neuropsychological deficits in the first several months after abstinence do not necessarily imply permanent deficit.

VARIABLES OF IMPORTANCE IN INTERPRETING NEUROPSYCHOLOGICAL TEST RESULTS

Parsons and Prigatano (1978) and Parsons and Farr (1981) provided detailed consideration of the variables that affect interpretation of neuropsychological test restuls. Other extensive discussions of this topic may be found in Filskov and Boll (1981). In brief, age and education have been shown to be quite significantly related to performance on most neuropsychological tests in normal individuals. The Wechsler Adult Intelligence Scale (WAIS) (Matarazzo, 1972), one of the most commonly used tests in neuropsychological examination, does provide an age correction as part of the process of obtaining the IQ and also provides age-corrected subtest scoring. The Halstead–Reitan Neuropsychological Battery (HRB) (Reitan & Davison, 1974), our most widely used and validated battery in neuropsychology, unfortunately does not provide age correction, so that the examiner has to rely on his general knowledge about studies investigating age and education effects on the overall level of impairment and subtest scores (e.g., Prigatano & Parsons, 1976). These problems are discussed elsewhere in this book.

The new Luria–Nebraska Neuropsychological Battery developed by Golden and his colleagues (Golden, 1981; Golden, Moses, Fishburne, Engum, Lewis, Wisniewski, Conley, Berg, & Graber, 1981) explicitly introduces age and education correction factors. If this test battery is validated in other laboratories, it will undoubtedly have a great methodological advantage over the tests that do not possess such corrections.

There are many other variables such as sex, type of occupation, and so forth, that may affect the results of neuropsychological examinations, but those effects are largely unknown at this time. Finally, there are specific variables associated with each drug that may affect the results. Consider the fact that about 40% of alcoholics have had some type of head injury (Parsons, 1977). Or consider the fact that many toxic impurities are found in street drugs. Are any obtained deficits in the alcohol or drug abuser due to head injury or drug impurities rather than to the drug itself? In subsequent sections we will consider some of these factors in more detail.

NEUROPSYCHOLOGICAL FINDINGS IN ALCOHOL AND DRUG ABUSERS

Alcohol Abusers

We initiate our discussion of this topic by considering the depressant drug alcohol as a prototypical abused drug. It is by far the most abused and has received more systematic study than any of the other abused drugs. Over the last decade there have been numerous reviews of neuropsychological findings in alcoholics (Eckardt & Ryback, 1981; Goldstein, 1976; Goodwin & Hill, 1975; Grant & Mohns, 1975; Kleinknecht & Goldstein, 1972; Miller & Savcedo, 1983; Parsons, 1977; Parsons & Farr, 1981; Parsons & Leber, 1981; Parsons & Leber, 1982; Ron, 1977; Tarter, 1975). There is a consensus in all of these reviews that (a) alcoholics have selective impairment of perceptual–cognitive intellectual functions and (b) the pattern of deficit performance is similar to that seen in other organic brain syndromes.

How impaired are alcoholics? Parsons and Farr (1981) and Parsons and Leber (1981) surveyed the world literature as to results of studies of the HRB. The HRB gives rise to an overall measurement of level of impairment (the Impairment Index) by calculating the ratio of the number of tests on which the individual scores in the impaired range to the total number of tests. An Impairment Index of .5 or above is considered in the impaired range. Parsons & Leber (1981) found that in 18 of 20 studies (90%), alcoholics had significantly higher scores on the Impairment Index than controls, but only in 67% of the studies was the Impairment Index .5 and above. This discrepancy between the comparisons with the controls and application of the Index cut-off point is due to the lack of correction for age, education, and general intelligence effects on the Impairment Index, a point that we made earlier. Nevertheless, the data suggest that the general level of impairment in alcoholics is probably mild to moderate when compared to nonalcoholic peers. What abilities are impaired? Parsons and Farr (1981) concluded that alcoholics had less efficient nonverbal abstracting and problem-solving abilities, visual–spatial and tactual–spatial difficulties, and slowed visuomotor performance. In contrast, verbal abilities as measured by the Verbal Scale of the WAIS were largely intact; almost all alcoholics studied are average to above average in verbal intelligence.

The specific tests on which alcoholics manifested deficit performance compared to controls or established norms are presented in Table 2. As any reader who is even cursorily conversant with neuropsychological studies of brain-damaged patients will recognize, these eight tests, with the possible exception of Picture Arrangement, have been shown repeatedly to be impaired in diverse groups of brain-damaged patients. In addition, in factor analytic studies of the combined WAIS and HRB in the same subjects, most of these tests load on one or two major

Table 2

WAIS and Halstead–Reitan Battery Tests on Which Alcoholics Are Impaired When
Compared to Nonalcoholic Controls[a]

Tests	Response requirement	Psychological process
WAIS		
Block Design	Reproduce visual spatial designs with blocks	Visual–spatial analysis and construction
Digit Symbol	Coding symbols to numbers	Visual–motor speed
Picture Arrangement	Rearrangement scrambled of cartoonlike pictures	Social judgment and sequential reasoning
Object Assembly	Assembly of jigsawlike puzzles	Ability to visualize and construct a gestalt in absence of concrete model
Halstead–Reitan Battery		
Category Test	Selection of attribute or organizing principle for series of visual–spatial stimuli	Nonverbal abstracting and problem solving
Tactual Performance Test— Time	Speed of fitting 10 geometric forms in form board while blindfolded with right hand, left hand, and both hands	Tactual–spatial speed and problem solving
Tactual Performance Test— Location	Drawing on a sheet of paper the location of forms on the form board	Tactual–spatial incidental memory
Trail Making—B	Drawing a line as rapidly as possible alternating between letters and numbers scattered over the page, e.g., 1 to A to 2 to B, etc.	Visual–motor speed and set flexibility

[a]Six of these eight tests (omitting Picture Arrangement and Object Assembly) comprise Reitan's (1973) Brain-Age-Quotient and are considered by him to be the most sensitive cognitive tests for measuring the effects of aging and brain damage.

factors corresponding to the Verbal and Performance Scale factor (Fabian, Parsons, & Silberstein, 1981; Goldstein & Shelly, 1971; Grant *et al.*, 1978).

Further, six of the eight tests (excluding Object Assembly and Picture Arrangement) have been identified by Reitan (1973) as the best measures of "current problem-solving ability" and the most sensitive to brain impairment. Reitan (1973) also has shown that these tests are quite sensitive to aging effects; that is, performance declines more rapidly over the decades on these six tests than on verbal tests such as WAIS, Vocabulary, Comprehension, and Similarities. In fact, he has developed a "Brain-Age-Quotient" (BAQ) based on these tests, which when corrected for age gives a score for which the normal value is 100. Both male and female alcoholics have significantly lower BAQs than controls. In a study of male alcoholics, the $\overline{X}$ BAQ was 88.1 compared to controls' 102.7 (Schau & O'Leary, 1977). In a study of female alcoholics, the $\overline{X}$ BAQ was 90 for the alcoholics and 100.4 for controls (Hochla, Parsons, & Fabian, 1982).

There seems to be little doubt that alcoholism results in mild but significant impairment in nonverbal abstracting, problem solving, and perceptual–motor speed. This is not to say that all verbal abilities are spared in alcoholics. Parsons and Leber (1981) have pointed out that while tests of verbal intelligence such as WAIS Vocabulary, Comprehension, and Similarities are typically intact in alcoholics, impaired functioning has been found on tests involving verbal memory, learning, problem solving, and abstracting. As abstracting tasks become more difficult or involve more problem-solving components, alcoholics are more prone to manifest deficits.

Do neuropsychological test results predict treatment course, outcome, and recovery? There is little data bearing on these questions. Only one study has been done to our knowledge in which the relationship between neuropsychological tests and treatment variables is examined. Leber and Parsons (1980) reported significant correlations between neuropsychological test performance and ratings by therapists as to behavior in therapy and prognosis. Alcoholics who had better perceptual–motor performance scores on tests such as Digit Symbol and Trails B were better participants in therapy, according to their therapist's ratings. Scores on the Block Design, Wisconsin Card Scoring Test, and Trails B were predictive of therapists' ratings of prognosis; patients with good prognosis performed better on these tests than patients with poor prognosis.

In the prediction of outcome of treatment and recovery, data are also sparse, although increasing attention to this question is visible in the literature. The first question to be addressed is whether there is recovery from neuropsychological deficits in abstinent alcoholics? Evidence favors a "yes" response but it is by no means an unqualified "yes." Parsons and Leber (1981) reviewed 22 studies of alcoholics who were initially tested in treatment programs and then retested at least once at a subsequent time. Improvement on retesting occurred in alcoholics in most studies, however, when control groups were also retested, they were frequently still significantly better than alcoholics (i.e., both groups improved but maintained the same differential). The one area of agreement seems to be that if alcoholics performed more poorly initially on verbal tests, they usually recovered to control levels by retesting. For nonverbal abstracting, problem solving, and perceptual–motor tests, results are varied (Parsons & Leber, 1981): Different studies find different patterns of recovery.

One of the problems in follow-up studies of alcoholics is that a certain number of the alcoholics resume drinking. There is evidence to suggest that these alcoholics perform more poorly on retest than those who abstain or have modest intake (Eckardt, Parker, Pautler, Noble, & Gottschalk, 1980). In an unpublished study in our laboratories, using a sample of male VA patients similar to Eckardt *et al.* (1980), we have also found that those alcoholics who resume drinking perform more poorly at retest 6 months later than do their abstinent peers, although both groups perform significantly more poorly than retested controls. In contrast, Schau, O'Leary, and Chavey (1980) found no differences between abstainers and modest resumers versus moderate to severe resumers.

Finally, do neuropsychological tests predict relapse? Again there is suggestive evidence beginning to accrue to indicate that such tests may be useful in prediction. Abbott and Gregson (1981) have shown that a "Patterned Cognitive Impairment Test" and a booklet form of the Rod and Frame Test predicted relapse weeks before relapse occurred in alcoholics at levels higher than most other social, demographic variables. Alcoholics who performed more poorly on these tests had significantly fewer weeks before resuming drinking. In our unpublished study referred to earlier, our male alcoholics who resumed drinking had poorer neuropsychological scores on measures of learning and memory on initial testing than did the abstainers. In a recent paper presentation (Parsons & Fabian, 1981) we have noted that a group of female alcoholics at one year follow-up who resumed drinking had significantly poorer neuropsychological test scores than those who remained abstinent.

In summary, we have considered the neuropsychological deficits associated with alcohol in some detail. There is little doubt that alcoholics have mild to moderate impairment in nonverbal abstracting problem solving and perceptual–motor speed, and that this impairment resembles that seen in other organic brain syndromes. There is increasing evidence that these deficits predict outcome; that is, those who are more impaired at initial testing are more likely to resume drinking. Also, there is preliminary data suggesting that the tests predict progress in the treatment situation. The examiner should be aware that the withdrawal reaction is poorly understood, and recent evidence suggests that it may last in certain alcoholics up to a month in the form of subtle neurophysiological changes. This fact coupled with the reports of recovery of functioning in abstinent alcoholics leads to a caution that cannot be overemphasized: Deficit performance obtained in alcoholics should not be regarded as a permanent loss of abilities.

Other Drug Abusers

Does chronic use of illicit drugs cause brain damage? We have all read in the newspaper or seen on television dramatic descriptions of how an individual under the influence of some illicit drug behaves bizarrely and in an uncharacteristic fashion. We have seen such individuals engaged in illegal activities, including vandalism while under the influence of drugs. Some of the drug education material distributed to high school students depict how LSD (d-Lysergic acid diethylamide) or PCP (Phencyclidine) can cause permanent brain damage in addition to the transient effects of the drug.

The psychiatric and neurological literature contains many individual case descriptions of patients who have used illicit drugs and have acquired documented organic brain damage (Kessler, Jortner, & Adapon, 1978; Rumbaugh, Bergeron, Fang, & McCormick, 1971). Autopsies on patients who died following heroin overdose demonstrate that 60% have demonstrated cerebral edema. A few studies utilizing pneumoencephalography (Von Zerssen, Fliege, & Wolf, 1970) and echoencephalography (Campbell, Evans, Thomson, & Williams, 1971) have reported brain damage in a small group of patients who have used illicit drugs. However, one cannot infer from a single case study or even a group of such studies that drug use causes brain damage because the brain damage may have some other etiology. Moreover, because brain damage may have occurred in one individual who used drugs does not imply that the population as a whole would experience brain damage if they chronically used drugs.

Few scientifically designed studies have been conducted investigating the chronic neuropsychological effects of illicit drugs on a large group of patients. Parsons and Farr (1981) reviewed the literature of all known studies that utilized the HRB to investigate the neuropsychological deficits found in drug abusers. These investigators reviewed eighteen such studies. They limited their review to those studies using the HRB because it is a standardized instrument widely used in clinical practice and measures a variety of perceptual, cognitive, memory, sensory, and motor behaviors. Moreover, HRB normative information is available from patients with known brain damage against which drug users' performance could be compared. Parsons and Farr (1981) reported a lack of consistent positive findings in their review. That is, when they compared various groups of drug abusers with normative information, the findings were far from conclusive in demonstrating a picture of consistent impairment in drug abusing patients. One may be somewhat surprised by this finding, for clinicians are repeatedly confronted with chronic drug users who have lowered intellectual functioning; however, clinical experience with individual cases is misleading when one attempts to extrapolate information gained in this fashion to the effects of chronic drug use in the whole population. The drug studies reviewed by Parsons and Farr (1981) will be discussed in the following section according to the primary drug or drugs used by subjects in these studies.

Marijuana

The five studies reviewed that investigated the effects of marijuana use on HRB performance all revealed a low average Impairment Index suggesting no documented neuropsychological deficits in marijuana users (Carlin & Turpin, 1977; Culver & King, 1974; Grant, Rochford, Fleming, & Stunkard, 1973; Mendelson & Meyer, 1972; Rochford, Grant, & LaVigne, 1977). The impairment indexes as indicated in Table 3 were in no case higher than .17. Thus the overall neuropsychological performance of marijuana-using subjects in these studies was in the normal range and was not suggestive of organic brain dysfunction. Obviously, this is not to say that there are not other effects accompanying chronic marijuana use such as the "A-Motivational" Syndrome (Cohen, 1980).

Opiates—Heroin

Two studies have reported HRB performance of heroin users (Fields & Fullerton, 1974; Hill, Reyes, Mikhael, & Ayre, 1978). Both of these studies found that heroin addicts' performance on the HRB was not suggestive of organic brain dysfunctioning.

Table 3
HRB Impairment Indexes, Age and IQ in Various Drug Abuser Groups[a]

Investigators	Drug	Impairment index[b]	Age	IQ or education
Carlin & Turpin (1977)	Marijuana	.15 (7)	24.1	122
Culver & King (1974)	Marijuana	.00 (7)	"20–25"	128
Grant et al. (1973)	Marijuana	.00 (4)	23	Medical student
Mendelson & Meyer (1972)	Marijuana	.17 (6)	22.0	117
Rochford et al. (1977)	Marijuana	.00 (3)	21.8	Medical student
Fields & Fullerton (1974)	Heroin	.24 (7)	25.0	109
Hill et al. (1978)	Heroin	.40 (5)	28.0	94
Trites et al. (1974)	Amphetamines	.30 (6)	19.4	105
Judd & Grant (1978)	Barbiturate	.38 (7)	25.7	108
Acord (1972)	LSD	.35 (7)	20.0	100
Acord & Barker (1973)	LSD	.50 (2)	21.5	2 years college
McGlothlin et al. (1969)	LSD	.33 (2)	40.0	College
Wright & Hogan (1972)	LSD	.14 (7)	20.0	109
Berry et al. (1977)	Inhalants	.36 (6)	18.6	90
Trites et al. (1974)	Inhalants	.40 (6)	16.5	95
Tsushima & Towne (1977)	Inhalants	.50 (2)	18.5	72
Adams et al. (1975)	Polydrugs[c]	1.00 (4)	26.7	99
Bruhn & Maage (1975)	Polydrugs	.50 (2)	23.1	110
Grant et al. (1976)	Polydrugs	.36 (7)	22.1	103

[a]An impairment index of .5 or above is considered to indicate impairment.
[b]Number in parentheses refers to number of the seven HRB tests (which comprise the impairment index) that were administered.
[c]Two other studies by Grant and Judd (1976) and Grant, Adams, Carlin, Rennick, Judd, Schooff, and Reed (1978) were not included because statistical analysis did not include presentations of $\bar{x}$'s.

Amphetamines and Barbiturates

One study of amphetamine users (Trites, Suh, Offord, Neiman, & Preston, 1974) and one study of barbiturate users (Judd & Grant, 1978) found that the HRB performance of patients using these drugs was not suggestive of organic brain dysfunction.

Hallucinogens (LSD)

The chronic effects of LSD ingestion on HRB performance was investigated by four studies (Acord, 1972; Acord & Barker, 1973; McGlothlin, Arnold, & Freedman, 1969; Wright & Hogan, 1972). For three of these studies the impairment indexes were in the unimpaired range suggesting no evidence of organic brain dysfunctioning. The remaining study (Acord & Barker, 1973), which reported an average impairment index suggesting a mild organic brain dysfunctioning (.50), used only two of the seven tests from the HRB; this fact, of course, would bring into question the reliability of these findings.

Inhalants

Three studies (Berry, Heaton, & Kirley, 1977; Trites et al., 1974; Tsushima & Towne, 1977) report neuropsychological test results of a group of subjects who had used inhalants chronically. Two of these studies found that the average performance of the individuals inhaling the drugs was in the unimpaired range. The third study (Tsushima & Towne, 1977), which used only two of seven Halstead battery tests, yielded an impairment index in the mildly impaired range.

Polydrugs

Polydrug users are those individuals who present with a history of multiple illicit drug use. Five studies have been conducted utilizing the HRB (Adams et al., 1975; Bruhn & Maage, 1975; Grant et al., 1978; Grant & Judd, 1976; Grant, Mohns, Miller, & Reitan, 1976) with polydrug users. Of these studies, three allowed for the computation of the impairment index, and of these three, two were in the impaired range and one was in the unimpaired range. Neither of the studies that found neuropsychological impairment in polydrug users utilized the complete HRB, and in one of the studies that found neuropsyhological impairment, the patients were tested only 48 hours after cessation of drug usage, which suggests that some of the patients may still be undergoing withdrawal effects.

Other Findings

While we have restricted our review to studies that employ the HRB, we should note one study of importance using another neuropsychological test battery.

Bergman, Borg, and Holm (1980) have examined a group of sedative and hypnotic (depressants) abusers for several years but who have not abused alcohol or other drugs. They were patients in a Swedish psychiatric clinic. There were 39 women and 16 men whose mean age was 47. They were compared with a group of control subjects matched on age, sex, mental status, and type of work. Subjects were given a battery of tests (for patients, 18 days after last drug ingestion) that had been used to measure impairment in alcoholic and brain-damaged patients: a synonyms test, the Thurstone Figure Classification Test, Koh's Block Design, a verbal learning test, the Trail-Making Test, and the Memory-For-Designs Test. No differences were found on the Synonyms (verbal reasoning) Test, but on all other tests the sedative and hypnotic abusers were significantly impaired at the $P < .001$ level. Using an overall clinical judgment, 68% of the abusers had mild or worse intellectual impairment compared with 16% of the controls ($P < .001$). Note that the battery used contains at least two of the tests we have described as most sensitive to alcohol effects (e.g., the Trail-Making Test and Block Design).

Methodological Issues in Studies of Chronic Drug Users

To further evaluate the findings concerning neuropsychological deficits in individuals who chronically use drugs, several important methodological considerations must be taken into account. One of the most important is that most drug users are not single drug users but use multiple drugs. For example, few individuals have exclusively used amphetamines without having experimented with barbiturates, marijuana, or alcohol. Most of the cited investigations studied patients who primarily used one drug, but the investigators did not systematically eliminate patients who had experimented with other drugs. Thus the findings are contaminated by the fact that patients in one particular subgroup of drug users may have in fact used multiple drugs.

Drugs obtained illegally on the street often contain substances unknown to the purchaser. Substances sold as marijuana or heroin generally do contain some of these drugs; however, substances purported to be mescaline and THC rarely prove to contain these drugs. Even if a drug illegally obtained contains the material it is supposed to contain, the percentage of purity can vary widely. In one study, heroin purchased on the street varied in purity between 0% and 17.5% by weight; the purity of Cocaine ranged from 0% to 100%, and samples of LSD contained absolutely no LSD to over 1,000 micrograms (Inaba, Way, Blum, & Schnoll, 1979).

A second methodological issue concerns the effects of the drug user's age. Many studies have demonstrated that Halstead Battery performance as summarized by the impairment index is highly correlated with age. The size of the correlation ranges from .50 to .60 (Golden & Schlutter, 1978; Prigatano & Parsons, 1976). The majority of patients studied in the drug studies are in their mid-20s or, in the case of the inhalant abusers, in their mid-teens (Table 3). Thus, these individuals are likely to have lower impairment indexes by virtue of their age in contrast to alcoholics whose mean age in the reported studies are in their 40s.

Efforts were not systematically made in the studies reported to control for the amount of the drug used and the duration of drug usage. There is some evidence, particularly in one study dealing with LSD (Cohen & Edwards, 1969) and another with heroin (Hill et al., 1978) to indicate that the longer that patients had used LSD or heroin, the more likely they were to show impairment in neuropsychological test performance.

Another methodological problem concerns the fact that intellectual functioning is correlated with HRB performance and that the magnitude of this correlation is rather high. The average IQ of subjects in the studies reviewed differed greatly (Table 3). For example, one study of marijuana users (Culver & King, 1974) found that the average full scale IQ of subjects was 128. The average full scale IQ of patients in one of the inhalant studies (Tshushima & Towne, 1977) was 72. Obviously if individuals who use inhalants are from a lower social economic status and have associated low IQ's, one cannot compare their performance with that of college students who have used marijuana. These two groups of patients may differ greatly in their premorbid performance, thus postdrug use measures would reflect not only changes that may occur due to drug use but also their premorbid intellectual capacities.

Several studies have demonstrated that patients with severe psychiatric problems as a group perform more poorly on neuropsychological tests than do nonpsychiatric controls (Adams & Jenkins, 1982). Many of the individuals who use certain types of drugs, particularly inhalants or amphetamines, are likely to present with an abnormal MMPI profile or psychiatric problem. Moreover, the longer the drugs are used, the greater the possibility of more severe psychiatric problems (McLellan, Woody, & O'Brien, 1979). This difference in psychopathology may also be related to poorer neuropsychological functioning independent of the integrity of the drug users' cerebral cortex.

Perhaps related to the lifestyle and psychopathology issue is the fact that many drug users, particularly polydrug users, reported a high incidence of traumatic head injuries (23%) (Grant et al., 1978). Obviously, if these drug-using patients have an increased incidence of head trauma, any change in their neuropsychological status may be due to the head injury rather than the illicit drug used. The presence of poor nutrition and medical problems related to drug use are also greater in drug abusers than in the normal population; for example, endocarditis, cotton fever (the street term for chills and fever following injection of particles or bacteria directly into the blood stream), tuberculosis, thrombophlebitis, hepatitis, allergic reaction to drugs, granulomatous lesions of the lung, pneumonitis, or other serious medical conditions that can be related directly to drug use but are not necessarily caused by the drug itself. The most frequently seen medical complication of intravenous drug usage is hepatitis. As many as 90% of hospitalizations for serum hepatitis result from parenteral drug use. One study of drug users cited by O'Brien, Wesson, and Schnoll (1976) indicated that fewer than 10% of heroin uses who "snorted" the drug showed abnormal liver functioning, whereas more than 35% of those who had used a needle had such findings.

If a patient overdoses on a drug, particularly heroin, he or she may well experience a coma, depressed respiration, tachycardia, and contracted pupils. The overdose obviously may be complicated by convulsive seizures, cardiorespiratory arrest, blindness (when quinine has been added to the heroin), or acute transverse myelitis.

As stated earlier, this review was limited only to studies utilizing the HRB. The possibility arises that if other neuropsychological tests were utilized, different findings would emerge.

Conclusions

What conclusions can be drawn from the studies of the chronic effects of drug abuse? Of the eight investigators who supplied mean impairment indexes for their samples of abusers, none were in the impaired range (Table 3). Ten other investigators presented data that allowed an estimate of impairment index from incomplete or transformed HRB findings. Of these 10 studies, 6 were in the impaired range. However, one must be very cautious here because some of these impairment indexes were based on as few as two of the seven Halstead–Reitan tests.

On the basis of currently available cutting scores (which of course a clinical neuropsychologist must use when presented with a single drug abuse patient), our review did not point to consistent neuropsychological deficits due to substance abuse other than perhaps polydrug abuse and possible other depressants such as sedative-hypnotics. Some studies found mild neuropsychological deficits and others found no deficits. No study however, reported neuropsychological deficits on the HRB with marijuana usage or amphetamines. For barbiturates, the one study that has reported deficits is strongly suggestive of deficit patterns similar to those found in alcoholic patients. Mixed findings were reported for users of hallucinogens, inhalants, and polydrug usage. When deficits were found, they tended to be on the same tests from the HRB as in alcoholism (Table 2).

CONSIDERATIONS IN TESTING ALCOHOL AND DRUG PATIENTS

Indications for Neuropsychological Testing

In a clinical situation, the clinical neuropsychologist and the referring physician must make decisions about whether neuropsychological tests would be appropriate for a given alcoholic or drug abusing patient. Ample reason for considering testing in alcoholics has been cited. Although the drug studies reviewed did not consistently find neuropsychological deficits among all chronic drug users, some studies did reveal that individual patients performed in the impaired range on neuropsychological tests.

Neuropsychological testing is expensive; it is clearly inappropriate to test all patients with a history of chronic alcoholic or drug usage. There are certain instances however, where neuropsychological testing is in order. If the patient voluntarily expresses a memory problem and states that this problem has interfered with his day-to-day functioning, then neuropsychological testing is advantageous. The purpose of this testing would be to document this subjective memory loss, but the data obtained from this testing could also serve as basis for memory rehabilitation. Neuropsychological testing is indicated if there is reason to believe that organic brain damage may have occurred, as in patients with histories of drug overdose, particularly if they have been in a coma, or if there is a history of seizures associated with his alcohol or drug use. Alcoholic patients with a history of delirium tremens are neuropsychological test candidates.

Neuropsychological testing may well assist the clinician in predicting which patients would be most likely to benefit from treatment. Several studies (Abott & Gregson, 1981; Berglund, Leijonquist, & Hörlén, 1977; Gregson & Taylor, 1977; Guthrie & Elliott, 1980; O'Leary, Donovan, & Chaney, 1978) have demonstrated that alcoholic patients who performed relatively well on neuropsychological testing did better in treatment than those who performed poorly. The criteria of treatment success varied from study to study, but in general outcome measures such as completion of treatment and decreased incidence of drinking after treatment served as the outcome measures. The most impressive predictive reports are those of Gregson and Taylor (1977) and Abbott and Gregson (1981) in New Zealand. In the first study, 90 male middle-aged lower socioeconomic level alcoholic inpatients were administered the Pattern Cognitive Impairment Test (PCIT). This test measures the ability to remember and process information in both short- and medium-term memory. A follow-up study conducted at 1, 3, and 6 months posttreatment revealed that the PCIT predicted both drinking and work behavior. In the second study, as we have noted earlier, they essentially corroborated their findings. Unfortunately, similar studies have not been conducted with drug-abusing patients. Thus it appears, at least from the few studies that have been done in the area, that alcoholic patients and presumably other drug abuse patients who have relatively intact neuropsychological functioning tend to do better in treatment and maintain abstinence in follow-up than do patients with poor performance on neuropsychological testing. Obviously much more research is needed in this area.

Another reason for neuropsychological testing, particularly in alcoholic patients with a long history of alcohol use, is to establish current base lines in neuropsychological functioning. If a patient continues to drink, the prediction is that the neuropsychological testing would deteriorate over time. Assessing neuropsychological status at a particular point in time would help the treatment staff in monitoring future possible neuropsychological deficits.

Selection of Neuropsychological Tests

Assuming that neuropsychological testing is required in a particular case, the next question one must ask is which neuropsychological tests would be appropriate to administer. From our experience and based upon current review of the literature, the HRB, especially as modified by Russell, Neuringer, and Goldstein (1970), is the most appropriate. The HRB tests most likely to demonstrate greater deficits among alcoholics and drug abusers are those comprising Reitan's (1973) Brain-Age-Quotient (Table 2). In our opinion, the greater the impairment on the Brain-Age-Quotient, the more likely the patient will have poor adaptation to life tasks, the less likely he is to complete treatment, and the more likely he is to resume drinking or abusing drugs. We also recommend the administration of the Wechsler Memory Scale as modified by Russell (1975). This test provides measures of immediate and delayed verbal and visuospatial memory. An alternative to the HRB is the Luria–Nebraska Neuropsychological Battery (Golden, 1981). However, only two studies on alcoholics have been reported to date (Chmielewski & Golden, 1980; DeObaldia, Parsons, & Leber, 1981). Both have found alcoholics to be mildly impaired compared to controls. Finally, the patient should be given personality tests, preferably the MMPI, to screen for other psychiatric problems that might influence test performance.

When to Administer Neuropsychological Tests

Deciding when to perform neuropsychological tests is the next important question to consider. Obviously, if a patient has not withdrawn from the drugs or is still undergoing detoxification from alcohol, testing would be inappropriate. Neuropsychological examination may be conducted whenever withdrawal symptoms have subsided for several days. To be on the cautious side, wherever possible, we would suggest that patients be drug-free at least a week before testing is undertaken. However, it should be noted that on outpatient units and many times on inpatient units it is difficult to know if patients are taking drugs illicitly even while in the treatment program. As noted earlier, a study by Grant et al. (1978) found that despite an elaborate procedure for examining behavioral indications of drug use, well trained examiners were unable to make accurate clinical judgments regarding the subjects' current drug use. Moreover, in a three-month follow-up study, they found that the incidence of positive drug urine findings was 42% and that these patients also performed significantly less well on the HRB than subjects with negative screening results. It may well be that some subjects did not volunteer for the blood test because they were fearful that the results would prove their drug usage; therefore the above incidence may be an underestimation of the actual number of subjects using drugs at time of testing.

Thus, a clinician performing neuropsychological examination of a drug abuser, particularly on an outpatient basis, should have a recent blood screen to insure that the patient is not using drugs at the time of the examination; otherwise the findings may be misleading. In any event, the psychological examiner should be particularly alert to any signs of drug or alcohol use present at the time of testing, particularly restlessness, irritability, tremulousness, anxiety, nystamus, dilated or pinpoint pupils, increased respiration rate, or excessive perspiration. For a detailed list of signs and symptoms associated with various drugs, the reader is referred to Peterson (1980).

In addition to formal neuropsychological examination, the clinical neuropsychologist should also conduct a thorough mental status examination, including an adequate drug history. The history should include an indication of what drugs have been used, year of their first use, the usual route of administration, the average daily dosage, and the most recent drug use. The patient should be queried as to history of drug overdose, coma, significant medical problems associated with drug use, head injury, "bad trips," or other significant medical or psychiatric history.

In attempting to provide a drug history, many times patients will use slang or street names for drugs, and at times it is quite difficult for the examiner to get an estimate for the actual drugs used. Included in Table 4 is a list of slang terms used for different types of drugs. However, as noted earlier, one should be cautious of the fact that many drugs obtained on the street are actually substances other than those purportedly purchased by the drug user.

The Neuropsychological Report: A Case Example

The neuropsychological examination culminates in a neuropsychological report. We exemplify our approach to report writing in the case presented below. We should note that because of the complexity of this case, the "Background Information" section is longer than our usual report. The data on which the report is based is presented in Table 5, following the report.

Report of Neuropsychological Examination

Identifying Information and Reason for Referral. This 45-year-old white divorced male with a history of polydrug use and alcoholism was seen for neuropsychological evaluation. We were asked for evidence of organic brain dysfunctioning.

Background Information. This patient presents with an approximate 8-year history of polydrug use. Given the patient's defensiveness and poor memory, a

Table 4
Slang Terms for Drugs[a]

Amphetamines

Beans, bennies, black beauties, blackbirds, black mollies, bumblebees, cartwheels, chalk, chicken powder, copilots, crank, crossroads, crystal, dexies, double cross, eye openers, hearts, jelly beans, lightning, meth, minibennies, nuggets, organces, pep pills, speed, roses, thrusters, truck drivers, turnabouts, uppers, ups, wake-ups.

Barbiturates

Barbs, block busters, bluebirds, blue devils, blues, christmas trees, downers, green dragons, marshmallow reds, Mexican reds, nebbies, nimbies, peanuts, pink ladies, pinks, rainbows, red and blues, redbirds, red devils, reds, sleeping pills, stumblers, yellow jackets, yellows

Cocaine

Bernice, bernies, big C., blow, C, coke, drean, flake, girl, gold dust, heaven dust, nose candy, paradise, rock, snow, white

Glutethimide

C.D., cibas

Hashish

Black russian, hash, kif, quarter moon, soles

Heroin

Big H, boy brown, brown sugar, caballo, Chinese red, chiva, crap, doojee, H, harry, horse, junk, Mexican mud, powder, scag, smack, stuff, thing

LSD

Acid, beast, big D, blue cheer, blue heaven, blue mist, brown dots, California sunshine, chocolate chips, coffee, contact lens, cupcakes, haze, mellow yellows, microdots, orange mushrooms, orange wedges, owsley, paper acid, royal blue, strawberry fields, sugar, sunshine, the hawk, wedges, white lightning, window pane, yellows

Marijuana

Acapulco gold, broccoli, bush, dry high, gage, ganga, grass, griffo, hay, hemp, herb, j, jay, Jane, Mary Jane, mota, mutah, Panama red, pod, pot, reefer, sativa, smoke, stick, tea, weed

MDA

Love drug

Mescaline

Beans, buttons, cactus, mesc, mescal, mescal buttons, moon

(continued)

Table 4 (*Cont.*)

Methamphetamines
Crystal, meth, speed
Methaqualone
Quas, quads, soapers, sopes
Morphine
Cube, first line, mocus, Mis Emma, morf, morpho, morphy, mud
Phencyclidine
Angel dust, DOA (dead on arrival), hog, killer weed (when combined with marijuana or other plant material), PCP, peace pill
Psilocybin/Psilocyn
Magic mushroom, mushroom

[a]From *Drugs of Abuse* (United States Department of Justice), Washington, D.C.: U.S. Government Printing Office, 1977.

valid detailed history could not be obtained. However, the patient apparently has misused many drugs, mainly barbiturates and narcotics. His barbiturate usage has been on a daily basis. He has only intermittently used narcotics, and from all available evidence was probably never physically addicted to the narcotics. The patient also admits to a long history of alcoholism, stating that he repeatedly drank up to 12 beers in an evening. He has consumed barbiturates and alcohol simultaneously, which obviously is a dangerous combination.

The patient has a history of two suicide attempts. In one of these attempts, the patient backed his car off a hill and had to be dragged unconscious from the burning vehicle. The patient remained unconscious for 6 hours and was hospitalized for approximately one month at that time. Another suicide attempt was made through an overdose. After taking large unknown quantities of barbiturates, the patient became comatose and was taken to the intensive care unit, where he stayed for a few days and was released.

The patient presents with a very sporadic work history, although at one period in his life he worked as a manager of a restaurant owned by his father. Approximately two years ago, following an argument with the father, the father committed suicide by shooting himself in the head with a pistol. The patient was present when his father killed himself, and reportedly the father's suicidal action stemmed from frustration with the patient. Following the father's death, the patient withdrew from those around him. He remained in his house and seldom went out. A housekeeper would stop by once a week to clean the house, pick up dirty linen, and bring in groceries. The housekeeper relates that it was not unusual for her to find the patient in what sounded like a semicomatose state, lying on the floor with empty barbiturate containers in evidence.

The patient is divorced, lives alone, is not working, and has no children. He supports himself on a small trust fund set up by his family. The patient is currently hospitalized on the drug treatment unit. He expressed a desire to undergo detoxification and in fact has remained drug-free on the unit for approximately three weeks.

Since being hospitalized, the patient has undergone a variety of tests including brain scan, electroencephalogram (EEG), echoencephalogram, skull x-rays, and CAT scan. All studies to date have been negative; however, his physical examination revealed some hyperactivity on his left lower extremity. Moreover, he has a questionable Babinski reflex on the left side.

Test Behavior and Test Administered. This patient is a grey-haired man who is clean-shaven but appears considerably older than his stated age due to his unkempt appearance and multiple scars over his forehead. He was wearing slippers and would shuffle his feet when walking. He continually smoked during testing. He had occasional difficulty pronouncing words, primarily when discussing his relationship with his father and his father's death. He was extremely respectful of the examiner and became easily frustrated over his recognizably poor test performance. As he became anxious over his test performance, the patient would move chairs into different positions and scoot his feet on the floor. The patient needed constant reassurance and encouragement from the examiner, particularly when he was performing poorly. The test results appear to be a valid estimate of the patient's current neuropsychological functioning. The patient was administered the Halstead Neuropsychological Battery, the Wechsler Memory Scale, and the MMPI.

Intellectual and Cognitive Functioning. This patient is functioning intellectually with a Full-Scale IQ of 95 (Verbal IQ = 107, Performance IQ = 87). It is noteworthy that the patient had a 20-point discrepancy between Verbal and Performance IQ. The patient performed best on tasks measuring his abstract generalizing ability and his ability to form appropriate similarities between word pairs. For example, he was able to give appropriate answers to such difficult word pairs as "praise" and "punishment," "poem" and "statue," "egg" and "seed." Depth and breadth of the patient's English vocabulary was good; he could define such words as "travesty," "impale," and "encumber." The patient's fund of general cultural information, arithmetic and numeric reasoning skills, and comprehension of social expectations and mores were all essentially within the normal range.

The patient, however, experienced difficulty in certain cognitive tasks. His psychomotor speed and hand coordinations were slow. The patient was not observant of his environment and had difficulty distinguishing significant from insignificant visual events. Moreover, the patient's social planning and anticipatory skills were limited. The patient's performance on Trail Making Test B indicated some difficulty visually scanning large amounts of information, focusing in on the most relevant aspects of that information, and performing associated psychomotor maneuvers. The patient experienced some mild difficulties when he attempted to discriminate subtle differences between word sounds of the "ee" variety.

Memory. This patient was oriented to month, day, year, and current location. The patient expressed some difficulty remembering two stories, each containing 23 bits of information. He remembered an average of nine bits of information from each of these two stories, a poor performance. The patient demonstrated even more significant deficits in his visual memory. Of the four Wechsler Memory designs, the patient recalled portions of only two.

Communicative Skills and Sensory–Perceptual Functions. The patient's reading, writing, and arithmetic skills were all grossly intact. He could read simple sentences without error but did experience problems pronouncing multisyllablic words. No marked signs of aphasia or agnosia were noted. On bilateral simultaneous stimulation, using tactual, auditory, and visual modalities, no suppressions were noted. No evidence of graphesthesia was noted. No evidence of dystereognosis was noted on the tactile performance test. The patient demonstrated marked construction dyspraxia in his attempt to draw the Greek cross and key.

Perceptual–Motor Functioning. The patient is right-handed and demonstrates right ocular dominance. Strength and grip was strong bilaterally as measured by the hand dynamometer. Finger oscillation speed was mildly impaired bilaterally. The patient's performance on the tactual performance test was more impaired with his left upper extremity than it was with his right. The patient also experienced bilateral difficulty integrating the necessary motor movements to place pegs in holes on the Purdue Peg Board.

Personality Test Results. The patient completed the MMPI in an honest, straightforward, and relatively nondefensive manner. Overall results suggest that this patient has difficulty controlling his impulses. He has more than the average amount of anger. He tends to act out aggressively and only later stop to contemplate the consequences of his action. He has a low energy level and has difficulty mobilizing his energy to perform the ordinary demands of his existence. Such individuals are likely to have a grouchy, complaining attitude toward life.

Summary and Conclusions. Overall results in neuropsychological testing were consistent with what we normally see in patients who have moderate to severe diffuse organic brain dysfunctioning. He has an impairment index of .9 (See Table 5). Moreover the patient's right hemisphere appears to be functioning less well than the left. The patient's pattern of performance on the various neuropsychological tests sensitive to right hemisphere functioning suggests that the

Table 5

Neuropsychological Findings for Patient GB on the Halstead-Reitan Battery

Hosp: VAH, inpt.	Referred by:		
Age: 44			
Birthdate: 05/02/28	Education: 13	Hdness: R	Sex: M
Occupation: Unemployed			

Purdue Peg Board:
LH 7   RH 8   BH (prs) 5

WRAT:
R: 12.8   S NA   A NA

Trails A   31"/0
Trails B   151"/0
Trails total   182"/0

Lateral Dominance Exam:
Hand   R 7 L 0
Eye   R 2 L 0
Foot   R 2 L 0
Name   R 8" L19"
Dynamic   R 36 L 31

MMPI:
? 0   PD 79
L 50   MF 57
F 46   PA 59
K 53   PT 50
HS 54   SC 44
D 53   MA 45
HY 56   SI 56

Wechsler Memory Scale:
MQ 89

WAIS:
VIQ 107
PIQ 87
FSIQ 95
Information 10
Comprehension 11
Arithmetic 10
Similarities 13
Digit Span 10
Vocabulary 13
Digit Symbol 5
Picture Completion 8
Block Design 9
Picture Arrangement 7
Object Assembly —

Sensory–Perceptual Examinations:
Suppressions

Tactile: RH 0 LH 0
        RH 0 LH 0
        RH 0 LF 0
Auditory: RE 0 LE 0
Visual: RV 0 LV 0
Finger ID: RH 0 LH 0
Finger-tip
Writing: RH 1 LH 0
Tactile Form
Recognition:
Time: RH NA LH NA
Errors: RH 0 LH 0

Category (errors)
1 (0)   2 (10)   3 (32)   4 (11)
5 (19)   6 (11)   7 (6)   79[a]

TPT:
RH 9.6
LH 9.9
BH 4.1   Time 23.6[a]
        Memory 4[a]
        Location 2[a]

Seashore Rhythm (errors) 3
Speech Perception (errors) 8[a]

Tapping:
RH 45   45[a]
LH 40

Impairment index: National 0.9[a]

[a]Scores beyond the cutting points for brain damage according to HRB national norms.

primary damage of the right hemisphere is most likely posterior in nature. The exact etiology of the patient's primary higher cortical dysfunctioning is unknown. However, the patient's repeated head injuries are probably the main cause, with drug-induced coma and barbiturate abuse and alcoholism playing a contributing role. The patient is in need of continued psychiatric treatment on discharge from the drug treatment unit.

SUMMARY

Alcohol and drug abuse are significant health problems in our society. All indications point to a continuation if not increasing prevalence of substance abuse in the future. Neuropsychological examinations provide important information on a variety of dimensions relevant to the alcohol and drug abuser's functioning (e.g., level of current cognitive–perceptual functioning; pattern of intact and impaired abilities; probability of brain dysfunction; potential for adapting to life tasks and rehabilitation potential). To be able to provide such information, the neuropsychologist needs background knowledge in organic brain syndromes, drug effects and pharmacological concepts, the natural history of drug abuse, empirical findings of neuropsychological research with alcohol and drug abusers and, of course, familiarity with the basic principles of neuropsychological examination.

The neuropsychological effects of alcohol abuse have been more thoroughly researched than any other drug. It is well established that alcoholics are mildly to moderately impaired in perceptual–cognitive functioning and that they are impaired on the tests of the HRB that are most sensitive to age and brain damage from other causes. These tests are the Halstead Category Test, the Tactual Performance Test—Time, and the Tactual Performance Test—Location Memory, the Trails B, and the WAIS Digit–Symbol and Block Design. Verbal abilities, at least as measured by the WAIS, are usually intact. More complex and demanding verbal tasks, however, are also impaired in alcoholics. The neuropsychological model that best fits the data is that of a mild generalized brain dysfunctional state. Whether alcoholics recover to normal neuropsychological functioning with abstinence is currently being investigated by a number of researchers; apparently some abilities do recover and others do not, but definitive conclusions are not possible at this time. Finally, there is some suggestive evidence that alcohol abusers who have greater neuropsychological impairment are more likely to resume drinking.

Neuropsychological impairment due to other drugs has been difficult to establish. There is little doubt from clinical reports that individuals abusing any one or more of a variety of drugs may have neuropsychological impairment and other medical evidence of brain dysfunction. However, our review of research studies indicates that, in contrast with HRB findings in alcoholics, HRB results with drug abusers are mainly in the nonimpaired range. There are suggestions that polydrug and sedative-hypnotic (depressants) users are more likely to manifest deficits than other drug abusers. When deficits are reported in drug abusers, they tend to be on the same tests as noted above for the alcoholics; however, there are many inconsistencies. Methodological problems in drug abuse research may be an important factor in the inconclusive results. Among these factors are: individuals tend to be polydrug users rather than users of exclusively one drug; street drugs are often impure or contain only a small amount, if any, of the presumed drug; amount and frequency of drug use is seldom accurately monitored; variations in age, education, and intelligence; degree and type of psychiatric disturbance; presence of head trauma, poor nutrition or other medical disorders (hepatitis); and history of overdosing.

Indications for neuropsychological testing include when the patient complains of cognitive difficulies, particularly in memory, or when there is a history of coma or seizures. Alcoholics who have had delirium tremens are prime candidates. Other indications include the need to establish assets and deficits for rehabilitation and/or baseline measurement. These findings then can be used for measuring treatment or recidivision effects.

Selection of an appropriate neuropsychological test battery depends in part on the questions being asked. We recommend the HRB as modified and extended by Russell et al. (1970) as the instrument of choice. It has the most extensive research history. The new Luria–Nebraska Neuropsychological Battery (Golden, 1981) may prove to be an acceptable alternate as research evidence accumulates. Whatever battery is used, neuropsychological testing should not commence until the acute drug intoxication and withdrawal symptoms have subsided; preferably at least a week after last drug ingestion. Drug screening analyses, particularly if the patient is not hospitalized, are desirable. If these are not available, the neuropsychological examiner should be familiar enough with the various behavioral signs of drug and alcohol use to incorporate possible drug toxicity or withdrawal as factors affecting the results of the neuropsychological evaluation. A mental status examination and thorough drug history are also advised.

The neuropsychological examination report should include identifying information and reason for referral. Background information should include particularly the history of drug ingestion and any other trauma or disease states that could have affected the brain, as well as any medical findings. The tests administered and behavior of the patient should be described followed by an evaluation of intellectual–cognitive skills, memory, communicative skills, sensory–perceptual and perceptual–motor functioning, and personality test results. A summary and conclusions containing specific answers to the referral question and recommendations for future testing or rehabilitation completes the report.

ACKNOWLEDGMENTS

We appreciate the patient efforts of Mrs. Joyce Robertson through the several drafts of this manuscript.

REFERENCES

Abbott, M. W., & Gregson, R. A. M. Cognitive dysfunction in the prediction of relapse in alcoholism. *Journal of Studies on Alcohol,* 1981, *43,* 230–243.

Acord, L. D. Halucinogenic drugs and brain damage. *Military Medicine,* 1972, *137,* 18–19.

Acord, L. D. & Barker, D. D. Hallucinogenic drugs and cerebral deficit. *Journal of Nervous and Mental Disease,* 1973, *156,* 281–283.

Adams, K., Rennick, P., Schooff, K. G., & Keegan, J. F. Neuropsychological measurement of drug effects: Poly-drug research. *Journal of Psychedelic Drugs,* 1975, *7,* 151–160.

Adams, R. L., & Jenkins, R. L. Basic principles of a neuropsychological examination. In Walker, C. E. (Ed.), *Clinical practice of psychology; A guide for mental health professionals.* New York: Pergamon, 1982.

American Psychiatric Association. *Diagnostic and statistical manual of mental disorders (DSM-III)* (3rd ed.). Washington, D.C.: Author, 1980.

Begleiter, H., & Porjesz, B. Persistance of a "subacute withdrawal syndrome" following chronic ethanol intake. *Drug and Alcohol Dependence,* 1979, *4,* 353–357.

Berglund, M., Leijonquist, H., & Hörlén, M. Prognostic significance and reversibility of cerebral dysfunction in alcoholics. *Journal of Studies on Alcohol,* 1977, *38,* 1761–1769.

Bergman, H., Borg, S., & Holm, L. Neuropsychological impairment and exclusive abuse of sedatives or hypnotics. *American Journal of Psychiatry,* 1980, *137,* 215–217.

Berry, G., Heaten, R. K., & Kirley, M. W. Neuropsychological deficits of chronic inhalant abusers. In B. H. Rumaek & A. R. Temple (Eds.), *Management of the poisoned patient.* Princeton: Science Press, 1977.

Bruhn, P., & Maage, N. Intellectual and neuropsychological functions in young men with heavy and long-term patterns of drug abuse. *American Journal of Psychiatry,* 1975, *132,* 397–401.

Campbell, A. M. G., Evans, M., Thomson, J. L. G., & Williams, M. J. Cerebral atrophy in young cannabis smokers. *Lancet,* 1971, *2,* 1219–1224.

Carlin, A. S., & Turpin, E. W. The effect of long-term chronic cannabis use and neuropsychological functioning. *International Journal of Addictions,* 1977, *12,* 617–624.

Chmielewski, C., & Golden, C. Alcoholism and brain damage: An investigation using the Standardized Luria–Nebraska Neuropsychological Battery. *International Journal of Neuroscience,* 1980, *10,* 99–105.

Cohen, S. Cannabis: Impact on motivation, Part II. *Drug Abuse and Alcoholism Newsletter,* 1980, *10*(1).

Cohen, S., & Edwards, A. E. LSD and organic brain impairment. *Drug Dependence,* 1969, *2,* 1–4.

Culver, C. M., & King, F. W. Neuropsychological assessment of undergraduate marijuana and LSD users. *Archives of General Psychiatry,* 1974, *31,* 707–711.

DeObaldia, R., Parsons, O. A., & Leber, W. R. Assessment of neuropsychological functions in chronic alcoholics using a standardized version of Luria's neuropsychological technique. *International Journal of Neuroscience,* 1981, *14,* 85–93.

Eckardt, M. J., Parker, E. S., Pautler, C. P., Noble, E. P., & Gottschalk, L. A. Neuropsychological consequences of post treatment drinking behavior in male alcoholics. *Psychiatry Research,* 1980, *2,* 135–147.

Eckardt, M. J., & Ryback, R. S. Neuropsychological concomitants of alcoholism. In M. Galanter (Ed.), *Currents in Alcoholism* (Vol. 8). New York: Grune & Stratton, 1981.

Fabian, M. S., Parsons, O. A., & Silberstein, J. A. Impaired perceptual–cognitive functioning in alcoholic women. *Journal of Studies on Alcohol,* 1981. *42,* 217–229.

Fields, F. R. J., & Fullerton, J. R. The influence of heroin addiction on neuropsychological functioning. *Veterans Administration Newsletter for Research in Mental Health & Behavioral Science,* 1974, *16,* 20–25.

Filskov, S. B., & Boll, T. J. *Handbook of clinical neuropsychology.* New York: Wiley, 1981.

Freedman, A. M. Opiate dependence. In H. I. Kaplan, A. M. Freedman, & B. J. Sadock (Eds.), *Comprehensive textbook of psychiatry* (Vol. 2, 3rd ed.). Baltimore: Williams & Wilkins, 1980.

Golden, C. J. A standardized version of Luria's neuropsychological tests: A quantitative and qualitative approach to neuropsychological evaluation. In S. B. Filskov & T. J. Boll, *Handbook of clinical neuropsychology* New York: Wiley, 1981.

Golden, C. J., & Schlutter, L. C. The interaction of age and diagnosis in neuropsychological test results. *International Journal of Neuroscience,* 1978, *8,* 61–63.

Golden, C. J., Moses, J. A., Fishburne, F. J., Engum, E., Lewis, G. P., Wisniewski, A. M., Conley, F. K., Berg, R. A., & Graber, B. Cross-validation of the Luria–Nebraska Neuropsychological Battery for the presence, localization and lateralization of brain damage. *Journal of Consulting and Clinical Psychology,* 1981, *49,* 491–507.

Goldstein, G. Perceptual and cognitive deficits in alcoholics. In G. Goldstein & C. Neuringer (Eds.), *Empirical studies of alcoholism.* Cambridge, Mass.: Ballinger, 1976.

Goldstein, G., & Shelly, C. H. Field dependence and cognitive, perceptual and motor skills in alcoholics: A factor analytic study. *Quarterly Journal of Studies on Alcohol,* 1971, *32,* 29–40.

Goodwin, D. W., & Hill, S. Y. Chronic effects of alcohol and other psychoactive drugs on intellect, learning and memory. In G. Rankin (Ed.), *Alcohol, drugs and brain damage.* Toronto: Addiction Research Foundation, 1975.

Grant, I., & Judd, L. L. Neuropsychological and EEG disturbances in polydrug users. *American Journal of Psychiatry,* 1976, *133,* 1039–1042.

Grant, I., & Mohns, L. Chronic cerebral effects of alcohol and drug abuse. *International Journal of Addictions,* 1975, *10,* 883–920.

Grant, I., Adams, K. M., Carlin, A. S., Rennick, P. M., Judd, L. L., Schooff, K., & Reed, R. Organic impairment in polydrug users: Risk factors. *American Journal of Psychiatry,* 1978, *135,* 178–184.

Grant, I., Mohns, L., Miller, M., & Reitan, R. M. A neuropsychological study of polydrug users. *Archives of General Psychiatry,* 1976, *33,* 973–978.

Grant, I., Reed, R., & Adams, K. M. Natural history of alcohol and drug related brain disorder: Implications for neuropsychological research. *Journal of Clinical Neuropsychology,* 1980, *2,* 321–332.

Grant, I., Rochford, J., Fleming, T., & Stunkard, A. A neuropsychological assessment of the effects of moderate marijuana use. *Journal of Nervous and Mental Disease,* 1973, *156,* 278–280.

Gregson, R. A. M., & Taylor, G. M. Prediction of relapse in men alcoholics. *Journal of Studies on Alcohol,* 1977, *38,* 1749–1759.

Grinspoon, L., & Bakalar, J. B. Drug dependence: Non-narcotic agents. In H. I. Kaplan, A. M. Freedman, & B. J. Sadock (Eds.), *Comprehensive textbook of psychiatry* (Vol. 2, 3rd ed.). Baltimore: Williams & Wilkins, 1980.

Guthrie, A., & Elliott, W. A. The nature and reversibility of cerebral impairment in alcoholism: Treatment implications. *Journal of Studies on Alcohol,* 1980, *41,* 147–155.

Hill, S. Y., Reyes, R. B., Mikhael, M., & Ayre, F. *A comparison of alcoholics and heroin abusers:*

Computerized transaxial tomography and neuropsychological functioning. Paper presented at the National Council on Alcoholism Meeting, St. Louis, April 1978.

Hochla, N. N., Parsons, O. A., & Fabian, M. S. Brain-age quotients in recently detoxified alcoholics, recovered alcoholics and non-alcoholic women. *Journal of Clinical Psychology*, 1982, *38*, 207–212.

Inaba, D. I., Way, E. L., Blum, K., & Schnoll, S. H. *Pharmacological and toxicological perspectives of commonly abused drugs* (Medical Monographs, No. 5, U.S. Public Health Service). Washington, D.C.: U.S. Government Printing Office, 1979.

Jaffe, J. H. Drug addiction and drug abuse. In L. G. Goodman & A. Gilman (Eds.), *The pharmacological basis of therapeutics* (5th ed.). New York: Macmillan, 1975.

Judd, L. L., & Grant, I. Intermediate duration organic mental disorders among polydrug abusing patients. Symposium on brain disorders: Clinical diagnosis and management. *Psychiatric Clinics of North America*, 1978, *1*, 153–167.

Kessler, J., Jortner, B. S., & Adapon, B. D. Cerebral vasculitis in a drug abuser. *The Journal of Clinical Psychiatry*, 1978, *39*, 559–564.

Kissin, B. Alcoholism and drug dependence. In R. C. Simons & H. Pardes (Eds.), *Understanding human behavior in health and illness.* Baltimore: Williams & Wilkins, 1977.

Kleinknecht, R. A., & Goldstein, S. G. Neuropsychological deficits associated with alcoholism. *Quarterly Journal of Studies on Alcohol*, 1972, *88*, 268–276.

Leber, W. R., & Parsons, O. A. *Neuropsychological functioning and clinical progress in alcoholism.* Paper presented at the 26th Annual Meeting of the Southwestern Psychological Association, Oklahoma City, 1980.

McGlothlin, W. H., Arnold, D. O., & Freedman, D. X. Organicity measures following repeated LSD ingestion. *Archives of General Psychiatry*, 1969, *21*, 704–709.

McLellan, A. T., Woody, G. E., & O'Brien, M. D. Development of psychiatric illness in drug abusers: Possible role of drug preference. *The New England Journal of Medicine*, 1979, *301*, 1310–1313.

Matarazzo, J. D. *Wechsler's measurement and appraisal of adult intelligence.* Baltimore: Williams & Wilkins, 1972.

Mendelson, J. H., & Meyer, R. E. Behavioral and biological concomitants of chronic marijuana smoking by heavy and casual users. *Technical papers of the first report of the national commission on marijuana and drug abuse.* Washington, D.C.: U.S. Government Printing Office, 1972.

Miller, W. R., & Saucedo, C. Neuropsychological impairment and brain damage in problem drinkers: A critical review. In C. J. Golden, J. A. Moses, Jr., J. Coffmann, W. R. Miller, & F. Strider (Eds.), *Clinical neuropsychology: Interface of neurological and psychiatric disorders.* New York: Grune Stratton, 1983.

O'Brien, C. P., Wesson, D. R., & Schnoll, S. H. *Diagnosis and evaluation of the drug abusing patient for treatment staff physicians* (Medical Monograph, No. 1, U.S. Public Health Service). Washington, D.C.: U.S. Government Printing Office, 1976.

O'Leary, M. R., Donovan, D. M., & Chaney, E. F. *The clinical utility of the brain–age quotient in alcoholism treatment.* Unpublished manuscript, 1978.

Parsons, O. A. Neuropsychological deficits in chronic alcoholics: Facts and fancies. *Alcoholism: Clinical and Experimental Research*, 1977, *1*, 51–56.

Parsons, O. A., & Fabian, M. S. Do recovered alcoholic women have perceptual–cognitive deficits? Paper presented at the National Council on Alcoholism Annual Meeting, New Orleans, 1981.

Parsons, O. A., & Farr, S. P. The neuropsychology of alcohol and drug abuse. In S. B. Filskov & T. J. Boll (Eds.), *Handbook of clinical neuropsychology.* New York: Wiley, 1981.

Parsons, O. A., & Leber, W. R. The relationship between cognitive dysfunction and brain damage in alcoholics: Causal, interactive or epiphenomenal? *Alcoholism: Clinical and Experimental Research*, 1981, *5*, 326–343.

Parsons, O. A., & Leber, W. R. Alcohol, cognitive dysfunction and brain damage. In National Institute on Alcohol Abuse and Alcoholism, *Biomedical processes and consequences of alcohol use* (Alcohol and Health Monograph 2). Rockville, Md.: The Institute, 1982. (DHHS Publ. No. (ADM) 82-1191)

Parsons, O. A., & Prigatano, G. P. Methodological considerations in clinical neuropsychological research. *Journal of Consulting and Clinical Psychology*, 1978, *46*, 608–619.

Peterson, G. C. Organic mental disorders. In H. I. Kaplin, A. M. Freedman, & D. J. Sadock (Eds.), *Comprehensive textbook of psychiatry*, III. Baltimore: Williams & Wilkins, 1980.

Prigatano, G. P., & Parsons, O. A. The relationship of age and education to Halstead Test performance in different patient populations. *Journal of Consulting and Clinical Psychology*, 1976, *44*, 527–533.

Ramsey, T. A. Opiate dependence. In A. Frazer & A. Winokur (Eds.), *Biological basis of psychiatric disorders*. New York: Spectrum Publications, 1977.

Reitan, R. M. Behavioral manifestations of impaired brain functioning in aging. Paper presented at the Annual Meeting of the American Psychological Association, Montreal, 1973.

Reitan, R. M., & Davison, L. A. (Eds.), *Clinical neuropsychology: Current status and applications*. Washington, D.C.: V. H. Winston & Son, 1974.

Rochford, J., Grant, I., & LaVigne, G. Medical students and drugs: Neuropsychological and use pattern considerations. *International Journal of Addictions*, 1977, *12*, 1057–1065.

Ron, M. A. Brain damage in chronic alcoholism: A neuropathological, neuroradiological and psychological review. *Psychological Medicine*, 1977, *7*, 103–112.

Rumbaugh, C. L., Bergeron, R. T., Fang, H. C. H., & McCormick, R. Cerebral angiographic changes in the drug abuse patient. *Radiology*, 1971, *101*, 335–344.

Russell, E., Neuringer, C., & Goldstein, G. *Assessment of brain damage: A neuropsychological key approach*. New York: Wiley, 1970.

Russell, E. W. A multiple scoring method for assessment of complex memory functions. *Journal of Consulting and Clinical Psychology*, 1975, *43*, 800–809.

Schau, E. J., & O'Leary, M. R. Adaptive abilities of hospitalized alcoholics and matched controls. *Journal of Studies on Alcohol*, 1977, *38*, 403–409.

Schau, E. J., O'Leary, M. R., & Chavey, E. F. Reversibility of cognitive defect in alcoholics. *Journal of Studies on Alcohol*, 1980, *41*, 733–748.

Seltzer, M. L. Alcoholism and alcoholic psychoses. In H. I. Kaplan, A. M. Freedman, & B. J. Sadock (Eds.), *Comprehensive textbook of psychiatry* (Vol. 2, 3rd ed.). Baltimore: Williams & Wilkins, 1980.

Smith, J. W. Neurological disorders in alcoholism. In N. J. Estes & M. E. Heineman (Eds.), *Alcoholism*. St. Louis, Mo.: C. V. Mosby, 1977.

Stinnett, J. L. Alcoholism. In A. Frazer & A. Winokur (Eds.), *Biological bases of psychiatric disorders*. New York: Spectrum Publications, 1977.

Tarter, R. E. Psychological deficit in chronic alcoholics: A review. *International Journal of Addiction*, 1975, *10*, 327–368.

Trites, R. L., Suh, M., Offord, D., Neiman, G., & Preston, D. *Neuropsychologic and psychosocial antecedents and chronic effects of prolonged use of solvents and methamphetamine*. Paper presented at the International Psychiatric Research Society, Ottawa, October, 1974.

Tsushima, W. T., & Towne, W. S. Effects of paint sniffing on neuropsychological test performance. *Journal of Abnormal Psychology*, 1977, *864*, 402–407.

United States Department of Justice. *Drugs of abuse*. Washington, D.C.: U.S. Government Printing Office, 1977.

Von Zerssen, D., Fliege, K., & Wolf, M. Cerebral atrophy in drug addicts. *Lancet*, 1970, *2*, 313.

Wright, M., & Hogan, T. P. Repeated LSD ingestion and performance on neuropsychological tests. *Journal of Nervous and Mental Disorders*, 1972, *154*, 432–438.

10

Normal Aging and the Concept of Dementia

GERALD GOLDSTEIN

This chapter will begin by stating the proposition that there is no substantial decline in intellectual function with advancing age except in the case of those elderly individuals who acquire diseases of the central nervous system. Thus, many elderly people may experience deterioration of intellectual functioning from a previously higher level, but not simply because they are elderly. The more fundamental reason is that, as one grows older, the probability of acquiring a disease of the central nervous system increases. The contrary view, also stated in an extreme form, is that following a peak period during early adulthood, intellectual abilities enter into a slow decline. This view was made popular through Wechsler's (1944) well-known curve of variations of intelligence scores and vital capacity with age. Thus, age may explain nothing or it may explain everything.

In examining these two divergent positions, it is important to make certain distinctions of a methodological nature. The terms age effects, age changes, age correlations, and age differences all sound about the same, but they really mean different things. An *age effect* is a phenomenon that can be directly associated with chronological age. To give a trivial example, the ability to identify a picture of an individual prominent during the early part of the twentieth century may be directly associated with age because people born after that individual was prominent cannot be expected to remember her or him. An *age change* has to do with an alteration of some function over time in the same individual. Age changes are

GERALD GOLDSTEIN • Research, Veterans Administration Medical Center, Pittsburgh, Pennsylvania 15206.

generally noted through some form of longitudinal study in which a cohort of individuals is studied over many years. An *age correlation* occurs when some function is related to chronological age at a statistically significant level. For example, there may be a significant correlation between chronological age and performance on a cognitive test. As we may recall from basic statistics, correlation does not imply causation, and so the noted association with age may have been produced by a variety of causative agents other than age itself. *Age differences* simply means that individuals of different ages perform at different levels on some task or function.

It is particularly important to note that an age difference and an age change are not at all the same thing. The term age change implies the presence of an observed change in some particular individual. While age differences may be established on the basis of a longitudinal study, more often than not they are established on the basis of cross-section studies consisting of comparisons between groups of different individuals of varying ages. For example, a group of 20-year-olds may be compared with a group of 70-year-olds on some test of cognitive ability. If the difference between groups in level of performance is statistically significant, then it is generally concluded that there is an age difference. However, the difference may have nothing to do with chronological age, and any inference suggesting that the difference noted is caused by the age difference would be scientifically indefensible. While careful investigators attempt to make comparison groups of this kind as comparable as possible with regard to factors that could effect performance on the dependent measure, attribution of causality remains questionable. For example, in studies of cognitive ability, most investigators attempt to equate groups for variables other than age that could effect performance such as education, sex distribution, socioeconomic status, and health status. However, that doesn't entirely do the job for many reasons. Just as an example, when one equates groups of different age brackets for education, one makes the assumption that x years of education in a 70-year-old is the same as x years of education in a 20-year-old. In other words, the education that people received during the second decade of the twentieth century is the same as the education received during the 1970s. Surely, that is unlikely to be the case.

These considerations might lead to the conclusion that in order to establish phenomena that are truly related to aging, it is best to do a longitudinal study. It is a better solution, but far from a perfect one. The difficulty with longitudinal studies of normal aging is that subjects become unavailable or ill, or they die. Therefore, as the study progresses over time, the sample becomes increasingly selective and decreasingly representative of the population from which it is drawn. Particularly when the more advanced age ranges are reached, one could be left with a relatively small sample of unusually healthy individuals, some of whom might in fact have acquired some undiagnosed medical condition that could affect their performance. There have been solutions proposed that deal with some of the methodological problems. For example, there is the problem of the so-called cohort or generational effect that haunts cross-sectional aging studies. The problem is that people who are of some particular age at one particular time or during one generation may be different in several respects from people who were the same age at some other point in time. Thus, in cross-sectional studies one is comparing not only different age groups but people brought up in different generations. Being brought up in different generations implies being brought up under different sociocultural conditions. Thus, the effects of age are inextricably confounded with the effects of being in a particular cohort. One proposed solution involves studying several cohorts longitudinally. Thus, for example, a group of people who were in their 20s during the 1940s could be followed over several years, but groups of people who were in their 20s during the 1960s and 1980s could also be followed. In this way, the investigator can examine the cohort effect by testing for differences among people who were in their 20s at different times, as well as the age changes through the longitudinal aspect of the design. Schaie and Labouvie-Vief (1974) undertook such a study and found that on certain tests there were striking generational differences while on other tests the age changes were much more pronounced than the cohort effects. However, even this very elegant kind of design does not answer questions concerning health status as a possible explanation for the longitudinal changes found.

The conclusion one might wish to draw on the basis of these methodological problems is that, while aging in and of itself might produce changes in level of cognitive function, it is essentially impossible to demonstrate this to be the case. Thus, in a scientific sense, chronological age becomes an unsatisfactory independent variable, and the investigator interested in the regularities of changes in cognitive function in an individual over time may do better by seeking other independent variables that can be studied with less ambiguity than is the case for chronological age. Those interested in evironmental effects might wish to focus on the extent to which the decrease in activity level and stimulation, which commonly seems to accompany aging, influences cognitive abilities. Those interested in medical issues might want to look at how changes in physiology, particularly as they impact on the central nervous system, affect cognition. Within this realm, neuropsychologists have looked at aging from the point of view of the interaction between chronological age and performance on tests used in the assessment of brain dysfunction. However, to the best of our knowledge, neuropsychologists have only looked at age differences and age correlations thus far. We know of no neuropsychological study of age changes, as defined above. In other words, there have been no longitudinal studies of normal individuals utilizing standard neuropsychological tests, unless one considers the Wechsler Adult Intelligence Scale to be a neuropsychological test. In any event, we know very little about changes in neuropsychological function over age in the same individual.

It is generally agreed that age-related changes in cognitive function do not affect all abilities equally. Generally, verbal abilities remain about the same throughout adult life, while abilities dependent upon psychomotor speed and perceptual abilities of various kinds deteriorate sharply with age. In initially bright people, the preservation of verbal ability is even more likely to occur. The age-associated changes that do occur do not become apparent until after 50 (Botwinick, 1978), not during the middle 20s as was thought by Wechsler (1944). Some investigators have suggested that "crystallized intelligence" does not deteriorate with age, while "fluid intelligence" does (Horn & Cattell, 1967). However, because tests of crystallized intelligence greatly resemble the WAIS verbal subtests while measures of fluid intelligence resemble the performance tests, the distinction contributes little more than does reference to what Botwinick (1978) has termed the "classic aging pattern": little if any decline in verbal ability with appreciable decline in psychomotor function. In this regard, even this distinction is somewhat ambiguous because psychomotor performance tests generally confound speed of performance with cognitive ability. The increasing slowness, with age, of information processing by the brain seems reasonably well established (Birren, 1964) and has been extensively studied with reaction time and related procedures.

Rather than using chronological age as the independent variable in studies of the relationship between aging and intellectual function, neuropsychological researchers now are seeking some way of measuring the age of the brain itself. As we know, the brain loses a multitude of neurons every day of its life, but consequences of this loss are not completely understood. It is, however, apparent that the brain cannot age at the same rate or even in the same way for all people. Because the passage of objective time is the same for everybody, it is also clear that there cannot be a perfect correlation between chronological age and the aging process that takes place in the brain. There are undoubtedly exogenous and endogenous sources of variability. Varying degrees of exposure to environmental toxins may have an effect, as may acquisition of some disease, personal habits, and genetic factors. Attempts to implement this concept have been made by Halstead and Rennick (1962), who used the term "Biological Age" to describe what we are talking about, and by Reitan (1973), who used the term "Brain Age." Reitan (1973) devised a method of computing a "Brain Age Quotient" in which "age" of the brain is compared with chronological age. The "Brain Age Quotient" is computed much like one would a mental age from the results of an intelligence test.

Another related line of investigation involves the development of an adequate brain model for aging. This question has typically been addressed indirectly through studies of individuals with some known disease entity and normal elderly individuals. As part of this approach, it is suggested that certain pathological entities produce premature aging of the brain. Perhaps the clearest and most direct studies involving this view have been accomplished in the area of alcoholism within the context of the attempt to test the so-called premature aging theory of alcoholism (Ryan & Butters, 1980). The methodology used in this research involves comparing alcoholics in a particular age range with carefully matched groups of nonalcoholics in an older range. It is generally found that the performance of the alcoholics is worse than that of their nonalcoholic age peers but comparable to normal people who are substantially older. Other investigators have been concerned with similarities and differences between brain damage in general and aging. Reed and Reitan (1963), for example, found that those neuropsychological tests that discriminate best between brain-damaged and non-brain-damaged individuals also discriminate best between old and young people. Goldstein and Shelly (1973) found that while there were similarities in test performance between normal elderly and diffusely brain-damaged individuals, the similarity was not complete. For certain abilities, they found a resemblance between the effects of normal aging and diffuse brain damage, but for other abilities they did not. Other research (Hallenbeck, 1964; Overall & Gorham, 1972) also suggests that the differences in cognitive abilities found between young and old people are not necessarily the same as those found between younger brain-damaged and non-brain-damaged people.

Kinsbourne (1980) has pointed out that there are three classes of pathological events that might affect the brain over the course of time. There may be a uniform process of neuronal depletion, a skewed process of neuronal depletion (which primarily affects the balance of various mutually inhibitory systems), or intense focal brain damage. Which of these events, or which combination of them, occurs obviously has a pronounced effect on what happens during the aging of a particular individual, and so one might expect to find a great deal of variability just with regard to the biological determinants of age-related changes. When one adds the environmental, sociocultural determinants, the potential for variability among individuals should increase substantially. It therefore becomes quite difficult to defend some particular simple rubric describing the effects of aging such as "crystallized versus fluid intelligence" or "verbal versus perceptual integrative skills." However, efforts to describe a variety of age-related phenomena in terms of some general concept such as selective attention (Kinsbourne, 1980) may be quite helpful.

Another way of dealing with the variability matter is the adoption of a syndrome approach in which it is assumed that a variety of changes may be associated with aging, but they can be conceptualized as occurring within a finite number of patterns or syndromes. Perhaps one of the more popular and controversial of the proposed syndromes has to do with the right or minor hemisphere. It is thought by some that the right hemisphere ages more rapdily than the left, as least in some individuals, and there have been some studies of that possibility (Goldstein & Shelly, 1981; Klisz, 1978). While no student of this matter seriously entertains the notion that the right cerebral hemisphere deteriorates physically more rapidly than the left, there is thought to be some possibility that the specific functions of the right hemisphere age more rapidly than do left hemisphere functions. Some critics of this view suggest that it only represents another way of saying that verbal abilities are relatively well preserved with age while performance abilities decline, since the left hemisphere is primarily responsible for the mediation of language skills while the right hemisphere controls perceptual–integrative or visual–spatial skills. However, Goldstein and Shelly (1981) and Gordon, Bentin, and Silverberg (1979) were able to demonstrate patterns of selective right hemisphere deterioration with aging that did not lend themselves to a simple verbal vs. perceptual-integrative interpretation. Goldstein and Shelly (1981) found that the discrepancy between performance times with the right and left hand on the Halstead Tactual Performance Test increased with age only in the direction of the left hand being worse than the right. In other words, an age difference was noted for relative dysfunction of the left hand (right hemisphere), but not of the right hand (left hemisphere). The Cognitive Laterality Battery used by Gordon, Bentin, and Silverberg (1979) assesses specialized functions of the two hemispheres utilizing cognitive measures that do not emphasize a contrast between verbal and performance abilities. Rather, the battery stresses differences between sequential processing, which is thought to be accomplished mainly by the left hemisphere, as opposed to simultaneous processing, thought to be primarily a right hemisphere function. Thus, there appears to be some evidence for selective right hemisphere functional deterioration that may not be readily explainable on the basis of the verbal versus performance dichotomy or the higher complexity level often associated with "right hemisphere" tests.

The other major viable alternative appears to be that the cognitive decline associated with aging may be described as a frontal lobe syndrome. The frontal lobe syndrome generally involves some combination of poor judgment and planning ability, diminished capacity to regulate impulses, apathy and changes in language function related to speech fluency, the ability to produce a spontaneous narrative, and the ability to use language in the regulation of behavior (Luria, 1973). Patients with frontal lobe structural brain damage often display one or more of these deficits in the form of lack of motivation, inability to maintain focused attention, poor impulse control, and impaired performance on complex cognitive tasks requiring abstraction, planning, and judgment. Unfortunately, the hypothesis that frontal lobe functions deteriorate more rapidly than functions associated with other regions of the brain has not been studied in a way comparable to what was done for the right hemisphere hypothesis.

The major difficulty seems to be that there are not as yet neuropsychological tests available that assess frontal lobe deficits in a specific and valid manner. While some neuropsychologists speak of "frontal lobe tests," such tests are often performed in a deficient manner by patients with nonfrontal lesions, and so lack sufficient specificity. Nevertheless, when one describes the clinical phenomenology of the frontal lobe patient, one can see the resemblances with what occurs with advanced age. The literature on problem solving and age (Botwinick, 1978) might also suggest to the neuropsychologist that the difficulties elderly people have with regard to shifting sets, implementing an orderly plan for problem solution, and filtering out irrelevant information while focusing on the relevancies, are much like what is seen in the case of the frontal lobe patient.

The syndromal approach to age-related cognitive changes as well as approaches that utilize various manifestations of a compiex construct such as selective attention, have the value of being able to explain at least to some extent the variability that is seen among elderly individuals. Perhaps the most accurate statement that can be made about this area is that as age increases, so does variability. Kinsbourne (1980) suggests that were it not for artifacts produced by the experimental designs and procedures used in aging research, this variability would become apparent. It is our view that at least some of this variability is contributed to by various health and physiological factors. There is evidence that the individual with a long history of alcoholism appears to age more rapidly than normal, and cardiovascular status, notably the maintenance of optimal blood pressure, appears to have a great deal to do with intellectual decline (Wilkie & Eisdorfer, 1971). The other significant factor is that a substantial portion of the elderly population acquires one of the progressive degenerative dementias. It is estimated that 5% to 7% of the population at age 65 have moderate to severe dementia, but that the probability of acquiring it increases with age (Miller & Cohen, 1981). Put in actual numbers, Ringler (1981) reports that there may be as many as 4 million people in the United States aged 65 or over who have at least mild dementia. It is now accepted by most authorities that dementia is an actual disease that one acquires or doesn't acquire, and not just the extreme end of the normal aging continuum. Thus, many consequences previously attributed to aging may in fact be the products of dementia, and it is that problem to which we will now turn our attention.

AGING AND DEMENTIA

Dementia represents a class of disorders in which *in vivo* definitive diagnosis is often not possible. The basic difficulty is that the brain cannot be directly seen, except when neurosurgery or biopsy is performed, and can only be visualized through indirect procedures, notably radiological ones. In order to confirm the diagnosis of certain progressive dementias, notably Alzheimer's and Pick's disease, it is necessary to directly examine brain tissue for characteristic pathological changes. These changes, which generally include senile plaques, neurofibrillary tangles, granulovacuolar degeneraton, and Pick bodies (in the case of Pick's disease), cannot be seen with even the most sophisticated radiological or nuclear medicine procedures. Thus, diagnosis of dementia is almost always a clinical rather than a pathological diagnosis. This technological problem, which may eventually be solved, provides a major difficulty in regard to achieving further understanding of the relationship between the aging process and cognitive function. The major problem is that as one goes up the age scale, in the form of a longitudinal or cross-sectional study, the probability of the occurrence of dementia increases. While the researcher interested in normal aging may attempt to eliminate subjects with dementia from the samples under investigation, when one gets into the more advanced age ranges, it is unlikely that this attempt will be entirely successful. The individual with mild and/or early dementia is particularly problematic because the diagnostic difficulties are most pronounced in those cases. Therefore, when one reaches the age range during which the most substantive cognitive changes begin to occur, one really can't say if a normally aging group is being studied or a group that contains an unknown percentage of individuals with dementia. The prevalence of dementia among the elderly makes the latter possibility a reasonably good one.

Thus, the neuropsychology of aging and the neuropsychology of dementia are borderlands in which clear distinctions cannot yet be made. However, there have been many studies of cognitive performance patterns in patients diagnosed as having dementia, some of which have been at least partially supported by autopsy data (Roth, 1980). If research of this type provides increasingly refined information about the specific changes characteristic of various subtypes of dementia, it will become increasingly possible to infer what actually occurs in normal aging. As indicated at the beginning of this chapter, we may find out that there are no substantial cognitive changes with normal aging, but we really don't know one way or the other yet.

Alzheimer's Disease

Alzheimer's disease is generally thought to be the most common of the progressive degenerative dementias. Its cause is generally accepted to be a neurochemical defect in which a central cholinergic deficiency appears, for presently unknown reasons. The progression of the disease is marked by gradual death of the neurons that provide receptor sites for choline, known as the cholinergic or choline neurons. Clinically, there is a presenile type, appearing in the middle 50s, and a senile type that appears during the 60s and later. Authorities are divided as to whether they are the same disease or not, but the brain pathology is the same in both cases. The course of the illness is marked by uniformly progressive intellectual deterioration, generally manifested first in the form of memory impairment, then by language and visual–spatial difficulties and finally by global deterioration of essentially all intellectual abilities. It is a terminal illness, with death generally occurring about 5 years after the onset of symptoms.

In his review of cognitive deficit in dementia, Miller (1981) divides the topic into the area of general intelligence (IQ), memory, language, perception, and other cognitive functions. The nature of the memory deficit is not fully understood, but is thought to involve both short-term and long-term memory. While clinical observation generally suggests that remote memories are better preserved than recent ones, experimental evidence suggests that there is significant impairment of both forms of memory. There is some evidence (Fuld, Katzman, Davies, & Terry, 1982) that patients with dementia make excessive intrusions, a phenomenon generally defined as inappropriate recurrence of a response to a preceding event. This finding would support the hypothesis that the capacity to suppress erroneous or inappropriate responses is disinhibited in dementia (Warrington & Weiskrantz, 1970). Because the effect is also seen in normal individuals when given scopolamine, a choline antagonist (Drachman & Leavitt, 1972), the finding would also support the cholinergic hypothesis of Alzheimer's disease. In any event, it would appear that the memory deficit in Alzheimer's disease is global, and apparently cannot be characterized in terms of such information processing categories as acquisition, encoding, storage, or retrieval; nor is it a specific short-term or long-term memory deficit.

The deterioration of language in Alzheimer's disease has recently become a matter of great interest. As a general summary statement, it can be said that the nature of the deterioration can be described as a gradual impoverishment of language. The size of the active vocabulary diminishes, as is manifested by increasing difficulties with word finding, and the ability to produce a narrative is reduced, sometimes to the point at which speech becomes unintelligible. Most authorities would now agree that Alzheimer's disease does not generally produce classic aphasic syndromes of the type commonly seen in stroke patients. Albert, Goodglass, Helm, Rubens, and Alexander (1981) point to the breakdown in logical associations, the naming deficit, the simplification of syntax, and the appearance of the symptoms of perseveration, echolalia, tangentiality, and intrusions of inappropriate material.

While patients with Alzheimer's disease do not generally develop primary visual or auditory perceptual deficits, visual–spatial difficulties are commonly observed. The capacity to make constructions, copy figures, read maps, or perform maze-type tasks may all be impaired. Attentional deficits have also been noted, particularly with regard to the presence of high susceptibility to distractions. Having made this point, however, it is nevertheless extremely important to evaluate visual and auditory acuity before drawing conclusions concerning cognitive ability in an elderly population.

In summary, Alzheimer's disease is characterized by a progressive wasting of the brain associated with correspondingly globally progressive intellectual impairment. The degree of correspondence has been documented by Blessed, Tomlinson, and Roth (1968), who obtained a $+.77$ correlation ($p < .001$) between the score on a dementia scale and senile plaque count obtained after death. The earliest cognitive deficits noted are generally in the area of short-term memory, but language, visual–spatial skills, and other cognitive abilities gradually deteriorate to the point of global, severe impairment and ultimate death. The cause of the disorder is now thought to involve a central cholinergic deficiency, but the reason for acquisition of the deficiency is as yet unknown.

Multi-Infarct Dementia and Focal Vascular Disease

In the past, it was thought that most dementia in the elderly was caused by cerebral arteriosclerosis, popularly known as "hardening of the arteries." Recent research has indicated that arteriosclerosis only involving the cerebral blood vessels in a diffuse way is quite rare, if it exists at all. Furthermore, it now seems that most dementia in the elderly is produced by Alzheimer's disease and not by vascular changes. However, there is a condition occurring in an estimated 12% to 20% of elderly demented individuals known as multi-infarct dementia (Rosen, Terry, Fuld, Katzman, & Peck, 1980). The condition exists primarily in hypertensive individuals who sustain multiple episodes of cerebral ischemia leading to cerebral infarcts that may be located in essentially any region of the brain. The course of the disorder is generally described as stepwise and patchy. It is stepwise because the course of the deterioration is dependent upon the occurrence of episodes of ischemia over time, and it is patchy because the infarcts can be distributed over various individual loci in the brain. However, the end result is a progressive dementia leading in some respects to the same kinds of neuropsychological deficits found in Alzheimer's disease. Indeed, the differential diagnosis between Alzheimer's disease and multi-infarct dementia is not always an easy one to make on clinical grounds.

By definition, the pattern of intellectual deterioration in multi-infarct dementia cannot be characterized in any specific way because of the great deal of variability caused by the episodic strokes appearing essentially anywhere in the brain. However, studies comparing age and education matched Alzheimer's disease patients with multi-infarct dementia patients, the Alzheimer's patients demonstrated substantially more impairment (Gainotti, Caltagirone, Masullo, & Miceli, 1980; Perez, Rivera, Meyer, Gay, Taylor, & Matthew, 1975). Apparently, the cognitive deficit associated with multi-infarct dementia is not as devastating as is the case for Alzheimer's disease. However, the physical and medical problems of multi-infarct patients are typically worse since they typically have heart disease and often have physical disabilities, such as hemiplegia or visual field defects, associated with their strokes.

Focal vascular disease is not generally classified as a form of dementia, but stroke is not at all an uncommon age-related phenomenon. We simply wish to point out here that the occurrence of a single major stroke can significantly alter the ongoing pattern of age-related cognitive changes. However, these alterations would be highly associated with the site and severity of the stroke. If the left hemisphere is primarily involved, the normally expected minimal changes in language function with age will not occur, and language may be significantly impaired for a greater or lesser period of time. If the stroke was in the right hemisphere, language changes might go through the normal aging process, but the expected decrement in visual–spatial and constructional difficulties may be greatly amplified. Thus, in the aging individual, the presence of a history of major stroke interacts very significantly with the aging process. However, unless the stroke victim develops multi-infarct dementia, the stroke in and of itself does not presage the acquisition of a progressive dementia. In other words, stroke patients may have specific neuropsychological deficits, but they do not necessarily have a progressive degenerative disease. It should be pointed out, however, that an estimated 16% to 20% of demented patients (Rosen *et al.*, 1980) have both Alzheimer's disease and multi-infarct dementia. Individuals with Alzheimer's disease may also have single major strokes. Thus, an individual patient may have symptomatologies associated with several disorders.

Aging and Alcoholism

There is a widely held view that alcoholism accelerates the aging process. Indeed, as we have already indicated, the changes associated with alcoholism may assist in providing a brain model for the normal aging process. Neuropathologists have reported that the pathological changes found in the brains of elderly individuals are often found in the brains of younger alcoholics (Brody, 1970; Courville, 1955; Ordy & Brizzee, 1975). Neuropsychological studies of the premature aging hypothesis have found that test performance of alcoholics looks in many respects like the performance of more elderly nonalcoholics. In the case of a study by Beck, Dustman, Blusewicz, and Cannon (1979), this finding was obtained despite a nearly 40-year age difference. Ryan and Butters (1980) have reported similar findings in the area of memory and learning. There is some evidence that the interaction between aging and alcholism, as related to intellectual deterioration, becomes accelerated with advancing years (Jones & Parsons, 1971).

The current diagnostic manual for mental disorders (DSM-III) contains the diagnosis of "Dementia Associated with Alcoholism." Dementia is defined with the same terms for this diagnosis as it is for other dementias, including those associated with aging. The only difference is that all causes have been excluded other than prolonged alcohol use. In order to rule out the acute effects of intoxication, the dementia must be present 3 weeks after the patient stops drinking. While there are doubtless significant neuropsychological differences between dementia associated with alcoholism and other dementias, they have not been systematically studied. We may note, however, that the language deficits frequently associated with Alzheimer's disease are not commonly seen in patients with alcoholism-related dementia. It may also be noted that the diagnosis of dementia associated with alcoholism is somewhat lacking in scientific respectability because it is usually exceedingly difficult to determine whether the dementia is indeed associated directly with alcohol abuse or with other conditions that commonly accompany alcohol abuse such as multiple head trauma, malnutrition, and liver disease.

From the point of view of the neuropsychology of aging, the effects of alcoholism are of particular interest because they dramatically represent a class of exogenous agents that interact with aging. The alcoholic may "become old before his or her time," or alcoholism may have a particularly deleterious effect on an aged brain. The extent to which other personal habits involving such matters as diet, drug use, and perhaps even exercise and smoking, influence the aging process would appear to be a matter of substantial significance.

Aging and Health

As we have already seen, the direct effects of the aging process, whatever they may be, interact with a variety of other influences in regard to determination of the type and degree of change in cognitive functioning. The issues related to dementia and well researched areas such as alcoholism have already been outlined, but there is another less well studied and understood area related to the influence of general physical health status on the aging process. The problem, put in its simplest form, is that perhaps following early childhood, the probability of acquiring an illness having consequences for the central nervous system increases with age. A multitude of diseases are age-related and are known to affect brain function. From a methodological standpoint, when we try to study normal aging, we try to study normal people. The difficulty is that as one gets into the more advanced years, it becomes increasingly difficult to, first of all, find normal subjects, and then to assure ourselves that they do not have a physical illness that could influence central nervous system function. In the elderly we see the long-term effects of a wide variety of factors that could be having significant influences, including but not restricted to lengthy periods of malnutrition, mild hypertension not associated with heart attack or stroke, chronic infection, long-term exposure to toxic substances in industrial settings, undiagnosed neoplastic disease, multiple head injury not sufficiently severe during any single episode to be brought to medical attention, and chronic pulmonary disease.

Documentation of the influence of health status on cognitive function in elderly people has been accomplished by Botwinick and Birren (1963) and by Correll, Rokosz, and Blanchard (1966). In both of these investigations, relationships were found between carefully evaluated health status and performance on cognitive tests. Wilkie and Eisdorfer (1971) found that subjects with high diastolic blood pressure showed more decline on the WAIS following a ten-year interval than did subjects with normal or borderline blood pressure.

There is also a growing neuropsychological literature concerning the relationships between physical disease entities, such as lead toxicity and chronic obstructive pulmonary disease, and cognitive function. In general, studies in these areas demonstrate relatively strong relationships. For example, Grant, Heaton, McSweeney, Adams, and Timms (1980) found that a large proportion of the chronic obstructive pulmonary disease patients they studied performed in the impaired range on the Halstead–Reitan battery. With regard to the specific role of aging, Jacobs, Alvis, and Small (1972) have suggested that many of the cognitive deficits seen among the elderly may be at least partially related to changes in cerebral oxygenation. Studies of individuals with systemic illnesses such as diabetes mellitus (Bale, 1973; Ryan, Vega, Drash, & Longstreet, 1982) have revealed similar relationships. Thus, it seems clear that health status may significantly influence cognitive function, and health status tends to decline as one gets into the more advanced age ranges. If one accepts these conclusions, the implications have both methodological and theoretical consequences.

Methodologically, in longitudinal studies of normal aging, changes in health status among members of the cohort under study tend to increasingly bias the sample. If subjects who develop health problems during the course of the study are dropped, the sample tends to consist of increasingly more individuals who are unusually healthy for their age. One finds oneself studying a group of "geriatric astronauts." If these subjects are not dropped, the sample remains more representative of what actually occurs to people as they get older, but the effects of aging and illness cannot be separated. In the case of cross-sectional studies, similar problems emerge. It is exceedingly difficult, from a practical standpoint, to obtain age samples that are equated for health status.

The theoretical implications of the aging and health matter bring us back to our initial thesis. There may, in fact, not be any neuropsychological changes associated in a meaningful way with chronological age alone. What associations exist may only be indirect ones related to the numerous changes in health status and physiological function that decline with age. Even such universally seen age-related changes as decline in memory ability (Botwinick, 1978) may be associated with corresponding decline in cardiovascular status as related to cerebral oxygenation. In any event, the task of the neuropsychologist might be defined in this area in terms of seeking associations between health status connected alterations in brain function as they may be related to aging and behavior.

Dementia and Pseudodementia

Wells (1979) has proposed that there is a group of elderly individuals who demonstrate symptoms of dementia but who do not have underlying brain disease. Rather, the dementia appears to be associated with a functional psychiatric disorder, generally depression. Thus, for example, patients with pseudodementia as opposed to actual dementia tend to complain about their cognitive losses, highlight their failures, and communicate a strong sense of distress. The extent to which dementia diagnosed in the elderly is really pseudodementia is not known, although there is evidence from epidemiological studies (Duckworth & Ross, 1975) that dementia in the elderly tends to be overdiagnosed, particularly in the United States.

The actual mechanism of pseudodementia is not fully understood. In that the syndrome does not appear to occur frequently in younger depressed patients, it probably represents some interaction between the effects of aging and depression. More specifically, Folstein & McHugh (1978) have suggested that the interaction involves biochemical changes associated with depression and the neuronal changes characteristic of aging. Thus, it is perhaps best characterized not as a pseudocondition but as a real dementia that is reversible. There are other types of reversible dementia, some of which may be associated with normal pressure hydrocephalus and some with various metabolic disorders. Perhaps the best diagnostic label is dementia syndrome of depression. In effect, many clinicians working in geriatric settings see patients who appear demented and who then recover in whole or part. However, the nature of the disorder that underlies this condition is not yet fully understood. At this point, considering our lack of knowledge, the term "pseudodementia" may seem somewhat gratuitous.

AN EXAMINATION OF THE CONCEPT OF DEMENTIA AND ITS RELATION TO THE NEUROPSYCHOLOGY OF AGING

Scientific Considerations

Until the term became somewhat more specifically defined, some neuropsychologists did not like to use the word dementia because it was viewed as synonymous with such other vagaries as "organic brain syndrome," "chronic brain syndrome," and "mental impairment." It remains an archaic term with a great deal of surplus meaning, but if its use is restricted to the progressive degenerative disorders of the brain, perhaps this situation has been remedied somewhat. However, the more important point is that the global nature of the term does not do full justice to the complex and varying patterns of brain-behavior relationships that characterize the various brain disorders we call dementia. As a possible analogy, the neuropsychologist might view calling all of these disorders "dementia" in a manner similar to how the oncologist might view the practice of calling all of the neoplastic diseases "cancer." In both cases, a more refined terminology is needed in order to make meaningful diagnoses, prognoses, and treatment plans. We will return to this point in our discussion of clinical considerations.

The major theoretical issues associated with the neuropsychology of dementia have to do with differences among different types of dementia, the nature of the neuropsychological deficits that characterize these disorders, and the possibly differing courses of the different disorders from the point of view of changes over time in pattern and level of cognitive function. Methodologically, a combined longitudinal and cross-sectional approach is required in order to investigate these matters. Longitudinal studies are required to trace the course of these disorders in individual patients, while cross-sectional investigations are needed to look at differences among the different diagnostic subgroups. It is possible that the further investigation of dementia may shed additional light on the normal aging process. Perhaps one way of putting the matter might be to raise the question of whether or not everybody would acquire a dementia if he or she lived long enough. If that is the case, then dementia might well be an accelerated aging process. If it is not the case, then the dementias are acquired diseases of the brain that are distinct from the morphological and neurochemical changes that take place over time in the normal brain. Current thinking about the dementias suggests that they are a number of disease entities and not a part of the normal aging process. However, the logical problem remains that we can never answer that question fully because we never know whether any particular individual would acquire the disease had he or she lived longer. Obviously, not all old people die demented, but that does not mean that they would not have become demented had they lived longer. Thus, it is not now possible to determine whether or not dementia is accelerated aging. However, were we to discover a biological marker for dementia that exists prior to acquisition of symptoms, we would be in a better position to answer the question. For example, if the central cholinergic deficiency thought to produce Alzheimer's disease is an inborn metabolic error, then some as yet unknown marker of that condition might exist from the time of birth. In the case of Alzheimer's disease, there is some hope that such a marker may be found in some characteristic of choline transport across the red blood cell membrane (Friedman, Sherman, Ferris, Reisberg, Bartus, & Schneck, 1981).

Another way of looking at the matter is that of determining whether or not the pattern of cognitive abilities seen in dementia resemble what is seen in the nondemented elderly. With regard to the dementia associated with Alzheimer's disease, a major difference would appear to lie in the matter of the dissolution of language. Language appears to be among our hardiest abilities and can sustain the ravages of time quite well. Indeed, we have noted an improvement in language ability over time in individuals without brain disease (Goldstein & Shelly, 1975). However, language can become significantly impaired with Alzheimer's disease. On the other hand, the relative absence of language impairment found in individuals with alcoholism related dementia (Parsons & Farr, 1981) give it a cognitive profile that is more similar to what is seen in normal aging than is the case for Alzheimer's disease. Thus, Alzheimer's disease may not represent accelerated aging but a different underlying process. The other major type of dementia, multi-infarct dementia, may or may not include language impairment, since that would depend on whether or not one of the strokes involves the speech area. It would seem apparent that multi-infarct dementia is not accelerated aging since it is so clearly related to the acquisition of cardiovascular disease. Furthermore, the course, clinical phenomenology, and associated symptoms of multi-infarct dementia typically do not resemble what is found in elderly people without known brain disease.

The nature of the neuropsychological deficits associated with dementia is far from well understood. In the case of Alzheimer's disease, it now seems apparent that there is little likelihood that a single rubric or dimension will provide a useful formulation of all the deficits noted. Neuropsychological research has provided extensive theoretical frameworks for a number of disorders such as the aphasias, Korsakoff's syndrome, and other specific syndromes. Thus, for example, the nature of the memory disorder in Korsakoff's syndrome is well understood in information processing terms (Butters & Cermak, 1980). However, such a level of theoretical understanding has not been reached for Alzheimer's disease. Attempts at such theorizing in the area of memory have led to the formulation of concepts related to intrusions, disinhibition, and defects in the encoding process. None of these attempts have really been successful, and the currently used memory theories involving multistage analysis and levels of processing have not revealed those particular aspects of the information processing chain that are defective in dementia.

In this regard, it seems to us that a distinction may be made between the unknown and the unknowable. While it is true that a great deal of memory research that could be done with Alzheimer's patients has not been done, there is some question as to how much of it is doable. A similar difficulty was noted many years ago in regard to schizophrenia research, where there eventually emerged a consensus of opinion that many of the cognitive deficits noted in schizophrenics were not in those realms that were being evaluated, but in the failure of the schizophrenic patient to attend to the task either because of high distractibility or insufficient motivation. Sometimes an unconventional attitude on the part of the patient was more a determinant of the outcome of the study than what is being sought by the experimenter. Perhaps the most powerful example of this phenomenon became apparent when Clark, Brown, and Rutschmann (1967) reported that the reduced flicker sensitivity of schizophrenics, reported in the literature on several occasions, was actually a response bias in the direction of increased cautiousness rather than a perceptual phenomenon.

In the case of Alzheimer's disease, much of the neuropsychological literature reflects profound impairment with a "bottoming out" on many of the standard neuropsychological tests. For example, in the study of Perez et al. (1975) the mean IQ for the Alzheimer's disease sample was 64.58 (S.E. = 5.21). When one considers that the mean age was 62.2, it is apparent that the average level of performance on any of the subtests was quite minimal. For example, the mean score for

Picture Completion was reported to be 2.18, with 10 being the mean score for the test standardization group. Obtaining 3 items correct out of the total 21 earns a scaled score of 3. In studies comparing Alzheimer's patients with patients suffering other forms of dementia, the Alzheimer's patients generally do significantly more poorly throughout. This generalized level of significantly impaired function provides substantial difficulty for neuropsychological analysis, and suggests that different types of assessment methods need to be developed before more can be learned. The difficulty is compounded further by the fact that neuropsychological studies done were obviously done with testable patients. The problem of testability becomes increasingly significant as the disorder progresses, and so we know very little about cognitive function during the late stages of the disorder.

Another difficulty regarding the study of Alzheimer type dementia has to do with the matter of variability in the neuropathology of the disorder. While in most cases the most prominent pathological changes are in the parietal lobes, there are cases in which frontal and limbic systems are mainly involved, or the speech region sustains the major damage. In these cases, personality and affective changes or language disorder may be the most prominent symptoms. Thus, while the pathological changes may be very similar from case to case, the location of those changes may vary substantially. It may therefore not be possible to line out a uniform course in the progression of Alzheimer's disease.

For all of the above reasons, while the pervasiveness and extent of the intellectual impairment found in Alzheimer's type dementia is well appreciated, its specific nature is not well understood. While the customary call for further research would seem to be appropriate at this point, what is more pertinent is a call for the development of new methods and techniques with which to do this research. It seems apparent that when a patient gets beyond the very early stages of Alzheimer's disease, administration of the standard neuropsychological clinical and experimental tests often cannot be accomplished in a manner capable of providing meaningful data. The solution seems to lie in the application of other methods. For example, Goodwin, Squires, and Starr (1978) proposed the use of an auditory evoked potential measure, prolonged P3 latency, as an objective indicator of dementia. Their dementia patients could cooperate for the evoked potential procedure, and most of them did develop a reliable P3 component. From an information processing standpoint, the inference can be made that prolonged latency may reflect slowness in the identification and processing of stimuli. This finding is of particular interest when one contrasts it with the P3 findings for schizophrenics who frequently do not show a reliable P3 response (Levit, Sutton, & Zubin, 1973). Thus, an objective physiological measure can shed some light on different information processing deficits in different diagnostic groups.

Another area that would appear to deserve further pursuit is language. Language can be assessed reasonably well without the necessity of formal testing. Simple stimulus situations, in which the patient may be asked, for example, to produce a narrative or answer a number of simple questions, can provide material that can be used for highly sophisticated linguistic analyses. Such analyses could provide valuable information concerning information processing in individuals who cannot cooperate for formal cognitive tests, or who can cooperate at such a minimal level that very little usable data are acquired. In general, perhaps some of our currently unanswered questions can be answered by asking them in an appropriate manner.

An information processing analysis of the progressive dementias cannot be accomplished in the same manner as one might conduct for more stable pathological processes such as aphasia simply because these disorders are progressive; what is true at one point in time may not hold on an indefinite basis. It is therefore ultimately necessary to add a longitudinal component to the model, allowing for some orderly method of observing change. Some early efforts have been made to conduct longitudinal studies of patients with dementia, and several of the textbooks describe a characteristic course, but very little has been verified on the basis of a systematic prospective study utilizing state-of-the-art procedures. While, for example, it is often said that short-term memory becomes impaired first, that inference is made on a retrospective, clinical basis and not on the basis of empirical investigation. We would suspect that, as in other areas, the course of the illness in Alzheimer's type dementia, while perhaps not as variable as might be found in multi-infarct dementia, is also substantially variable, and the early signs may not be the same for all patients.

It is our view that, at present, dementia as defined as a progressive degeneration of the brain with corresponding progressive intellectual impairment, is a scientifically respectable concept. However, we do not yet have a sufficiently refined taxonomy for it such that it is possible to classify the variability that clearly exists, nor do we know much about the nature of the cognitive deficits involved. Memory impairment seems to be the most prominent and well studied symptom, but the nature of the memory deficit is not understood to the extent it is in the purer amnesic disorders such as alcoholic Korsakoff's syndrome. We also do not know much about the course of the disorder, particularly in regard to the progression of cognitive impairment. Recent neurochemical findings strongly suggest that Alzheimer's disease is a disease in the true sense and not simply an extreme point along the aging continuum. The reason for its development in susceptible individuals is not yet known, but the presence of a central cholinergic deficiency as the immediate cause of the brain pathology seems well established.

Clinical Considerations

There is no curative treatment for the progressive dementias, and so clinical concerns are somewhat different from what is the case in reversible disorders and diseases in which the arrest of the pathological process is at least possible. The progressive dementias clearly cannot presently be reversed, nor is there any good evidence that the process can be arrested. One can therefore raise issues concerning the clinical needs of patients with these disorders beyond nursing-oriented, humane health care. The way in which this question is currently answered involves several points. First, and perhaps most optimistically, there have been reports that certain chemical agents can improve cognitive function in demented patients, at least minimally and temporarily. There is evidence that physostigmine can produce a brief improvement in memory in Alzheimer's disease patients, and numerous investigations have taken place involving the use of lecithin and choline. While the results of this research have been largely negative, they have been instructive in regard to providing a direction for ongoing pharmacological research. Perhaps one of the more important aspects of this direction has to do with making proper diagnoses, since the effects of various compounds may be quite specific to particular types of dementia. Also, in the case of Alzheimer's disease, it is becoming clear that the choline neuron depletion is related to a cell membrane transport problem, and simply loading the system with a choline precusor or with choline may not be effective if these substances do not actually get into the neurons.

A second clinically relevant point is that while there may be no curative treatment for dementia, there are effective treatments available and other treatments that may be made effective in the future. The effective treatments available are largely associated with the often significant secondary symptoms of dementia. For example, depression may be successfully treated with antidepressant medication. Various forms of psychosocial management and treatment can surely improve the quality of life of the demented patient, can possibly increase longevity, and can permit maximal comfort and productiveness during the patient's remaining years. Aside from these considerations, the possibility that specific retraining in certain cognitive skills, mainly memory, can be effective is currently under intensive investigation. It is because of this latter possibility that it becomes particularly important to know about the nature of the cognitive deficits found in the different dementias. For example, if language therapy is to be effective, it is important to know more than we do at present about the specifics of language dissolution in dementia. The same holds true for memory. The nature of the memory deficit needs to be understood before it can be remediated.

SUMMARY

The general tenor of our remarks here can be summarized in terms of our initial proposition concerning the lack of intellectual deterioration with normal aging. We have shown that research with exceptionally healthy elderly individuals, as compared with individuals somewhat less healthy (Botwinick & Birren, 1963; Correll *et al.*, 1966) demonstrated that health is a very significant factor in regard to intellectual decline. The most specific health-related matter appears to concern whether or not the elderly individual acquires a dementing illness. Perhaps the fairest summary statement to make is that while intellectual decline can accompany normal aging, it is essentially impossible to demonstrate this to be the case. Thus, chronological age is really not a satisfactory independent variable for neuropsychological research. Surely, chronological age has strong implications for health and psychosocial status, and such factors should be considered by the clinical neuropsychologist. There is no question that as people get older they are more susceptible to a variety of illnesses and are increasingly likely to develop psychiatric disorders and difficulties in living associated with alienation, turning inward, rejection, economic deprivation, and related matters. However, the particular focus of the neuropscyhologist is on the brain, and on the relationship between brain function and behavior. In that regard, chronological age alone tells us very little about the status of an individual's brain and brain functions. It is our view that this matter has highly significant clinical and social relevance for the elderly, because the assumption is often made that simply on the basis of age there has been sufficient depletion of neurons to produce dementia. Such an assumption may have had the unfortunate consequence of viewing elderly people with functional psychiatric disorders as demented, and thus not providing them with appropriate treatment. The whole issue of depressive pseudodementia became an issue because of this frequently observed difficulty in the treatment of elderly people. Thus, putting the matter bluntly, while we may speak of the neuropsychology of aging, there is in principle no such thing. However, there can be a neuropsychology of the brain disorders of the elderly encompassing the areas of dementia and the role of health status in regard to determining level of intellectual function.

The most devastating cognitive deficits associated with the aging process are generally seen in people who acquire dementia, particularly if it is of the Alzheimer type. There is an expanding neuropsychology of dementia involving basic studies of cognitive function, assessment and diagnostic procedures, and treatment and management methods. The underlying mechanism for Alzheimer's disease seems reasonably well established, but the reason for the development of this mechanism in vulnerable individuals is not yet understood. Further discoveries in this area may ultimately lead to the development of curative or process arrest level treatment, but such treatments are not yet available. Aside from the dementias, it is becoming clear that maintenance of good health throughout life has implications for the degree of intellectual decline one may experience in old age. Steps such as maintenance of optimal blood pressure, prevention and adequate treatment of pulmonary disease, and moderation in regard to use of alcohol and related chemicals may all promote minimization of cognitive decline. Thus, unless one is unfortunate enough to acquire one of the progressive dementias, the relationship between cognitive function and chronological age does not necessarily represent an inexorable process, but seems open to the benevolent impact of adequate health care and maintenance.

REFERENCES

Albert, M. L., Goodglass, H., Helm, N. A., Rubens, A. B., & Alexander, M. P. *Clinical aspects of dysphasia.* New York: Springer-Verlag/Wein, 1981.

Bale, R. N. Brain damage in diabetes mellitus. *British Journal of Psychiatry,* 1973, *122,* 337-341.

Beck, E. C., Dustman, R. E., Blusewicz, M. J., & Cannon, W. G. Cerebral evoked potentials and correlated neuropsychological changes in the human brain during aging: A comparison of alcoholism and aging. In J. M. Ordy & K. Brizzee (Eds.), *Sensory systems and communication in the elderly.* New York: Raven Press, 1979.

Birren, J. E. *The psychology of aging.* Englewood Cliffs, N.J.: Prentice-Hall, 1964.

Blessed, G., Tomlinson, B. C., & Roth, M. The association between quantitative measures of dementia and senile change in the cerebral grey matter of elderly subjects. *British Journal of Psychiatry,* 1968, *114,* 797-811.

Botwinick, J. *Aging and behavior: A comprehensive integration of research findings.* New York: Springer, 1978.

Botwinick, J., & Birren, J. E. Mental abilities and psychomotor resonses in healthy aged men. In J. E. Birren, R. N. Butler, S. N. Greenhouse, L. Sokoloff, & M. Yarrow (Eds.), *Human aging: A biological and behavioral study.* Washington, D.C.: U.S. Government Printing Office, 1963.

Brody, H. Structural changes in the aging nervous system. *Interdisciplinary Topics in Gerontology,* 1970, *7,* 9-21.

Butters, N., & Cermak, L. S. *Alcoholic Korsakoff's syndrome: An information processing approach to amnesia.* New York: Academic Press, 1980.

Clark, C., Brown, I., & Rutschmann, J. Flicker sensitivity and response bias in psychiatric patients and normal subjects. *Journal of Abnormal Psychology,* 1967, *72,* 35-42.

Correll, R. E., Rokosz, S., & Blanchard, B. M. Some correlates of WAIS performance in the elderly. *Journal of Gerontology,* 1966, *21,* 544-549.

Courville, C. *Effects of alcohol on the central nervous system.* Los Angeles: San Lucas Press, 1955.

Drachman, D. A., & Leavitt, J. Memory impairment in the aged: Storage versus retrieval deficit. *Journal of Experimental Psychology,* 1972, *93,* 302-308.

Duckworth, G. S., & Ross, H. Diagnostic differences in psychogeriatric patients in Toronto, New York and London. *Canadian Medical Association Journal,* 1975, *112,* 847-851.

Folstein, M. F., & McHugh, P. R. Dementia syndrome of depression. In R. Katzman, R. D. Terry, & K. L. Bick (Eds.), *Alzheimer's disease: Senile dementia and related disorders.* New York: Raven Pess, 1978.

Friedman, E., Sherman, K. A., Ferris, S. H., Reisberg, B., Bartus, R. T., & Schneck, M. K. Clinical response to choline plus piracetam in senile dementia: Relation to red-cell choline levels. *New England Journal of Medicine,* 1981, *304,* 1490-1491.

Fuld, P. A., Katzman, R., Davies, P., & Terry, R. D. Intrusions as a sign of Alzheimer dementia: Chemical and pathological verification. *Annals of Neurology,* 1982, *11,* 155-159.

Gainotti, G., Caltagirone, C., Masullo, C., & Miceli, G. Patterns of neuropsychological impairment in various diagnostic groups of dementia. In L. Amaducci, A. N. Davison, & P. Antuono (Eds.), *Aging of the brain and dementia.* New York: Raven Press, 1980.

Goldstein, G., & Shelly, C. H. Similarities and differences between psychological deficit in aging and brain damage. *Journal of Gerontology,* 1975 *30,* 448-455.

Goldstein, G., & Shelly, C. Does the right hemisphere age more rapidly than the left? *Journal of Clinical Neuropsychology,* 1981, *3,* 65-78.

Goodwin, D. S., Squires, K. C., & Starr, A. Long latency event-related components of the auditory evoked potential in dementia. *Brain,* 1978, *101,* 635-648.

Gordon, H. W., Bentin, S., & Silverberg, R. *Asymmetrical cognitive deterioration in demented and Parkinsonian patients.* Paper presented at Second INS European Conference, Noordwijkerhout, Holland, 1979.

Grant, I., Heaton, R. K., McSweeney, A. J., Adams, K. M., & Timms, R. M. Brain dysfunction in COPD. *Chest*, 1980, *77*, 308–309.

Hallenbeck, C. E. Evidence for a multiple process view of mental deterioration. *Journal of Gerontology*, 1964, *19*, 357–363.

Halstead, W. C., & Rennick, P. Toward a behavioral scale for biological age. In C. Tibbitts & W. Donahue (Eds.), *Social and psychological aspects of aging.* New York: Columbia University Press, 1962.

Horn, J. L., & Cattell, R. B. Age differences in fluid and crystallized intelligence. *Acta Psychologia*, 1967, *26*, 107–129.

Jacobs, E. A., Alvis, H. J., & Small, S. M. Hyperoxygenation: A central nervous system activator? *Journal of Geriatric Psychiatry*, 1972, *5*, 107–121.

Jones, B. M., & Parsons, O. A. Impaired abstracting ability in chronic alcoholics. *Archives of General Psychiatry*, 1971, *24*, 71–75.

Kinsbourne, M. Attentional dysfunctions and the elderly: Theoretical models and research perspectives. In L. W. Poon, J. L. Fozard, L. S. Cermak, D. Arenberg, & L. W. Thompson (Eds.), *New directions in memory and aging.* Hillsdale, N.J.: Lawrence Erlbaum Associates, 1980.

Klisz, D. Neuropsychological evaluation in older persons. In M. Storandt, I. C. Siegler, & M. F. Elias (Eds.), *The clinical pychology of aging.* New York: Plenum, 1978.

Levit, A. L., Sutton, S., & Zubin, J. Evoked potential correlates of information processing in psychiatric patients. *Psychological Medicine*, 1973, *3*, 487–494.

Luria, A. R. *The working brain.* New York: Basic Books, 1973.

Miller, E. The nature of the cognitive deficit in dementia. In N. E.Miller & G. D. Cohen (Eds.), *Clinical aspects of Alzheimer's disease and senile dementia.* New York: Raven Press, 1981.

Miller, N. E., & Cohen, G. D. *Clinical aspects of Alzheimer's disease and senile dementia.* New York: Raven Press, 1981.

Ordy, J. M., & Brizzee, K. R. *Neurobiology and aging.* New York: Plenum, 1975.

Overall, J. E., & Gorham, D. R. Organicity versus old age in objective and projective test performance. *Journal of Consulting and Clinical Psychology*, 1972, *39*, 98–105.

Parsons, O. A., & Farr, S. P. The neuropsychology of alcohol and drug use. In S. B. Filskov & T. J. Boll (Eds.), *Handbook of clinical neuropsychology,* New York: Wiley, 1981.

Perez, F. I., Rivera, V. M., Meyer, J. S., Gay, J. R. A., Taylor, R. L., & Matthew, N. T. Analysis of intellectual and cognitive performance in patients with multi-infarct dementia, vertebrobasilar insufficiency with dementia and Alzheimer's disease. *Journal of Neurology, Neurosurgery and Psychiatry*, 1975, *38*, 533–540.

Reed, H. B. C., & Reitan, R. M. A comparison of the effects of the normal aging process with the effects of organic brain-damage on adaptive abilities. *Journal of Gerontology*, 1963, *18*, 177–179.

Reitan, R. M. Behavioral manifestations of impaired brain functions in aging. In J. L. Fozard (Chair), *Similarities and differences of brain-behavior relationships in aging and cerebral pathology.* Symposium presented at the meeting of the American Psychological Association, Montreal, Canada, 1973.

Ringler, R. L. Aging Perspectives. In N. E. Miller & G. D. Cohen (Eds.), *Clinical aspects of Alzheimer's disease and senile dementia.* New York: Raven Press, 1981.

Rosen, W. G., Terry, R. D., Fuld, P. A., Katzman, R., & Peck, A. Pathological verification of ischemic score in differentiation of dementias. *Annals of Neurology*, 1980, *7*, 486–488.

Roth, M. Senile dementia and its borderlands. In J. O. Cole & J. E. Barrett (Eds.), *Psychopathology in the aged.* New York: Raven Press, 1980.

Ryan, C., & Buters, N. Learning and memory impairments in young and old alcoholics: Evidence for the premature-aging hypothesis. *Alcoholism: Clinical and Experimental Research*, 1980, *4*, 190–198.

Ryan, C., Vega, A., Drash, A., & Longstreet, C. *Neuropsychological changes associated with juvenile-onset insulin-dependent diabetes.* Paper presented at 10th Annual International Neuropsychological Society Meeting, Pittsburgh, Pennsylvania, February 1982.

Schaie, K. W., & Labouvie-Vief, G. Generational versus ontogenetic components of chnage in adult cognitive behavior: A fourteen-year cross-sequential study. *Developmental Psychology,* 1974, *10,* 305–320.

Warrington, E. K., & Weiskrantz, L. Amnesic syndrome: Consolidation or retrieval? *Nature,* 1970, *228,* 628–630.

Wechsler, D. *Measurement of adult intelligence.* Baltimore: Williams and Wilkins, 1944.

Wells, C. E. Pseudodementia. *American Journal of Psychiatry,* 1979, *136,* 895–900.

Wilkie, F., & Eisdorfer, C. Intelligence and blood pressure in the aged. *Science,* 1971, *172,* 959–962.

11

Neuropsychological Effects of General Medical Disorders

RONA ARIEL and MARY ANN STRIDER

Traditionally, neuropsychologists have been mainly concerned with the evaluation and study of neurological conditions creating impairment in intellectual functioning. They have tended to concentrate largely on the brain itself and have viewed most problems of concern to them as occurring within the cranium. However, neuropsychologists are becoming increasingly involved in the evaluation of patients who suffer from diseases that may affect any part of the body.

Although the brain and other parts of the body are separate in terms of anatomy, they function as an integrated whole. Thus, when other organ systems are affected by disease, the brain may also become impaired. This impairment may result from damage to brain tissue from the disease process itself. Alternatively, brain dysfunction may occur as a secondary effect of the disease elsewhere in the body, such as a lowering of cognitive function due to failure of other organ systems to provide necessary nutrients to the brain. The idea of multiple interactive systems is primary to the discussions of the disease concepts and conditions presented here. There is no single causality; nothing in the body functions in total independence. Although this is easy to acknowledge on one level, the concept is pervasive in understanding brain–body relationships.

In the assessment of patients who have medical problems, however, it is essential to consider more than a single cause for any neuropsychological dysfunction. Not only their medical condition, but psychiatric and social problems

RONA ARIEL • Department of Psychology, Indiana State University, Terre Haute, Indiana 47809. MARY ANN STRIDER • Department of Psychiatry, University of Nebraska Medical Center, Omaha, Nebraska 68106.

may influence a patient's behavior and functioning. The determination of the presence and severity of any brain effects thus requires knowledge of the possible contribution of many factors—the disease itself, the organ systems affected, the phase of the illness, the treatments for it, premorbid personality and coping capacity of the patient, the patient's estimated level of cognitive functioning prior to illness, and so forth.

In many disease conditions, brain effects have only been assumed because of reported changes in the mental or behavioral state of some patients with the disease. Relatively little research has been published on neuropsychological assessment of individuals suffering from many nonneurological diseases. Even when central nervous system (CNS) effects are reported as being possible or frequent, there is as yet little understanding as to the types of cognitive deficits occurring or likely to occur with different disease processes, and even less is understood about recovery patterns or residual dysfunction.

This chapter will be divided into two sections. The first section will discuss the functioning of each major organ system in the body and the ways in which its malfunction may affect the brain, including descriptions of some disease types specific to that organ system. The next section will then describe some common medical conditions and disorders that tend to have "systemic" effects throughout the body. Throughout the chapter, we will present hypotheses regarding patients' cognitive and emotional functioning derived from the published studies of neuropsychological assessment. Where research data is not available, we will describe clinical symptoms that implicate possible neuropsychological deficits.

Throughout our discussion we will refer frequently to the central nervous system, but this will most often focus on the brain and not the spinal cord or peripheral nervous system.

THE BODY AS A COMPLEX SYSTEM—AN OVERVIEW

The human body is composed of approximatetly 100 trillion cells (Brobeck, 1979), which are organized into structures that perform a variety of different tasks. Each cell, and the structure of which it is a part, is oriented toward maintaining a *homeostatic* or stable condition of the body. Some of the larger structures are called *organs,* and organs that work together to perform a unified function are often called *systems* (for example, the heart and blood vessels make up the circulatory system). Maintenance of homeostasis occurs through a reciprocal interplay of all structures in the body. When one or more of these functional structures loses its ability to contribute its share to maintaining homeostasis, all the cells of the body suffer to some degree, and the resulting dysfunction may lead to death of the organism or to illness.

An important concept to remember throughout this chapter is that the different parts of the body operate in *harmony*. All cells have some functions in common: all require oxygen and nutrients; all must convert these substances into energy in order to perform their own specialized tasks; and all must deliver their products and waste materials into their surroundings for delivery to other parts of the body. In order for these cellular functions to be carried out, the proper concentrations of many constituents must be maintained in the fluid surrounding the cells. The various systems of the body work together to ensure that this occurs, and they make continual adjustments to changes in any conditions.

Our primary focus is to describe how illness affects the central nervous system, most specifically the brain. An understanding of the causes and consequences of such effects, however, must arise from an understanding of the general functions of each organ system in a healthy body and the ways these interact with the brain. In the body, the smooth operation of all systems is accomplished by means of complex control systems. There are thousands of these throughout the body. Every body cell is both an initiator and receptor of the "messages" that trigger these control systems (e.g., "Provide more oxygen," "There's too much water here," "Where's my breakfast?!!").

In addition, there are a number of substances important to the functioning of all cells, which we shall refer to periodically in our discussion. *Electrolytes* are inorganic chemicals used for initiating, maintaining, and terminating various cellular metabolic reactions and control mechanisms. They act on the cell membrane, allowing it to transmit electrochemical impulses or to select which substances can be passed back and forth across it. *Water* constitutes 70–85% of every cell and is an important medium in which various substances can be dissolved or suspended. Its unique physical properties make it the best fluid for transmission of particles. *Proteins* are organic substances that hold cell parts together (fibrous proteins) or help initiate various chemical reactions occurring inside the cells (enzymes). There are also *nucleoproteins,* which contain the DNA codes for hereditary transmission and for regulation of cell duplication. *Lipids* are substances soluble in fat solvents, which combine with structural proteins to make cell membranes impervious to any but the most chosen guests. *Carbohydrates* are the nutritional fuel for the cells. Various gases provide combustion in chemical reactions *(oxygen)*, maintain tension and pressure inside the cell, and are also an end product of many metabolic reactions *(carbon dioxide)*.

The Brain and Central Nervous System

Brain structure and functions have been reviewed in other sections of this book. We are most concerned here with the functions of the brain in relation to other body processes. The brain has unusual energy requirements. Although it comprises only 2% of total body weight, it receives about 15% of the cardiac output and accounts for 20% of the body's oxygen consumption (Freedman, Kaplan, & Sadock, 1976). As a consequence of this high energy demand, brain cells are extremely sensitive to alterations in their supply of energy sources, mainly oxygen and glucose. Even mild energy deficits can impair the function and integrity of the brain cells.

In the normal brain, energy is obtained mainly by oxidation of glucose to carbon dioxide and water. This energy is then expended for the transportation of ions and other compounds across cell membranes and for the synthesis of various cell constituents. Since oxygen and glucose are transported by the blood to the brain cells, adequate cerebral blood flow is a crucial factor in brain metabolism. Adequate availability of nutrients, such as glucose and proteins, is dependent upon proper functioning of the digestive system.

When parts of the brain are damaged, other organ systems may or may not be disrupted. If damage occurs in cortical areas, usually only a person's cognitive and sensory–motor skills are affected. Damage to some subcortical areas may disrupt the "automatic" functioning of other systems, however, such as heart beat, blood pressure regulation, breathing, hormonal balance, water regulation, or immune response. This often leads to further disability and possibly to more brain damage.

If nerves peripheral to the brain are damaged, generally only the area served by those nerves is impaired. However, if a major organ system is involved, it may begin to function improperly, creating imbalances in other systems. If the damage occurs to nerves in the limbs, the individual can generally survive. However, the reduction in movement places the person at high risk for developing many serious conditions, as some body movement is essential for regulation of digestive, lymphatic, and blood circulation processes.

Thus we can see that all parts of the body in some way contribute to maintaining brain function and vice versa. A disruption in one system is likely to create disturbances elsewhere.

The Hemolytic System

The primary function of the hemolytic or blood system is to perform a carrier and delivery service of transporting oxygen from lungs to tissues and returning carbon dioxide, conveying foodstuffs from the alimentary canal to tissues, and returning waste products to the kidneys. It also has other important duties, such as maintaining the water content of the tissues, harboring the body's defense cells, carrying hormones that regulate body functions, and performing a meterological service by helping to regulate body temperature. Blood is composed of plasma and cells.

Plasma

The plasma portion of blood contains water and various solid particles such as proteins, electrolytes, nonprotein organic substances (acids, fats, and sugars), antibodies, and hormonal secretions. *Water balance* is extremely important, both for maintaining the proper concentrations of chemical substances in and around cells and for providing the means of transporting these around the body. Such interchanges are accomplished by means of osmotic and hydrostatic pressures. *Osmotic pressure* is the force exerted upon water molecules by substances in solution inside the cell. The amount of pressure is determined by the concentration of these dissolved particles, and this in turn is dependent upon the properties of the particular cell membrane that separates the water and solubles, as though asking water to "come in" when the solid concentration gets too high, and to "go out" when it gets too low. *Hydrostatic pressure* is that which flowing blood exerts upon the capillary walls in relation to the pressure of fluids outside the walls. Pressure at the artery end of the capillaries is always higher, forcing fluid into the spaces around the cells; at the venous end the pressure is lower, drawing up fluid and its solids into the vessels. Changes in blood pressure thus affect the water concentration around the cells.

The *proteins* in the plasma help to initiate and inhibit blood clotting, and help to maintain normal blood pressure by providing the necessary thickness. They produce some nourishment for blood cells and also serve as a reserve of protein for other body tissues when food intake is insufficient. They also serve as "carriers" for some immune substances which react to foreign agents. The various non-protein organic particles and inorganic constituents are those being carried to tissues for use or are waste products of metabolism.

Blood Cells

Blood cells come in three types. *Red blood cells* contain hemoglobin, which is specially built to carry oxygen. These cells are manufactured in the bone marrow and then stored in the spleen until needed. Abnormal increases in the number of red blood cells can cause problems by clumping together and creating "traffic jams" that slow blood flow and impede circulation. One such abnormal condition is *polycythemia vera*, a dysfunction of the bone marrow that causes it to produce too many red cells. Blood flow then slows considerably. Even though there is plenty of oxygen, the person has difficulty breathing and may become cyanotic. The spleen enlarges because of the extra storage of blood, and many hemorrhages occur in small vessels because of the changes in blood pressure. The result to the brain may be a lowering of function due to insufficient circulation or blockage of a cerebral vessel. Other pathological increases in red cells can result from emphysema, heart disease, chronic carbon monoxide poisoning, some chemical poisonings, or repeated small hemorrhages.

An abnormal decrease in red cells is called *anemia*. This may occur from continued bleeding or from actual destruction of the red cells by infection, poisons, or abnormalities in their structure causing them to disintegrate. Defective red cells can develop because of nutritional deficiencies, bone marrow abnormalities, or toxic agents that modify bone marrow functioning. Another defect in hemoglobin formation in red cells occurs with an inherited condition called sickle cell disease. The red cells become rigid, inflexible, and entangled with one another, blocking the capillaries. The result is oxygen deprivation to cells, hemorrhage, thrombosis, and severe anemia.

White blood cells serve defensive and clean-up functions by attacking and ingesting foreign particles, building walls around damaged tissues, and helping to remove clots or dead tissue for later disposal. They come in many shapes and sizes, each having its own prescribed functions. White cells will increase normally whenever an infection is present, and the relative proportions of the different types of cells can sometimes be used to determine what the infection is. Diseases that create an abnormal increase in white cells, such as leukemia, Hodgkin's disease, and infectious mononucleosis, often result in large-scale destruction of healthy cells. Many diseases can also lower their numbers abnormally (called leukopenia), reducing the body's ability to fight infections.

Platelets are blood cells that assist in the clotting function needed to seal leaks in capillaries and set up a "dam" against blood loss from larger vessels by narrowing the channel opening. They have a tendency to clump together around any rough surfaces or foreign matter. Whenever a clot forms within a vessel, partially or completely closing its channel, it is called a *thrombus*. Usually this occurs in a vein. If the clot or any portion of it detaches and then plugs another vessel some distance away, it is called an *embolus*. The resulting insufficient blood flow creates *ischemia* or starvation of tissue, and if death or damage to cells occurs it is called an *infarction*. Thrombi tend to form whenever there is injury to a vessel wall or from abnormal clumping of platelets. The latter may sometimes occur during or after an operation due to some reaction to the injections used or to immobility following anesthesia.

Effects on the Brain

Thrombus formation anywhere in the body is serious because of the high tendency for emboli to pass through the heart and be carried to the lungs or brain. Emboli can also plug heart vessels, reducing pumping efficiency and increasing the risk of further thrombus formation. Emboli to the brain often cause cerebral infarctions (see Chapter 7).

Neurological symptoms are commonly reported in diseases in which there is an excess of red cells or platelets (Aita, 1964). These include headaches, dizziness, visual and hearing problems, and parasthesias. Patients who hemorrhage easily may show more severe focal deficits, such as aphasia and hemiparesis, or exhibit a progressing dementia as more and more brain tissue is destroyed by repeated hemorrhages.

Anemia can produce variable CNS effects. Chronic anemia may result in overall lowering of brain function because of cerebral hypoxia. Convulsions, diffuse organic brain syndromes, focal vascular lesions, hemorrhages, and blindness have been reported in severe cases, such as patients with sickle cell anemia (Aita, 1964).

A severe reduction of platelets or defects in coagulation factors often results in spontaneous bleeding. This can be a primary disease (e.g., thrombocytopenia purpura) or it can be secondary to another process, such as leukemia, toxic chemicals, irradiation, infection, or massive blood transfusion. If such hemorrhage occurs within the brain, it may be single or multiple, small or large, and may resemble a focal stroke or a progressing dementia (Aita, 1964).

Unfortunately, very few studies have been published that have investigated neuropsychological functioning in patients with primary blood diseases. Generally these disorders accompany other diseases, such as leukemia or connective tissue diseases, and this complication confounds the research interpretation problem. One study reported evaluation of 20 children with chronic thrombocytopenia (Matoth, Zaizov, & Frankel, 1971) after noting that a large number of these patients had learning and behavior problems when compared to rheumatic fever and abdominal pain patients. All patients were given Bender Visual–Motor Gestalt, WISC, and Human Figure Drawing tests. No statistical differences showed up between the groups, and not test patterns differentiated the groups; all patients had average IQ's. Over two-thirds of the thrombocytopenic group exhibited "soft" neurological signs of "minimal brain dysfunction." However, over 50% had mild diffuse abnormal EEG's, compared to only 15% of the other groups. In this investigation, neuropsychological testing was not diagnostically helpful. The groups were small, however, and the tests used may not have been sensitive enough to detect differences. Results with children, who are still undergoing brain development, may differ from those with adults. Thus, hypotheses about the effects of chronic thrombocytopenia are as yet inconclusive.

The Digestive System

The digestive process takes place in the digestive canal, which is essentially a tube with openings at each end—the mouth and anus. Digestion begins in the mouth, where three pairs of glands excrete saliva that mixes with chewed food, aids swallowing and begins to break starch down into sugars.

The chewed semiliquid food is swallowed through the esophagus and enters the stomach. The stomach is the widest and most muscular section of the digestive canal. Upon contact with the stomach wall, food is covered with highly acidic gastric secretions. This gastric juice primarily breaks down proteins. The stomach also produces the intrinsic factor, a substance required for vitamin B12 absorption.

Food passes in small increments into the small intestine. Here the major proportion of digestion occurs and absorption takes place. The small intestine receives substances from the liver, gall bladder, and pancreas to aid its digestive function.

The liver is the main chemical factory of the body and essential to life. Structurally the liver is a series of lobules that are constructed around a central vein, the hepatic vein, which leads to the right side of the heart. In addition to its role in digestion, it plays a vital part in the formation and destruction of red blood cells.

The liver is the detoxication center for any chemical that cannot be metabolized for nutrition. It modifies drugs so they can be readily excreted by the kidneys. Alcohol has a toxic action on liver cells and will interfere with the organ's ability to inactivate drugs, especially central nervous system depressants. If liver tissue is destroyed in its detoxication work, the cells are replaced with fat and connective tissue. This condition, "fatty liver," may progress to cirrhosis and greatly reduces liver function. Alcohol is only metabolized by the liver and is one of the primary causes of cirrhosis. Many poisons, solvents, and pesticides can also cause liver damage.

The liver stores vitamins A, D and B_{12}. It also manufactures plasma proteins and forms urea from the deamination (nitrogen removal) of amino acids. The liver is also important in maintaining blood glucose level. Liver insufficency will lead quickly to low blood glucose levels and fatal hypoglycemia.

Because of the liver's essential role and varied processes, its malfunction has significant impact on the body and brain through its toxicity of unmetabolized intestinal nitrogenous compounds. Hepatic encephalopathy as a syndrome has been reported in association with chronic and acute liver disease. It has been clinically described as involving impaired intellectual functioning, reduced consciousness, slowed reaction, and emotionality. Elsass, Lund, & Ranek (1978) gave selected tests to 30 cirrhotic patients, comparing their performance to patients showing diffuse brain impairment. They concluded that the hepatic patients were similar to the diffuse brain-damaged group in some subtests but had an attentional deficit not seen in the diffuse group. Rehnstrom and colleagues (Rehnstrom, Simert, Hansson, Johnson, & Vang, 1977) assessed 41 liver disease patients. They reported marked intellectual impairment regardless of the etiology of the cirrhosis. More important, they noted that some impairments found in psychological testing would likely not be detected in an ordinary medical investigation. Baseline assessment in the early stages of liver disease is thus recommended to enable later changes to be more validly interpreted. There is variability in liver disease, with rapid changes in a patient's functioning. This must be considered in timing and length of testing carried out.

The liver continually secretes a bile that contains bile salts for the breaking down of fats. The bile is stored in the gall bladder until triggered by the presence of fat in the small intestine. The bile duct is also joined by the pancreatic duct from the pancreas. The constitutents of bile may precipitate out to form gallstones. If such stones block the bile duct, jaundice will develop and the person will become ill. The function of the pancreas in digestion is to assist in reducing the acid from the stomach and further digest fat, protein, and starch. The pancreatic juice contains essential enzymes for each type of food digestion as well as considerable bicarbonate ion for neutralizing acid.

After mixing with the bile and pancreatic juice in the duodenum, the food is moved into the lower part of the small intestine where millions of small villi cover the inner intestinal lining. At the end of this stage the food has been broken down into the basic substances, which are absorbed into the blood and serve as the basic units for metabolism of substances when assimilated into tissue structures.

The lower section of the small intestine is the major site of food absorption. Absorption occurs through active transport and by diffusion (osmosis) into the blood, which is then carried into the liver. The liver filters out any foreign debris and removes excess glucose and amino acids. The excess glucose is converted to fat and stored in a type of connective tissue. At the same time that absorption is occurring for fats, proteins, and carbohydrates, the rate of absorption of electrolytes from ingested minerals will be influenced. Sodium, potassium, chloride, nitrate, and bicarbonate electrolytes are easily absorbed, while calcium, magnesium, and sulfate are more poorly absorbed.

Disorders of the small intestine are comparatively few. The most common is probably due to gallstones blocking bile secretion and causing inadequate absorption of fatty acids. Another cause of abnormal digestion is a failure of the pancreas to secrete its juice into the small intestine.

After food passes through the small intestine, it proceeds to the large intestine, also called the colon. Essentially no digestion takes place in the colon. The colon's function is the absorption of water and electrolytes from the food mixture and the storage of fecal matter until it can be expelled. If the colon is infected, food may be quickly passed through with little water absorbed. Feces are then watery (diarrhea), which can cause debilitating loss of body water and electrolytes. Because water is the basic solvent of the body, its utilization needs special note.

Dissolved in the water of the body are many compounds that contribute to control system factors of pH water concentration, and the volume of circulating blood. Fluids within a cell hold particularly potassium and phosphate. Extracellular fluid contains mostly sodium chloride and bicarbonate. Transferences and exchanges of these substances occur frequently to maintain homeostasis. Dehydration, where there is a water loss either from between cells or within cells, can occur because of lack of adequate water intake or because of vomiting, diarrhea, excessive perspiration, heat stroke, or respiratory difficulties. The person has symptoms of thirst, decreased perspiration, a dry tongue, and personality changes.

It can progress to a confusional mental state and on to delirium collapse, convulsions, and coma (Aita, 1964).

A less common situation is water excess, which can also disrupt the elctrolyte balance. Water excess affects the proper transport of blood and creates brain swelling. This can progress to an acute brain syndrome.

Vitamins, especially B complex, and mineral salts are also necessary to adequate nutrition. Much interest in CNS problems center around several of these substances.

Vitamin B complex represents a group of water-soluble vitamins that include B_1 (thiamine), niacin, B_2 (riboflavin), and B_{12} and folic acid. Components of this complex are known to be essential in brain metabolism, serving as coenzymes for nerve impulse transmission. Severe thiamin deficiency produces Wernicke's encephalopathy and is suspected to cause some of the confusional states in elderly arteriosclerotic patients. The initial symptoms of Wernicke's encephalopathy are difficulty in concentration and disturbed sleep, followed by confusional states, staggering gait, and vision problems, and possibly terminating in stupor or coma. This most frequently occurs in association with chronic alcoholism and severe malnutrition.

Victor, Adams, & Collins (1971) have reported follow-up on survivors of the acute stage of Wernicke's encephalopathy. Within 1 to 2 months following treatment, most vision abnormalities improved. Gait problems were reversible in only one half of the patients. Global confusion always recovered but memory deficits remained, with 84% of the 186 patients developing a Korsakoff psychosis. The extent of recovery in severe thiamine deficiency awaits adequate neuropsychological study, especially in cases where alcoholism, with its likely liver impairment, is not involved. Pathological changes have been documented involving many small hemorrhages in the thalamus, hypothalamus, and gray matter in the upper part of the brain stem in vitamin B_1 deficiences. (Aita, 1964; Victor *et al.,* 1971).

Niacin is found in liver and kidney yeast. Deficiency of niacin leads to skin changes and brain damage leading to dementia. Vitamin B_{12}, which is absorbed from the small intestine, requires a substance—the intrinsic factor—which is produced in the gastric mucosia. Defective absorption due to any disease of the small intestine can thus cause its deficiency. Impaired brain function in pernicious anemia is supported by abnormal EEG records in over 60% of cases seen by Walton *et al.* (1954). Shulman (1967) found memory deficits in 75% of the patients. Some patients diagnosed as suffering presenile dementia have been found to have low vitamin B_{12} serum, which responds to vitamin treatment (Hunter, Jones & Matthews, 1967). If the condition is long standing, a less favorable response is expected and permanent brain deficits are likely (Strachan & Henderson, 1965; Roos 1974; Roos & Willanger, 1977).

Vitamin B_{12} and folic acid are essential for red blood cell development in bone marrow. A deficiency leads to anemia and a degeneration of the spinal cord. Vitamin C is a water-soluble vitamin and its deficiency leads to a condition called scurvy, characterized by hemorrages. Vitamin C is hypothesized to be involved in the formation of connective tissue, and its absence prolongs wound healing. Vitamin D and its products are crucial to the absorption of calcium from the digestive tract. A deficiency leads to soft bones.

Mineral salts refer mainly to sodium and potassium salts necessary for adequate electrolyte balance. Aita (1964) reports various symptoms found in mineral deficiencies. An excess of potassium in the body fluids can produce heart changes and respiratory changes, listlessness, cold in the extremities, and muscular paralysis. Potassium depletion may produce muscle weakness, paralysis, or occasional mental states, and coma can occur from potassium loss coupled with hypertension, renal disease, extensive surgery, or trauma as from burns. Calcium deficit can produce tetany and convulsions. Calcium excess may produce renal dysfunction and muscular weakness, bone and muscular pain, and, in severe cases, acute brain syndrome.

In general, electrolyte imbalance can affect brain functioning by causing edema, reduced neuronal firing, or seizures and coma. It is not possible in reality to specify the particular effects from one type of ion change because of the close interplay among a number of electrolytes. The above descriptions are clinical ones because no neuropsychological data yet exist that address these conditions.

The Cardiovascular System

The main functions of the cardiovascular system are: to pump blood through the body; to pick up and deliver fluids, gases, chemicals, and nutritive substances; and to increase or decrease blood flow in response to activity levels. The structures comprising this system are the heart, large arteries and veins, smaller arterioles and venules, and the tiny capillaries. In traveling through the system, blood moves from the right side of the heart to the lungs to pick up oxygen. It returns to the left side of the heart and is then pumped to the rest of the body, branching into smaller and smaller vessels (arteries). After fluid exchange with the tissues, blood flows into the venous end of the circulation, merging into larger and larger vessels (veins) to the right side of the heart. The manner of blood flow and the way it is regulated by the vascular system are crucial principles to the understanding of cardiovascular function.

Blood Flow and Pressure

Blood traveling through vessels exerts different pressures and moves at different speeds according to the size of the vessel. The heart works very hard to maintain a limited range of pressures and velocities in the vessels. Thus, any increase in friction, such as occurs with blockages, narrowing, or roughness along the vessel walls, increases the workload of the heart and can eventually lead to heart failure.

Blood emerges from the heart into the arteries at very high pressure. As it branches into the smaller arterioles, the greater surface area of the small vessel network creates greater friction, and the pressure gradually decreases. Pressure is maintained at a fairly constant level in the capillaries, where the exchange of fluids and solids takes place with the tissue cells. Blood then enters the venous vessels, where velocity gradually increases and friction decreases with each merger into a larger vessel, resulting in a gradual increase of venous blood pressure as well.

A number of factors contribute to the maintenance of normal pressure in the system: the amount of blood expelled from the heart; the quantity or *volume* of blood in the entire system; the ability of the vessel walls to expand and rebound (elasticity) to maintain pressure between heart pumps; the thickness or *viscosity* of blood, which affects the amount of force needed to push it through the system; and the peripheral or small vessel resistance to blood flow. When any one of these factors changes, the others make adjustments in an attempt to maintain a normal range of pressures in the system.

Blood pressure in the veins is also maintained partially by subatmospheric pressure within the chest cavity, which acts to expand the veins and thereby help "suck" the blood up into the cavity toward the heart. Flow through venous vessels must overcome the effects of gravity, and if the pressure-regulating factors fail, then blood will likely accumulate in the lowest parts of the body, resulting eventually in blockage.

Many different conditions can cause or result from abnormal variations in blood pressure. An abnormal increase in blood pressure is called *hypertension*. Most forms of hypertension are probably due to a generalized constriction of the smaller vessels. This can result from a reduced oxygen supply to the nerve centers regulating constriction and dilation of the small vessels, if there is insufficient blood flow to the brain. An overactive thyroid increases output of the heart and can also produce hypertension if uncontrolled. A restriction of adequate blood flow to the kidneys causes them to malfunction and release a substance that brings about constriction of peripheral vessels, eventually leading to hypertension, enlargement of the heart, and degenerative changes in the arteries. This is called hypertension secondary to renal disease. In all forms of hypertension there is an increased risk of eventual heart dysfunction or of cerebral hemorrhage.

The Heart

The heart pumps blood by contracting and relaxing in rhythmic cycles, with the rate changing in relation to demands made by the rest of the body. The heart is composed of four chambers, muscle, nerves, its own blood vessels, valves, and sheaths (the *pericardial sacs*) which enclose and protect it.

The heart requires adequate blood pressure to supply its own tissues with oxygen and essential nutrients. It can draw from its own stores of nutrients in emergencies, but cannot run without a continual supply of oxygen and some electrolytes. There are special nerve tissues placed strategically within each chamber, which initiate and regulate its contractions. If any of these become damaged, contractions become irregular and pumping efficiency is reduced or even stopped. Between the heart chambers and on entrance to the large vessels are valves that may become deformed from disease, causing impaired flow of blood. The pericardial sacs protect and lubricate the muscle, preventing overstretching on expansion.

Heart action is influenced by nerve impulses and chemical "messages" transmitted from other parts of the body. These interact with one another in regulating the pace and rhythm of heart beats, and are in turn influenced by such things as exercise, emotional state, metabolic balance, and drugs. If heart tissue becomes diseased, then *hypertrophy* or enlargement is a means of compensating. The heart must dilate to a greater extent to liberate the needed amount of energy, and this repeated stretching promotes growth in the size of the muscle fibers. Hypertrophy is most commonly caused by hypertension and valve disese, but can also result from disease in the heart vessels, an overactive thyroid, anemia, congenital heart defects, and deformation in the walls of the large vessels (called an aneurism). Infection or disease in the pericardial sacs creates inflammation and *edema* (fluid build-up), which restricts heart action and lowers its efficiency. Some infections may invade the heart and cause damage to muscle, nerves, vessels, or valves.

When the heart is overworked for long periods, chronic heart failure develops. Such a condition is most often brought about by chronic infections or disease, excessive muscular effort and prolonged rapid heart action, or large increases in the total volume of blood, such as during massive transfusions. The end result is that blood flow slows down everywhere and "log jams" occur, raising the pressure, reducing adequate oxygen intake, congesting and enlarging the liver and spleen, disrupting the kidneys, and generally creating edema thoughout the body.

The Vessels

Dilation and constriction of the smaller blood vessels are controlled by *vasomotor* nerves. These arise in the spinal cord but have connections in the hypothalamus and the prefrontal and orbitofrontal cortex of the brain. The nerves are reflexive and respond to even minute changes in temperature, sensation, deep air inhalation, hormones, or drugs in their attempts to maintain blood pressure at the peripheral level. Blood gases, specifically oxygen and carbon dioxide, influence blood pressure but have opposite effects in the large and small blood vessels. Low oxygen/high CO_2 tension will cause constriction of the large vessels and raise blood pressure, but will dilate the tiny peripheral vessels. High oxygen/low CO_2 tension will dilate the large vessels and lower blood pressure, while constricting the tiny vessels. These oppositional effects help regulate the oxygen/CO_2 balance around the tissue cells, as well as protect the smaller, more vulnerable vessels from being damaged by extreme variations in blood pressure. Nerve disorders of the peripheral vascular network or diseases that damage the vessel walls tend to disrupt the maintenance of blood pressure and gas balance, causing blood starvation of local tissues.

Effects on the Brain

Disease anywhere in the cardiovascular system initiates a vicious cycle of adjustments, and the heart works harder and harder to compensate for these changes, resulting in further damage. A compromised heart eventually leads to a compromised brain. Although the brain will demand a greater share of materials needed by the body, prolonged heart dysfunction will lower the amount available to the brain cells. Insufficient oxygen and nutrients are likely to produce results of diffuse neuropsychological dysfunction. The individual is likely to have cognitive deficits in many skill areas, although these may be mild unless the damage to the heart (or reduction of blood flow) has been severe. Many of the cognitive deficits in heart patients may not even be noticed because their other symptoms are more disabling and demand more attention. Mild deficits that are noticeable are often temporary and thus of less immediate concern.

When circulation to the heart itself is blocked and tissue is damaged (commonly called a "heart attack"), there is often an extreme drop in blood pressure. This may produce symptoms of dizziness or massive mental changes such as delirium or dementia. The lack of oxygen to brain tissue may produce focal deficits such as aphasia, sensorimotor disturbances, or visual difficulties, and these effects can be either temporary or permanent. A cerebral hemorrhage may occur from the increased pressure and destruction to cerebral vessels, producing either diffuse or focal effects that are usually more permanent. Because all of these deficits are more disrupting to the individual's ability to function, they are likely to cause more concern to the patient and the doctor, and are often the symptoms that lead to a neuropsychological evaluation. If such diseases progress slowly, then compensation usually occurs, and these patients may appear to have normal cognitive function.

Another outcome of cardiac disease may be the development of bacterial endocarditis, an infection of the heart tissue wherein bacteria collect in damaged valves or in the pericardial sacs. As well as creating inflammation and edema, the bacteria find it easier to spread through the circulation to other areas of the body. If they enter the brain, the result is usually a *septic embolism* (a blockage creating infection in that area), widespread meningitis, or development of a focal brain abscess. Neuropsychological effects can be quite variable, ranging from focal deficits that resemble a stroke, to a diffuse encephalopathy (widespread inflammation). The variations possible make it a difficult condition to diagnose. Neuropsychological evaluations should be repeated on follow-up visits to determine if further damage is occurring and to assess the extent of residual impairment.

The development of hemorrhages in the brain from hypertensive destruction of vessels also produces variable effects. Hemorrhages generally result in focal deficits, but these can be singular or multiple, and depending on where they occur, can cause mild or severe disruption of cognitive functional systems. Acute hypertensive encephalopathy (generalized inflammation) may produce massive edema and pressure effects leading to severe diffuse deficits, convulsions, decerebrate rigidity, coma, or death from cerebral hemorrhage.

Hypotension, or low blood pressure, generally has only mild or unnoticeable effects on brain functioning, but can produce diffuse impairment of moderate to severe degrees as well. The patient may complain of amnesia, excessive fatigue, fainting, convulsions, or loss of specific cognitive abilities, all of which indicate that ischemia to brain tissue has occurred. As the results are variable and often fluctuating, the diagnosis of brain damage or permanent impairment is a difficult one to make.

Cardiovascular problems can also modify blood constituents, producing brain ischemia because of the alteration in blood flow or inability of the cells to carry oxygen. Many such problems may first be labelled as "psychiatric" or emotional disorders, because the patient exhibits depression or thought disorder as the first symptoms. In elderly patients especially, psychiatric disturbance may be related to use of diuretic medications (to reduce water retention), which sometimes produce electrolyte imbalances when taken chronically and may mimic psychiatric or organic disorders such as depression and paranoia (Taylor, 1979).

Cardiovascular surgery has its own risks. Brain circulation may become impaired while the patient is connected to an "artificial" heart. Thrombosis, embolism, anoxia, or toxic/allergic reactions to anesthesia or injected medications may occur. Infections can develop that spread to brain tissue, or the heart may simply fail to regain its normal rhythm after surgery. All of these may cause cognitive deficits of varying degree and location.

Studies using EEG tracings have indicated that heart surgery patients show more abnormalities after heart surgery than before (Brobeck, 1979), and if these do not return to normal within 3 to 4 weeks it is likely that cerebral damage has occurred. Studies utilizing neuropsychological tests indicate that signs of cerebral dysfunction *prior* to surgery place the person at higher risk for development of later cerebrovascular problems and also for death during surgery (Kilpatrick, Miller, Allan, & Lee, 1975).

A number of neuropsychological studies have been conducted on patients who undergo surgery for occlusions or narrowing of the internal carotid arteries. Such patients are often diagnosed because they experience transient ischemic attacks (TIA's) with such symptoms as dizziness, memory loss or disorientation, mild speech problems, visual changes, or mild sensorimotor deficits. Symptoms last for only short periods, but they warn of impending cerebral stroke, which occurs in about one-third of these patients if left untreated (Thompson, Patman, & Talkington, 1978).

Studies have been conducted to determine if surgery also improved intellectual functioning as well as preventing strokes. The majority of investigators used the WAIS, the Halstead–Reitan Battery, or a mixed variety of spatial, memory, visual–motor, and abstract reasoning tests. Of the studies reporting improvement in intellectual or sensory-motor functioning, there was a wide variation in results when the same measures were used (Bornstein, Benoit, & Trites, 1981; Goldstein, Kleinknecht, & Gallo, 1970; Haynes, Gideon, King, & Dempsey, 1976; Horne & Royle, 1974; Jacques, Garner, Tager, Rosenstock, & Fields, 1978; King, Gideon, Haynes, Dempsey, & Jenkins, 1977; Owens, Pressman, Edwards, Tourtellotte, Rose, Stern, Peters, Stabile, & Wilson, 1980; Perry, Drinkwater, & Taylor, 1975). Other studies reported either deterioration or no significant cognitive changes following surgery (Drake, Baker, Blumenkrantz, & Dahlgren, 1968; Matarazzo, Matarazzo, Gallo, & Weins, 1979; Murphy & Maccubbin, 1966; Williams & McGee, 1964). The Matarazzo study analyzed results on an individual as well as group basis and compared the results to previous studies using the same tests. They concluded that most of the improvement was an artifact of test-retest practice effects and not really representative of better brain functioning. Most individuals who had cognitive deficits prior to surgery continued to exhibit the same or more deficits on long-term follow-up. Despite the large number of studies done on this particular group of patients, the issue still appears to be controversial.

Personality changes, such as depression, paranoia, irritability, anxiety, and psychosis also occur with some frequency in cases where heart or vessel disease has lead to some cognitive impairment (Lishman, 1978). These changes are often noticed before actual intellectual deficits appear and may be attributed to the patient's inability to adjust to illness factors. In many cases these changes may be the outcome of injury to the brain tissue, and this possibility needs to be thoroughly evaluated.

Respiratory System

Carbon atoms from food digestion need oxygen (O_2) atoms from inspired air to produce heat and energy, and form carbon dioxide (CO_2) as a waste product. The function of the lung is this essential gas exchange.

The lung is a pair of elastic structures that completely fills the thoracic cavity in the chest. The lung takes in oxygen, gives off carbon dioxide, and assists in the regulation of the acidity (pH) of the blood. The composition of the lung wall is a semipermeable membrane that forms a blood/gas barrier that allows diffusion of gases. Air is pulled in on the interior side by ventilation, while pulmonary circulation from the heart brings blood past the exterior side and O_2 and CO_2 exchange places across the lung membrane. This diffusion occurs because gases will flow from a higher pressure to a lower pressure. Because the lungs have a reserve oxygen supply of less than 2 minutes, a continual renewal of air is necessary.

Respiratory movements are under the control of the respiratory center in the medulla, which signals the respiratory muscles. Damage to the brain's respiratory center would necessitate the use of artificial means of respiration. A loss of lung elasticity causes poor expiration. This rigidity most frequently occurs from chronic bronchitis or coughing, but aging alone results in some tissue stiffness. Asthma, lung edema, and membrane thickening will also impair elasticity. Emphysema occurs when there is dilation of the lung air vesicles, usually due to atrophy of the walls, and expiration is greatly reduced. Fluid or air between the lung and chest wall will impair respiration. Anything that causes blocked airways, like asthma or bronchitis, will reduce respiration rate. The lung can become inflamed, as in pneumonia, and then fluid forms within the lobes, thus reducing oxygen exchange.

Brain–Lung Relationship

The main interest in lung function is the high metabolic need of the brain for oxygen carried in blood. Blood oxygen is carried in two forms, dissolved and in combination with hemoglobin. Oxygenated hemoglobin is bright red, while reduced hemoglobin is more purple. This is why a person looks blueish (cyanotic) when arterial oxygen saturation is low. Carbon monoxide, which has about 250 times the affinity of oxygen for hemoglobin, interferes greatly with the oxygen transport function of blood. In the healthy person, fresh oxygen is continually added to the blood flowing from the heart through the lungs, and delivered to tissues in the body and organs. Carbon dioxide is picked up by the blood and brought to the lung, where it is expired.

An adequate level of carbon dioxide is also required for control of blood pH and healthy body functioning. Blood pH must remain within a limited range to maintain a viable medium for body protein and enzyme activity. The respiratory center has the main role in controlling blood pH in association with the kidneys. The carbon dioxide blood level cues the respiratory center to increase breathing if carbon dioxide is high or to reduce respiration if the level is low. A low carbon dioxide level induces increased excitability in nerves and muscles, and can bring about spontaneous spasms. This state is known as tetany. Carbon dioxide is a vasodilator; therefore a low CO_2 level will reduce cerebral blood flow and the person will feel dizzy and have trouble thinking.

Asphyxia is where there is oxygen lack and CO_2 excess in the body. Anoxia is a state of oxygen shortage alone; when less severe, it is called hypoxia. Anoxia affects the brain, especially the cortex and higher centers that are involved in evaluation and judgment. In anoxia the person become disoriented and passes quickly into coma.

There are several types of anoxia (Barcroft, 1920; Lishman, 1978). *Anoxic anoxia* is due to lack of oxygen in the inspired air, or is the result of lung diseases such that available oxygen cannot enter the blood. A second type is called *anaemic anoxia* and is due to a deficiency of hemoglobin. This is most frequently caused by a state of anaemia, but it may also be the result of carbon monoxide poisoning or abrupt blood loss as in gastrointestinal hemorrhage. Smith and Brandon (1973) assessed carbon monoxide victims and found that almost half had memory impairment at follow-up, and irritability and impulsiveness occurred commonly in one-third of patients. Symptoms may remain for up to a year.

A third type of anoxia, *stagnant anoxia,* results from blood flow difficulties; despite adequate oxygen content, oxygen tension, and hemoglobin carrying capacity, blood flows at such a slow rate that it does not supply tissues with enough oxygen to meet their needs. Another type is *histotoxic anoxia* (metabolic). In this condition there is a failure in the tissue cells to extract oxygen from the blood. This occurs in cyanide or carbon disulphide poisoning and with hypoglycemia. *Overutilization anoxia* occurs locally in epileptic seizures due to the high demand on the blood supply.

The body can only survive complete anoxia for 6 minutes. The cerebral cortex and the myocardium are most vulnerable to anoxia. It appears that in anything less than total oxygen deficit, brain cells may continue to survive but will cease neuronal firing. With improved nutrition and restored oxygen, some cells may recover, although they will remain weakened and vulnerable.

Actual neuropsychological research in the area of brain damage in lung disorders is quite limited. Chronic obstructive pulmonary disease (COPD) has been studied mainly by physiological and biochemical means. Studies by Krop, Block, and Cohen (1973) and Block, Castle, and Keitt (1974) have used some neuropsychological measures in assessing COPD patients; they report that depressed neuropsychological functioning was prevalent, although comparisons to normal control groups were not used.

Persons with impaired lung function are likely to be more cerebrally vulnerable to any other event that can alter brain metabolism. They may react with severely acute symptoms to even mild brain trauma, drug influence, or alcohol use.

Urinary System

The kidneys are bean-shaped organs located against the posterior wall of the abdomen. Their principal function is to assist in the maintenance of water balance, blood pH, and electrolyte balance. The functional unit of the kidney is a nephron, which is a huge mass of filter tubes. There are estimated to be about 1 million nephron units in each kidney (Green, 1978).

Blood goes to the kidneys directly from the aorta by way of the renal arteries. The renal arteries divide into a net of intertwined capillaries shaped into a tiny ball. This coil ball of capillaries is called the glomerulus. The blood returns from the kidney via the renal vein. Blood flow is slowed as it goes through the glomerulus, giving time for water ions and small molecules like urea to diffuse outward. These substances are "filtered," and unwanted material is passed on to the bladder. Some substances, such as glucose, are returned to the blood stream for further use.

The ability of the kidney to reabsorb water is regulated by a hormone released by the pituitary gland (ADH). The bladder serves as a storage space for the urine until elimination occurs. Presence of any abnormal constituents in the urine can offer clues to underlying disorders in the kidneys and elsewhere in the body.

Damage to the kidney is termed nephrosis. Infections (nephritis) may also impair the functioning of the kidneys. When kidney function is impaired and urine production is reduced, the waste products that are usually excreted are retained in the body, leading to potentially fatal disorders. Diet may be used to control such problems up to a point, but eventually dialysis may be required. In dialysis, the blood of the patient is filtered through an artificial kidney. Dialysis treatments may take up to 6 hours three times a week.

Severe psychological as well as neuropsychological complications are known to arise from dialysis. Depression is common, both as a function of the body dysfunction as well as stress on the patient. The patient may then be unable to follow the necessary medical regimen, further exacerbating the disease. Other phenomena, however, show that some symptoms and behavior can be related to interference with nervous system functioning (Marshall, 1979).

It is well known that cognitive functioning is severely impaired in uremia. Characteristic symptoms such as sluggish mentation, lethargy, anorexia, nausea and vomiting, tremors, sleepiness, or convulsions have been widely documented (Ginn, 1975; Raskin & Fishman, 1976). These symptoms are relieved by dialysis. It is important to note that there is a time lag between treatment on dialysis and subsequent improvement or deterioration of the patient's behavior or mental status changes. Lewis, O'Neil, Dustman, and Beck (1980) found performance on tests of visual–motor speed and accuracy was best 24 hours after dialysis. The reason for this lag is not known, although it is hypothesized to represent a delay in cellular recovery or in distribution of toxic agents.

It is now well recognized that an encephalopathy called *dialysis disequilibrium syndrome* may be a consequence of the dialysis procedure (Marshall, 1979). This syndrome has a characteristic course. Over 2–3 months the patient develops intermittent slowing speech with stuttering and word-finding problems. Symptoms usually are more predominant during or right after dialysis. This progresses to difficulty in producing sentences, and myoclonus and dyspraxic movements occur. Severe memory loss, concentration probems, and at times overt psychosis develops. Other symptoms appear toward the end of the dialysis run and may subside over several hours, but the delirium, when it appears, may persist for several days. Evidence suggests that shifts of sodium and potassium, with movement of water into the brain (edema), may cause the disequilibrium syndrome (Raskin & Fishman, 1976). It is still unclear which toxic metabolites or end products are responsible for the documented changes.

There is also a *dialysis dementia*, an ultimately fatal encephalopathy seen in long-term dialysis (Alfrey, Mishell, Burks, Contigaglia, Lewin, & Holmes, 1972; Mahurkar, Dhar, & Salta, 1973). It is first characterized by a disturbance in speech, with facial grimacing, convulsions, and eventually dementia. The symptoms would initially occur during the dialysis and clear after a period of time, but eventually these remissions no longer occur and the syndrome progresses. The pathogenesis of this order remains unknown and no successful treatment has been found.

There is the report of subdural hematomas in dialysis patients (Talalla, Halbrook, Barbour, & Kurze, 1970). This appears to be related to two possibilities. Many of these patients are given anticoagulant drugs so that they can maintain their shunts against thrombosis. Secondly patients with kidney failure can have abnormal bleeding. The symptoms may look similar to the dialysis disequilibrium syndrome and sometimes are very difficult to clinically differentiate. However, the persistence or worsening of symptoms between dialysis runs would alert one to consider a subdural hematoma as opposed to the disequilibrium syndrome, and neuropsychological assessment can aid in documenting the patient's functional level.

The main problem in kidney transplant is the possiblity of immune rejection of the new organ. The hormones of the adrenal cortex have ability to suppress allergic responses, and cortisols have been employed to help suppress organ rejection in transplants.

Assessment of mental status and neuropsychological functioning in uremic patients can provide useful treatment recommendations. Obtaining good baseline measures early in the diagnosis of renal disease will allow more valid assessment of any later deterioration and response to dialysis when initiated. The timing of neuropsychological assessment of dialysis patients must be considered. Patients fluctuate greatly at periods in dialysis regimen. It appears that metabolic effects, which modulate brain functioning, vary widely and produce different performance patterns.

Ryan, Souheaver, and DeWolff (1981) reported comparative neuropsychological assessments on chronic hemodialysis patients, undialyzed uremic patients, and medically–psychiatrically ill patients. On the Halstead–Reitan Battery, significant differences were found between the kidney patient group and the comparison group of medical–psychiatric patients. Dialysis patients did perform better than uremic patients on some tasks but were impaired relative to the medical–psychiatric group. A valuable aspect of this study was the clear indication that chronic hemodialysis patients cannot be considered essentially normal in their neuropsychological functioning.

Endocrine System

The endocrine system consists of the following glands; pituitary, thyroid, four parathyroids, two adrenals, the pancreas, two gonads, the placena in pregnancy, and the thymus. Hormones are chemical substances produced by the endocrine glands and are secreted directly into the blood. The hormones circulate in the blood and influence the activity of distant organs.

The *pituitary* gland lies in a bony cavity at the base of the skull, suspended from the hypothalamus. Its two sections have quite different functions. The posterior pituitary is directly behind the chiasma of the optic nerve. A tumor of the pituitary can, from pressure, cause some visual field defects or complete blindness. The posterior pituitary produces two hormones; antidiuretic hormone (ADH) and oxytocin. ADH has as its function the regulation of reabsorption of water by the kidney tubules. It also causes vasoconstiction of blood vessels and, if present in large amounts, hypertension. Oxytocin is important in pregnant women because it produces contractions of the uterus and facilitates lactation.

The anterior pituitary gland, which is thought to be controlled by inhibiting and releasing factors from the hypothalamus, releases six hormones: human growth hormone, thyrotropic hormone, ACTH (adrenocorticotrophic hormone), prolactin, and two gonadotrophic hormones. The human growth hormone (somatotropin) reacts on body tissue generally. During childhood it stimulates the growth of bone and muscle tissue, and an overactivity may lead to giantism, while underactivity produces dwarfism. It does not appear essential to nervous system development and therefore low production produces undersized but not retarded individuals.

The *thyroid* gland has two pear-shaped lobes moulded to the sides of the trachea. Thyroid hormones stimulate metabolism. They act in all cells of the body, increasing the rate at which food is converted into heat and energy. The functioning of the thyroid gland requires iodine in the diet, and people who are deficient in iodine may develop an iodine deficiency goiter or swelling of the thyroid gland. This results in underactivity of the gland. A goiter, however, may also be due to a tumor that may result from overactivity of the gland.

Underactivity of the thyroid gland (called hypothyroidism) will result in the lowering of the body's metabolism. This condition in adulthood is called myxoedema. When such a condition occurs in children it may produce a cretin (a mentally retarded dwarf). In underactivity of the thyroid, the patient develops lowered body temperature, a lowered heart rate, sluggish activity, and generalized edema. The patient appears lethargic and has slow cognitive functioning. Appetite is reduced and hearing, taste, and smell may be impaired as mucoid material is deposited (Lishman, 1978). Depression is a frequently entertained diagnosis because myxoedema has an insidious onset it may exist for several months before striking symptoms demand attention. Psychosis with mental confusion, paranoia, auditory hallucinations, and delirium features can develop. In some cases a dementia picture is seen. Coma, when it occurs, carries a high mortality rate. Where hypothyroidism had been undiagnosed for long periods, intellectual and memory deficits may remain (Jellinek, 1962). In such suspected cases, repeat assessment of functioning is called for.

Should the thyroid gland be overactive, this is called hyperthyroidism. Metabolic rate increases, temperature may rise, faster heartbeat is maintained, and the patient may complain of difficulties staying asleep. Patients with overactive thyroids may present as very nervous and irritable, overactive, and possibly paranoid. They may lose weight and have an anxious, staring expression with possible protrusion of the eyeballs. The hyperarousal can produce concentration problems due to distractibility, and persons may be diagnosed as manic. An acute reaction of delirium and organic psychoses occasionally accompany hyperthyroidism. Accurate diagnosis and treatment of thyroid disorders usually yields good results.

The two *adrenal glands* are situated on each side of the kidneys. The central part of the adrenal gland releases mainly adrenalin and noradrenalin, called catecholamines, and is triggered by sympathetic nervous stimulation. Excessive production of catecholamines can result in high blood pressure. When present in excess, aldosterone will cause sodium and water retention and a loss of potassium. The adrenal cortex also produces several corticosteroids.

The functions of the adrenal cortex are complex. It has antiallergic and antiinflammatory properties and is also involved in protein metabolism. A high blood cortical level will favor the use of protein for heat and energy production and lead to diabetes mellitus. The excess of cortisol with the resulting edema, increased blood pressure, and blood glucose gives rise a condition called Cushing's disease. Cushing's disease may present with personality changes, complaints of fatigue and wakefulness, and menstrual irregularities. Psychiatric difficulties, usually depression, have been reported in about half of the diagnosed cases; 15% or more show psychosis (Michael & Gibbons, 1963). Treatment of the endocrine disorder is highly effective in reversing the symptoms. Whelan *et al* (1980) found varying degrees of diffuse cerebral dysfunction in two-thirds of the group. Impairment was more frequent and severe in nonverbal, visual–ideational, and visual–memory measures.

Underactivity of the adrenal gland is called *Addison's disease.* It can occur because of atrophy, or the gland may be destroyed by tuberculosis. The patient has increased vulnerability to infections and a low blood sugar. The patient may comment on a salt craving and personality changes may be observed. The patient becomes more quiet and seclusive, unexpressive, and apathetic, exhibits psycho-motor retardation, and may show depressive and paranoid aspects. Psychotic behavior may occur with paranoid delusions, agitation, and even hallucinations. Memory deficits are quite common (Michael & Gibbons, 1963). Psychological abnormalites common to chronic exhaustion are seen, fostering a diagnosis of depression or dementia. Clinical reports hold that recovery is highly successful, but neuropsychological studies are not available.

There are four *parathyroid* glands, which are situated close to the thyroid gland. They produce parathormone, which helps maintain plasma calcium level. Reduction of the parathyroid gland leads to a low plasma calcium. The result of this is excitability of nerves and neuromuscular junctions, ultimately leading to tetany. Similar increased excitability of nerve cells in the brain may lead to convulsions.

The *pancreas,* the digestive role of which has already been mentioned, also has an endocrine function. It produces insulin in the beta cells of the islets of Langerhans; insulin regulates carbohydrate metabolism and facilitates the entry of glucose into cells, thus lowering blood sugar. The alpha cells of the islets of Langerhans secrete glucagon, which tends to elevate blood sugar. The level of blood sugar itself stimulates the alpha or beta cells to secrete their hormones.

If damage to the beta cells occurs, inadequate insulin is secreted and the con-dition called diabetes mellitus results. Carbohydrate metabolism is abnormal and glucose accumulates in the blood (hyperglycemia). When glucose cannot enter the cells and be oxidized for energy, fat and protein are metabolized. This gives rise to ketone bodies, which are toxic to brain cells. If ketone bodies reach a high blood level, coma may result. The symptoms of ketosis appear more slowly than hypo-glycemic symptoms seen in hyperinsulism.

In cases of hyperinsulinism, where there is an overproduction of the hor-mone, the result is *hypoglycemia,* when the blood sugar falls precipitously and brain cells suffer a glucose deficit. Stages of hypoglycemia are similar to stages of anesthesia. A person will initially show emotional instability and personality changes before more definite mental confusion occurs. The patient feels weak with tachycardia, feelings of anxiety, and tremors. These persons may appear manic or intoxicated and show temper outbursts or extreme lethargy and apathy. This pro-gresses to mental confusion and later loss of consciousness and deep coma.

There is wide nervous system involvement in diabetes mellitus. Thirty per-cent of the patients with diabetes are at risk for functional brain impairment from repeated comas and hypoglycemia episodes. Neuropsychological functioning can vary greatly in diabetes mellitus patients, depending on their state of diabetic con-trol. The examiner must be sensitive to the patient's endocrine status in inter-preting the acuteness or chronicity of any found deficits. Repeated evaluations are required to assess residual damage.

The Lymphatic System

The lymphatic system, often referred to as the immune system, is similar to the hemolytic and cardiovascular systems in structure, but differs in function. Its primary purposes are to defend against invasion by injurious agents, to gather up and destroy worn-out cells, and to make antibodies, which keep watch for foreign substances. It also stores extra red cells and produces hormonal substances that help regulate development of new red cells. The lymphatic system is composed of the spleen, lymph vessels and nodes, lymph fluid, and defensive cells.

Spleen

The spleen is the main storage center for new red cells and the destruction center for old ones. It also makes some types of white cells (the lymphocytes). In emergencies such as during exercise or bleeding, the spleen dumps large numbers of red cells into the blood stream to ensure an adequate supply of oxygen.

Lymph Vessels

The lymph system has its own tiny vessels, which drain fluid from the tissue spaces. These vessels form into larger ducts, which eventually merge into the blood stream. Situated strategically along the byways are the lymph nodes, which act as "toll barriers," preventing large particles or foreign cells from entering the blood stream. Lymph cells in the nodes are fairly effective in combating most foreign organisms except viruses. Ducts and nodes are found almost everywhere in the body except the central nervous system. Lymph capillaries are placed such that practically anything that enters the body through skin or mucosal linings must first bypass the lymph system. Lymph vessels are really dumping streams for the body, removing the large proteins and particulate matter that accumulate in the extracellular spaces. Overaccumulation would disrupt water and electrolyte balance, increase pressure on the capillaries, shut down blood flow, and eventually result in death.

Lymph Fluid

Lymph fluid is similar to blood but contains mostly white lymphocytes and has only a few red cells, amino acids, and electrolytes. Fluid interchange with tissues operates by the same principles as with the cardiovascular system, with the exception that substances pass through the lymph before entering the venous circulation. Thus lymph flow is increased whenever capillary pressure is raised.

Lymph fluid is formed in the liver, intestine, and lymph system. The fluid is kept moving through the channels from the action of pressure on the lymph vessels during muscle contraction, passive body movements, arterial pulsations, and compression of body tissues from the outside. Valves keep the fluid moving in only one direction. Without body motion, however, the flow is not maintained effectively, and this is one of the reasons why patients are kept as active as possible when they are confined to bed.

Lymph Cells

White cells of the immune system that eat invading organisms are called *phagocytes*. Other immune cells called *lymphocytes* carry substances that react directly with invading cells or toxins. Some of these immune cells are "happy to meet" only very specific bacteria or parasites, and have been programmed to say "hello" on sight. This natural immunity was established early in life by the thymus gland, which made all of the patterns from which immune cells are produced when needed. Immunity can also be developed against unfamiliar organisms, but only after a first exposure. These sensitized lymphocytes are called *antibodies,* and the agents they are taught to recognize and attack are termed *antigens*. The only disadvantage of this nifty protection process is that it takes a long time for the body to first develop these antibodies after learning the antigen code. Some infections can manage to do a great deal of damage before antibody factories are geared up for production. However, any second attack will usually be repelled because the body subsequently keeps plenty of the new cell types around. Slowly developing infections also usually give the immune system sufficient time to make specific antibodies for them, and these types of infections are usually not as destructive.

Immune–Neuroendocrine Interactions

The CNS and endocrine system both play important roles in the regulation of the immune response. This is particularly true under conditions of stress. Stress first has most effect in terms of the individual's cogitive interpretation of events and their meaning. This then influences the action of the endocrine system, which produces hormones triggering reactive effects throughout the body. Cells respond in an attempt to adapt to the imbalances caused by the stress. The hypothalamus and pituitary secrete hormones that influence the adrenal gland. This in turn releases other hormones that modulate various immune responses, stimulating or suppressing particular immune cell production or activity level.

Glucocorticoids appear to have a suppressing effect on inflammation and provide resistance to infection and the symptoms of autoimmune diseases. Various biogenic amines and other neurotransmitters also influence immune responses, although their effects are less well understood and are only implicated because of their association with various immune disorders. The secretions of the various endocrine glands appear to be released in rather complex combinations to modulate immune responses, and these interactions are currently an active area of research (Ader, 1981).

Immune Diseases

Although the immune cells are very adament about eliminating foreign substances, they generally respect and avoid the body's own cells. In some diseases, however, this recognition ability fails and the person's own cells are attacked by the immune system, causing inflammation and widespread destruction to healthy tissues. Such a condition is known as *autoimmunity*. Although not yet well understood, it appears to result from different types of processes: possibly defects in the manufacture of some of the cell recognition codes (like mistypes on manuscripts), or errors in duplication of the body's own proteins such that they are no longer identified as family. Invading agents may also mimic the body's own proteins so well that these proteins are then attacked by the immune cells along with the unwelcome guest. Many types of nonspecific diseases are now believed to be related to autoimmune processes. Examples of some of these are the connective tissue diseases of middle and later life, such as rheumatoid arthritis and systemic lupus erythematosus (discussed later in this chapter).

Connective Tissue System

Connective tissue refers to fibrous tissues that provide support for holding cells together and form a protective covering around the body and internal organs. Connective tissue cells are found everywhere in the body, but large amounts of them are found in bones and joint tissues. The connective tissue system is composed of ligaments, tendons, and cartilage, the skin, blood vessels, internal membrane linings, and sheath coverings of organs and muscles. These cells also constitute a large portion of organs such as the eyeballs, lungs, heart, kidneys, and liver (American Rheumatism Association Committee, 1973).

Basic Structures

Connective tissues are built to withstand different tensional stresses, and thus take many forms. Regardless of form, there are three basic types of fibers, all made of long chains of proteins and different amounts of other materials such as carbohydrates and acids. *Collagen* is the dominant structural material, and its cells make up about 25% of total body protein. It is found mostly in the skin, tendons and ligaments, and sheath coverings. *Reticulin* is made up of fine branching filaments, and is mostly found around blood vessels and muscle fibers and in solid organs such as the liver, kidney, and spleen. *Elastin* fibers are very stretchable and are found abundantly in blood vessels, ligaments, and eyes, and in lesser amounts throughout the body.

All connective fibers are imbedded in *ground substance,* a gelatinous mixture of proteins and large sugar molecules. These sugars, or glycosaminoglycans, can bind large amounts of water and help to regulate fluid balance. The connective cells and ground substance also perform essential repair functions for healing wounds.

Bones are important because they provide a rigid framework for organ attachments and leverage for body movements, and also contain the marrow needed to produce blood cells. The joints are the connections between bones and are composed of different tissues that allow various degrees of separation and movement. The thick fluid in the joints is a liquid ground substance that acts as a lubricant and source of nutrient for the joint linings.

Disorders of Connective Tissue

Disorders of connective tissue can either be inherited or acquired. The genetic maladies are rare and will not be discussed here. The acquired conditions generally include rheumatoid arthritis, systemic lupus erythematosus (SLE), progressive systemic sclerosis (PSS), polymyositis and dermatomyositis, Sjogren's syndrome, amyloidosis, various forms of vasculitis, and rheumatic fever. Although different in terms of severity and the age groups affected, these diseases all display features associated with inflammation and destruction or alteration of connective tissues. Because so many structures in the body can be affected, the diseases are considered to be "systemic." Common symptoms include fatigue, fever, muscular weakness, joint swelling and pain, skin lesions, gastrointestinal erosions with hemorrhages, peripheral vascular dysfunctions, neuropathies, and blood cell disorders such as anaemia and thrombocytopenia. The course of the illness may vary greatly from patient to patient, with periods of remission and exacerbation, a chronic mild illness, severe and rapidly progressing deterioration, or fluctuations between mild and severe episodes. Some patients with these diseases may become severely disabled due to crippling joint deformities or loss of function in a major organ, such as the kidneys. The initial symptoms can mimic many other diseases because they are so variable, and thus they are difficult to diagnose and treat.

CNS Effects

Comprehensive neuropsychological research has been meagerly reported in connective tissue disease patients. Medical literature would indicate that the effects on the brain and central nervous system from these diseases are variable and generally unpredictable. The small vessel inflammation and destruction can produce focal ischemic lesions in many organs, causing them to malfunction and reduce their support to the brain. Vessels in the brain may also be affected, although pathological studies have been inconsistent in confirming this with most of the disease types except giant cell arteritis (American Rheumatism Association Committee, 1973). Hypertension is a frequent outcome of these diseases. Its affects have been described in the cardiovascular section of this chapter. Compression effects or ischemia may produce peripheral neuropathy, with sensory or motor losses in digits and limbs. Diffuse or focal cerebral infections may occur due to the suppresson of immune responses from the drugs taken for treatment.

Although evidence of the disease process itself occurring within the brain has not been confirmed, studies have indicated the presence of immune complexes associated with connective disease processes in the choroid plexus of the brain (Atkins, Kondon, Quismorio, & Friou, 1972; Bresnihan, Hohmeister, Cutting, Travers, Waldburger, Blacj, Jones, & Hughes, 1979; Breshnihan, Oliver, Grigor, & Hughes, 1977; Winfield, Lobo, & Singer, 1978). Psychoses, severe depression, and mental confusion have been reported frequently in patients. Reactions to corticosteroids, antihypertensives, antidiuretics, anti-inflammatory agents, and other treatment drugs may produce changes in emotional or mental state, although it is often difficult to separate this from effects of the disease itself.

CNS effects have most frequently been reported with SLE, including emotional disorders, convulsions, chorea, and cerebrovascular accidents with focal neurological deficits. These usually occur in patients with highly active and severe disease, and they account for up to 25% of the fatalities because of cerebral hemorrhage or seizures. In early stages of the disease, CNS effects may be mild and transient, or may so resemble a psychiatric disorder that the patient is given a diagnosis such as psychosis or depression (Bennett, Bong, & Spargo, 1978; Hughes, 1979).

EFFECTS OF SYSTEMIC DISEASES

Very little is known about neuropsychological deficits in general medical diseases, although hypotheses can be developed from the available medical and psychiatric literature. Generally, all diseases have systemic *effects* to some degree, but "systemic" diseases are those in which the disease process itself invades many organ systems simultaneously or in progression. In the following section we will present the known and hypothesized neuropsychological effects of some common diseases, not because these are the most likely ones to be encountered by a neuropsychologist, but because they provide a broad conceptual *framework* of the ways in which these conditions can produce brain impairment.

Many treatments for various diseases also have their own inherent risks and difficulties. Drugs, chemotherapy, and irradiation may produce neurological side effects that are more disabling to the patient than the disease itself, especially if they remain permanent. Separating the relative contributions of disease and treatment to any cognitive dysfunction is a complex, difficult, and sometimes impossible task. Periodic assessments when patients are both on and off treatment may help to sort out the relative effects.

Malignant Disorders

Evidence of cancer anywhere in the body presents a risk that it may have metastasized or spread to the brain. This is particularly true of some types of cancers that develop in the lungs, gastrointestinal tract, and reproductive system, because they can easily be carried to the brain through the circulatory system. When tumors occur in the brain after originating elsewhere, they have effects similar to growths developing originally in the brain. Although most tumors develop in a localized area, some spread diffusely throughout brain tissue. Even localized tumors are difficult to diagnose, since the cancerous process not only destroys the local tissue, it also raises intracranial pressure, disrupts normal circulation, and creates compression on brain tissue in remote locations (Lishman, 1978). These may then appear as a diffuse process. Alternatively, the tumor may develop very slowly and, depending on where it grows, may be adequately compensated for and reveal few or no neurological or intellectual deficits until it has spread extensively. When neurological or neuropsychological signs are observed in patients with various forms of cancer, the possibility of intracerebral metastases needs to be considered and radiographic or biopsy examinations made.

A large number of patients who develop cerebral cancer exhibit emotional and behavioral symptoms that precede or parallel neurological evidence of a disease. These may appear as "personality changes" and take the form of alterations in affect, thinking, or behavior, mimicking almost any psychiatric disorder. Such symptoms are as important to recognize and glean from the patient's history during the neuropsychological examination as is their testing performance. One needs to consider that these may be either effects of cerebral involvement, or the patient's individual emotional and cognitive reaction to a life-threatening illness.

Most malignant cancers invade deep brain tissue rather than the dura or skull, although all types are possible. Once tumors have developed in the brain, a variety of effects may occur. Raised intracranial pressure disturbs the brain stem reticular formation and its projections to areas of the cortex, hinders circulation, and restricts drainage of cerebral spinal fluid. The resulting build-up of fluid creates edema and direct compression and damge to brain tissue in areas other than the site of the tumor. The slowed circulation creates ischemia and the metabolic disturbances may produce electrolyte and cell function imbalances, further lowering cognitive functioning (Aita, 1964). Thus patients with localized tumors may show localized effects, but often will also exhibit diffuse deficits, making their condition difficult to diagnose.

Malignant cancer may not invade the brain directly but may create effects elsewhere that disrupt brain functioning. Neoplasms in the digestive tract may restrict absorption of needed nutrients; in the endocrine glands, they may create severe disorders in immune and regulatory metabolic processes; in the liver and kidneys, they may create biochemical and electrolyte changes affecting blood exchange and waste disposal; and in the vascular system, they may disrupt blood pressure and flow. Toxic reactions that are possibly metabolic or immunologic may produce diffuse symptoms resembling multifocal encephalopathy. All of these conditions are likely to disrupt brain functioning to some degree. If the cancer can be treated, some of these effects are usually reversible, although in some cases the damage has been severe and will likely show persistent deficits, such as those resulting from metastatic emboli, ischemia, and severe seizures.

Sometimes the therapy for malignant cancers has its own damaging effects. Surgery carries a risk of respiratory or circulatory problems affecting the brain even if the surgery is performed on another organ, and certainly contributes to damage when performed on the brain. Cytotoxic chemotherapy (drug treatment toxic to particular cell types) not only disrupts metabolic processes on a wide scale, but also may alter immune resistance and leave the person open to bacterial or fungal infections. Radiation therapy may damage the central nervous system directly, but these effects are often latent, occurring months or years after the treatment (Aita, 1964).

Metastatic neoplasms are an abnormal proliferation of singular cell types, which spread to parts of the body other than where they originated. Neoplastic disorders of the lymphatic and hemolytic systems result in some type of neurological involvement in an estimated 15–50% of patients (Aita, 1964). Hodgkin's disease and lymphosarcoma are somewhat similar in their effects. Neoplastic accumulations of lymph cells collect in the spaces around the spinal cord and at the base of the brain, creating compression effects, impedance of blood flow, ischemia, and increased risk of infection. These can appear as focal deficits, convulsions, or a diffuse dementing process. Myeloma is a cancerous disease originating in bone marrow. Abnormal plasma cells grow rapidly and spread throughout the bone, destroying and replacing bone tissue, depressing production of red cells, and disrupting blood chemistry. Renal damage frequently occurs, with its own consequent effects. In the central nervous system, spinal compression, seizures, and focal cerebral deficits from invasion of dural areas, and subcortical syndromes from lower brain compression frequently occur.

Leukemia is an abnormal proliferation of white blood cells. These cells then often infiltrate the bone marrow, spleen, liver, and lymph nodes, creating anaemia. Effects on the brain are usually diffuse. Blood vessels become clogged with leukemic cells anywhere in the brain, creating occlusions, ischemia, hemorrhages, and edema. The individual becomes susceptible to infections and toxic reactions, which further lower brain function. The condition may be acute and then is usually rapidly fatal, or may be chronic and continue for years. Neuropsychological effects are likely to be variably focal or diffuse, both across individuals and within one individual over time.

Leukemia is one disease that has received a greater share of attention in neuropsychological research, primarily because it is a disease devastating to children. Many of these studies have investigated the differential effects of the disease and treatments given for it. Use of irradiation and chemotherapy are still considered controversial when used prophylactically, since there is some question as to whether these may not cause more damage or produce delayed development. Follow-up studies ranging from 2 to 4 years after irradiation therapy have showed variable results.

A representative example of such studies is that done by Soni, Marten, Pitner, Duenas, and Powazek (1975), which used school achievement tests and IQ tests to compare patients with acute lymphocytic leukemia (ALL) and controls who received body irradiation for other reasons. They found no real differences between the groups, but unfortunately did not control for age differences between the groups. Other studies using the Weschler Intelligence Scale for Children have found differences. Moss, Nannis, & Poplack (1981) compared ALL patients to their healthy siblings and found significantly lower IQ's in the ALL group. Patients who received irradiation at younger ages showed greater decrements in intellectual functioning than those who were older when they were given the treatments. Eiser (1978) found that children receiving irradiation within 2 months after initial diagnosis tended to perform more poorly than those receiving 6 months or more after diagnosis, but the deficits occurred mainly with quantitative and speeded tasks rather than with language skills. Studies comparing ALL children with solid tumor patients (Eiser, 1980), looking at the incidence of CNS impairment in chemotherapy patients (Meadows & Evans, 1976), and comparing long-term ALL survivors with newly diagnosed patients (Goff, Anderson, & Cooper, 1980) all found the ALL patients to score lower on various tasks.

These studies concluded that younger children are particularly at risk for developing brain dysfunction when given such treatments at early ages. It is possible, however, that toxic treatments are given to such children because they are also at higher risk for dying from the disease. It is also difficult to parcel out the effects of chronic illness on a child's development, since these children frequently experience long breaks from school and family while hospitalized, and they undergo painful treatments on a frequent basis when the disease is exacerbated. The use of repeated neuropsychological assessments has been valuable in indicating the different aspects of the controversy, and in clarifying the relationship of age to the use of toxic treatments. Whether these relationships hold for adult-onset leukemia is still an unanswered question.

Toxic Substances

Ingestion or infiltration of toxic substances into the body create a variety of CNS effects, depending on the substance and the amount of its accumulation. Some toxic agents leave a severe residual effect, even after very minute doses, while others may not show effects until after large amounts have entered the body. Humans generally are exposed to such agents by consuming contaminated food-stuffs or water, or by exposure in occupational settings where heavy chemicals are present. They may also be exposed by breathing polluted air such as industrial fumes or sprayed insecticides.

There appear to be wide individual variations in response to some chemicals, while others generally have the same effect on everyone. CNS effects due to non-drug chemical poisoning are often extremely difficult to diagnose. Heavy metal exposure (lead, mercury, manganese, arsenic, thallium, methyl bromide, carbon disulphate) is usually quite serious, even in small amounts. Along with damage to kidneys, liver, heart, or lungs, the brain is almost always affected. Most of these substances produce motor or visual difficulties, and in many cases these are permanent. Confusion, coma, and severe psychiatric symptoms, such as psychoses, depression, emotional reactiveness, and aggression, also predominate (Lishman, 1978).

Lead poisoning is most commonly found in children who live in areas where lead-based paints have been used (which they consume) or where there is a high concentration of industrial fumes. Neuropsychological sequelae in chronic exposure are often permanent, and are expressed in school difficulties or behavior problems. In adults with mild exposures, peripheral limb disorders are most common. In serious cases, severe and permanent intellectual impairment occurs. The CNS effects are believed to be caused from edema, vascular destruction, and ischemia from raised intracranial pressure. Significant cerebral atrophy is also common (Lishman, 1978).

Mercury poisoning usually occurs in industrial workers and in persons who consume large amounts of seafood from areas where the chemical has been dumped. Mercury intoxication has also been associated with consumption of over-the-counter laxatives containing mercurous chloride (Davis, Wands, Weiss, Price, & Girling, 1974). The usual effects on the brain of this substance are motor tremors and various emotional disorders. Manganese and carbon disulphate poisoning are generally rare and occur from occupational exposure. Emotional disturbances, sensorimotor problems, and visual impairment are the usual effects, and are likely to be permanent.

Arsenic and thallium are generally very toxic, and are absorbed by inhalation of industrial contaminants or by ingestion of unwashed foods treated with insecticides. Both lower brain functioning, but thallium produces long-term residuals such as seizures and severe motor or visual problems (Lishman, 1978). Inhalation of paint thinner, glue sniffing, and gasoline sniffing have more recently become problems with young adults. Long-term effects of these substances are not well known, but evidence of severe brain degeneration is accumulating (Escobar & Aruffo, 1980).

Effects of carbon monoxide poisoning are also less well known. Inhalation of coal gas, car exhaust, or welding fumes in nonaerated enclosures are common causes. Severity of long-term effects is usually dependent upon the length of exposure, but effects may be variable across individuals. There is usually recovery in mild cases, but in some severe cases a relapse will occur months later, with confusion, coma, tremors, and other symptoms becoming long-lasting (Walton, 1977).

SUMMARY—DISEASE PROCESSES AND BRAIN DYSFUNCTION

We have attempted to provide a broad overview of body processes and their relationship to brain function, as well as indicate the ways in which dysfunction anywhere in the body may produce brain impairment. The multiple and complex factors involved in understanding these relationships serve to emphasize the importance of being knowledgeable about the physiological functioning of individuals when one becomes involved in the evaluation of medical patients. Acquiring such knowledge is a lengthy and studious process, often extending years beyond one's basic training and involving experience with a variety of medical patients.

Neuropsychologists whose primary interest is research currently have an "open field" in general medicine in which to investigate a great many unanswered questions. Effects of most diseases have not been adequately researched, and methodologies need to be improved to account for the many factors that can influence results. The challenge for professionals working in this area is not only its complexity, but also in keeping up with advances in medical information, which make such research easier to complete.

REFERENCES

Ader, R. (Ed.). *Psychoneuroimmunology*. New York: Academic Press, 1981.

Aita, J. A. *Neurologic manifestations of general diseases*. Springfield, Ill.: Charles C Thomas, 1964.

Alfrey, A. C., Mishell, J. M., Burks, J., Contigaglia, R. H., Lewin, E., & Holmes, J. H. Syndrome of dyspraxia and multifocal seizures associated with chronic hemodialysis. *Transactions. American Society for Artificial Internal Organs*, 1972, *18*, 257–261.

American Rheumatism Association Committee, G. P. Rodnan (Ed.). *Primer on the rheumatic diseases* (7th ed.). Atlanta: Arthritis Foundation, 1973.

Atkins, C. J., Kondon, J. J., Quismorio, F. P., & Friou, G. J. The choroid plexus in systemic lupus erythematosus. *Annals of Internal Medicine*, 1972, *76*, 65–72.

Barcroft, J. Anoxemia. *Lancet,* 1920, *2,* 485–489.

Bennett, R. M., Bong, D. M., & Spargo, B. H. Neuropsychiatric problems in mixed connective tissue disease. *American Journal of Medicine,* 1978, *65,* 955–962.

Block, A. J., Castle, J. R., & Keitt, A. S. Chronic oxygen therapy treatment of chronic obstructive pulmonary disease at sea level. *Chest,* 1974, *65,* 279–288.

Borstein, R. A., Benoit, B. G., & Trites, R. L. Neuropsychological changes following carotid endarterectomy. *Canadian Journal of Neurological Science,* 1981, *8,* 127–132.

Bresnihan, B., Hohmeister, R., Cutting, J., Travers, R. L., Waldburger, M., Blacj, C., Jones, T., & Hughes, G. R. The neuropsychiatric disorder in systemic lupus erythematosus: Evidence for both vascular and immune mechanisms. *Annals of the Rheumatic Diseases,* 1979, *38,* 301–306.

Bresnihan, B., Oliver, M., Grigor, R., & Hughes, G. R. V. Brain reactivity of lymphocytotoxic antibodies in systemic lupus erythematosus with and without cerebral involvement. *Clinical and Experimental Immunology,* 1977, *30,* 333.

Brobeck, J. R. (Ed.). *Best & Taylor's physiological basis of medical practice* (10th ed.). Baltimore: Williams and Wilkins, 1979.

Davis, L. E., Wands, J. R., Weiss, S. A., Price, D. L., & Girling, E. F. Central nervous system intoxication from mercurous chloride laxatives. *Archives of Neurology,* 1974, *30,* 428–431.

Drake, W., Baker, M., Blumenkrantz, J., & Dahlgren, H. The quality and duration of survival in bilateral carotid occlusive disease: A preliminary survey of the effects of thromboendarterectomy. In J. Toole, R. Siekert, & J. Whisnant (Eds.), *Cerebral vascular disease.* New York: Grune & Stratton, 1968.

Eiser, C. Intellectual abilities among survivors of childhood leukemia as a function of CNS irradiation. *Archives of Diseases of Children,* 1978, *53,* 391–395.

Eiser, C. Effects of chronic illness on intellectual development. A comparison of normal children with those treated for childhood leukemia and solid tumors. *Archives of Disease in Children,* 1980, *55,* 766–770.

Elsass, P., Lund, V., & Ranek, L. Encephalopathy in patients with cirrhosis of the liver: A neuropsychological study. *Scandanavian Journal of Gastroenterology,* 1978, *13,* 241–247.

Escobar, A., & Aruffo, C. Chronic thinner intoxication: Clinico-pathologic report of a human case. *Journal of Neurology, Neurosurgery, and Psychiatry,* 1980, *43,* 986–994.

Freedman, A. M., Kaplan, H. I., & Sadock, B. J. *Modern synopsis of comprehensive textbook of psychiatry* (Vol. 2). Baltimore: Williams and Wilkins, 1976.

Ginn, H. E. Neurobehavioral dysfunction in uremia. *Kidney International.* 1975, *7,* 217–221.

Goff, J. R., Anderson, H. R., Jr., & Cooper, P. F. Distractability and memory deficits in long-term survivors of acute lymphoblastic leukemia. *Journal of Developmental and Behavioral Pediatrics,* 1981, *2,* 29–34.

Goldstein, S. G., Kleinknecht, R. A., & Gallo, A. E., Jr. Neuropsychological changes associated with carotid endarterectomy. *Cortex,* 1970, *6,* 308–322.

Green, J. H. *Basic clinical physiology.* Oxford: Oxford University Press, 1978.

Haynes, C. D., Gideon, D. A., King, G. D., & Dempsey, R. L. The improvement of cognition and personality after carotid endarterectomy. *Surgery,* 1976, *80,* 699–704.

Horne, D. J., & Royle, J. P. Cognitive changes after carotid endarterectomy. *Medical Journal of Australia,* 1974, *1,* 316–317.

Hughes, G. V. R. *Connective tissue diseases* (2nd ed.). Oxford: Blackwell Scientific, 1979.

Hunter, R., Jones, M., & Matthews, D. M. Post-gastrectomy vitamin-B12 deficiency in psychiatric practice. *Lancet,* 1967, *1,* 47.

Jacques, S., Garner, J. T., Tager, R., Rosenstock, J., & Fields, T. Improved cognition after external carotid endarterectomy. *Surgery and Neurology,* 1978, *10,* 223–225.

Jellinek, E. H. Fits, faints, coma and dementia in myxoedema. *Lancet,* 1962, *2,* 1010–1012.

Kilpatrick, D. G., Miller, W. C., Allan, A. N., & Lee, W. H. The use of psychological test data to predict open-heart surgery outcome: A prospective study. *Psychosomatic Medicine*, 1975, *37*, 62–73.

King, G. D., Gideon, D. A., Haynes, C. D., Dempsey, R. L., & Jenkins, C. W. Intellectual and personality changes associated with carotid endarterectomy. *Journal of Clinical Psychology*, 1977, *33*, 215–220.

Krop, H. D., Block, A. J., & Cohen, E. Neuropsychological effects of continuous oxygen therapy in chronic obstructive pulmonary disease. *Chest*, 1973, *64*, 317–322.

Lewis, E. G., O'Neil, W. M., Dustman, R. E., & Beck, E. C. Temporal effects of hemodialysis on measures of neural efficiency. *Kidney International*, 1980, *17*, 357–363.

Lishman, W. A. *Organic psychiatry: The psychological consequences of cerebral disorder.* Oxford: Blackwell Scientific, 1978.

Mahurkar, S. D., Dhar, S. K., & Salta, R. Dialysis dementia. *Lancet*, 1973, *1*, 1412–1415.

Marshall, J. Neuropsychiatric aspects of renal failure. *The Journal of Clinical Psychiatry*, 1979, *40*, 81–85.

Matarazzo, R. G., Matarazzo, J. D., Gallo, A. E., Jr., & Weins, A. N. IQ and neuropsychological changes following carotid endarterectomy. *Journal of Clinical Neuropsychology*, 1979, *1*, 97–116.

Matoth, Y., Zaizov, R., & Frankel, J. J. Minimal cerebral dysfunction in children with chronic thombocytopenia. *Pediatrics*, 1971, *47*, 698–706.

Meadows, A. T., & Evans, A. E. Effects of chemotherapy on the central nervous system. A study of parenteral methotrexate in long-term survivors of leukemia and lymphoma in childhood. *Cancer*, 1976, *37*, 1079–1085.

Michael, R. P., & Gibbons, J. L. Interrelationships between the endocrine system and neuropsychiatry. *International Review of Neurobiology*, 1963, *5*, 243–302.

Moss, H. A., Nannis, E. D., & Poplack, D. G. The effects of prophylactic treatment of the central nervous system on the intellectual functioning of children with acute lymphocytic leukemia. *American Journal of Medicine*, 1981, *71*, 47–52.

Murphy, F., & Maccubbin, D. A. Carotid endarterectomy: A long-term follow-up study. In J. Shillito (Ed.), *Clinical neurosurgery* (Vol. 13). Baltimore: Williams and Wilkins, 1966.

Owens, M., Pressman, M., Edwards, A. E., Tourtellotte, W., Rose, J. G., Stern, D., Peters, G., Stabile, B. E., & Wilson, S. E. The effect of small infarcts and carotid endarterectomy on postoperative psychological test performance. *Journal of Surgical Research*, 1980, *28*, 209–216.

Perry, P. M., Drinkwater, J. E., & Taylor, G. W. Cerebral dysfunction before and after carotid endarterectomy. *British Medical Journal*, 1975, *4*, 215–216.

Raskin, N. H., & Fishman, R. A. Neurologic disorders in renal failure. *The New England Journal of Medicine*, 1976, *294*, 204–210.

Rehnstrom, S., Simert, G., Hansson, J. A., Johnson, G., & Vang, J. Chronic hepatic encephalopathy: A psychometrical study. *Scandanavian Journal of Gastroentrology*, 1977, *12*, 305–311.

Roos, D. Neurological complications in a selected group of partially gastrectomized patients with particular reference of B12 deficiency. *Acta Neurologica Scandanavica*, 1974, *50*, 719–752.

Roos, D., & Willanger, R. Various degrees of dementia in a selected group of gastrectomized patients with low serum B12. *Acta Neurologia Scandanavica*, 1977, *55*, 363–376.

Ryan, J. J., Souheaver, G. T., & DeWolff, A. S. Halstead–Reitan test results in chronic hemodialysis. *Journal of Nervous and Mental Disease*, 1981, *169*, 311–314.

Shulman, R. Psychiatric aspects of pernicious anaemia: A prospective controlled investigation. *British Medical Journal*, 1967, *3*, 266–270.

Smith, J. S., & Brandon, S. Morbidity from acute carbon monoxide poisoning at three-year follow-up. *British Medical Journal*, 1973, *1*, 318–321.

Soni, S. S., Marten, G. W., Pitner, S. E., Duenas, D. A., & Powazek, M. Effects of central nervous system irradiation on neuropsychological functioning of children with acute lymphocytic leukemia. *New England Journal of Medicine,* 1975, *293,* 113–118.

Strachan, R. W., & Henderson, J. G. Psychiatric syndromes due to avitaminosis B12 with normal blood and marrow. *Quarterly Journal of Medicine,* 1965, *34,* 303–317.

Talalla, A., Halbrook, H., Barbour, B. H., & Kurze, T. Subdural hematoma associated with long-term hemodialysis for chronic renal disease. *Journal of the American Medical Association,* 1970, *212,* 1847–1849.

Taylor, J. W. Mental symptoms and electrolyte imbalance. *Australian and New Zealand Journal of Psychiatry,* 1979, *13,* 159–160.

Thompson, J. E., Patman, R. D., & Talkington, C. M. Carotid surgery for cerebrovascular insufficiency. *Current Problems in Surgery,* 1978, *15,* 1–68.

Victor, M., Adams, R. D., & Collins, G. H. *The Wernicke–Korsakoff syndrome.* Oxford: Blackwell Scientific, 1971.

Walton, J. N. (Ed.). *Brain's diseases of the nervous system* (8th ed.). Oxford: Oxford University Press, 1977.

Walton, J. N., Kiloh, L. G., Osselton, J. W., & Farrall, J. The electroencephalogram in pernicious anemia and subacute combined degeneration of the cord. *Electroencephalography and Clinical Neuropsychology,* 1954, *6,* 45–64.

Whelan, T. B., Schteingart, D. E., Starkman, M N., & Smith, A. Neuropsychological deficits in Cushing's syndrome. *Journal of Nervous and Mental Disease,* 1980, *168,* 753–757.

Wilimas, J., Goff, J. R., Anderson, H. R., Jr., Langston, J. W., & Thompson, E. Efficacy of transfusion therapy for one to two years in patients with sickle cell disease and cerebrovascular accidents. *Journal of Pediatrics,* 1980, *96,* 205–208.

Williams, M., & McGee, T. Psychological study of carotid artery occlusion and endarterectomy. *Archives of Neurology,* 1964, *10,* 293–297.

Winfield, J. B., Lobo, P. I., & Singer, A. Significance of anti-lymphocyte antibodies in systemic lupus erythematosus. *Arthritis and Rheumatism,* 1978, *21,* 215.

12

Neuropsychological Evaluation of Children and Adolescents with Psychopathological Disorders

MICHAEL G. TRAMONTANA

Clinical observations and research reports strongly suggest that brain impairment is at least a contributing factor in the functional and behavioral difficulties displayed by many children and adolescents with psychopathological disorders (e.g., Hertzig & Birch, 1968; Seidel, Chadwick, & Rutter, 1975; Tramontana, Sherrets, & Golden, 1980). Apart from any direct relationship between brain impairment and pscyhopathology, its presence during childhood or adolescence appears to place the affected youngster at particularly high risk for developing emotional and behavioral difficulties, far more so than with other physical handicaps (Seidel *et al.,* 1975).

The functional limitations of the brain-impaired child may set the stage for increased exposure to stress and psychonoxious reactions from the environment, including parental responses ranging from overprotection to scapegoating, and thus may predispose the youngster to emotional and behavioral disturbance in time (Rutter, 1977). The precise mechanisms are unknown, but the effects do appear to persist and to influence many areas of adjustment and adaptability, including frustration tolerance, coping style, and school performance (Hertzig & Birch, 1968; Milman, 1979; Rutter, 1977). It is important, therefore, that the

MICHAEL G. TRAMONTANA ● Psychology Department, Bradley Hospital, Section of Psychiatry and Human Behavior, Brown University, East Providence, Rhode Island 02915.

functional limitations of the brain-impaired child or adolescent be comprehensively assessed, with early and accurate detection at least being the first step in reducing the risk for the development or progression of psychopathological disturbance.

Although there is an unusually high incidence of brain impairment among children and adolescents with psychopathological disorders, it often goes undetected in the routine neurological examinations performed in mental health facilities. For example, Hertzig and Birch (1968) found a 34% rate of neurological abnormality in a careful examination of psychiatrically hospitalized adolescents, a rate which far exceeded the less than 5% rate of abnormality found in a normal comparison group. However, only 6% of those found to be neurologically impaired had actually been so identified by hospital staff. Tramontana *et al.* (1980) found a 60% rate of abnormality in a comprehensive neuropsychological evaluation of hospitalized child and adolescent psychiatric patients whose neurological examinations on admission were all within normal limits. Estimates of incidence obviously vary as a function of the methods and criteria used in identifying brain impairment, and in terms of differences in the subject samples selected. It is not uncommon, however, for brain impairment to exist in child or adolescent patients despite the absence of positive findings in a neurological examination, electroencephalogram, or review of history (Rutter, 1977). Accurate detection in this population evidently requires the use of more comprehensive assessment procedures than are customarily employed.

The nature and extent of brain impairment, as well as the role it plays in failures of adjustment, can vary considerably among disturbed youngsters for whom it is actually a contributing factor. Besides detection, it is important in the individual case to determine precisely *how* brain impairment is related to existing psychopathology and difficulties in adjustment, to determine the kinds of situations in which the youngster would tend to be more or less limited, and to specify conditions that are most likely to help maximize existing capabilities and adjustment potential. This is the task of clinical neuropsychology when applied to this population. Being a direct and comprehensive appraisal of brain function, a standardized neuropsychological evaluation can be used to specify the behavioral effects of known brain damage, to reveal undetected abnormalities in brain function that may nonetheless impede the youngster's adaptability and response to therapeutic efforts or, conversely, to reveal areas of functional potential that perhaps would not otherwise be apparent.

Neuropsychological diagnosis may be viewed as a *hypothetical construct* out of which testable predictions regarding prognosis and treatment of the individual can be derived (Tramontana, 1983). By relating behavioral and functional deficits to the brain, and by doing this in a way that draws upon the theory and science of brain-behavior relationships, an integrated perspective is obtained that permits the tying together of otherwise discrete behavioral observations into clusters of related symptoms for which certain interventions are theoretically likely to be beneficial. Such predictions can then be tested through programmatic implementation, and thereafter modified in relation to actual outcome. Thus, when incorporated into a more complete diagnostic evaluation, a neuropsychological evaluation can provide an important perspective in understanding the disturbed child or adolescent's difficulties, and in suggesting where and how intervention might most profitably proceed.

This chapter focuses on neuropsychological assessment in the diagnostic evaluation of children and adolescents with psychopathological disorders. The use of various single-test assessments (e.g., the Bender Motor Gestalt Test) will not be discussed, as the drawbacks in relying upon single, all-purpose measures of "organicity" have been well documented (e.g., Golden, 1978, Reitan, 1974a). Not only is there the dual problem of false positives and false negatives in diagnosing brain dysfunction on the basis of a single test, there is also the problem that no single test could ever provide the kind of detailed and comprehensive appraisal of brain function necessary for treatment planning. A battery of neuropsychological tests is needed for this. As will be seen, however, little attention has been given to the systematic application of standardized neuropsychological test batteries in the evaluation of psychopathologically disturbed children and adolescents. The chapter should thus be viewed more as a proposal for future directions rather than a review of past efforts in this area. It begins with an overview of existing neuropsychological research on children and adolescents, and outlines various interpretive problems and issues involved in the neuropsychological evaluation of children and adolescents with psychopathological disorders. Applications are illustrated through selected case examples covering a range of psychopathology, and guidelines for research and practice with this population are discussed.

NEUROPSYCHOLOGICAL RESEARCH ON CHILDREN AND ADOLESCENTS

Research on standardized neuropsychological test batteries has been far less extensive with children and adolescents than with adults. Perhaps this is so mainly because of the greater number of potentially confounding factors that can obscure and complicate the appraisal of brain-behavior relationships in childhood or adolescence (Boll, 1974). Factors such as maturation and developmental changes in the organization of brain function, assorted environmental factors, distinguishing onset when pathology is involved, and age-specific constraints on how abilities are assessed—especially for the very young—contribute to the relatively greater complexity involved in studying the child or adolescent. The Luria–Nebraska Neuropsychological Battery (Golden, Hammeke, & Purisch, 1980; Golden, Purisch, & Hammeke, 1979) has been standardized on adults, and can be extended downward only with considerable caution to persons as young as 12 years of age (Golden, 1980). A children's version of the battery for youngsters aged 8 to 12 has been developed (Golden, 1981), but basic normative and validational studies are just in progress. A similar set of procedures based also on Luria's neuropsychological examination (Christensen, 1975), and suitable for use with adolescents 12 years of age and older, was recently introduced by Majovski and his colleagues (Majovski, Tanguay, Russell, Sigman, Crumley, & Goldenberg, 1979a, 1979b) but has not yet received validational study. By far, existing research on youngsters below the age of 15 has been with the test procedures collectively known as the Halstead–Reitan Neuropsychological Battery. These include the Reitan–Indiana Neuropsychological Test Battery for Children (ages 5 through 8) and the Halstead Neuropsychological Test Battery for Children (ages 9 through 14), along with various supplemental tests that are commonly incorporated into each of the two versions of the battery (see Reitan & Davison, 1974, for a complete description).

The Halstead–Reitan Neuropsychological Battery has been shown to distinguish accurately between normal youngsters and variously composed groups with confirmed brain damage, both in the 5 to 8 age range (Klonoff & Low, 1974; Reitan, 1974b) and in the 9 to 14 age range (Boll, 1974; Klonoff & Low, 1974; Reed, Reitan, & Klove, 1965). Comparative results have been reported for youngsters with minimal cerebral dysfunction (Klonoff & Low, 1974), mental retardation (Matthews, 1974), and learning disability (Selz & Reitan, 1979; Tsushima & Towne, 1977). In the study by Selz and Reitan (1979), the validity of an actuarial system of neuropsychological rules for classifying youngsters aged 9 to 14 as normal, learning disabled, or brain damaged was assessed. The system consisted of 37 empirically derived rules, which were based on normative test data on the battery and which incorporated Reitan's four methods of inferring impaired brain function (i.e., level of performance, pattern of performance, right–left differences, and pathognomonic signs; see Reitan & Davison, 1974). Each rule transformed the subject's raw data to a score of 0 to 3, with 0 representing adequate performance, 1 for performance that was slightly below normal, 2 for probably abnormal performance, and 3 for definitely abnormal performance. Scaled scores were then summed to yield a total score for the subject; the higher the sum of scale scores, the greater was the evidence of brain impairment. Based on optimal cutoffs for the sum of scaled scores that best discriminated their groups, Selz and Reitan were able to classify their subjects as normal, learning disabled, or brain damaged with an overall accuracy of 73.3%. Misclassifications were almost entirely in the direction of false negatives, as the system evidently tended to underestimate dysfunction in the learning-disabled and brain-damaged subjects in their study. However, the hit rate rose to 87% when the investigators excluded the learning-disabled group and simply classified their subjects as either brain damaged or normal.

In the first of a series of studies devoted to a comprehensive assessment of brain impairment among children and adolescents with psychopathological disorders, Tramontana and his colleagues (Tramontana *et al.*, 1980) applied the Selz–Reitan system of rules in a neuropsychological evaluation of a mixed sample of psychopathologically disturbed youngsters. Twenty hospitalized child and adolescent psychiatric patients without known brain damage who ranged from 9 to 15 years of age were administered the Halstead–Reitan Neuropsychological Battery and were then classified as normal, learning disabled, or brain damaged according to the cutoffs established by Selz and Reitan. Consecutive admissions in this age range were selected if there was neither a history of brain damage, no positive findings on an admitting neurological examination, nor any other evidence of a neuropathological condition. Four subjects were left-handed, and no subject had a primary diagnosis of mental retardation or learning disability. IQ ranged from 70 to 128 ($M = 92.9$, $SD = 15.3$) but the sample was unevenly distributed with respect to sex (there were 16 boys and 4 girls). The sample was heterogeneous in terms of severity and chronicity of psychopathological disturbance, with roughly equal numbers of subjects falling in the broad diagnostic categories of adjustment reaction, neurosis, conduct disorder, and psychosis. Moreover, half of the sample was classified as chronic based on an arbitrary cutoff of 2 years since estimated time of onset (i.e., when treatment was first sought).

Table 1 shows the overall results for the psychopathological youngsters in relation to the Selz and Reitan groups. The psychopathological group had a mean sum of scaled scores (SSS) that was significantly higher than the Selz and Reitan normals, significantly lower than their brain-damaged group, but that did not differ significantly from their learning-disabled group. Using the SSS cutoffs established by Selz and Reitan, 40% of the psychopathological subjects were neuropsy-

Table 1

Comparative Performance[a] of Psychopathological Youngsters on
Selz–Reitan Sum of Scaled Scores

Group	Sum of scaled scores[b]			
	N	M	SD	Range
Tramontana, Sherrets, & Golden (1980):				
Psychopathological	20	25.50	13.20	6 to 60
Selz & Reitan (1979):				
Normal	25	10.60	6.62	1 to 25
Learning disabled	25	24.44	9.61	8 to 43
Brain damaged	25	40.60	18.51	11 to 74

[a]$P < .001$ for psychopathological versus normal and for psychopathological versus brain-damaged means, but no significant differences between the psychopathological and learning-disabled groups.

[b]The higher the score, the greater was the evidence of brain dysfunction.

chologically classified as normal (SSS of 19 or less), 35% were classified as learning disabled (SSS of 20 to 35), and 25% were classified as brain damaged (SSS of 36 or more). Thus, altogether, 60% of the disturbed youngsters demonstrated some degree of dysfunction according to the rules system, despite the relatively conservative criteria for subject selection that had been applied. Their overall performance reflected an intermediate level of neuropsychological impairment quite similar to the Selz and Reitan learning-disabled group, except that the psychopathological group was more variable and had twice the percentage of subjects classified as brain damaged. Impaired performance was much more likely among the youngsters whose psychopathological disorders were at least 2 years in duration and who showed a lag of 2 grades or more in academic achievement. Moreover, IQ correlated significantly with overall performance ($r = -.65$), and there was a tendency for the younger subjects in the psychopathological group to perform more poorly, but the trend did not reach statistical significance ($r = -.38$).

The particular difficulties displayed by the psychopathological group on the Halstead–Reitan Neuropsychological Battery are shown in Table 2. This shows the scaled score mean and standard deviation on each Selz–Reitan rule, the percentage of subjects demonstrating impaired performance on it, and the correlation between rule score and the sum of scaled scores. With few exceptions, performance tended to be poorer in the more complex perceptual and cognitive tasks than in relatively simple sensory and motor tasks. For example, there were more errors in Fingertip Number Writing and Tactile Form Recognition than in Tactile Finger Recognition; performance was poorer on the Category Test in comparison to Tapping. At least half of the sample showed impaired performance on the Category Test, Fingertip Number Writing, and on various items of the Aphasia Screening Test (rules 26, 28, 30, 31, and 32). However, the difficulties on rules

Table 2

Results of Psychopathological Youngsters ($N = 20$) on Selz–Reitan
Neuropsychological Rules[a]

| | Scaled score[b] | | | |
Rule	M	SD	% Impaired[c]	r^d
Level of performance				
1. Category Test—errors	1.70	0.98	.55	.64[f]
2. Tactual Performance Test (TPT)—total time	0.75	0.97	.15	.43
3. TPT—memory	0.60	1.14	.20	.38
4. TPT—localization	0.45	1.00	.15	.47[f]
5. Trails A—time	0.85	0.67	.15	.63[f]
6. Trails B—time	0.85	1.18	.30	.69[f]
7. Speech—errors	0.90	1.12	.25	.65[f]
8. Rhythm—correct	1.15	1.09	.45	.53[f]
9. Verbal IQ	0.65	0.81	.20	.68[f]

(*continued*)

Table 2 (*Cont.*)

Rule	Scaled score[b]		% Impaired[c]	r^d
	M	SD		
10. Performance IQ	0.50	0.89	.15	.63[f]
11. Full Scale IQ	0.55	0.76	.15	.69[f]
12. Tapping—preferred hand	0.70	1.13	.20	.56[f]
13. Tapping—nonpreferred hand	0.80	1.11	.30	.56[f]
Pattern				
14. Pattern IQ	0.40	0.60	.05	.34
Right–Left differences				
15. Tapping	1.05	1.05	.25	.17
16. Grip	1.05	1.28	.30	.18
17. TPT	0.70	0.80	.20	−.18
18. Name Writing—preferred hand	0.40	0.60	.05	.11
19. Name Writing—difference	0.20	0.52	.05	.03
20. Tactile Finger Recognition, right hand errors— left hand errors	0.10	0.31	.00	.08
21. Fingertip Number Writing, right hand errors— left hand errors	0.30	0.73	.05	.31
Pathognomonic signs				
22. Imperception errors	—	—	—	—
23. Tactile Finger Recognition errors	0.35	0.75	.15	.20
24. Fingertip Number Writing errors	1.50	1.24	.50	.68[f]
25. Tactile Form Recognition errors	1.25	1.16	.40	.50[f]
Aphasia battery:[e]				
26. Constructional dyspraxia			.50	.51[f]
27. Dysnomia			.10	.39
28. Spelling dyspraxia			.85	.27
29. Dysgraphia			.40	.56[f]
30. Dyslexia			.60	.38
31. Central dysarthria			.70	.59[f]
32. Dyscalculia			.80	.55[f]
33. Right–left confusion			.45	.62[f]
34. Auditory verbal dysgnosia			.00	.00
35. Visual number dysgnosia			.00	.00
36. Visual letter dysgnosia			.00	.00
37. Body dysgnosia			.05	.31

[a]From "Brain Dysfunction in Youngsters with Psychiatric Disorders: Application of Selz–Reitan Rules for Neuropsychological Diagnosis" by M. G. Tramontana, S. D. Sherrets, and C. J. Golden, *Clinical Neuropsychology*, 1980, *2*, 118–123. Copyright 1980 by *Clinical Neuropsychology*. Reprinted by permission.

[b]Scaled scores ranged from 0 to 3: 0 = normal or better; 1 = slightly below normal; 2 = probably impaired; 3 = definitely impaired.

[c]Subjects with a scaled score of 2 or 3.

[d]Correlation of rule score with sum of scaled scores.

[e]Means were not computed because of the dichotomous method of assigning scaled scores for performance on the Aphasia battery.

[f]$P < .05$ or better.

28 and 30 (i.e., spelling and reading), although rather common in the sample (having occurred at rates of 85% and 60%, respectively), were not necessarily associated with more general neuropsychological impairment. That is, scores on neither of these aphasia tasks were significantly correlated with SSS. Moreover, the correlations between individual rule scores and SSS indicated that, of Reitan's four methods of inference, pattern of performance (rule 14) and right–left differences (rules 15 to 21) contributed little to the overall neuropsychological classification of the psychopathological youngsters.

The development of the Selz–Reitan rules for neuropsychological diagnosis should facilitate further clinical and research applications of the Halstead–Reitan Neuropsychological Battery to older children and younger adolescents. The system has merit despite the objections raised by Amante (1980) on matters pertaining mainly to the subject-selection criteria used by Selz and Reitan in their validation study—especially their operational definition of learning disability. The system facilitates interpretation by the inclusion of approximate norms, by the incorporation of multiple methods of inference, and by the use of a uniform scoring scale that permits direct comparisons among the various scores within an individual's profile. The use of scaled scores rather than raw scores should also have the effect of reducing error variance, and thereby improve discriminative power in research comparisons of different subject groups. These are seemingly basic considerations, but they are welcome innovations nonetheless. The system will obviously require cross-validation with larger samples, more specific age-norms must be developed (rather than the single set of normative standards that now exists for the entire 9 through 14 age range), and several technical problems pertaining to scoring must be addressed (see Tramontana et al., 1980).

With respect more specifically to the evaluation of psychopathologically disturbed children and adolescents, the results obtained by Tramontana et al. (1980) raise some important questions. Can it be that so many disturbed youngsters are actually brain impaired despite the absence of positive findings on a neurological examination and review of history? It was already indicated that the accurate detection of brain impairment in this population—especially when it is of a subtle nature—requires the utilization of more intensive and comprehensive assessment procedures than are customarily employed (cf. Rutter, 1977). Thus, the neuropsychological evaluation may have been sensitive to abnormalities in the psychopathological youngsters that had been missed in the routine neurological examination.

On the other hand, just because the performance of many of the disturbed youngsters fell in the impaired range on the basis of existing norms, does not necessarily mean that it signified *brain* impairment. This becomes especially true when it is considered that classification was ultimately independent of both pattern of performance and right–left differences—as methods of inference. Lacking adequate norms for psychopathologically disturbed, non-brain-damaged youngsters, it is not known to what extent emotional, motivational, or behavioral factors may produce impaired performance on the Halstead–Reitan and other commonly used neuropsychological test batteries, without brain impairment being implicated. This question is being addressed by research currently in progress by Tramontana and his colleagues in which the performance of psychopathological youngsters on both the Halstead–Reitan Neuropsychological Battery and the children's version of the Luria–Nebraska Neuropsychological Battery is being compared with results obtained through computed tomography. In the meantime, their initial study serves to underscore the risk of false-positive diagnosis, which may exist in this population when dysfunctional neuropsychological performance in emotionally or behaviorally disturbed youngsters is simply interpreted as reflecting brain impairment. This problem and other interpretive issues that complicate the neuropsychological evaluation of children and adolescents with psychopathological disorders are discussed more fully in the next section of the chapter.

INTERPRETIVE PROBLEMS AND ISSUES

In the absence of appropriate norms, and in the absence of localizing signs in the performance profile, many rival interpretations exist in evaluating the abnormal neuropsychological performance of the psychopathologically disturbed child or adolescent. In most cases, the major interpretive problem involves distinguishing the effects of *deficit versus disturbance versus delay* in the neuropsychological results.

Abnormal performance may be the result of brain impairment, but alternatively may reflect the disruptive and regressive effects of emotional and motivational factors in the youngster's disturbed psychological adjustment. A debilitating psychopathological disturbance in childhood or adolescence, in the absence of brain damage, may itself be enough to produce a generalized impairment on a host of neuropsychological tests. To some extent, impaired performance could result from the disruptive effects of anxiety, depression, or psychogenically based problems with impulse control and attention. In cases of early onset, moreover, such conditions would not only disrupt present functioning, but also could have impeded the past attainment and development of various skills and abilities that are prerequisite to adequate or age-appropriate neuropsychological performance.

It was seen in the Tramontana *et al.* (1980) study, for example, that although spelling and reading difficulties were rather common within their sample of disturbed youngsters, neither was significantly correlated with a composite index of neuropsychological impairment. For this population, therefore, difficulties in academically related areas such as these may not necessarily constitute pathognomonic signs—at least not in the neuropsychological sense of the term—in that they may often be associated with factors besides brain dysfunction (e.g., long-term motivational problems in school). It was also seen that performance tended to be more impaired in complex rather than simple tasks. This too could be explained without necessarily inferring brain impairment, in that psychopathological conditions that interfere with focused or sustained attention are more likely to take their toll on performance as task demands are increased (McGhie, 1970).

In addition to developmental delays that are secondary to the effects of a prolonged psychopathological condition, delayed or irregular development can also be a function of physiological variations in the rate of brain growth and maturation. The literature shows that there is a rather wide range of nonpathological variation in maturational rates underlying various areas of neurological development—including the establishment of laterality—and that the presence of "soft" neurological signs in youngsters can often be attributed to maturational lags that are unrelated to structural damage to the brain (Schain, 1977). This appears to be a particularly important etiological factor, for example, with many youngsters diagnosed as having minimal cerebral dysfunction (e.g., Klonoff & Low, 1974). Whether attributable to a psychopathological condition or atypical brain maturation, however, the delayed youngster's performance may certainly appear deficient in relation to standards based on chronologic peers, but it need not signifiy brain damage.

It is perhaps this issue, in particular, which makes neuropsychological evaluation with youngsters generally so much more complex than with adults. If an adult with an unremarkable premorbid history begins to demonstrate difficulties in reading or writing, there are relatively few plausible explanations to compete with the impression that this probably relects a loss of function associated with an acquired brain lesion. With a child or adolescent, however, onset may be unclear, and it may be difficult to discern whether such difficulties represent a loss of function or are instead due to arrested, interrupted, or delayed development. Furthermore, if development is delayed, why is this so? Is it a product of chronic brain impairment? Does it instead point toward an abnormally slow or irregular rate of maturation of an otherwise intact brain? Or, in the case of disturbed youngsters, does it reflect developmental impediments secondary to the cumulative effects of the psychopathological condition, *per se?*

Inferring brain impairment is obviously simplified and strengthened when there are indications of lateralized deficits or other localizing features in the test profile, rather than when differential diagnosis is based simply on defective levels of performance or on pathognomonic signs that are of questionable significance with this population. Whereas an emotional disturbance may produce a relatively general interference with present performance and perhaps past achievement, it is implausible that only certain functions or only those involving one side of the body would mainly be affected. Thus, brain impairment essentially becomes implicated by default, when neither disturbance nor delay—as rival interpretations—can fully account for the obtained neuropsychological findings. Once brain impairment is identified, evaluation then entails determining the role that it has probably played in the youngster's disturbed adjustment, and its relative significance in conjunction with other contributing factors. In many cases there will most likely be a complex interaction of diverse contributing factors—including the combined effects of deficit, disturbance, and delay—producing the difficulties in performance and adjustment exhibited by the psychopathologically disturbed child or adolescent.

A related interpretive issue with this population involves distinguishing the *direct versus indirect* effects of abnormal brain function. In some cases, brain dysfunction may be directly responsible for the particular psychopathological symptoms and failures in adjustment exhibited by the child or adolescent. For example, disinhibitory symptoms, distractibility, and problems with impulse control and foresight in an adolescent may be directly tied to frontal lobe dysfunction. In other cases, however, brain dysfunction may play more of an indirect etiological role, one that essentially sets the stage for other factors to come into play, which themselves act to produce an emotional or behavioral disturbance and perhaps further aggravate existing functional difficulties. For example, a child might be experiencing a mild impairment of parietal–occipital functions of the left cerebral hemisphere, an impairment that would tend to impede the youngster's acquisition of basic academic skills in reading, arithmetic, and perhaps spelling upon entry into school. If undetected, however, and if educational plans and expectations are not appropriately modified, the child would probably encounter repeated failure and frustration in the learning process and may, in turn, develop a general aversion to school. The relatively specific nature of the child's disabilities may eventually become obscured by a general pattern of underachievement brought about by a defensive orientation to the educational process, and manifested either in withdrawal, resignation and disinterest, or outright oppositionality and misconduct. Parents and teachers, moreover, may come to view the youngster as lazy, apathetic, or otherwise difficult, and may themselves generate expectations of the youngster that would only serve to perpetuate the existing problems. If this state of affairs were to go unchecked, the problems could conceivably "snowball," so that by the time of adolescence some fairly serious behavior problems and academic deficiencies may have become well established. Whereas in this example brain dysfunction served to "get the ball rolling," and caused the youngster to get off to a poor start, it was mainly its indirect effects and poor management that brought about an end result far more serious than the initial problem. Retrospective accounts similar to this have emerged in recent neuropsychological investigations of juvenile delinquents and other behavior-disordered adolescents (see Chapter 13).

Brain dysfunction is ordinarily associated with both direct and indirect effects. It is important for these to be distinguished or—in the case of recent injuries—to anticipate what the indirect effects would likely be, so that appropriate preventive interventions may be applied promptly to offset or curtail reactive problems that could otherwise become chronic in time. Although differences will exist—depending on the nature and severity of brain dysfunction and any compensatory changes that have occurred—the more chronic the brain dysfunction, and the earlier its onset, the greater will be the range and extent of indirect effects that it would likely produce. This is because of the relatively greater toll that the impairment would take on subsequent development and achievement, and probably accounts for why youngsters with chronic brain damage generally exhibit more extensive neuropsychological impairment than those with acute injuries (Klonoff & Low, 1974).

Lastly, another important issue with this population involves distinguishing *damage versus dysfunction* when interpreting abnormal neuropsychological results. It was indicated before that dysfunctional performance on a neuropsychological evaluation can result not only from brain damage, but also can occur with serious psychopathological disturbances for which there may be no evidence of structural damage to the brain. A distinction between brain damage and brain dysfunction is implied; that is, whereas brain damage is one cause of brain dysfunction, brain dysfunction can occur from factors other than the destruction of brain tissue. It can be rather variable in psychoses—perhaps secondarily to neurophysiological and biochemical abnormalities—waxing and waning in conjunction with the exacerbation and remission of manifest symptoms. It is this variability, coupled with the presence of nonspecific attentional disturbances, that often serves to distinguish dysfunctional performance that is not necessarily associated with brain damage in psychopathological patients.

Review of the more extensive adult literature on this topic shows that earlier efforts to distinguish between brain damage and a serious mental disturbance such as schizophrenia on the basis of neuropsychological results had proved to be largely unsuccessful. Indeed, discrimination rates were often no better than chance, especially among chronics (Heaton, Baade, & Johnson, 1978; Hevern, 1980). More recent work has shown that this can in fact be done with acceptable accuracy with either the Halstead–Reitan Battery (Golden, 1977) or the Luria–Nebraska Battery (Purisch, Golden, & Hammeke, 1978; Moses & Golden, 1980), and that although there is a high rate of neuropsychological abnormality among non-brain-damaged schizophrenics, the pattern of findings is distinctive. For example, pathological elevations on the Rhythm, Receptive Speech, Memory, and Intelligence scales of the Luria–Nebraska Battery is a pattern of dysfunctional performance commonly found in schizophrenics, but is not necessarily associated with brain damage (Purisch *et al.,* 1978). Here, the neuropsychological abnormalities in acoustic discrimination, language comprehension, memory, and complex intellectual operations appear to be secondary to the disturbances in attention and thinking associated with schizophrenia, and tend to improve as psychotic symptoms are reduced.

Whereas dysfunction is certainly present, it is not necessarily of the chronic nature that would tend to exist with brain damage, and is perhaps reversible to the extent that improvement in the psychosis can be achieved. Thus, in reexamining the patient after a period of time and upon clinical remission, the neuropsychological evaluation becomes more specifically an appraisal of potential reversibility, by distinguishing the areas of dysfunctional performance that are more or less likely to persist despite improvement in psychopathological symptoms. This same rationale and model of practice may be applied to psychotic youngsters, especially when there appears to be a sudden onset or a fluctuating course in the manifestation of the psychosis.

The foregoing should serve to underscore the main interpretive problems and issues involved in the neuropsychological evaluation of children and adolescents with psychopathological disorders. Prognosis and treatment selection for the individual case will depend on a variety of factors, of course. Neuropsychological diagnosis provides one perspective, one that can perhaps have an important effect in guiding predictions and treatment decisions in ways that are positively related to the child or adolescent's clinical outcome and general adjustment. For this to be done with clarity, however, it is necessary to distinguish the differential effects of deficit versus disturbance versus delay in the neuropsychological findings, the direct versus indirect effects of any existing brain dysfunction, as well as whether it is dysfunction versus damage, *per se,* that is reflected in abnormal results. These interpretive issues are illustrated in the following case examples, albeit with varying emphasis, as neuropsychological findings are presented on three youngsters who differ not only with respect to the type of brain dysfunction manifested, but also in terms of the contributing role it has apparently played in their psychopathology and difficulties in adjustment.

CASE EXAMPLES

In some cases a neuropsychological evaluation may be used to delineate the precise effects of known brain damage. Being a direct and comprehensive examination of brain function, the neuropsychological evaluation serves to specify the functions that are most impaired and those that are relatively spared by a brain lesion that has been documented through independent neurodiagnostic methods. Such was the case in the first example to be discussed, a case described by Newlin and Tramontana (1980), in whom a confirmed subcortical lesion played a direct role in producing a set of symptoms closely resembling the syndrome of hyperactivity.

Subcortical Brain Pathology in a Hyperactive Adolescent

N. B. was a 16-year-old-boy who was psychiatrically hospitalized for behavioral and mental changes coinciding with the onset of a malignant subcortical brain tumor approximately 2 years earlier. A computed tomography (CT) scan had been performed at that time, which had revealed an area of high density within the right-anterior portion of the basal ganglia, occupying the head of the caudate nucleus on the right side, and extending into the internal capsule. This is shown in Figure 1. Figures 2 and 3 further illustrate the location of the lesion and the anatomical structures involved. Another CT scan was performed 1 year later, after chemotherapy and radiation treatment, and is shown in Figure 4. This revealed an apparent resolution of the tumor but also showed bilateral atrophy that was probably secondary to the radiation treatment, with some enlargement of the ventricles and widening of the sulci.

The personality changes induced by the tumor persisted, however. N. B.'s clinical picture at the time of psychiatric admission was characterized by hyper-arousal and a general breakdown in the regulation of goal-directed behavior, cognition, and affect. Symptoms included vocal perseveration together with clang associations and rapid speech. Short-term and recent memory were impaired, and

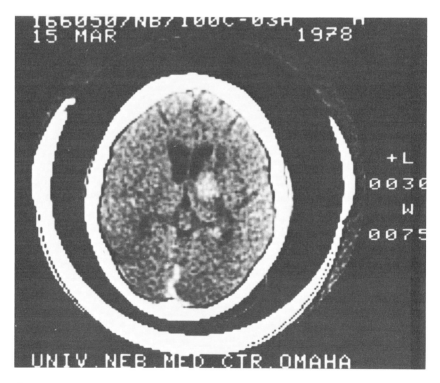

Figure 1. CT scan (slice 3A) showing the tumor within the right-anterior portion of the basal ganglia. (From "Neuropsychological Findings in a Hyperactive Adolescent with Subcortical Brain Pathology" by D. B. Newlin and M. G. Tramontana, *Clinical Neuropsychology*, 1980, *2*, 178–183. Copyright 1980 by *Clinical Neuropsychology*. Reprinted by permission.)

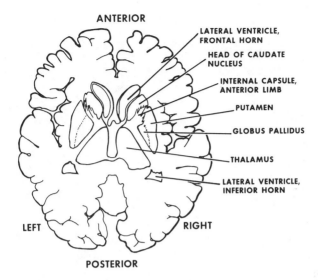

Figure 2. Identification of selected subcortical structures corresponding to the CT scan slice shown in Figure 1. (From "Neuropsychological Findings in a Hyperactive Adolescent with Subcortical Brain Pathology" by D. B. Newlin and M. G. Tramontana, *Clinical Neuropsychology*, 1980, *2*, 178–183. Copyright 1980 by *Clinical Neuropsychology*. Reprinted by permission.)

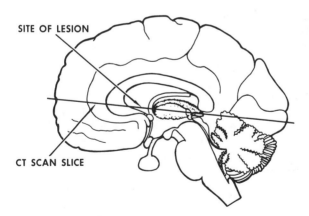

Figure 3. Lateral perspective locating the site of the lesion and the level from which the CT slice was drawn. (From "Neuropsychological Findings in a Hyperactive Adolescent with Subcortical Brain Pathology" by D. B. Newlin and M. G. Tramontana, *Clinical Neuropsychology*, 1980, *2*, 178–183. Copyright 1980 by *Clinical Neoropsychology*. Reprinted by permission.)

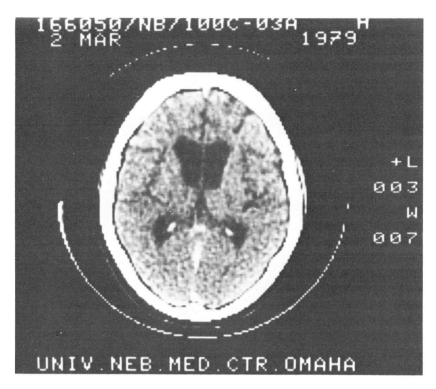

Figure 4. Subsequent CT scan (slice 3A) showing resolution of the tumor after treatment. (From "Neuropsychological Findings in a Hyperactive Adolescent with Subcortical Brain Pathology" by D. B. Newlin and M. G. Tramontana, *Clinical Neuropsychology,* 1980, *2,* 178–183. Copyright 1980 by *Clinical Neuropsychology.* Reprinted by permission.)

he showed a tendency to confabulate in recalling details of his distant past. He displayed a superficially outgoing, friendly, and carefree manner but exhibited considerable motor restlessness and distractibility. In many ways his symptoms were similar to those of a hyperactive child. Treatment with Ritalin was, in fact, tried; it resulted in apparent improvement in his attention span. Additional findings included a history of obesity and chronic enuresis. Moreover, he was still prepubescent at the age of 16—a condition possibly related to the proximity of his tumor to the pituitary gland. For the most part, however, his premorbid history had been unremarkable.

N. B.'s results on the Luria–Nebraska Neuropsychological Battery, which were obtained during his psychiatric hospitalization, are shown in Figure 5, where his performance on the various scales of the battery is depicted in terms of a *T*-score profile with a mean of 50 and a standard deviation of 10. Adjusting for age

and education, a critical level of approximately 59 was used in his case in desig-
nating scale elevations falling in the brain-damaged range (see Golden *et al.,*
1980). Basic motor, sensory–perceptual, and spatial functions appear to have been
largely intact, judging by the absence of significant elevations on the Motor, Tactile, and Visual scales in his profile. There was a *T*-score difference of approximately 10 points between the Left Hemisphere and Right Hemisphere scales, but
this probably underestimated the relative impairment of the right cerebral hemisphere (i.e., considering that the patient was left-handed, and that these scales
were standardized on primarily a right-handed population). The greater elevation
of the Motor scale compared to the Tactile scale, and of Expressive Speech over
Receptive Speech, in contrast, pointed toward predominately anterior impairment.
Moreover, inspection of the individual items on the Motor scale revealed a specific
dysfunction of the left upper extremity, and—assuming right-hemispheric speech

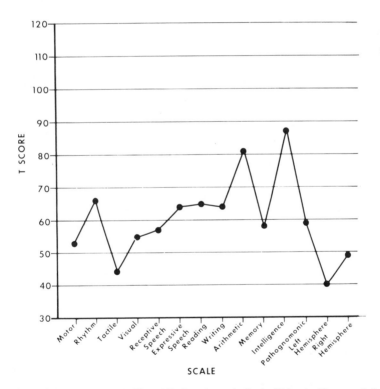

Figure 5. *T*-score profile (*M* = 50, *SD* = 10) of results on the Luria–Nebraska Neuropsychological
Battery for N. B. Critical level = 59. (From "Neuropsychological Findings in a Hyperactive Adolescent with Subcortical Brain Pathology" by D. B. Newlin and M. G. Tramontana, *Clinical Neuropsychology.* 1980, *2*, 178–183. Copyright 1980 by *Clinical Neuropsychology.* Reprinted by
permission.)

dominance because of the patient's noninverted, left-handed writing posture (Levy & Reid, 1976)—his impaired performance on the Expressive Speech scale could be viewed as compatible with other indications of right-frontal involvement.

Other findings included very pronounced elevations on the Arithmetic and Intelligence scales as well as lesser elevations on Rhythm, Reading, Writing, and Memory. It is unlikely that these primarily reflected the effects of diffuse cortical damage, especially in considering the only modest elevation of the Pathognomonic scale (which serves as a general indicator of brain damage). Rather, in the context of the other findings, it seems more likely that much of the patient's problem here resulted from a breakdown in the regulatory and inhibitory functions of attention, making him susceptible to interference and distraction in tasks requiring highly focused attention or the efficient execution of higher mental functions. Accordingly, this would implicate prefrontal cortical impairment (especially in light of his very poor performance on the Intelligence scale), and also raises the possibility of subcortical involvement.

Table 3 shows N. B.'s raw scores and Selz–Reitan conversions on the Halstead–Reitan Neuropsychological Battery, as well as his results on the Wechsler Adult Intelligence Scale. His performance was quite poor on Fingertip Number Writing and on the Localization component of the Tactual Performance Test. However, his excellent performance on both Tactile Finger Recognition and Tactile Form Recognition would argue against an interpretation of parietal dysfunction. The bilateral nature of his errors on Fingertip Number Writing and the relative complexity of both this task and the Tactual Performance Test suggested that problems in sustaining attention were instead largely responsible for his difficulty on these particular tactile tasks. This may likewise account for his moderately impaired performance on Rhythm. However, his failure to show an expected superiority with his preferred (left) hand on Tapping, his performance decline on the third trial of the Tactual Performance Test with the reintroduction of his left hand, together with his apparent difficulty in maintaining and shifting mental set on both the Category Test and on Trails A and B, pointed toward the likelihood of right-frontal involvement. His low-average performance on the Wechsler, moreover, probably reflected a decline from at least an average level of intelligence, judging from his premorbid academic achievement and his performance on the Similarities subtest.

Apart from providing generally less indication of impairment and in not giving any indication of a difficulty in expressive speech, the Halstead–Reitan results corresponded rather well to those found with the Luria–Nebraska. Together, the neuropsychological evaluations pointed toward a general breakdown in the regulatory functions of attention and to the likely involvement of the right frontal lobe, perhaps particularly prefrontal areas.

Theory (e.g., Luria, 1966, 1973) and research (e.g., Gorenstein & Newman, 1980; Pribram & McGuinness, 1975) posit a nonspecific, regulatory function for

Table 3
Raw Scores and Selz–Reitan Conversions[a] on Halstead–Reitan Battery for N. B.[b]

Wechsler Adult Intelligence Scale			Tapping		
Information	9		Preferred (left)	38.0	(0)
Comprehension	6		Nonpreferred (right)	38.8	(0)
Arithmetic	6		Difference		(1)
Similarities	10		Grip Strength		
Digit Span	6		Preferred (left)	25 kg	
Vocabulary	7		Nonpreferred (right)	21 kg	
Digit Symbol	6		Difference		(0)
Picture Completion	8		Tactile Finger		
Block Design	9		Recognition—errors		(0)
Picture Arrangement	7		Left	1	
Object Assembly	6		Right	0	
Verbal IQ	90	(0)	Difference		(0)
Performance IQ	83	(1)	Fingertip Number		
Full Scale IQ	86	(1)	Writing—errors		(3)
Pattern IQ		(0)	Left	11	
Category Test—errors	58	(2)	Right	9	
Tactual Performance Test			Difference		(0)
Preferred (left)	200 sec		Tactile Form		
Nonpreferred (right)	112 sec		Recognition—errors		(0)
Both hands	157 sec		Left	0	
Difference		(0)	Right	0	
Total time	469 sec	(1)	Sensory Imperception—errors		(0)
Memory	4	(1)	Aphasia Screening Test		
Localization	0	(3)	Constructional dyspraxia		(2)
Trails-time			Spelling dyspraxia		(1)
Part A	30 sec	(2)	Dysgraphia		(2)
Part B	70 sec	(2)	Visual letter dysgnosia		(3)
Speech—errors	9	(0)	Sum		(27)
Rhythm—correct	17	(2)			

[a]Shown in parentheses: (0) = normal or better; (1) = slightly below normal; (2) = probably impaired; and (3) = definitely impaired.
[b]From "Neuropsychological Findings in a Hyperactive Adolescent with Subcortical Brain Pathology" by D. B. Newlin and M. G. Tramontana, *Clinical Neuropsychology*, 1980, *2*, 178–183. Copyright 1980 by *Clinical Neuropsychology*. Reprinted by permission.

a variety of subcortical structures that, when impaired, tend to be manifested through abnormalities in general arousal and attention. In some respects such a condition could resemble the generalized disturbance in performance often seen in cases of either diffuse cortical damage or frontal lobe dysfunction and—in terms of neuropsychological results—may be rather difficult to distinguish. Newlin and Tramontana (1980) have discussed the particular features in the preceding case which served to implicate subcortical impairment. Briefly, they suggest that the possibility of subcortical involvement should at least be considered in cases who otherwise appear to show frontal lobe dysfunction, especially when hyperarousal and distractibility are highly salient features in the history and test performance but evidence of motor impairment is largely absent. In the case of N. B., however, the indications of prefrontal and right premotor involvement in his neuropsychological results further suggested that the subcortical tumor had actually infiltrated or exerted significant pressure effects on these cortical areas, and that descending pathways between frontal lobe and anterior limbic structures—pathways that inhibit or otherwise regulate emotion and arousal—had probably been disturbed or destroyed, with a resultant loss of inhibitory control. Thus, the proximity of the lesion to both frontal lobe and anterior limbic structures in the case of N. B. serves to illustrate the intimate relationship between these neuroanatomical regions in the regulation of goal-directed behavior, cognition, and affect, and points toward their possible role in disinhibitory psychopathology such as hyperactivity.

A neuropsychological conceptualization of the case would suggest that some improvement in symptoms could perhaps be achieved by efforts aimed at reducing the boy's net level of stimulation, either medically or through environmental modifications. Care would also have to be taken to devise a rehabilitation program in which complex tasks and demands are broken down into simpler components, and in which feedback and reinforcement contingencies are not presented over an extended time frame. Prognosis, of course, would depend on continued stabilization of his neurological status. In terms of the interpretive issues raised earlier, this youngster exemplifies a case in whom there was essentially a direct relationship between brain damage, *per se,* and psychopathological disturbance. Moreover, of the various factors that can contribute to abnormal neuropsychological performance in disturbed youngsters—i.e., deficit, disturbance, and delay—deficit was by far the most critical factor in his case.

There are other cases, however, for whom a neuropsychological evaluation may reveal otherwise undetected abnormalities in brain function, which significantly impede the youngster's adaptability and response to therapeutic efforts. Both direct and indirect effects may be involved, and the factors of disturbance and delay may compound the problems produced by deficits in brain function. These are exemplified in the next case example, a schizophrenic boy with an inferred impairment of the left cerebral hemisphere.

Left-Hemispheric Impairment in a Childhood Schizophrenic

R. L. was a 13-year-old-boy with a history of difficulties dating back to about the age of two. He had been in treatment for much of this period, carrying diagnoses ranging from hyperactivity to childhood schizophrenia, but failed to show a satisfactory response to either psychotherapeutic intervention or treatment with a variety of psychotropic medications. He was in an engineered class prior to his most recent hospitalization, but although placed in the seventh grade his overall academic achievement fell at less than a third-grade level, with particular difficulties in the areas of reading comprehension and math. Hospitalization was precipitated by a recent deterioration in his behavior, manifested by temper outbursts, increased withdrawal and preoccupation with themes of torture and aggression, and by noncompliance with rules at home and at school. His mental status examination on admission revealed distractibility, generally bland affect, autistic preoccupations, a lack of spontaneous speech, and replies that were sometimes so inappropriate that it was unclear as to whether he had actually comprehended the questions asked. The diagnosis of Childhood Schizophrenia appeared to be appropriate at the time.

Additional findings revealed a history of possible birth trauma and a number of congenital anomalies. He was prepubescent and his bone-age films and height were comparable to that of a 10-year-old. There was a delay of approximately another 2 years predicted before he would reach puberty. In the absence of endocrine abnormalities, however, his short stature and maturational delays were judged to be familial in nature. He was left-handed, and there were reported complications in the patient's delivery, but there was never confirmation of any actual period of perinatal anoxia. There were also reports of abnormal findings on an earlier electroencephalographic examination, but a subsequent examination during his recent hospitalization was judged to be within normal limits.

Table 4 shows R. L.'s results on the Wechsler Intelligence Scale for Children–Revised (WISC-R). His difficulty on primarily the verbal subtests is quite apparent, as evidence in the very striking difference between his Verbal IQ of 64 and his Performance IQ of 92. School-related difficulties may have been partly involved in his poor performance on Information and Arithmetic, but observed difficulties in formulating logical verbal responses were more likely responsible for his outstandingly poor performance on both Vocabulary and Comprehension. Although he was distractible, this alone could not account for his difficulty in these areas, especially in light of his rather good performance on both Block Design and

Table 4
WISC-R[a] Results for R. L.

Verbal subtests[b]		Performance subtests			
Information	4	Picture Completion	9	Verbal IQ	64
Similarities	7	Picture Arrangement	7	Performance IQ	92
Arithmetic	5	Block Design	14	Full Scale IQ	76
Vocabulary	2	Object Assembly	12		
Comprehension	2	Coding	3		
Digit Span	5				

[a]Wechsler Intelligence Scale for Children—Revised.
[b]Subtest values are scaled scores with $M = 10$ and $SD = 3$.

Object Asembly. Rather, a specific difficulty in processing words and symbols was probably involved, an interpretation that is further supported by his conspicuously poor performance on Coding.

His results on the Luria–Nebraska Neuropsychological Battery are shown in Figure 6, where a critical level of about 65 is used in the case of his age and education in evaluating scale elevations on the T-score profile. Motor, sensory–perceptual, and spatial functions were essentially intact, judging by the absence of significant elevations on the Motor, Rhythm, Tactile, and Visual scales in his profile. Pronounced elevations were instead found on Receptive Speech, Arithmetic, Memory, and Intelligence. Taken by themselves, these scale elevations would not provide convincing evidence of brain damage because, as already indicated, similar elevations are commonly found in non-brain-damaged schizophrenic adults due to their distractibility and disrupted thought processes (cf. Purisch *et al.*, 1978). Likewise, the patient's elevations on Reading, Writing, and Arithmetic could be viewed as indications of disrupted academic achievement brought about

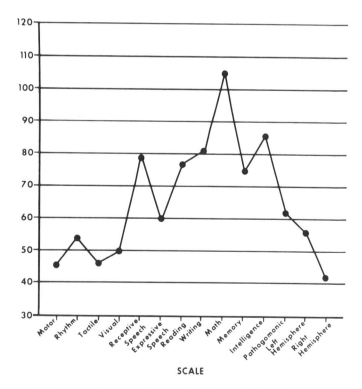

Figure 6. T-score profile ($M = 50$, $SD = 10$) of results on the Luria–Nebraska Neuropsychological Battery for R. L. Critical level = 65.

by his long-standing psychopathological disturbance, and thus would not necessarily be indicative of cerebral impairment. His Pathognomonic scale did approach the critical level, but it is perhaps mainly on the basis of his particular pattern of performance on the various scales that an inference of brain impairment emerges. These include the 14-point higher elevation of the Left Hemisphere scale in comparison to the Right, a difference which is all the more remarkable when it is considered that elevations on these scales depend on impaired motor or tactile performance with the contralateral hand, but—as indicated—R. L.'s overall performance on the Motor and Tactile scales was within normal limits. However, inspection of the individual items on the Motor scale did reveal a specific difficulty in positioning with the right hand. These findings, together with his relatively good performance in nonverbal, acoustic discrimination and in visual–spatial perception, as opposed to tasks of a more verbal nature, pointed toward a lateralized impairment of the left cerebral hemisphere. Moreover, his much poorer performance on Receptive Speech in comparison to Expressive Speech suggested a primarily posterior locus of dysfunction within the left cerebral hemisphere.

Inspection of the individual items within the Receptive Speech scale showed difficulties mainly with the sequential organization and logical–grammatical structure of language, and in dealing with relational concepts such as "on top of," "before," and so forth. These difficulties, in turn, appeared to contribute to much of his poor performance on the Intelligence scale, as well as on Reading and Writing—where difficulties in phonemic discrimination were also involved. His impairment in the analysis of what-follows-what in language tasks was also manifested on the Arithmetic scale, both in his failures in comprehending multiple-digit numbers and in the sequential analysis involved in more complex arithmetic problems. Taken together, the neuropsychological results yielded the inference of a focal impairment of temporal–parietal areas within the left cerebral hemisphere, resulting primarily in a receptive language disorder.

Computed tomography results were not available, but the findings in a subsequent pediatric neurological evaluation corresponded precisely to the neuropsychological diagnosis. The patient's left-handedness was judged to be pathological in nature, given the reduced length and width of his right upper extremity and the posturing of his right arm as he would walk. From a structural standpoint, there appeared to be a static insult to the left temporal–parietal region, which was probably neonatal in origin. The neuropsychological findings would suggest, however, that despite the patient's apparent reversal of handedness and the likelihood of early onset, there evidently had not been a compensatory reversal of hemispheric dominance for speech with the injury of the left cerebral hemisphere.

The relation of R. L.'s possible anoxia at birth to his unilateral brain damage is uncertain, but invites speculation. Although perinatal anoxia does not invariably lead to chronic impairment (Schain, 1977), indications are that the hemispheres differ with respect to their vulnerability to oxygen deficiency. Cerebrovascular asymmetries are such that the left hemisphere is likely to be affected sooner and more severely (Bruens, Gastaut, & Gione, 1960; Carmon, Harishanu, Louringer, & Lavy, 1972; LeMay & Culebras, 1972).

Psychotic conditions such as autism and childhood schizophrenia are often associated with major abnormalities in language performance and development (Quay & Werry, 1979). An impairment of the speech-dominant, left-cerebral hemisphere may be involved, but its detection can often be obscured by the seemingly nonspecific nature of the child's problems, and by the fact that a psychotic process in childhood—unrelated to brain damage—may produce highly disturbed performance in a variety of language tasks. Alternative factors such as self-preoccupation and interpersonal withdrawal, inadequate socialization, or motivational factors such as pronounced oppositionality—to name a few—could instead account for the apparent failure of many psychotic children to acquire or use language appropriately. Valid neuropsychological diagnosis in these broadly defined populations requires that, besides poor language performance, other localizing signs must be present in the test results to support an inference of left hemispheric impairment.

Differential diagnosis was facilitated in the case of R. L. by the presence of localizing features in his neuropsychological results. Psychosis alone could not have accounted for the obtained pattern of findings. Then again, neither could brain damage, considering that his dysfunction in a number of areas exceeded the apparent degree of brain damage present. His dysfunctional performance and highly disturbed adjustment most probably reflected the combined effects of brain impairment, psychosis, and atypical maturation, or, put differently, the combined effects of deficit, disturbance, and delay. For whatever reasons, however, the neuropathological condition had gone undetected prior to the neuropsychological evaluation, with its cumulative effects over the years resulting both in specific learning disabilities and in a general impediment in being understood, and in understanding the verbal communications of others. These problems had evidently been attributed to the psychosis alone and treated accordingly, albeit without success. Detection of the receptive language disorder in his case was obscured, no doubt, by the resemblance of his discontinuities in speech and distorted comprehension to what is often seen in psychosis. One can only wonder whether much of the boy's eventual autistic withdrawal, hostility, oppositionality, and apparent frustration (i.e., indirect effects) could have been avoided or at least reduced had his language disorder been promptly detected, and appropriate intervention provided. This, together with emphasizing expression in his areas of relative strength, may have had the effect of fostering a sense of contact with a reality in which mastery is possible.

There are other cases for whom dysfunctional performance is observed in the neuropsychological results but indications of brain damage, *per se*, are highly equivocal. Irregular or delayed maturation may constitute a plausible inference in accounting for the results, and the role of brain dysfunction in the youngster's disturbed adjustment may be reflected mainly through its indirect effects. These are seen in the next case example, a behavior-disordered and learning-disabled adolesent with an apparent neurodevelopmental delay.

Neurodevelopmental Immaturity in a Behavior-Disordered Adolescent with Learning Disabilities

M. C. was a 12-year-old boy with a history of difficulties in academic performance, frustration tolerance, and attention span. He had been identified as specific learning disabled in the second grade, and was subsequently diagnosed as hyperactive and treated with Ritalin. He reportedly had been adjusting well to the special educational services being provided, but although in the sixth grade, his overall academic achievement still fell at less than a fourth grade level—with his greatest difficulty being in reading comprehension. He was referred for outpatient treatment by his school because of a pronounced deterioration in his conduct over the preceding year, manifested in disruptive classroom behavior, fighting with his peers, and noncompliance at home and at school.

Additional findings at that time included an apparent history of delayed or irregular maturation, particularly in motor development. Bone-age films were not available, but an earlier physical therapy evaluation showed M.C. to be functioning substantially below age level in gross motor skills, in strength and balance, and in differentiating and coordinating the two sides of his body. There was also the problem of an unstable home environment that was reportedly taking an emotional toll on the boy, in that his parents were currently undergoing a divorce. Provisional diagnoses at the time of referral included Attention Deficit Disorder with Hyperactivity, Developmental Dyslexia, and Adjustment Reaction with Mixed Disturbance of Emotions and Conduct.

M.C.'s results on the WISC-R are shown in Table 5. Perhaps the most con-

Table 5
WISC-R[a] Results for M. C.

Verbal subtests[b]		Performance subtests			
Information	9	Picture Completion	10	Verbal IQ	97
Similarities	10	Picture Arrangment	10	Performance IQ	102
Arithmetic	9	Block Design	13	Full Scale IQ	100
Vocabulary	10	Object Assembly	14		
Comprehension	10	Coding	5		
Digit Span	11				

[a]Wechsler Intelligence Scale for Children—Revised.
[b]Subtest values are scaled scores with $M = 10$ and $SD = 3$.

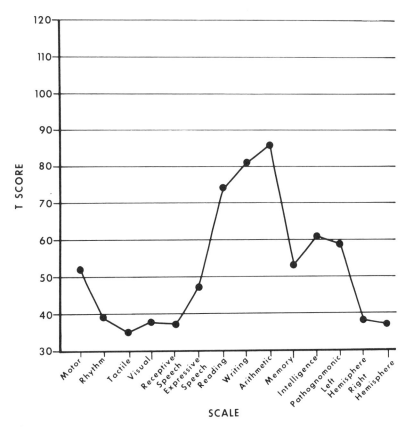

Figure 7. *T*-score profile ($M = 50$, $SD = 10$) of results on the Luria–Nebraska Neuropsychological Battery for M. C. Critical level = 67.

spicuous finding here—apart from his overall average intelligence—was his very poor performance on the Coding subtest. This stood in striking contrast to his rather good performance on both Block Design and Object Assembly, and thus would rule out visual- motor difficulties or a general problem with speeded tasks as being primarily responsible. Rather, problems either with the symbol-processing component of the task or with the mental "flexibility" required in shifting efficiently between the two types of stimulus input were more likely involved.

Figure 7 shows his results on the Luria–Nebraska Neuropsychological Battery. The patient was right-handed. Using a critical level of about 67, impaired performance was found on only the Reading, Writing, and Arithmetic scales in his profile. His Pathognomonic scale, although elevated, did not reach the critical value, and there was no evidence of lateralized impairment when measured in terms of motor and tactile performance with the contralateral hand. These findings would tend to weaken a general impression of brain damage. Moreover, judging by his excellent performance on the Rhythm, Tactile, Visual, and Receptive Speech scales, it is doubtful that distractibility or other nonspecific disrupting factors alone played an important role in his difficulties on Reading, Writing, and Arithmetic. Rather, ongoing or residual problems with the particular mental functions underlying these complex skills were probably involved.

There are several ways in which these results can be further interpreted. M. C.'s elevation on the Writing scale was due mainly to severe spelling difficulties. Item analysis also revealed that whereas visual-letter recognition and auditory-phonemic discrimination were each intact, the integration of these cross-modality processes constituted a particular problem for M. C., and largely accounted for his observed impediments in reading and spelling. This would implicate the tertiary or integrating zone for sensory cortex within the left cerebral hemisphere—an area corresponding approximately to the left angular gyrus—where temporal, parietal, and occipital pathways intersect (Luria, 1966, 1973). A similar localization of dysfunction may have accounted for his difficulties in arithmetic operations as well. It is possible that the connecting pathways in this region that are responsible for the integration of visual and auditory information had been selectively destroyed, or perhaps never fully developed, making it difficult for M. C. to visualize the words he would hear, and to sound-out the ones he would see. The possibility of arrested or incomplete development is all the more plausible when a tertiary cortical zone is involved, given the relative duration of its maturation and the hierarchical progression of its development.

A related interpretation emerges, one that postulates delayed frontal lobe development as also involved. Past reports of M. C.'s significantly delayed motor development would be compatible with this, as perhaps would his history of hyperactivity and poor attention span. His elevation on the Motor scale—although certainly not at a level indicative of current impairment—conformed to a pattern suggestive of a frontal locus of dysfunction, and possibly represented vestiges of what were once more substantial difficulties in motor performance. Mild problems were, in fact, still evident in coordinated movement and fine motor control, and in occasional word-finding difficulty and slurred speech. Qualitative analysis also revealed mild difficulties with the speech regulation of motor acts and the suppression of ongoing response tendencies or principles of action when having to switch to new ones, particularly on the concept formation items of the Intelligence scale. Likewise, in the absence of an impairment in visual recognition or receptive language, the poor performance seen before on Coding probably stemmed from a difficulty with the flexible but controlled regulation of mental set and motor output required in the task—in a fashion similar to what is involved with the Trail Making Test—Part B. These findings would implicate the tertiary or prefrontal region of the frontal lobes (Luria, 1966; Milner, 1964; Teuber, 1964).

Brain maturation—including myelinization—proceeds roughly along a posterior to anterior axis, with the prefrontal region of the frontal lobes being the last to achieve full development. This is a gradual process in which maturation of the prefrontal region typically begins by about the age of 4 and is nearing completion by adolescence (Burr, 1960; Conel, 1959). Myelinization of some forebrain structures actually extends well beyond puberty and into adulthood before full maturity is achieved (Yakovlev & Lecours, 1967). In some cases, however, this process is significantly delayed. For the schoolage child, this may be reflected in problems with self-regulated behavior and perhaps difficulties in academic learning as well—especially when accompanied by delayed development of posterior tertiary zones. This may have accounted for the history of behavioral problems and learning disabilities in the case of M. C. For the adolescent, however, accumulated academic deficiencies may exist, but the delay may be manifested primarily through disordered behavior. Behavior disorders in adolescents have multiple determinants, of course, but neurodevelopmental immaturity of the frontal lobes appears to be a contributing factor in some instances (Pontius, 1972; Pontius & Ruttiger, 1976). Unlike the child, the adolescent is ordinarily expected to display greater impulse control and flexibility, to show greater capacity to delay responding, to utilize foresight and planning, to anticipate long-range consequences for present actions, and to evaluate behavior according to appropriate principles of conduct. The adolescent who is delayed in terms of prefrontal development would obviously have substantial difficulty in adjusting to these kinds of age-appropriate demands and expectations placed on chronologic peers. With respect to the case of M. C., this may have contributed to his reported behavioral deterioration prior to referral, in that it coincided with the approach of adolescence.

Thus, the last case exemplifies a youngster for whom dysfunctional neuropsychological performance may reflect the residual and accumulated effects of neurodevelopmental delay. Similar patterns of findings are fairly common among behavior disordered youngsters (see Chapter 13 by Sherrets in this volume), and may be taken to suggest delayed brain development when evidence of brain damage, *per se,* is largely equivocal but there is independent evidence of atypical physical maturation. The direct effects of this condition may be apparent in the form of underdeveloped abilities and poor behavioral regulation, but it is perhaps the accumulation of its indirect effects over the years that weighs more heavily in the youngster's later functioning and adjustment. Early identification of these youngsters is quite important, for even if they should eventually "catch up" and reach neurological maturity, chronic behavior problems and persistent underachievement could have already become established along the way by their having to adjust to situations for which they were not ready.

SUMMARY: GUIDELINES FOR RESEARCH AND PRACTICE

The preceding case examples should provide some idea of the kinds of interpretive problems and issues that arise in the neuropsychological evaluation of children and adolescents with psychopathological disorders. The application of comprehensive neuropsychological methods with this population has been a fairly recent undertaking, and indications are that much work will be needed to assure their valid use in decisions pertaining to diagnosis, prognosis, and treatment. There are, however, a number of guidelines for research and practice that appear to be particularly relevant at this time.

As indicated before, more complete normative data are needed for psychopathologically disturbed, non-brain-damaged children and adolescents to reduce the risk of false-positive diagnosis with this population. Standardized neuropsychological test batteries such as the Halstead–Reitan and the Luria–Nebraska are each a comprehensive set of procedures of proven sensitivity in detecting even subtle degrees of impairment in cortical functions. It is perhaps precisely this sensitivity, however, which may lead to errors in diagnosis when dysfunctional performance in non-brain-damaged, disturbed youngsters is mistakingly interpreted as reflecting brain damage. Not knowing the extent to which psychopathological conditions during childhood and adolescence can produce abnormal levels of performance on various neuropsychological tests—without brain impairment being involved—it is imperative that diagnosis not be based on defective levels of performance alone. In the absence of appropriate norms, inferences of brain impairment and differential diagnosis must be supported by other features in the neuropsychological results (i.e., the pattern of performance, right–left differences, and pathognomonic signs).

Differential diagnosis in some cases might also make use of repeated or follow-up neuropsychological assessments. This would be helpful, for example, with youngsters for whom dysfunctional performance appears to stem mainly from attentional and motivational problems or other psychogenically based aspects of their psychopathological condition. A repeated evaluation upon clinical improvement or remission may yield results that are within normal limits or, instead, may reveal areas of dysfunction that persist despite improvement in psychopathology and that must be taken into account as limiting factors in the child or adolescent's eventual adjustment. Follow-up assessments—albeit over a more extended period—would also be useful with cases for whom developmental delays are inferred. This could help to determine whether earlier disabilities have, in fact, subsided with subsequent maturation and achievement, and might provide a basis for revising intervention plans when this appears appropriate.

A related matter has to do with the need for longitudinal studies in research investigations of outcome as a function of neuropsychological diagnosis. As already discussed, a complex interaction of diverse contributing factors is most likely involved in the failure in adjustment of the psychopathologically disturbed child or adolescent. Neuropsychological diagnosis provides one perspective, one which often leads to predictions regarding immediate and long-range prognosis, the kinds of situations in which the youngster will be more or less limited, as well as the characteristics that a program of intervention should include. Such predictions, however, are usually based on theoretical consideration, as research on outcome as a function of neuropsychological diagnosis is largely lacking at this time. It will be important to determine how predictions derived from this particular diagnostic perspective actually correspond to the child or adolescent's eventual adjustment.

The incorporation of independent neurodiagnostic methods in conjunction with neuropsychological assessment is clearly needed, not only for the sake of validational research on neuropsychological diagnosis with this population, but also to assure valid diagnosis for the individual case. No single neurodiagnostic procedure can capture the full range of ways in which brain impairment can be manifested. An integrated and comprehensive appraisal is possible only through a multimethod approach that incorporates recent refinements and developments in noninvasive neurodiagnostic technology. These various procedures fall along a structural–functional continuum with respect to the particular perspective provided, with a neuroanatomical focus provided through computed tomography, a neurophysiological focus with both the electroencephalogram and regional cerebral blood-flow analysis, and the highest level of functional analysis provided through the neuropsychological evaluation. Correspondencies among specific patterns of neuroanatomical, neurophysiological, and neuropsychological abnormality will differ, depending on the particular type of brain pathology involved.

Lastly, a case-study approach might provide a useful adjunct to research in this area. Validational studies have begun, and it is important that others follow. Neuropsychological reports on selected cases with relevant accompanying data can certainly complement this effort by underscoring particular problems and issues that arise, and by offering tentative guidelines in the neuropsychological evaluation of children and adolescents with psychopathological disorders.

REFERENCES

Amante, D. A critique of a proposed set of neuropsychological rules. *Journal of Consulting and Clinical Psychology,* 1980, *48,* 525–527.

Boll, T. J. Behavioral correlates of cerebral damage in children aged 9 through 14. In R. M. Reitan & L. A. Davison (Eds.), *Clinical neuropsychology: Current status and applications.* New York: Wiley, 1974.

Bruens, J. H., Gastaut, H., & Gione, G. Electroencephalographic study of the signs of chronic vascular insufficiency of the Sylvian region in aged people. *EEG Clinical Neurophysiology,* 1960, *12,* 283–295.

Burr, H. S. *The neural basis of human behavior.* Springfield, Ill.: Charles C. Thomas, 1960.

Carmon, A., Harishanu, Y., Louringer, E., & Lavy, S. Asymmetries in hemispheric blood volume and cerebral dominance. *Behavioral Biology,* 1972, *7,* 853–859.

Christensen, A. L. *Luria's neuropsychological investigation manual.* New York: Spectrum, 1975.

Conel, J. L. *The postnatal development of the human cerebral cortex.* Cambridge: Harvard University Press, 1959.

Golden, C. J. Validity of the Halstead–Reitan Neuropsychological Battery in a mixed psychiatric and brain-injured population. *Journal of Consulting and Clinical Psychology,* 1977, *45,* 1043–1051.

Golden, C. J. *Diagnosis and rehabilitation in clinical neuropsychology.* Springfield, Ill.: Charles C Thomas, 1978.

Golden, C. J. Personal communication, 1980.

Golden, C. J. The Luria–Nebraska Children's Battery: Theory and form. In G. Hind & J. Obrzut (Eds.), *Neuropsychological assessment and the school-aged child.* New York: Grune & Stratton, 1981.

Golden, C. J., Hammeke, T. A., & Purisch, A. D. *The Luria–Nebraska neuropsychological battery: Manual* (Revised). Los Angeles: Western Psychological Services, 1980.

Golden, C. J., Purisch, A. D., & Hammeke, T. A. *The Luria–Nebraska neuropsychological battery: A manual for clinical and experimental uses.* Lincoln: University of Nebraska Press, 1979.

Gorenstein, E. E., & Newman, J. P. Disinhibitory psychopathology: A new perspective and a model for research. *Psychological Review,* 1980, *87,* 301–315.

Heaton, R. K., Baade, L. E., & Johnson, K. L. Neuropsychological test results associated with psychiatric disorders in adults. *Psychological Bulletin,* 1978, *85,* 141–162.

Hertzig, M. E., & Birch, H. G. Neurological organization in psychiatrically disturbed adolescents. *Archives of General Psychiatry,* 1968, *19,* 528–537.

Hevern, V. W. Recent validity studies of the Halstead–Reitan approach to clinical neuropsychological assessment: A critical review. *Clinical Neuropsychology,* 1980, *2,* 49–61.

Klonoff, H., & Low, M. Disordered brain function in young children and early adolescents: Neuropsychological and electroencephalographic correlates. In R. M. Reitan & L. A. Davison (Eds.), *Clinical neuropsychology: Current status and applications.* New York: Wiley, 1974.

LeMay, M., & Culebras, A. Human brain-morphologic differences in the hemispheres demonstrable by carotid arteriography. *New England Journal of Medicine,* 1972, *287,* 168–170.

Levy, J., & Reid, M. Variations in writing posture and cerebral organization. *Science,* 1976, *194,* 337–339.

Luria, A. R. *Higher cognitive functions in man.* New York: Basic Books, 1966.

Luria, A. R. *The working brain.* New York: Basic Books, 1973.

Majovski, L., Tanguay, P., Russell, A., Sigman, M., Crumley, K., & Goldenberg, I. Clinical neuropsychological screening instrument for assessment of higher cortical deficits in adolescents. *Clinical Neuropsychology,* 1979, *1,* 3–8. (a)

Majovski, L., Tanguay, P., Russell, A., Sigman, M., Crumley, K., & Goldenberg, I. Clinical neuropsychological evaluation instrument: A clinical research tool for assessment of higher cortical deficits in adolescents. *Clinical Neuropsychology,* 1979, *1,* 9–19. (b)

Matthews, C. G. Applications of neuropsychological test methods in mentally retarded subjects. In R. M. Reitan & L. A. Davison (Eds.), *Clinical neuropsychology: Current status and applications.* New York: Wiley, 1974.

McGhie, A. Attention and perception in schizophrenia. In B. Maher (Ed.), *Progress in experimental personality research* (Vol. 5). New York: Academic Press, 1970.

Milman, D. H. Minimal brain dysfunction in childhood: Outcome in late adolescence and early adult years. *Journal of Clinical Psychiatry,* 1979, *40,* 371–380.

Milner, B. Some effects of frontal lobectomy in man. In J. M. Warren & K. Akert (Eds.), *The frontal granular cortex and behavior.* New York: McGraw-Hill, 1964.

Moses, J., & Golden, C. J. Cross validation of the effectiveness of the Luria–Nebraska Neuropsychological Battery in discriminating between schizophrenic and neurological populations. *International Journal of Neuroscience,* 1980, *10,* 121–128.

Newlin, D. B., & Tramontana, M. G. Neuropsychological findings in a hyperactive adolescent with subcortical brain pathology. *Clinical Neuropsychology,* 1980, *2,* 178–183.

Pontius, A. A. Neurological aspects in some type of delinquency especially among juveniles: Toward a neurological model of ethical action. *Adolescence,* 1972, *7,* 289–308.

Pontius, A. A., & Ruttiger, K. F. Frontal lobe system maturational lag in juvenile delinquents shown in narratives test. *Adolescence,* 1976, *11,* 509–518.

Pribram, K. H., & McGuinness, D. Arousal, activation, and effort in the control of attention. *Psychological Review,* 1975, *82,* 116–149.

Purisch, A. D., Golden, C. J., & Hammeke, T. A. Discrimination of schizophrenic and brain-injured patients by a standardized version of Luria's neuropsychological tests. *Journal of Consulting and Clinical Psychology,* 1978, *46,* 1266–1273.

Quay, H. C., & Werry, J. S. *Psychopathological disorders of childhood (2nd ed.). New York: Wiley, 1979.*

Reed, H. B., Reitan, R. M., & Klove, H. The influence of cerebral lesions on psychological test performances of older children. *Journal of Consulting Psychology,* 1965, *29,* 247–251.

Reitan, R. M. Methodological problems in clinical neuropsychology, In R. M. Reitan & L. A. Davison (Eds.), *Clinical neuropsychology: Current status and applications.* New York: Wiley, 1974. (a)

Reitan, R. M. Psychological effects of cerebral lesions in children of early school age. In R. M. Reitan & L. A. Davison (Eds.), *Clinical neuropsychology: Current status and applications.* New York: Wiley, 1974. (b)

Reitan, R. M., & Davison, L. A. *Clinical neuropsychology: Current status and applications.* New York: Wiley, 1974.

Rutter, M. Brain damage syndromes in childhood: Concepts and findings. *Journal of Child Psychology and Psychiatry,* 1977, *18,* 1–21.

Schain, R. J. *Neurology of childhood learning disorders* (2nd ed.). Baltimore: Williams & Wilkins, 1977.

Seidel, U. P., Chadwick, O. F., & Rutter, M. Psychological disorders in crippled children: A comparative study of children with and without brain damage. *Developmental Medicine and Child Neurology,* 1975, *17,* 563–573.

Selz, M., & Reitan, R. M. Rules for neuropsychological diagnosis: Classification of brain function in older children. *Journal of Consulting and Clinical Psychology,* 1979, *47,* 258–264.

Teuber, H. L. The riddle of frontal lobe function in man. In J. M. Warren & K. Akert (Eds.), *The frontal granular cortex and behavior.* New York: McGraw-Hill, 1964.

Tsushima, W. T., & Towne, W. S. Neuropsychological abilities of young children with questionable brain disorders. *Journal of Consulting and Clinical Psychology,* 1977, *45,* 757–762.

Tramontana, M. G. Application of neuropsychological methods in the evaluation of coexisting mental retardation and mental illness. In F. J. Menolascino & B. M. McCann (Eds.), *Mental health and mental retardation: Bridging the gap.* Baltimore: University Park Press, 1983.

Tramontana, M. G., Sherrets, S. D., & Golden, C. J. Brain dysfunction in youngsters with psychiatric disorders: Application of Selz–Reitan rules for neuropsychological diagnosis. *Clinical Neuropsychology,* 1980, *2,* 118–123.

Yakovlev, P. I., & Lecours, A. R. The myelogenetic cycles of regional maturation of the brain. In A. Minkowski (Ed.), *Regional development of the brain in early life.* Oxford: Blackwell, 1967.

13

Neuropsychology and Behavior Disorders in Children and Youth

STEVEN D. SHERRETS

Estimates of the incidence of behavior disorders in school-aged populations varies from a high of 20% to 30% to a low of 1.5% to 3% (Wood & Zabel, 1978). One has but to read the daily newspaper or hear the latest statistics on juvenile delinquency to realize this is a growing problem. Arrests of youth for all crimes rose 138% from 1960 to 1974, and 254% for the violent crimes of murder, rape, robbery, and aggravated assault (Federal Bureau of Investigation, 1974). Certainly not all behavior-disordered youth appear in the criminal statistics. Numerous laws, the most recent of which is P.L. 94-142 (The Education of All Handicapped Children's Act of 1975), mandate educational programs for all children regardless of handicapping condition. This has resulted in many behavior-disordered individuals being returned or maintained in the public school classroom and the development of a growing concern for understanding the causes and treatments of behavioral problems. Despite the high frequency of occurrence, serious research into either etiologies or treatment of this group of children did not occur with any frequency until the end of World War II (Rie, 1971). Even then, the primary concern was for individuals labeled as juvenile delinquents. In fact, there was no specific medical or psychological diagnosis even available for this group until 1968 (*Diagnostic and Statistical Manual of Mental Disorders* American Psychiatric Association, 1968). Over time the estimates have suggested that behavior problems are increasing in frequency. One must bear in mind, however, that there are

STEVEN D. SHERRETS • Director of Day Hospital, Bradley Hospital, Section of Psychiatry and Human Behavior, Brown University, East Providence, Rhode Island 02915.

numerous possible reasons for such a report other than increases in the behavior itself. For example, since World War II there has been a proliferation of service facilities and providers (Rhodes & Ensor, 1979), which may have increased referrals for existing but underserved populations. Moreover, the expanded service network may not only be a reflection of increased knowledge (such as in pharmacological treatment of these problems), but an indication of changing attitudes as well.

Historically, the concern over most problems of childhood has developed concurrently with the concept of childhood itself. According to Rie (1971), the study of behavior-disordered children has been essentially ignored until contemporary times because of an inclusive development of the concept of childhood prior to these times. In fact, Aries (1962) points out that in medieval times children who no longer required constant care from their mother were considered part of adult society, and that before such a time livestock took precedence over wives and children (Despert, 1965). While by the mid-eighteenth century the child had obtained a tenuous foothold within the family, the odds *against* surviving past 5 years of age were three to one, and survival could still mean later abandonment (Aries, 1962). This impoverished attitude toward childhood appears to be the foundation for the almost total absence of concern for emotional disorders of children prior to the eighteenth century (Kanner, 1962). Several authors (Kanner, 1962; Lewis, 1959; Lowrey, 1944; Rubinstein, 1948) have observed the absence of published literature regarding behavior-disordered children even as late as 1930.

Still, the mid-eighteenth century was a period of positive change, and philosophers such as Rousseau and Pestalozzi began to place much greater emphasis upon the importance of childhood and the necessity of an educational environment (Nakosteen, 1965). However, subsequent recognition was not altogether positive, at least not initially. The mentally ill, the behavior disordered, the aged, and the orphaned were all lumped together and often treated as criminals (Felix, 1967). It wasn't until the nineteenth century that this attitude began to change, in part because of the development of theories and of scientifically based facts about possible causes (Paine, 1964).

As research and theories on problems of childhood emerged, they mirrored the prevailing social and political attitudes toward children (Rie, 1971). Frequently, in fact, research and opinion have been closely aligned and at times indistinguishable from one another. Nowhere has this been more true than in the area of childhood behavior disorders. Environmental explanations of behavior disorders have been dominant for many years, in guiding both research and popular opinion. Because of the overwhelming evidence that social/environmental factors were frequent companions of behavior disorders and the prevailing attitude that society would have a greater chance of successfully intervening with such factors, evidence to support the alternative explanations offered by the biological theories was not aggressively pursued. Biology was viewed rather narrowly and it was felt that to accept a biological theory one had to reject the role of learning and motivation (Merton & Nisbet, 1961).

It would appear that science is far from detached of the influence of prevailing cultural attitudes. Boring (1950) pointed this out in noting that scientific progress is slowed not only by ignorance—each discovery being dependent upon its predecessor—but also by the " . . . habits of thought that pertain to the culture of any period; an idea too strange or preposterous . . . may be readily accepted as true only a century or two later" (p.7). While early theories suggested that behavior disorders were caused by demonic possessions, excessive masturbation, parasites, episodes of fright or defective digestion (Spitzka, 1890), in recent years we have examined the role played by the environment. Concern over environmental issues may have led us into a "habit of thought" that, while more valid that Spitzka's views, may nevertheless have resulted in ignoring other potential influences on the behavior of children.

Surely behavior disorders must have multiple determinants, for no single etiological factor can apply in all cases. Once having begun to receive due attention, early authors pointed out their beliefs that the primary causes included an improperly developed super-ego to sufficiently inhibit the pressures of the id (Cohen, 1955; Healy & Bronner, 1936; Stott, 1950), while others have pointed to role theory (Tannenbaum, 1938), culture conflict (Sellin, 1938), and social disorganization (Shaw & McKay, 1929), association theory (Cohen & Short, 1958), improper learning (Miller, 1958), and finally psychobiological causes (McCord, 1958). The literature abounds with volumes written on the sociological aspects of behavioral disorders, and numerous studies, many with conflicting results, have considered psychological theories as well (Peterson, Quay, & Cameron, 1959). Sheldon's (1949) system of detailing behavior as a function of human physique was widely recognized and considered by some to be a biological theory, but here no direct causal link was proposed. However, until recently few researchers have taken the biological theories seriously.

Many early biological theories were vague, opinionated, and too all-encompassing with the tendency toward overgeneralization, which led serious researchers to appropriately reject them as inadequate. To quote an early text (Merton & Nisbet, 1961), which contained a critical review of this area: "Behavior becomes a direct manifestation of some underlying condition in the glands, the nervous system, or more vaguely, 'the constitution'" (p. 91).

Nash (1978) has struck a serious and hopefully fatal blow, however, at the separatist view that the behavior of humans is due to either nature or nurture. For the first time we seem now to be able to explore the interaction of these two factors and to disregard the criticism that research or theorizing with one variable necessarily means we are rejecting the other. Consistent with this view are the conclusions of Rutter (1977), who in reviewing the available literature, including his own research, reports that brain-damaged individuals may be more susceptible to the development of behavior problems within certain environments. Other authors have reported numerous findings that are suggestive of an interaction between environmental conditions and the presence of brain dysfunction. One may cause the other or each may interact to exacerbate the effects taken singly or together (Clark, 1970; Cravioto & Delicardie, 1970; Lewis & Balla, 1976; Pasamanick, 1956, 1961; Stott, 1962). In 1937 Julian Huxley called for research of an interactive nature such as this because of what he saw was the current trend toward such intensive specialization that each branch of science was reduced to a condition of meaninglessness. It has taken over 40 years for us to realize that behavior disorders must have multiple determinants, many of which interact with each other.

For many years, little has been offered to explain behavior disorders based upon improper brain functioning, although many of the very early theorists such as Bender (1947), Lombroso (1911), and Mills (1890) believed that some form of dysfunction within the nervous system must be present in the behaviorally disordered. Approaches such as these were frustrated, however, by a lack of knowledge of the nervous system and of technology with which to test theories and by the prevailing attitude that environmental approaches offered more hope of successful intervention.

The emphasis placed upon environmental approaches led to a lack of concern about differentiating among various types of behavior disorders. The fact that behavior disorders were not even considered as separate psychiatric diagnoses until 1968 (*Diagnostic and Statistical Manual of Mental Disorders*, American Psychiatric Association, 1968) bears this out. Even to date most investigations utilizing juvenile delinquents as subjects make little attempt to differentially describe their subject populations. Partly because of inadequate subject description, available research has largely produced inconclusive and inconsistent results when considering the role of individual differences in personality characteristics of the behaviorally disordered. Peterson *et al.* (1959) have pointed out that: "Most investigations of personality factors in crime and delinquency have begun with a legally defined sample of offenders, proceeded with comparisons of a matched group of non-offenders, and ended with ambiguous results" (p. 395). After reviewing 113 such comparisons, Scheussler and Cressey (1950) stated that: "The doubtful validity of many of the obtained differences, as well as the lack of consistency in the combined results, makes it impossible to conclude from these data that criminality and personality elements are associated" (p. 478).

Peterson *et al.* (1959) have suggested that the negative findings may reflect an actual lack of individual differences between offenders and nonoffenders or may be the result of inappropriate methodology. The first conclusion is not entirely untenable, for as Merton and Nisbet (1961) have observed, almost any child could be defined as a delinquent at one time or another in his life due to the broad legal definitions of delinquency.

A problem has arisen because it has been generally assumed there are two kinds of children, delinquent and nondelinquent, and this broad division has not been precise enough to illuminate differences. Compounding the problem is the fact that research tools are often subjective, and terminology used to describe the behavior of acting-out children has been frequently inappropriate. Such terms as "frivolous, carefree, devil-may-care extroversion" (Pierson & Kelly, 1963, p. 443) and "childish naughtiness . . . strong self-assertive tendencies, abnormal habits and attitudes and character defects . . ." (Desai, 1970, p. 75) imply a strong evaluative component but offer little in the way of operational definitions.

It appears clear that, without the availability of an acceptable taxonomy of behavior problems little can be accomplished in research or service approaches based upon any individual differences, including brain dysfunction. The use of such a taxonomy is a critical first step in differentially investigating etiologies, treatments, or prognosis. Historically, the most commonly used classification systems (e.g., the American Psychiatric Association's DSM-II, 1968) are based upon narrative descriptions of disorders that are not operationally defined and are generally found to have low reliability and validity (Beitchman, Dielman, Landis, Benson, & Kemp, 1978; Freeman, 1971; Tarter, Templer, & Hardy, 1975.) There is no evidence that these systems differentiate as to etiology, prognosis, or differential response to treatment (Edelbrock, 1979).

Considerable advances, however, have recently been made in the empirical classification and differentiation of behavior-disturbed children and adolescents. Achenbach and Edelbrock (1978) provide an extensive review of parent and teacher rating scales of children's behavior disorders. In an effort to improve on the previous work of others in this area, Achenbach and Edelbrock (1978, 1979) and Achenbach (1978) have developed a rating scale that provides descriptions of both narrow and more general patterns of behavior. They have developed reliable rating scales and norms for both males and females in the age groups of 4 to 5, 6 to 11, and 12 to 16. The scales were developed by factor analyzing a diverse array of behavior problems as checked by parents or parent surrogates. The initial checklist was constructed from a survey of the literature and case histories of 1,000 child psychiatric patients. Later factor analyses and norms were developed from administrations to over 1,200 normal and psychiatric youngsters from various scoioeconomic levels, racial groups, and settings on the east coast. Differential etiologies and treatments can be delineated only after careful attention is given to descriptions of individual subject variables such as history, developmental levels, sex, and above all, operationally defined behavioral descriptions. Many of the historically equivocal and contradicting results of past studies can be avoided by more complete and objective descriptions of both subject populations and their behavior problem patterns. The availability of scales such as this coupled with recent advances in neuropsychology have considerably brightened the prospects of investigating individual neurological differences in behavior-disordered populations.

RESEARCH IN NEUROPSYCHOLOGY AND BEHAVIOR DISORDERS

Neuropsychology, while a relatively young science, has experienced remarkable growth in recent years (Benton, 1969). Its application to research with behavior-disordered individuals promises a number of significant breakthroughs in understanding etiologies and potentially even the development of new treatments for these individuals. However, in its early history, the application of neuropsychology to behavior problems was often ignored or complicated by numerous problems.

Werner and Strauss (1940), Lombroso (1911), Mills (1890) and Strauss and Lehtinen (1947) were among the first to suggest that neurological factors played a significant role in behavior disorders. Strauss and Lehtinen were the first to coin the terminology "minimal brain damage" in referring to mentally retarded children with behavior problems. Their suggestion of the presence of subtle brain damage broke ground that allowed the seeds of this type of research to grow. Since this time a number of studies have recognized that apparent brain dysfunction of various types is found in a large percentage of children with severe behavior disorders.

In one survey of 150 behavior-disordered children, some form of brain dysfunction was found in 59% (Hanvik, Nelson, Hanson, Anderson, Dressler, & Zarling, 1961). The incidence of neurological dysfunction varies with the particular diagnosis, but hospitalized adolescent psychiatric patients have been found to exhibit such dysfunction four to eight times more frequently than matched normal controls (Hertzig & Birch, 1966). Whether such dysfunction is simply a correlate of behavior problems or, as some authors believe, an etiological factor in this behavior (e.g., Anderson, 1974; Clements, 1966) remains an open question. There is considerable variability reported in the published literature regarding the extent and nature of neuropsychological dysfunctions.

To date, most of the research investigating brain dysfunction in behaviorally disturbed children has not tended to find focal or localizing signs of damage or improper development in specific areas of the brain. Generally, the conclusions indicate that nonlocalizing, "soft" neurological signs simply occur more frequently in the disordered group (e.g., Berman, 1972; Hertzig, 1969; Kennard, 1960; Larsen, 1964; Pollack, 1969; Wikler, Dixon, & Parker, 1970). Others have found perceptual problems, which can be construed as "soft" signs (Close, 1973), to be present in behaviorally disturbed children more frequently than in controls (Clements & Peters, 1962; Diller & Weinberg, 1968; Stevens, Boydstun, & Dykman, 1967).

The major problem with this research is that the results are "seductively suggestive" but lacking in any definitive conclusions. The findings have occurred consistently enough to warrant further research; however, historically the quantity of the available studies has far surpassed the quality. Many of the procedures used are of low or questionable reliability and are influenced by a variety of unrelated functions and factors (Langhorne, Loney, Paternite, & Beckholdt, 1976; Paine, Werry, & Quay, 1968; Werry, 1968). Werry (1979) pointed out that diagnosis of brain dysfunction was no more than a guess. Werry (1979) and an earlier article by Pond (1961) further state that there has usually been no way of proving such dysfunction is causally related to the problem behavior even when its existence can be documented. Another glaring deficiency in this area has been the lack of any theoretical or conceptually based relationship between behavior disorders and brain function.

Many investigations have been little more than descriptions of neuropsychological factors in behavior-disordered samples with no use made of controls. Frequently in those comparative studies utilizing controls, performance on single trial/unitary tasks are compared between the two groups. However, the tasks utilized have been empirically devised and are not pure measures of brain damage. Rutter, Graham, and Jule (1970) and Werry (1979) point out that, except within broad limits, behavioral manifestations of particular brain injuries cannot be predicted. Herbert (1964), in reviewing the available psychodiagnostic techniques applied to children to discriminate between brain-damaged and normal subjects, cites numerous problems with the techniques and concludes they can by no means be used as the sole criterion for diagnoses of cerebral pathology. The empirically devised battery by Reitan (Reitan & Davison, 1974) and his colleagues and the theoretically and empirically based battery by Golden, Hammeke, and Purisch (1978) each provide considerable promise for improving the measurement problems that have historically plagued this research. However to date only two studies (Sherrets, 1980; Tramontana, Sherrets, & Golden, 1980) have applied these batteries to populations including behavior disordered individuals. These will be reviewed later in this chapter.

Certainly the problems with investigating such a relationship have been multiple. Many professionals remain committed to social learning theory explanations of behavior disorders and have resisted research of this type. The primary impediments, however, have been with the lack of adequate theory and with improper methodology and measurement ability within neuropsychology, although additional problems of major proportions have rested with the difficulty in classifying behavioral disorders.

POSSIBLE RELATIONSHIPS BETWEEN NEUROLOGICAL FUNCTIONING AND BEHAVIOR DISORDERS

Many authors have become quite polarized in their views on the possible link between the brain and behavior disorders. Unfortunately, those who are highly critical would apparently have us ignore the growing body of literature that strongly suggests some form of age-specific improper brain function is at least a corollary, if not a causal agent or a factor exacerbating the behavior symptoms. If we recognize the complexity of brain function and the number of possible explanations for behavior disorders, we can surely see this is an entangled area to research. There exist three possible links between brain function and behavior disorders. First is the presence of actual neurological damage, where once healthy tissue has been damaged by physical or infectious insult, anoxia, tumors, or severe nutritional deficiency. Obviously such factors must have occurred after the developmental period for the particular brain structure.

Secondly, there is the possibility of neurological dysfunction, in which case the tissue is no more or less inoperative than in the case of brain damage, but the cause differs. There is no history of damage to once healthy tissue, but instead we have improper function because one or more areas of the brain necessary for efficient functioning have failed to form. The influence is not simply a delay in development but represents the absence of development. This may be due to genetic influences, anoxia, nutritional deficiency, lack of stimulation, or even infectious insult to the embryo.

Thirdly, we may experience a neurological developmental delay. In this case, the apparent dysfunction in the brain is present only when we consider expectations for age-specific development and abilities. Actually there is no evidence of brain damage or even dysfunction, but only a more slowly growing nervous system. For many years we have known that males generally take longer for neurological development than females, yet we do not infer that all males are brain damaged or neurologically dysfunctional. It would appear to be relatively easy to extend our view of this differential rate of development to individuals as well. We accept the idea of delays or irregular patterns of development in language, motor skills, social/emotional development, physical growth, and so on. Consequently, it seems reasonable to adopt a similar view for the maturation of the nervous system.

Behavior disorders themselves can be related to multiple neurologically based problems from any of these three sources. The influence may be a direct cause, as with temporal lobe epilepsy or dysfunction in behavior control mechanisms such as the limbic system or frontal lobes, as well as indirect causes due to diminished sensory input, improper processing of information, or the inability to properly express oneself and even memory deficits. The latter influences account for the possible link between educational deficits and behavior problems (Murray, 1976).

In no case, whether the cause is direct or indirect, need a predetermined behavior problem develop as a result of a dysfunctional nervous system. Factors such as severity, chronicity, age, sex, concommittant problems, the presence or absence of familial support systems, various environmental influences, and even the historical quality of stimulation and brain function will be determining factors in the delineation of the type and severity of behavior disorders that develop or even determine if such a problem develops at all.

Many of the potential sources of neurological dysfunction have been found to interact with environmental influences. Clark (1970) noted these connections in his report on crime in America. For example, Cravioto and Delicardie (1970) call attention to the role of proper nutrition in developing the ability to read and write properly.

Improper perinatal care and insult from disease or trauma are also factors in neurological dysfunction. Pasamanick (1961) found a greater prevalence of such factors in behaviorally disturbed children. Stott (1968) also has extensive research in this area suggesting that a variety of factors, including stress in the mother during pregnancy, can result in long-term effects. Stott (1962) stresses how children with early central nervous system trauma are often more vulnerable to the effects of nonsupportive families and chaotic environments. Lewis and Balla (1976) report that such may be the case even with late childhood central nervous system insults. Rosenzweig (1976) reports how a lack of proper stimulation can produce improper brain development. These authors, supported by data from numerous animal studies, point out the likelihood that a lack of sufficient stimulation can, in particular, cause late maturation of the nervous system. Rutter (1977) and Thomas and Chess (1975) each discuss brain/environment interactions that can operate in reciprocal fashion. That is, environmental influences being responsible for the development of a behavior problem in a neurologically predisposed individual as well as how some neurologically dysfunctional individuals may fail to properly cope with less fortunate environments or fail to receive the full benefit of even positive environments.

Premature and low birth weight infants appear to be at greater risk for development of both neurological deficits and behavior problems (Drillien, 1964, 1970; Kawi & Pasamanick, 1958). Apparently of lesser importance are birth injuries (Benaron, Tucker, Andrews, Boshes, Cohen, Fromm, & Yacorzynski, 1960), although cerebral anoxia at birth has been identified, at least retrospectively, as a factor (Towbin, 1971).

Wender (1972), Morrison and Stewart (1971), and Cantwell (1972, 1975) all report a possible genetic transmission of vulnerability to central nervous system dysfunction. This is particularly true in problems associated with hyperactivity. Genetic transmission is also a possible factor in the development of temperaments that could predispose a child to a behavior problem (Thomas, Chess, & Birch, 1968; Thomas & Chess, 1980).

The same environmental factors that have been found to be related to the development of sociopathic behavior (Glueck & Glueck, 1962) have also been found to be related to the development of the capacity to form attachments. The Harlow (1971) experiments taught us that, in the absence of proper care, love, and stimulation, particularly within the first year of life (see Lamb, 1977, for research with humans), we apparently lose the capacity for attachment, have improper brain development, and exhibit a move toward sociopathic behavior.

Many positive environmental influences are important to insure complete brain development. In their absence the brain fails to develop as programmed or develops more slowly. The brain dysfunction and brain delay hypotheses appear to be the best explanations of the majority of studies considering brain function and behavior disorders. The preponderance of the literature appears to support the developmental delay hypothesis. Such a hypothesis argues that behavioral problems are more acceptable in younger children but are not tolerated when they persist into later childhood (Satz & Fletcher, 1980). In fact, the "soft neurological signs" that are so often reported with behavior-disordered populations are generally indications of age-specific neurological immaturities. Evidence for a delay in neurological development among behavior-disordered children was obtained by Dykman, Ackerman, Clements, and Peters (1971) and Peters, Romine, and Dykman (1975). Denckla and Rudel (1977) and Oettinger, Majovski, Limbeck, and Gauch (1974) also report evidence for an underlying physiological immaturity. The latter authors, in investigating the effects of stimulants on children diagnosed as having Minimal Brain Dysfunction, found that bone age and height were immature prior to treatment with the drug and that they continued to grow for a longer period than their noninvolved counterparts.

The timing of cerebral specialization may be influenced by the presence of the sex hormones that influence the age of puberty onset (Waber, 1976). This may account for some sex differences in brain organization, differential maturation rates for males and females, and the persistence of "soft neurological signs." This could also help to explain the controversial link between the XYY karyotype syndrome and criminality. Forssman and Hambert (1967) found that this genetic combination, which results in additional male sex hormones, occurred more frequently in criminals who have a history of childhood behavior problems than in a comparison group of criminal men without such a history.

Ellingson (1954) reports EEG abnormalities in 45% to 58% of sampled populations of adult criminals and sociopaths, although he indicates the rates for behavior-problem children are somewhat lower, possibly because of a tendency to be more conservative when interpreting results with this population. His conclusion that no relationships have been established between specific EEG abnormalities and specific types of behavioral symptoms in children still appears valid; however, evidence here continues to support a general neurological developmental delay theory.

EEG abnormalities, primarily slow wave activity that exceeds expected levels by age, are common among children with behavior disorders (Anderson, 1963; Beshai, 1971; Forssman & Frey, 1953; Green, 1961; Gross & Wilson, 1974; Hill, 1952; Kellaway, Crawley, & Maulsby, 1965; Kennard, 1960; Klinkerfuss, Lange, & Weinberg, 1965; Laufer, Denhoff, & Solomons, 1957). In reviewing EEG studies, Stamm (1978) reports several abnormal findings occuring much more frequently in behavior-disordered children. Occipital or diffuse slow wave activity are the most common findings (Gross & Wilson, 1974; Hughes & Park, 1969; Ingram, Mason, & Blackburn, 1970; Satterfield, 1973; Wikler, Dixon, & Parker, 1970). These are of particular interest since these wave forms have been shown to decline with age (Gibbs & Gibbs, 1950; Satterfield, 1973).

A number of authors have also shown immature wave patterns in this population when using auditory or visual evoked potentials (Buchsbaum & Wender, 1973; Dustman & Beck, 1969; Ounsted, 1969; Satterfield, 1973; Serafetinides, 1965; Treffert, 1964).

While the relationship between behavior problems and seizure disorders is frequently called into question (Gunn & Bonn, 1971), behavior problems are sometimes thought to be seizure related. These types of problems are most likely to occur with a temporal lobe foci of abnormality (Ervin, Epstein, & King, 1955).

In one sample of clinic-referred delinquents, 6% demonstrated psychomotor epileptic symptoms (Lewis & Balla, 1976). This compares with a .3% to .4% rate in the general population (Ervin, 1975). Of course, accidents, poisoning, drug abuse, child abuse, and infection can all result in neurological anomalies as well (Schain, 1977).

FUNCTIONAL NEUROANATOMY

With the recent improvements in neuropsychological theory and measurement, we should be able to proceed toward greater sophistication with investigations into brain–behavior relationships to better understand behavior-disordered individuals. As previously indicated, behavior problems can develop directly from specific lesions or more indirectly from general dysfunction or neurodevelopmental delays. Practically any neurological structure could be directly or indirectly related to behavior problems; therefore only those structures with the most probable relationship to the educational and behavioral problems of this population are reviewed herein. For purposes of clarity, subcortical and cortical areas will be discussed separately; however, growing evidence suggests that cortical inhibition is supplied for ipsilateral subcortical arousal and emotional processes (Tucker, 1981). Therefore a clear demarcation between cortical and subcortical functioning is not entirely possible.

Subcortical Structures

Since Papez (1937) first pointed out the role of the limbic system in emotion and behavior, knowledge has been continuing to accumulate strongly suggesting the relationship between these structures and behavior disorders. While parts are considered to be "transitional cortex," these highly interconnected structures are among the phylogenetically oldest and most central parts of the brain for emotional and behavioral control. Glasser and Pincus (1969) report various limbic structures that are associated with behavioral problems. Components of the limbic system control or influence memory, learning, anxiety, rage, placidity, and alertness, endocrine responses, aggressive behavior, and sexual activity. As Papez predicted, following stimulation of particular limbic structures, there are after-discharges that spread throughout the limbic system (MacLean, 1952, 1954). Medial portions of the temporal lobes are associated with the amygdala, hippocampus, hippocampal formation, and uncus. These areas are particularly susceptible to subacute and chronic forms of encephalitis (Pincus & Tucker, 1978). The amygdala appears to be the controlling mechanism for the fight-or-flight syndrome. Stimulation can cause fear reactions and even rage. Acting out in response to intense emotions can be triggered by the amygdala and the posterior hypothalamus (Watts, 1975). Deficits within the septal region, where the sense of pleasure is generated, can exacerbate problems with an amygdaloid origin (Watts, 1975).

Apparent behavioral problems secondary to memory deficits can be related to lesions within the hippocampal area. Numerous investigators have demonstrated the importance of this limbic structure in memory (Corkin, 1965; DeJong, Itabashi, & Olson, 1969; Douglas & Pribram, 1966; Isaacson, 1972; Penfield and Milner, 1958; Scoville & Milner, 1957).

A nonlimbic structure located within the brain stem, the reticular formation, may be implicated in persons with attentional deficits and in those individuals who are over- or underaroused (Lindsley, 1958). This structure works closely with cortical areas, including the frontal lobes, and has many widespread connections to auditory, visual, olfactory, somotasensory, proprioceptive, sympathetic, and vagal connections (Smith, 1972).

The thalamus is a relay station for sensory and motor impulses to and from the cerebral hemispheres. Lesions here tend to be short lived but can result in reduced scores on verbal tasks (left thalamic lesions) (Bell, 1968; Ojemann, 1971; Ojemann & Ward, 1971; Vilkki & Laitinen, 1974) or deficits in spatial ability (right thalamic lesions).

The two cerebral hemispheres communicate with each other through the corpus callosum. Apathy, violence, an inability to concentrate, forgetfulness, delusions, and hallucinations can all develop from lesions within the corpus callosum (Toglia, 1961).

Cortical Structures

The four lobes on each side of the cerebral hemispheres are essential for proper intellectual and behavioral functioning for all tasks that are integrative, complex, or demand sustained or continuing concentration (Borkowski, Benton, & Spreen, 1967; Chedru, Leblanc, & Lhermitte, 1973; Coheen, 1950; Dee & Van Allen, 1971; DeRenzi, Faglioni, & Scotti, 1970; Kahn, Pollack, & Fink, 1960; McDonald, 1964; McDonald & Burns, 1964; Olbrich, 1972; Reitan, 1959). Within a normally developing brain, the two hemispheres are asymmetrical in size, blood flow, and function (Golden, 1978). Specialization of function within each of the hemispheres is important to ensure optimal, noncompetitive operations within the cortex as a whole. A lack of complete dominance and specialization frequently produce reading and spelling dyslexias (Springer & Deutsch, 1981), which are so common with behavior-disordered populations. Here left–right distinctions are confused and mirror-image letters and numbers are reversed; they may spell backwards or have inconsistent spelling with the correct letters being present but placed in an improper sequence. Delayed or absent specialization can cause disorders in speech, reading, and spelling as well as increased sensitivity to stress and temperamental instability.

Figure 1 (p. 354) presents the order of cortical myelination. The myelination is an index of the state of maturation of neuronal systems (Conel, 1939). As can be seen from Figure 1, the frontal cortex and the angular gyrus are among the last areas to mature. The latter structure is extremely important in the integration of audiovisual information. Visual language must be translated to auditory language before it can be understood. This translation takes place within the angular gyrus located within the parietal lobe along the border of the occipital/temporal lobe (Watts, 1975). This area is also responsible for the reverse process, translating a verbal word to a visual one so it can be spelled. Connections exist between the frontal lobes and the angular gyrus, and frequently both areas show a uniform dysfunction, especially when the cause is a neurodevelopmental delay.

Figure 2 (p. 355) presents a diagram of the cortical areas. While many areas of the brain may be involved in various aspects of behavioral disorders, no single cortical structure offers as much promise in understanding behavioral disorders as does the frontal cortex. It is within this area of the brain that Luria's theoretical views can be most clearly demonstrated. This highly sophisticated structure regulates and mediates many subcortical systems to produce the complexity of behavior that humans are capable of (Milner, 1958). Numerous behaviors that frequently occur in behaviorally disordered individuals are influenced by the frontal lobes. Table 1 presents the major functions of the motor, premotor, and prefrontal areas of the frontal lobes.The importance of this area of the brain in higher cognitive functioning has been known since the early nineteenth century, but its com-

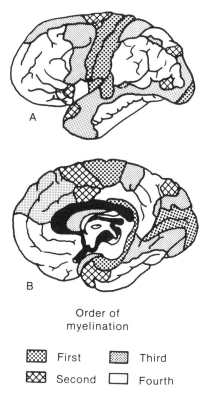

Order of
myelination

First   Third
Second   Fourth

Figure 1. Maturation and order of myelination of the human cortex. Part A shows the left hemisphere. Part B is a section of the median plane showing the right hemisphere. The white areas are the last to myelinate. (Adapted from Meine myelogenetische Hirnlehre mit biographischer Einleitung by P. Flechsig, Berlin, Springer Verlag, 1927.)

plexity and interconnections to subcortical areas eluded detection by early researchers (Gross & Weiskrantz, 1964).

Presentation of a sampling of the frontal lobe functions quickly demonstrates their potential role as an etiological factor in behavior disorders. Maturation of this area produces the ability to self-regulate behavior and perform complex chains of actions controlled by intrinsic intentions or by verbal instruction (Luria, Pribram, & Homskaya, 1964). Control of impulsivity and inhibiting and delaying selected responses are a major responsibility of this area (Milner, 1970; Rosvold & Szwarcbart, 1964). While overall intelligence test scores do not tend to be affected by damage to the frontal lobes (Hebb & Penfield, 1940), the ability to satisfactorily complete several cognitive tasks is impaired, as are planning and having foresight, considering choice situations (making a decision), solving verbal problems (particularly arithmetical problems requiring shifts from one operation

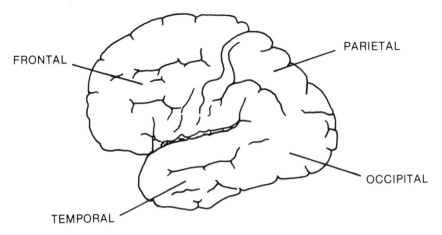

FRONTAL

PARIETAL

OCCIPITAL

TEMPORAL

Figure 2. Lobes of the human cortex.

to another) (Luria, 1973), and logical reasoning and creative thinking (Smith, 1972).

Dysfunction in the frontal lobes can produce numerous emotional and behavioral effects as well. Impairment is seen in the inability to anticipate future consequences of behavior, failing to evaluate current behavior with respect to a goal, indifference to one's behavior, simple, silly joking, emotional incontinence (crying and laughing in rapid alternation), inability to orient actions to the social and ethical standards of the community, hyperactivity, and apathy (Golden, 1978;

Table 1

Frontal Lobe Functions

Cognitive and emotional	Motor	Behavior
1. Creative thinking 2. Anticipation of consequences 3. Goal-directed behavior 4. Logical reasoning and planning 5. Solution of complex verbal problems 6. Maintainance of social and ethical standards 7. Lesions may produce: emotional incontinence, apathy; simple, silly joking; loss of verbal commands.	1. Control of voluntary movements 2. Expressive speech 3. Lesion may produce: gait disorders; jerky motor movements; loss of conjugate eye movements; slow, garbled, or even loss of speech.	1. Self-recognition of behavior (insight) 2. Verbal control of behaviors 3. Coordination of complex chains of behavior 4. Inhibition and delaying of responses 5. Control of perseveration 6. Lesions may produce: hyperactivity; loss of coordinated movements; distractibility; impulsivity.

Luria, 1973; Pincus & Tucker, 1978). Individuals with frontal lobe dysfunction may be impulsive, distractible, perseverative, and presumably incapable of responding according to rules that they can nevertheless verbalize (Milner, 1970). Verbal commands may not be retained and are replaced by more habitual and firmly established actions (Luria, 1973).

A variety of motor and speech symptoms are possible in some cases. Gait disorders and increased muscle tone may occur, and there may be interference with conjugate eye movements (Smith, 1972). Jerky movements replace smooth skilled behavior, and speech may be slowed or garbled. The loss of all expressive speech may even occur (Golden, 1978).

Such deficits in cognition, motor control, emotion, and behavior may be due to developmental delays rather than damage *per se*. The frontal lobes themselves are among the last area of the brain to develop. Brain maturation proceeds along a posterior to anterior axis with the frontal areas being the last to achieve full development. This is a gradual process that is typically nearing completion during adolescence (Burr, 1960) and may even continue for two decades (Flechsig, 1927; Yakovlev & Lecours, 1967). In comparison to the child, the adolescent is expected to display greater impulse control, a greater capacity to delay responding, to utilize both insight and foresight, to anticipate long-range consequences for present actions, and so forth. Because these are the very functions mediated by the frontal lobes, adolescents with developmental delays in this area will appear neurologically and behaviorally more like a child. Such a hypothesis is also consistent with the fact that males experience a greater likelihood of both neurologically delayed development and overrepresentation in populations of behaviorally disordered adolescents (Pollack, 1969; Werry & Quay, 1971). Such a delay hypothesis could well explain why many behavior-disordered children seem to "grow out of it" (Coleman, 1964; Reckless, 1967).

Moving in a posterior and clockwise direction from the frontal lobes, one finds the parietal lobe, which is responsible for processing somatosensory input from the body. About one-fifth of the anterior cells in this area direct motor output as well (Luria, 1973). These areas work in close unison with the frontal lobes for major motor activity.

The left parietal lobe is closely involved with speech and writing (Luria, 1966). Here, lesions can interfere with the smoothness of speaking and produce disorders in writing with similar letters such as L and K.

Damage to the left parietal/occipital region can result in difficulties with spelling as well in spatial deficits (Kinsbourne & Warrington, 1964; Luria & Tsvetkova, 1964). This area is also involved in the ability to understand and manipulate arithmetic symbols (Benson & Weir, 1972).

Damage to the right parietal lobe tends to produce problems similar to those of the left, only less severe. The right lobe in this area is responsible for attention, awareness of left-side movements (McFie & Zangwill, 1960), recognition of faces

(Luria, 1973), and classifying nonverbal material (Warrington & Taylor, 1973). The right parietal area also plays a role in the basic spatial abilities required for drawing or assembling objects (DeRenzi & Faglioni, 1967).

Continuing to move in a posterior direction in the cortex, the occipital lobe is found. The left occipital lobe is involved in the combining of visual input into patterns (Luria, 1973). Damage here may produce deficits in visual scanning or failure to direct attention to important details (Cumming, Hurwitz, & Perl, 1970). Deficits in this region can result in inability to read or recognize letters or numbers (Greenblatt, 1973). Visual memory can also suffer (Benson, Segarra, & Albert, 1974). Right occipital damage results in spatial problems, such as in the inability to remember faces, or to interpret complex, unfamiliar visual patterns (Golden, 1978).

Finally, the last structure is the temporal region. The temporal lobes receive information from the auditory system (Luria, 1964). The majority of information received by each ear goes to the opposite side of the brain (Kimura, 1961). Visual and auditory hallucinations can be caused by damage to the anterior-medial area of the temporal lobe (Mullan & Penfield, 1959). Temporal lobe epilepsy can result in depression (Weil, 1959), distortions of time and space (Williams, 1968), and loss of memory (Meyer & Yates, 1955).

The left temporal lobe is involved in the decoding of speech (Zurif & Ramier, 1972). "Word deafness" (subject cannot understand speech), with no accompanying deficit in writing or reading, can be caused here (Yamadori & Albert, 1973). Verbal memory and recall is also a function of the left temporal lobe (Meyer, 1959), and damage to the temporo-occipital region can result in dyslexia (Denckla & Bowen, 1973).

The right temporal lobe is involved in decoding complex nonverbal patterns. This includes musical abilities such as pitch and rhythm (Milner, 1958). Dysfunction here can also interfere with remembering complex visual stimuli (Rubino, 1970).

PROBLEMS IN INVESTIGATING A NEUROPSYCHOLOGICAL DELAY

The preceding review strongly suggests that neurodevelopmental delays are more likely related to behavior disorders than clear indications of brain damage. In fact, it is relatively rare to find only 1% or less of the cases of specific brain pathology (damage) that will have a direct effect of lowering inhibitory controls in juvenile delinquents. However, it would appear to be a mistake to ignore the preponderance of evidence that has accumulated over the years suggesting that some form of neuropsychological problems exist within this population. Tramontana, Sherrets, and Golden (1980) applied the Halstead–Reitan Neuropsychological battery to hospitalized psychiatric patients without known brain damage ranging in age from 9 to 15 years of age and found 60% of the subjects indicating some form of neuropsychological dysfunction. While this population was not made up of only behavior-disordered individuals, a large percentage of the sample could have been so classified. Utilizing the Selz–Reitan rules for neuropsychological diagnosis (Selz & Reitan, 1979), 40% of the youngsters were classified as normal, 35% as learning-disabled, and 25% as brain-damaged. A large percentage of the learning-disabled group as well as many of the brain-damaged individuals appeared to be experiencing either a neuropsychological delay or some form of dysfunction rather than localizable brain damage. In a larger study, which is as yet unpublished, utilizing only behavior-disordered individuals, both from a psychiatric facility and an institution for juvenile delinquents, Sherrets (1980) found a similar rate of impairment with 62 male subjects between 12 and 16 years of age on the Luria–Nebraska Neuropsychological Battery. The impairment rate was somewhat higher in the psychiatric as opposed to delinquent subjects. Consistent with a delay hypothesis, neuropsychological performance was found to be a function of age. The findings indicated curvilinear rather than linear data in that younger and older subjects evidenced fewer age-specific dysfunctions. Use of the localization scales indicate that much of the dysfunction was located largely within the cortical areas of the frontal lobes and within the junction of the parietal/occipital/temporal lobes (angular gyrus). These locations are exactly what would be expected with a delay hypothesis. Curvilinear data represents only one of the problems that surfaced within this particular investigation, however.

Many individuals who take a developmental approach in explaining behavior disorders as a function of brain dysfunction or immaturity appear to be arguing for curvilinearity of the data. However, not one previous investigation reports a test for such a function. Therefore, depending upon the particular age of the subjects, such a relationship may be evident only at particular developmental periods. At this point, it would appear that the greatest amount of age-specific indications of dysfunction or immaturities occur between 9 to 13 years of age. In the case of younger subjects, inadequate norms and a lack of methodology to quantify brain function pose difficult problems. Obviously the curvilinearity of the data presents many troublesome statistical issues since most of our significance tests are sensitive to linear as opposed to curvilinear relationships.

Another serious flaw in all the research reported to date, including the above-mentioned studies, is that they have not completed longitudinal investigations. The delay hypothesis can only be adequately investigated with longitudinal designs, which consider changes across time. Longitudinal data are particularly difficult to obtain with this subject population; however, an investigation is currently underway by Sherrets and his colleagues. Longitudinal research into brain function are confounded by the fact that we expect to see a regression to the mean as well as improvement of chronic disorders because of plasticity and recovery of function.

In doing correlational studies, looking at brain function and behavior disorders, one has to be cautious in assuming a unitary etiology across the developmental period considered. Individuals with a longstanding history of behavior problems may find it difficult to act any other way; even though the initial etiology (some form of brain dysfunction or delay) may diminish with age, the behavior problems themselves become habitual. The behavior problems may become less frequent and impulsive but considerably more deliberate and, unfortunately in some cases, illegal. One possible explanation for the habitual nature of the behavior problems lies in the "learned helplessness" research. Any child who continually attempts to make an adjustive demand but for whatever reason finds it impossible, soon learns to be helpless and to not attempt further adjustments. What may be happening with these children is similar to what the early research on learning-disabled children found. Such children were initially excited about attending school but later became behavior problems and appeared to be amotivated with many, if not most, being convinced that they were unable to achieve educationally.

As previously stated, with younger subjects in particular, we have a lack of conclusive norms. With additional research and applications of the neuropsychological batteries with younger children, additional normative data will be obtained. However, with younger subjects, conclusive norms for individual cortical areas will never be equivalent to those with adults since such subjects have less specific brain function. Additionally, independent verification of a delay is a problem. We have subtle symptoms indicating a neurodevelopmental delay, which itself can only be indirectly confirmed. Autopsy research of brain development, Luria's theory, and the available empirical research appear to confirm the presence of the neurodevelopmental delay or some form of neuropsychological dysfunction; however, at present both remain hypothetical constructs. The immature EEG patterns, the findings of greater deficits in higher than lower cognitive functions, the fact that most behavior-disordered individuals show some improvement with age, frequent findings of small or nonexistent left/right differences, diminished age-specific behavior control, frequent findings indicating an absence of clearly established cerebral dominance, concomitant developmental delays such as enuresis, reduced bone age, immature language or motor development, and greater deficits in expressive rather than receptive vocabulary, all lend support for the construct of a neurodevelopmental delay, but definitive verification may not at present be possible.

The verification problem is further exacerbated by the fact that there can be multiple causes of such delays or dysfunction as well as competing explanations for the behavior and performance on neuropsychological batteries. Hopefully we have reached the point where we can stop taking a unitary view of nature–nurture influences and can observe how the two interact with each other. However, at present there are multiple possible causes of neuropsychological delays including:

improper nutrition; maternal stress during pregnancy; genetic factors; lack of sufficient patterned stimulation early in life; prematurity at birth, plus birth complications including toxemia, forcep delivery, and prolonged labor; cerebral anoxia; alcohol and drug use; physical infections; cerebral insult; and even possibly hypoglycemia.

In addition to statistical problems with the curvilinearity of the relationships and the methodological issues already indicated, other statistical problems will frequently be encountered. Because of the frequent extreme behavior, a restricted range in the data results in reducing the size of the correlation coefficients. In investigating any type of developmental delay, large variations in individual performance are also frequently found. These statistical factors, coupled with the above-mentioned methodological issues, greatly reduce the sensitivity of our statistical tests for either correlational studies or control group comparisons, which expect to find significant between-group differences.

Future research should take into account the complexity in investigating potential relationships among the many variables. Historically most of the criticisms that have been levied at this area of research have been valid. However, as suggested earlier in this chapter, it often appears that they go well beyond the theoretical and methodological issues involved and are intended to perpetuate the mind-body arguments that have gone on since Aristotle. Brain function not only influences environmental adaption, but environmental conditions influence brain functioning. The two act in a reciprocal fashion. Investigators into this area need not offer support for either side of the controversy but instead should seek an integration of the two positions that will ultimately produce a greater understanding of the children labeled as behavior disordered.

REFERENCES

Achenbach, T. M. The child behavior profile: I. Boys aged 6 through 11. *Journal of Consulting and Clinical Psychology,* 1978, *46,* 478–488.

Achenback, T. M., & Edelbrock, C. S. The child behavior profile: II. Boys aged 12–16 and girls aged 12–16. *Journal of Consulting and Clinical Psychology,* 1979, *47,* 223–233.

Achenbach, T. M., & Edelbrock, C. S. The classification of child psychopathology: A review and analysis of empirical efforts. *Psychological Bulletin,* 1978, *84,* 1275–1301.

Anderson, R. M., Jr. Wholistic and particulate approaches in neuropsychology. In W. B. Weimer & D. S. Palmera (Eds.), *Cognition and the symbolic processes.* Hillsdale, N.J.: Lawrence Erlbaum, 1974.

Anderson, W. The hyperkinetic child: A neurological appraisal. *Neurology,* 1963, *13,* 371–382.

Aries, P. *Centuries of childhood: A social history of family life.* New York: Vintage Books, 1962.

Beitchman, J., Dielman, T., Landis, J., Benson, R., & Kemp. P. Reliability of the group for advancement of psychiatry diagnostic categories in child psychiatry. *Archives of General Psychiatry,* 1978, *35,* 1461–1466.

Bell, D. S. Speech functions in the thalamus inferred from the effects of thalamotomy. *Brain,* 1968, *91,* 619.

Belmont, I., Benjamin, H., Ambrose, J., & Restuccia, R. D. Effect of cerebral damage on motivation in rehabilitation. *Archives of Physiological and Medical Rehabilitation,* 1969, *50,* 507.

Benaron, H. B., Tucker, B. E., Andrews, J. P., Boshes, B., Cohen, J., Fromm, E., & Yacorzynski, G. K. Effect of anoxia during labor and immediately after birth on the subsequent development of the child. *American Journal of Obstetric Gynecology,* 1960, *80,* 1129–1142.

Bender, L. Childhood schizophrenia. *American Journal of Orthopsychiatry,* 1947, *17,* 40–56.

Benson, D. F., Segarra, J., & Albert, M. L. Visual agnosia—prosopagnosia. *Archives of Neurology,* 1974, *30,* 307.

Benson, D. F., & Weir, W. F. Acalculia: Acquired anarithmetica. *Cortex,* 1972, *8,* 465.

Benton, A. L. (Ed.). *Contributions to clinical neuropsychology.* Chicago: Aldine, 1969.

Berman, A. Neurological dysfunction in juvenile delinquents: Implications for early intervention. *Child Care Quarterly,* 1972, *1,* 264–271.

Beshai, J. A. Behavioral correlates of the EEG in delinquents. Reprinted from American Psychological Association, *Proceedings, 79th Annual Convention,* 1971, 459–460.

Boring, E. G. *A history of experimental psychology.* New York: Appleton-Century-Crofts, 1950.

Borkowski, J. G., Benton, A. L., & Spreen, O. Word fluency and brain damage. *Neuropsychologia,* 1967, *5,* 135.

Buchsbaum, M., & Wender, P. Average evoked responses in normal and minimally brain dysfunctioned children treated with amphetamine. A Preliminary Report. *Archives of General Psychiatry,* 1973, *29,* 764–770.

Burr, H. S. *The neural basis of human behavior.* Springfield, Ill.: Charles C Thomas, 1960.

Cantwell, D. P. Psychiatric illness in the families of hyperactive children. *Archives of General Psychiatry,* 1972, *27,* 414–417.

Cantwell, D. P. *The hyperactive child: Diagnosis, management and current research.* New York: Spectrum Publications, 1975.

Chedru, F., Leblanc, M., & Lhermitte, F. Visual searching in normal and brain damaged subjects: Contribution to study of unilateral inattention. *Cortex,* 1973, *9,* 94.

Clark, R. *Crime in America.* New York: Simon and Schuster, 1970.

Clements, S. D. *Minimal brain dysfunction in children—Terminology and identification* (NINDB Monograph No. 3). Washington, D.C.: U.S. Public Health Service, 1966.

Clements, S. D., & Peters, J. E. Minimal brain dysfunctions in the school age child. *Archives of General Psychiatry,* 1962, *6,* 185–197.

Close, K. Do young children need educational care? In J. Frost (Ed.), *Revisiting early childhood education: Readings.* New York: Holt, Rinehart & Winston, 1973.

Coheen, J. J. Disturbances in time discrimination in organic brain disease. *Journal of Nervous and Mental Diseases,* 1950, *112,* 121.

Cohen, A. *Delinquent boys.* Chicago: Free Press, 1955.

Cohen, A., & Short, J. Research in delinquent subcultures. *Journal of Social Issues,* 1958, *14,* 20–37.

Coleman, J. *Abnormal psychology and modern life.* Glenview, Ill.: Scott, Foresman & Company, 1964.

Conel, J. L. *The postnatal development of the human cerebral cortex.* Cambridge, Mass.: Harvard University Press, 1939.

Corkin, S. Tactually guided maze learning in man. Effects of unilateral cortical excisions and bilateral hippocampal lesions. *Neuropsychologia,* 1965, *3,* 339.

Cravioto, J., & Delicardie, E. R. Mental performance in school age children: Findings after recovery from early severe malnutrition. *American Journal of Disabled Children,* 1970, *120,* 404–410.

Cumming, W. J. K., Hurwitz, L. J., & Perl, N. A. A study of a patient who had alexia without agraphia. *Journal of Neurology, Neurosurgery and Psychiatry,* 1970, *33,* 34.

Dee, H. L., & Van Allen, M. W. Simple and choice reaction time and motor strength in unilateral cerebral disease. *Acta Psychiatrica Scandanavica,* 1971, *47,* 315.

DeJong, R. N., Itabashi, H. H., & Olson, J. R. Memory loss due to hippocampal lesions: Report of a case. *Archives of Neurological Psychiatry*, 1969, *20*, 339.

Denckla, M. B., & Bowen, F. B. Dyslexia after left occipitotemporal lobectomy: A case report. *Cortex*, 1973, *9*, 321.

Denckla, M. B., & Rudel, R. *Anomalies of motor development in hyperactive boys without traditional neurological signs. Annals of Neurology*, 1978, *3*, 231–233.

DeRenzi, E., & Faglioni, P. The relationship between visuo–spatial impairment and constructional apraxia. *Cortex*, 1967, *3*, 327.

DeRenzi, E., Faglioni, P. & Scotti, G. Hemispheric contribution to exploration of space through the visual and tactile modalities. *Cortex*, 1970, *6*, 191.

Desai, H. Factors relating to juvenile delinquency. *Indian Educational Review*, 1970 *5*, 74–83.

Despert, J. L. *The emotionally disturbed child—Then and now.* New York: Brunner, 1965.

Diagnostic and statistical manual of mental disorders (1st ed.) (DSM-I). Washington, D.C.: American Psychiatric Association, 1968.

Diller, L., & Weinberg. J. Attention in brain-damaged people. *Journal of Education*, 1968, *150*, 20–27.

Douglas, R. J., & Pribram, K. H. Learning aids and limbic lesions. *Neuropsychologia*, 1966, *4*, 197.

Drillien, C. M. *The growth and development of the prematurely born infant.* Baltimore: Williams & Wilkins, 1964.

Drillien, C. M. Fresh approaches to prospective studies of high risk infants. *Pediatrics*, 1970, *45*, 7–8.

Dustman, R., & Beck, E. The effects of maturation and aging on the wave form of visually evoked potentials. *Electroencephalography and Clinical Neurophysiology*, 1969, *26*, 2–11.

Dykman, R. A., Ackerman, P. T., Clements, S. D., & Peters, J. E. Specific learning disabilities: An attentional deficit syndrome. In H. R. Myklebust (Ed.), *Progress in learning disabilities* (Vol. 2). New York: Grune & Stratton, 1971.

Edelbrock, C. Empirical classification of children's behavior disorders: Progress based on parent and teacher ratings. *School Psychology Digest*, 1979, *8*, 355–369.

Education for all Handicapped Children Act. Public Law 94-142. U.S. Congress, November 29, 1975.

Ellingson, R. J. The incidence of EEG abnormality among patients with mental disorders of apparently non-organic origin: A critical review. Reprinted from *The American Journal of Psychiatry*, 1954, *3*, 263–275.

Ervin, F. Organic brain syndrome associated with epilepsy. In A. M. Freedman, H. I. Kaplan, & B. J. Sadock (Eds.), *Comprehensive textbook of psychiatry* (2nd ed.). Baltimore: Williams & Wilkins, 1975.

Ervin, F., Epstein, A. W., & King, H. E. Behavior of epileptic and nonepileptic patients with "temporal spikes." *Archives of Neurology and Psychiatry*, 1955, *74*, 488.

Federal Bureau of Investigation, United States. *Uniform crime reports for the United States.* Washington, D.C.: Government Printing Office, 1974.

Felix, R. H. *Mental illness—Progress and prospects.* New York: Columbia Univeristy Press, 1967.

Flechsig, P. *Meine myelogenetische Hirnlehre mit biographischer Einleitung.* Berlin: Springer, 1927.

Forssman, H., & Frey, T. Electroencephalograms of boys with behavior disorders. *Acta Psychiatrica*, 1953, *28*, 61–73.

Forrsman, H., & Hambert, G. Chromosomes and antisocial behavior. *Exceptor Criminology*, 1967, *7*, 113–117.

Freeman, M. A reliability study of psychiatric diagnosis in childhood and adolescence. *Journal of Child Psychology, Psychiatry, and Allied Disciplines*, 1971, *12*, 43–54.

Gibbs, E., & Gibbs, F. Electroencephalographic changes with age during sleep. *Clinical Neurophysiology*, 1950, *2*, 355.

Glasser, G. H., & Pincus, J. H. Limbic encephalitis. *Journal of Nervous and Mental Disorders,* 1969, *59,* 149.

Glueck, S., & Glueck, E. *Family environment and delinquency.* Boston: Houghton, Mifflin, 1962.

Golden, C. J. *Diagnosis and rehabilitation in clinical neuropsychology.* Springfield, Ill.: Charles C Thomas, 1978.

Golden, C. J., Hammeke, T. A., & Purisch, A. D. Diagnostic validity of a standardized neuropsychological battery derived from Luria's neuropsychological tests. *Journal of Consulting and Clinical Psychology,* 1978, *46,* 1258–1265.

Green, J. Association of behavior disorder with an electroencephalographic focus in children without seizures. *Neurology,* 1961, *11,* 337–344.

Greenblatt, S. A. Alexia without agraphia or hemianopsia: Anatomical analysis of an autopsied case. *Brain,* 1973, *96,* 307.

Gregory, I. Psychiatric syndrome due to acute reversible brain disorders. *Journal of Lancet,* 1961, *81,* 270–275.

Gross, C. G., & Weiskrantz, L. Some changes in behavior produced by lateral frontal lesions in the macaque. In J. M. Warren & K. Akert (Eds.), *The frontal granular cortex and behavior.* New York: McGraw-Hill, 1964.

Gross, M. D., & Wilson, W. C. *Minimal brain dysfunction.* New York: Brunner/Mazel, 1974.

Gunn, J., & Bonn, J. Criminality and violence in epileptic prisoners. *British Journal of Psychiatry,* 1971, *118,* 337.

Hanvik, L. J., Nelson, S. E., Hanson, H. B., Anderson, A. S., Dressler, W. H., & Zarling, V. R. Diagnosis of cerebral dysfunction in children. *American Journal of Disordered Children,* 1961, *101.* 364–375.

Harlow, H. *Learning to love,* San Francisco: Albion, 1971.

Healy, W., & Bronner, A. *New light on delinquency and its treatment.* New Haven: Yale University Press, 1936.

Hebb, D. O., & Penfield, W. Human behavior after extensive bilateral removals from the frontal lobes. *Archives of Neurology and Psychiatry,* 1940, *44,* 421–438.

Herbert, M. The concept and testing of brain damage in children: A review. *Journal of Child Psychology and Psychiatry,* 1964, *5,* 197–216.

Hertzig, M. Neurologic findings in children educationally designated as "brain-damaged." *American Journal of Orthopsychiatry,* 1969, *39,* 437–446.

Hertzig, M., & Birch, H. Neurological organization in psychiatrically disturbed adolescents. *Archives of General Psychiatry,* 1966, *19,* 528–537.

Hill, D. EEG in episodic psychotic and psychopathic behavior. *Electroencephalography and Clinical Neurophysiology,* 1952, *4,* 419–442.

Hughes, J. Infant death rates. *Journal of the American Medical Association,* 1971, *216,* 1481–1482.

Hughes, J., & Park, G. Electro-clinical correlations in dyslexic children. *Electroencephology and Clinical Neurophysiology,* 1969, *26,* 119.

Huxley, J. *Ends & means,* New York: Harper, 1937.

Ingham, S. Cerebral localization of psychological processes occurring during a two-minute experience. *Journal of Nervous and Mental Disorders,* 1948, *107,* 388.

Ingram, T., Mason, A., & Blackburn, I. A retrospective study of 82 children with reading disability. *Developmental Medicine and Child Neurology,* 1970, *12,* 271–281.

Isaacson, R. Hippocampal destruction in man and other animals. *Neuropsychologia, 1972,* **10,** *47.*

Kahn, R. L., Pollack, M., & Fink, M. Figure-ground discrimination after induced altered brain function. *Archives of Neurology,* 1960, *2,* 547.

Kanner, L. Emotionally disturbed children: A historical review. *Child Development,* 1962, *33,* 97–102.

Kawi, A. A., & Pasamanick, B. Association of factors of pregnancy with reading disorders in childhood. *Journal of the American Medical Association,* 1958, *166,* 1420–1423.

Kellaway, P., Crawley, J., & Maulsby, R. The electroencephalogram in psychiatric disorders in childhood. In W. Wilson (Ed.), *Applications of electroencephalography in psychiatry.* Durham, N.C.: Duke University Press, 1965.

Kennard, M. Value of equivocal signs in neurologic diagnosis. *Neurology,* 1960, *10,* 753–764.

Kimura, D. Some effects of temporal lobe damage on auditor perception. *Canadian Journal of Psychology,* 1961, *15,* 156.

Kinsbourne, M., & Warrington, E. K. Disorders of spelling. *Journal of Neurology, Neurosurgery, and Psychiatry,* 1964, *27,* 224.

Klinkerfuss, G., Lange, P., & Weinberg, W. Electroencephalographic abnormalities of children with hyperkinetic behavior. *Neurology,* 1965, *15,* 883–891.

Lamb, M. E. The development of mother–infant and father–infant attachments in the first year of life. *Child Development,* 1977, *48,* 167–181.

Landauer, T. K., & Whiting, J. W. M. Infantile stimulation and adult stature of human males. *American Anthropologist,* 1964, *66,* 1007–1028.

Langhorne, J., Loney, J., Paternite, C., & Beckholdt, H. Childhood hyperkinesis: A return to the source. *Journal of Abnormal Psychology,* 1976, *85,* 201–209.

Larsen, V. Physical characteristics of disturbed adolescents. *Archives of General Psychiatry,* 1964, *10,* 55–64.

Lashley, K. S. *Brain mechanisms and intelligence.* Chicago: University of Chicago Press, 1929.

Lashley, K. S. Functional determinants of cerebral localization. *Archives of Neurological Psychiatry,* 1937, *38,* 371.

Laufer, M., Denhoff, E., & Solomons, G. Hyperkinetic impulse disorder in children's behavior problems. *Psychosomatic Medicine,* 1957, *19,* 38–49.

Levin, H. S. Motor impersistence in patients with unilateral cerebral disease: A cross validational study. *Journal of Consulting Clinical Psychology,* 1973, *41,* 287.

Lewis, D. O., & Balla, D. A. *Delinquency and psychopathology.* New York: Grune & Stratton, 1976.

Lewis, Nolan D. C. American psychiatry from its beginnings to World War II. In S. Arieti (Ed.), *American handbook of psychiatry* (Vol. 1). New York: Basic Books, 1959.

Lindsley, D. B. The reticular system and perceptual discrimination. In K. H. Jasper, L. D. Proctor, R. S. Knighton, W. C. Noshay, & R. C. Costello (Eds.), *Reticular formation of the brain.* Boston: Little, Brown, 1958.

Lombroso-Ferrero, G. *Criminal man according to the classifications of Cesare Lombroso.* New York: Putnam, 1911.

Lowrey, L. G. Psychiatry of children. *American Journal of Psychiatry,* 1944, *101,* 375–388.

Luria, A. R. Neuropsychology in the local diagnosis of brain injury. *Cortex,* 1964, *3,* 1.

Luria, A. R. *Higher cortical functions in man.* New York: Basic Books, 1966.

Luria, A. R. *The working brain.* New York: Basic Books, 1973.

Luria, A. R., & Tsvetkova, L. S. The programming of constructive activity in local brain injuries. *Neuropsychologia,* 1964, *2,* 95.

Luria, A. R., Pribram, H., & Homskaya, F. D. An experimental analysis of the behavioral disturbance produced by a left frontal arachnoidal endothelioma (meningioma). *Neuropsychologia,* 1964, *2,* 257.

MacLean, P. Some psychiatric implications of physiological studies on fronto-temporal portion of limbic system. Electroencephalogram. *Clinical Neurophysiology,* 1952, *4,* 407.

MacLean, P. The limbic system and its hippocampal formation. Studies in animals and their possible relation to man. *Journal of Neurosurgery,* 1954, *11,* 29.

McCord, W. The biological basis of juvenile delinquency. In J. Roucek (Ed.), *Juvenile delinquency.* New York: Philosophical Library, 1958.

McDonald, R. D. Effect of brain damage on adaptability. *Journal of Nervous and Mental Disease,* 1964, *138,* 241.

McDonald, R. D., & Burns, S. B. Visual vigilance and brain damage: An empirical study. *Journal of Neurological Neurosurgery and Psychiatry*, 1964, *27*, 206.

McFie, J. & Zangwill, O. L. Visual constructive disabilities associated with lesions of the left cerebral hemisphere. *Brain*, 1960, *83*, 243.

McKay, S., & Golden, C. J. Empirical derivation of experimental scales for localizing brain lesions using the Luria–Nebraska Neurosychological Battery. *Clinical Neuropsychology*, 1979, *1*, 19–23.

Merton, R. K., & Nisbet, R. A. (Eds.). *Contemporary social problems*. New York: Harcourt, Brace & World, 1961.

Meyer, V. Cognitive changes following temporal lobectomy for relief of temporal lobe epilepsy. *Archives of Neurological Psychiatry*, 1959, *81*, 299.

Meyer, V., & Yates, A. J. Intellectual changes following temporal lobectomy for psychomotor epilepsy. *Journal of Neurology, Neurosurgery, and Psychiatry*, 1955, *18*, 44.

Miller, W. Lower class culture as a generating milieu of gang delinquency. *Journal of Social Issues*, 1958, *14*, 5–19.

Mills, C. K. Hysteria. In J. M. Keating (Ed.), *Cyclopaedia of the diseases of children—Medical and surgical*. Philadelphia: Lippincott, 1890.

Milner, B. Psychological defects produced by temporal lobe excision. *Research Publications of the Association for Research on Nervous and Mental Disease*, 1958, *36*, 244–257.

Milner, M. *Physiological psychology*. New York: Holt, Rinehart and Winston, 1970.

Montagu, A. *The nature of human aggression*. New York: Oxford University Press, 1976.

Morrison, J. R., & Stewart, M. A. A family study of the hyperactive child syndrome. *Biological Psychiatry*, 1971, *3*, 189–195.

Mullan, S., & Penfield, W. Illusions of comparative interpretation and emotion. *Archives of Neurological Psychiatry*, 1959, *81*, 269.

Murray, C. A. *The link between learning disabilities and juvenile delinquency*. Washington, D.C.: Law Enforcement Assistance Administration, 1976.

Nakosteen, M. *The history and philosophy of education*. New York: Ronald Press, 1965.

Nash, J. *Developmental psychology: A psychobiological approach* (2nd ed.). Englewood Cliffs, N.J.: Prentice-Hall, 1978.

Oettinger, L., Majovski, L. V., Limbeck, G. A., & Gauch, R. Bone age in children with minimal brain dysfunction. *Perceptual and Motor Skills*, 1974, *39*, 1127–1131.

Ojemann, G. A. Alteration in non-verbal short term memory with stimulation in the region of the mammillothalamic tract in man. *Neuropsychologia*, 1971, *9*, 195.

Ojemann, G. A., & Ward, A. A. Speech representation in the ventrolateral thalamus. *Brain*, 1971, *94*, 669.

Olbrich, R. Reaction time in brain damaged and normal subjects to variable preparatory intervals. *Journal of Nervous and Mental Disease*, 1972, *155*, 356.

Ounsted, C. Aggression and epilepsy rage in children with temporal lobe epilepsy. *Journal of Psychosomatic Research*, 1969, *13*, 237–242.

Paine, R. S. The contribution of neurology to the pathogenisis of hyperactivity in children. *Clinical Proceedings of the Children's Hospital*, 1964, *19*, 235–247.

Paine, R., Werry, J., & Quay, H. C. A study of "minimal cerebral dysfunction." *Developmental Medicine and Child Neurology*, 1968, *10*, 505–520.

Papez, J. W. A proposed mechanism of emotion. *Archives of Neurology and Psychiatry*, 1937, *38*, 725.

Pasamanick, B. Pregnancy experience and the development of behavior disorders in children. *American Journal of Psychiatry*, 1956, *112*, 613–617.

Pasamanick, B. Epidemiological investigations of some prenatal factors in the production of neuropsychiatric disorders, In P. H. Hoch & J. Zubin (Eds.), *Comparative epidemiology for mental disorders*. New York: Grune & Stratton, 1961.

Penfield, W., & Milner, B. Memory deficit produced by bilateral lesions in the hippocampal zone. *Archives of Neurological Psychiatry*, 1958, *79*, 475.

Peters, J. E., Romine, J. S., & Dykman, R. A. A special neurological examination of children with learning disabilities. *Developmental Medicine and Child Neurology*, 1975, *17*, 63–78.

Peterson, D., Quay, H., & Cameron, G. Personality and background factors in juvenile delinquency as inferred from questionnaire responses. *Journal of Consulting Psychology*, 1959, *23*, 395–399.

Pierson, G., & Kelly, R. Anxiety, extroversion, and personality idiosyncrasy in delinquency. *The Journal of Psychology*, 1963, *56*, 441–445.

Pincus, J. H., & Tucker, G. J. *Behavioral neurology*. New York: Oxford University Press, 1978.

Pollack, M. Suspected early minimal brain damage and severe psychopathology in adolescence. *Adolescence*, 1969, *4*, 361–384.

Pond, D. Psychiatric aspects of epileptic and brain-damaged children. *British Medical Journal*, 1961, *2*, 1377–1382, 1454–1459.

Reckless, W. *The crime problem*. New York: Meredith, 1967.

Reitan, R. M. *Manual for administration of neuropsychological test batteries for adults and children*. Indianapolis, privately mimeographed, 1959.

Reitan, R. M., & Davison, L. A. (Eds.). *Clinical neuropsychology: Current status and applications*. Washington, D.C.: V. H. Winston & Sons, 1974.

Rhodes, W. C., & Ensor, D. R. Community programming. In H. C. Quay and J. S. Werry (Eds.), *Psychopathological disorders of childhood* (2nd ed.). New York: Wiley, 1979.

Rie, H. E. (Ed.). Historical perspective of concepts of child psychopathology. In *Perspectives in child psychopathology*. Chicago: Aldine-Atherton, 1971.

Riese, W. The sources of Jacksonian neurology. *Journal of Nervous and Mental Disorders*, 1956, *124*, 125.

Rosenzweig, M. R. Effects of environment on brain and behavior in animals. In E. Schopler and R. J. Reichler (Eds.), *Psychopathology and child development*. New York: Plenum, 1976.

Rosvold, H. E, & Szwarcbart, M. K. Neural structures involved in delayed-response performance. In J. M. Warren & K. Akert (Eds.), *The frontal granular cortex and behavior*. New York: McGraw-Hill, 1964.

Rubino, C. A. Hemispheric lateralization of visual perception. *Cortex*, 1970, *6*, 102.

Rubinstein, E. Childhood mental disease in America: A review on the literature before 1900. *American Journal of Orthopsychiatry*, 1948, *18*, 314–321.

Rutter, M. Brain damage syndromes in childhood: Concepts and findings. *Journal of Child Psychology, Psychiatry, and Allied Disciplines*, 1977, *18*, 1–21.

Rutter, M., Graham, P., & Jule, W. *A neuropsychiatric study in childhood clinics in development*. London: SIMPL Heinemann, 1970.

Satterfield, J. EEG issues in children with minimal brain dysfunction. *Seminars in Psychiatry*, 1973, *5*, 35–46.

Satz, P., & Fletcher, J. M. Minimal brain dysfunctions: An appraisal of research concepts and methods. In H. E. Rie & E. D. Rie (Eds.), *Handbook of minimal brain dysfunctions*. New York: Wiley, 1980.

Schain, R. J. *Neurology of childhood learning disorders* (2nd ed.). Baltimore: Williams & Wilkins, 1977.

Scheussler, K., & Cressey, D. Personality characteristics of criminals. *American Journal of Sociology*, 1950, *44*, 476–484.

Scoville, W. B., & Milner, B. Loss of recent memory after bilateral hippocampal lesions. *Journal of Neurological Neurosurgical Psychiatry*, 1957, *20*, 11.

Sellin, T. *Culture conflict and crime*. New York: Social Science Research Council, 1938.

Selz, M., & Reitan, C. Rule for neuropsychological diagnosis: Classification of brain function in older children. *Journal of Consulting & Clinical Psychology*, 1979, *47*, 258–264.

Serafetinides, E. A. Aggressiveness in temporal lobe epileptics and its relation to cerebral dysfunction and environmental factors. *Epilepsia,* 1965, *6,* 33–42.

Shaw, C. L., & McKay, H. *Juvenile delinquency in urban areas.* Chicago: University of Chicago Press, 1929.

Sheldon, W. *Varieties of delinquent youth.* New York: Harper, 1949.

Sherrets, S. D. *Behavior disorders in adolescents: Neuropsychological and behavioral correlates.* Unpublished doctoral dissertation, University of Nebraska, 1980.

Smith, C. U. M. *The brain towards an understanding.* New York: Capricorn Books, 1972.

Spitzka, E. C. Insanity. In John M. Keating (Ed.), *Cyclopaedia of the diseases of children: Medical and surgical.* Philadelphia: Lippincott, 1890.

Springer, S. P., & Deutsch, G. *Left brain, right brain.* San Francisco: W. H. Freeman, 1981.

Stamm, J. Minimal brain dysfunction: Psychological and neurophysiological disorders in hyperkinetic children. In M. Gazzaniga (Ed.), *Handbook in neuropsychology.* New York: Plenum, 1978.

Stevens, D., Boydstun, J., & Dykman, R. Presumed minimal brain dysfunction in children; relationship to performance on selected behavioral tests. *Archives of General Psychiatry,* 1967, *16,* 281–285.

Stott, D. H. *Delinquency and human nature.* Dunfermline, Fife, Scotland: The Carnegie United Kingdom Trust, 1950.

Stott, D. H. Evidence for a congenital factor in maladjustment and delinquency. *American Journal of Psychiatry,* 1962, *118,* 781–794.

Stott, D. H. *Studies of troublesome children.* New York: New York Humanities Press, 1968.

Strauss, A. A., Lehtinen, L. E. *Psychopathology of the brain-injured child.* New York: Grune & Stratton, 1947.

Tannenbaum, F. *Crime and the community.* New York: Ginn, 1938.

Tarter, R., Templer, D., & Hardy, C. Reliability of the psychiatric diagnosis. *Diseases of the Nervous System,* 1975, *36,* 30–31.

Thomas, A., & Chess, S. A longitudinal study of three brain damaged children. *Archives of General Psychiatry,* 1975, *32,* 457–465.

Thomas, A., & Chess, S. *The dynamics of psychological development.* New York: Brunner/Mazel, 1980.

Thomas, A., Chess, S., & Birch, H. *Temperament and behavior disorders in children.* New York: New York University Press, 1968.

Toglia, J. U. The corpus callosum. *Diseases of the Nervous System,* 1961, *22,* 428.

Towbin, A. Organic causes of minimal brain dysfunction. Perinatal origin of minimal cerebral lesions. *Journal of the American Medical Association,* 1971, *217,* 1207–1214.

Tramontana, M. G., Sherrets, S. D., & Golden, C. J. Brain dysfunction in youngsters with psychiatric disorders: Application of Selz–Reitan rules for neurosychological diagnosis. *Clinical Neuropsychology,* 1980, *2,* 118–123.

Treffert, D. A. The psychiatric patient with an EEG temporal lobe focus. *Archives of General Psychiatry,* 1964, *12,* 278–286.

Tucker, M. Lateral brain function, evolution and conceptualization. *Psychological Bulletin,* 1981, *89,* 19–46.

Vilkki, J., & Laitinen, V. Differential effects of left and right ventrolateral thalamotomy on receptive and expressive verbal performances and face matching. *Neuropsychologia,* 1974, *12,* 11.

Waber, D. Sex differences in cognition: A function of maturation rate? *Science,* 1976, *192,* 572–573.

Warrington, E. K., & Taylor, A. M. The contribution of the right parietal lobe to object recognition. *Cortex,* 1973, *9,* 152.

Watts, G. O. *Dynamic neuroscience: Its application to brain disorders.* Hagerstown, Md.: Harper & Row, 1975.

Weil, A. A. Ictal emotions occuring in temporal lobe dysfunction. *Archives of Neurology,* 1959, *1,* 87.

Wender, P. A. The minimal brain dysfunction syndrome in children. I. The syndrome and its relevance for psychiatry. II. A psychological and biochemical model for the syndrome. *Journal of Nervous Mental Disorders,* 1972, *155,* 55–71.

Werner, H., & Strauss, A. A. Causal factors in low performance. *American Journal of Mental Deficiency,* 1940, *45,* 213–218.

Werry, J. Studies on the hyperactive child. IV. An empirical analysis of the minimal brain dysfunction syndrome. *Archives of General Psychiatry,* 1968, *19,* 9–16.

Werry, J. Organic factors. In H. Quay & L. Werry (Eds.), *Psychopathological disorders of childhood* (2nd ed.). New York: Wiley, 1979.

Werry, J., & Quay, H. The prevalence of behavior symptoms in younger elementary school children. *American Journal of Orthopsychiatry,* 1971, *41,* 136–143.

Wikler, A., Dixon, J. F., & Parker, J. B. Brain function in problem children and controls: Psychometric, neurological, and electroencephalographic comparisons. *American Journal of Psychiatry,* 1970, *127,* 94–105.

Williams, D. Man's temporal lobe. *Brain,* 1968, *91,* 639.

Wood, F. H., & Zabel, R. H. Making sense of reports on the incidence of behavior disorders/emotional disturbance in school-aged populations. *Psychology in the Schools,* 1978, *15,* 45–51.

Yakovlev, P. I., & Lecours, A. R. The myelogenetic cycles of regional maturation in the brain. In A. Minkowski (Ed.), *Regional development of the brain in early life.* Oxford: Blackwell, 1967.

Yamadori, A., & Albert, M. L. Word category aphasia. *Cortex,* 1973, *9,* 112.

Zurif, E. B., & Ramier, A. M. Some effects of unilateral brain damage on the perception of dichotically presented phoneme sequences and digits. *Neuropsychologia,* 1972, *10,* 103.

14

Neuropsychology and Exceptional Children

MARK SCHACHTER

The neuropsychological study of exceptional children is an expanding field. Recent developments have included particularly strong growth in the study of learning disabilities, and less rapid expansion in the neuropsychological exploration of such conditions as mental retardation, cerebral palsy, and other central nervous system disorders. In these respective conditions, neuropsychological assessments may provide much more detailed analyses of learning problems than traditional psychological assessments. This leads to linkage between neuropsychologists and educators. Neuropsychological methods and test results can become important in designing individualized educational plans and in choosing effective methods for rehabilitating exceptional children to their fullest potential.

Before discussing neuropsychology and the various exceptionalities in children, it is important for the reader to be aware of both the strengths and limitations of clinical neuropsychology with children. Just as with many other fields, studying neuropsychological deficits in children has been an offshoot of studying deficits in adults. Many of the tests used in the neuropsychological assessment of children, for example, are simplifications of tests already designed for use with adults. This may have been an expedient but inappropriate tactic, for as Teuber and Rudel (1962) have demonstrated, brain-damaged children and brain-damaged adults differ in their performances on the same psychological tasks even when

MARK SCHACHTER ● Robert Warner Rehabilitation Center, Children's Hospital, Department of Pediatrics and Department of Psychology, State University of New York at Buffalo, Buffalo, New York 14209.

site of lesion is the same across these groups. Therefore, it may become necessary to develop neuropsychological testing techniques that can take into account the qualitative differences between children and adults, which is apparent both in the cognitive organization of normal persons of different ages and in their recovery and deficit patterns after brain damage.

Boll (1974) points out that in children many more factors interfere with neuropsychological assessment than is the case in adulthood. For example, age of the child, age of onset of the problem, developmental rate, and chronicity of the brain lesion are factors that complicate the study of brain behavior relationships in childhood. Reitan (1974) matched brain-damaged and control children and then tested them on the Reitan–Indiana Neuropsychological Test Battery. His findings suggested that brain damage affects children by putting a rather global limit on normal development, leading to a general depression of adaptive abilities. This was contrasted with findings in adults suggesting that much more specific deficits would be found in analogous lesions. Similar results had earlier been reported by McFie (1961) in children undergoing hemispherectomy before the first year of life. He reported a limit on the IQ ultimately attained by these children and an inferiority of verbal IQ relative to performance IQ regardless of which hemisphere had been removed.

Lenneberg (1967) has advanced the viewpoint that a critical periods concept is best suited to explain the developmental aspect of cerebral damage. He cites such examples as hypothyroidism and rubella, which can cause brain damage in the fetus but not in the adult. He also notes that hemiplegias acquired in adulthood are often associated with language disorders when the injury is to the left hemisphere. However, infantile hemiplegias are not often associated with aphasic speech disorders.

Neuropsychology has been hampered by the tremendous difficulties inherent in conducting longitudinal studies of brain-damaged children and controls. With few exceptions, research has come to focus on cross-sections of the age span rather than following any one group throughout its developmental process. The state of the art is also compromised by the use of the same tests in children as those used to study adults, even though qualitative differences between these groups have been demonstrated. Ultimately, it may become necessary to develop batteries of neuropsychological instruments that are specifically designed to assess brain functioning at different age levels. At the present time, however, such instruments as the Reitan Neuropsychological batteries, the new Luria–Nebraska, and other specific tests coming from the human experimental tradition in neuropsychology are the extent of our repertoire.

The linkage between neuropsychology and special education is an old one. Strauss and Werner (1943) studied children who they described as being exogenously brain damaged, that is, nongenetically based and inflicted by outside agents. These researchers utilized neuropsychological concepts that had first been expounded by Kurt Goldstein (1936), and presented in the earlier chapter on history.

Strauss and Lehtinen (1947) extended Goldstein's (1942) work into the area of exceptional children. He adopted a unitary dysfunction view of the effects of brain damage while describing a behavioral syndrome in children, which he labeled "the brain injured child." The brain-injured child category is the forerunner of later classifications that include minimal brain dysfunction, attentional deficit disorder, and learning disability.

By the late 1940s, innovators such as Halstead (1947), using batteries of tests, were studying more specific effects of brain damage. Halstead's student, Ralph Reitan, would later refine the techniques involved in this test battery, expanding them to include a wider range of adaptive abilities and revising some of the tests for use with children. The Halstead–Reitan tradition has become one of the cornerstones of neuropsychological assessment.

In addition, there is the experimental human neuropsychology framework that is exemplified by the work of Benton and Hecaen (1970), Teuber and Rudel (1962), and others involving more in-depth analysis of the functioning of specific brain regions following damage. Both the clinical and experimental traditions may be found in neuropsychological studies of exceptional children of various types. Benton (1974) indicates that most neuropsychological research with exceptional children has focused on learning disabilities. Difficulty in researching other groups, such as the mentally retarded, has been due to other complications, such as limitations in the ability of retarded children to follow instructions and severity of motoric handicaps leading to difficulties in responding. However, there has been neuropsychological research conducted with children suffering not only from learning disabilities but also from mental retardation, cerebral pasly, seizure disorders, and other conditions adversely affeting the central nervous system.

Based on neuropsychological reearch and clinical practices, the neuropsychologist can become a valuable asset in diagnosing and assessing both severity and types of deficits exhibited by exceptional children. Valuable contributions to academic, cognitive, and social adaptation may be made through the use of broadly based neuropsychological evaluations, which can assess the child's relative strengths and weaknesses across sensory, motoric, and cognitive abilities.

DIAGNOSING BRAIN DAMAGE IN CHILDREN

Much as with adult neuropsychology, some work with exceptional children has focused on the issue of the ability of psychological tests to discriminate brain-damaged children from controls. This is an important issue in two respects. First, from a psychometric perspective, it is important to have an idea of how accurate our tests really are. Secondly, from a clinical perspective, brain damage may interact and, in fact, be a contributing factor to psychiatric disorders in children. Rutter (1977), in his Isle of Wight study, discovered that, while the locus of brain lesion was not associated with psychiatric disorder, the severity of brain damage was associated with an increaed incidence of psychiatric symptoms in children. Conceivably, appropriate identification of children with or without brain dysfunction would lead to different case management in these two instances.

Particularly with the Reitan battery, neuropsychologists have collected normative data to assist in discriminating brain-damaged from nondamaged children. Knights (1970) has prepared smoothed normative data on tests for evaluating brain damage in children. This set of norms includes most of the Reitan battery and additional normative data on motor steadiness tests and other measures. Spreen and Gaddes (1969) collected developmental norms on 15 neuropsychological tests used in evaluation of children aged 6 through 15. Trites (1977) has collected data on a population of learning-disabled children using the Halstead–Reitan battery in its various adaptations for children, as well as other neuropsychological measures. In everyday clinical practice, these norms are a valuable asset to the neuropsychologist in determining the relative standing of a child in comparison to his age mates.

A number of neuropsychological studies have compared children with known brain damage to controls and/or to learning-disabled children. These studies have attempted to establish the effectiveness of certain tests to discriminate between such groups. One example of such a study was conducted by Selz and Reitan (1979). Using tests from the Reitan battery, subjects were divided into normal, learning-disabled, and brain-damaged groups. On 11 of 13 neuropsychological measures, significant differences were obtained across these three groups. Generally, controls did best, brain-damaged children did worst, and learning-disabled children fell between these two groups. Tsushima and Towne (1977) compared children suspected of brain damage on this basis of history with control subjects not suspected of brain damage. They found that 10 neuropsychological variables differentiated the two groups and that a discriminant function analysis composed of 5 variables accurately classified 72.6% of the subjects. The 10 most discriminating variables included: grip strength for dominant and nondominant hand, finger tapping rate for dominant and nondominant hand, Purdue pegboard on nondominant hand, performance IQ, picture completion, block design, full scale IQ, and the object assembly subtests. Unfortunately, no control for IQ level was included in this research.

Reed, Reitan, and Klove (1965) compared 50 brain-damaged children, ranging in age from 10 through 14 years, with 50 control children. Using the WISC and the Reitan Neuropsychological Tests, significant differences were obtained between groups on all measures employed. Typically, subjects with brain lesions were more frequently impaired on tests dependent upon language functions than on tests dependent upon other skills. Reitan (1974) notes many differences between the abilities lost by children following brain damage and those impaired in adults.

As mentioned previously, there is disagreement as to the adequacy of using the same measures to diagnose brain dysfunction in children as used in adults. Even the study by Reed *et al.* (1965) indicates different patterns of deficits across the age span using the Reitan battery. It should be pointed out, however, that Rourke (1975) found greater similarities between deficit patterns between his sample of children and adults than some of the authors already cited, who may have used younger subjects. The overall trend in this line of research has been to establish the validity of neuropsychological tests, particularly many of those used by Reitan and his co-workers to differentiate brain-damaged and control subjects. Additional studies relevant to this area include those of Reitan (1974) and Boll (1974), as well as Selz and Reitan (1979).

LEARNING DISABILITIES AND NEUROPSYCHOLOGY

Having established the ability of neuropsychological tests to discriminate brain-damaged from control subjects, the next section of this chapter explores neuropsychological studies of learning-disabled children. It should be recalled that the learning disabilities classification grew out of Strauss and Lehtinen's (1947) original work with children that he labeled "brain injured." In addition, children with learning disabilities may be labeled in some clinics as suffering from minimal brain dysfunction or attention deficit disorders, with or without hyperactivity. This collection of terms may imply to some that learning-disabled children are therefore brain-injured or suffer from brain dysfunction. However, there are certainly other opinions on this matter. These include the theories that learning-disabled children may suffer from developmental delays, genetic predisposition towards reading or learning problems, and emotionally based learning difficulties (Bannatyne, 1976). As we shall see, neuropsychological studies of learning-disabled children using Reitan methods tend to imply a deficit model, (i.e., that learning problems are based upon cerebral dysfunctions). In contrast, studies coming from the experimental neuropsychology tradition may be interpreted as supporting either deficit or delay formulations as to the etiology of these problems.

Rourke (1976) has explored the differing implications of a lag versus a deficit theory to account for reading retardation. He notes that, if reading retardation is caused by a lag in the maturation of the left hemisphere, as theorized by some authors, then it would be logical to expect affected children to ultimately catch up to their peers in reading proficiency. In contrast, adherence to the position that learning disabilities and reading retardation, in particular, are caused by cerebral defects would not assume that children would ultimately catch up. However, adhering to a defect position would not necessarily be a pessimistic point of view in that special educational methods might enlist other neuronal structures in learning to read than those usually employed. In this way, children with brain dysfunction might ultimately develop adequate reading skills despite the initial handicap.

Use of Reitan's methods in investigations of children with learning disabilities dates back to the late 1960s. Doehring (1968) studied patterns of impairment in children with specific reading disabilities. He included many measures from the Reitan battery along with independent measures of aphasia, visual–motor, and visual–verbal perception. Reading-disabled subjects performed below the mean of the matched control group on all but five measures, all of which required somesthetic perception. Significantly, more experimental subjects were judged by raters to have cerebral dysfunction on the basis of the test protocols than were the controls. The dysfunctions tended to be limited to the left hemisphere. This may have been due to the fact that only emotionally nondisturbed children with performance IQs higher than verbal IQs were included in the experimental group. A later study by Rourke, Dietrich, and Young (1973) indicated that verbal–performance IQ discrepancies on the WISC could be indicative of neuropsychological profiles in young children. Children with low verbal, higher performance IQs did poorly on measures, such as the Speech Sounds Perception Test, that reflect left hemisphere functions. Conversely, those with performance IQ below verbal IQ did poorly on right hemisphere tasks like mazes and the Purdue pegboard. Rourke's (1975) research project on children with learning disabilities indicated that verbal–performance IQ discrepancies may be predictive of neuropsychological test battery findings suggesting right or left hemisphere dysfunction in older children as well.

Several other investigators have used Reitan tests in assessing children with learning problems and/or minimal brain dysfunction (MBD). For example, Knights and Hinton (1967) followed 50 children diagnosed as suffering from minimal brain dysfunction. This group averaged 10.6 years of age and 105 IQ. According to these authors, only nine of the MBD children had normal neuropsychological profiles. Frequently, the MBD children had deficits on the aphasia screening examination, Purdue pegboard, reasoning, and spatial tests. The groups referred to clinic for reading problems did poorest on the Tactual Performance Test, which measures spatial abilities. If the chief complaint was distractibility, they did poorest on the pegboard. The group with poor concentration did poorest on aphasia screening, while hyperactive children did poorest on the Trail Making Test.

Byron Rourke's (1975) research project on brain-behavior relationships in children with learning disabilities has examined both the academic and neuropsychological characteristics of this group. Rourke's (1975) research program indicates that the overall pattern of results on a neuropsychological test battery is a better predictor of performance in academic skills than the simple level of scores on the individual neuropsychological test. His data also indicate that cerebral dysfunction is present in many retarded readers. Sensory–motor integration problems were common among the younger children in Rourke's (1975) reading-disabled groups, while higher conceptual skill deficits, such as the Categories Test, were more common among the older children. Rourke (1975) argues that reading disability is a nonspecific deficit associated with different patterns of ability impairment across the range of children. For example, Rourke and Finlayson (1975) reported on the neuropsychological significance of variations in the pattern of performance on the trail making tests for older children with learning disabilities. Trail Making Test A requires the child to connect numbered circles in sequence, while Trail Making Test B requires the child to alternate between numbered and lettered circles. These authors found that children with impaired performance on Trail Making, Part B, tended to have lower verbal than performance IQs. In contrast, children with poor performance on both Part A and Part B tended to suffer from poor visual–spatial skills.

Sweeney and Rourke (1978) investigated the significance of phonetically accurate versus phonetically inaccurate spelling errors in younger and older children classified as retarded spellers. Children with spelling problems but who made phonetically accurate mistakes differed from normal children on very few variables. However, there were many differences between normal children and those making inaccurate phonetic mistakes. Phonetically inaccurate spelling was correlated with WISC verbal IQ 15 points inferior to performance IQ and retardation in both spelling and reading, suggesting a pervasive language deficit.

Rourke (1976) reports further research in which reading-disabled children were retested 2, 3, and 4 years after initial evaluations during grades one and two. Sensory–motor integration problems were common among the younger children aged 7 to 8 in Rourke's (1976) longitudinal study of reading-disabled groups, while higher conceptual skill deficits, such as on the categories test, were more common as the subjects got older, 2, 3, and 4 years later. His results suggest that a developmental lag is accountable for the results on simple visual–spatial, visual–motor, and verbal expression tests. However, these results are thought to be based upon tests not primarily subserved by the left hemisphere's functioning. Probable neuropsychological deficits are found in left hemispheric tests, and Rourke (1976) believes that, unless reading-retarded children do in fact catch up to normals, a simple deveopmental lag proposal cannot be supported by his data.

Reed (1967a) established a relationship between finger agnosia and reading achievement. In subjects at a chronological age of 10 years, the group with more right-handed errors in localizing fingers read more poorly than the group making more left-handed errors. However, this relationship did not obtain in the group of 6-year-olds also included in the study. Reed (1967b) also reported that, at a chronological age of 10 years, more poor readers had performance IQs 15 points or more greater than their verbal IQs than had higher verbal than performance IQs.

Some of the findings discussed in the previous section point to the possibility of identifying subgroups of reading- or learning-disabled children based upon neuropsychological test batteries. Reading is a very complex skill, requiring visual, auditory, and motoric abilities. In addition, conceptual skills and integration of information across modalities is necessary for successful reading skill development. As Luria (1973) points out, any cognitive ability can be disrupted through brain damage or dysfunction. However, the more complex the skill, the greater the number of cerebral areas involved in its execution. Luria (1973) further states that damage to any one of the areas involved in completing a complex process will disrupt the process in a unique manner. Applying this theoretical framework to reading and learning problems, we must wrestle with the possibility that reading- and language-disabled children may represent several distinct subgroups. In each group, the complex function of reading may have been disrupted in some particular manner. Relevant research on this question has typically been of two types. The first type examines a group of reading- or learning-disabled children on a battery of neuropsychological tests and then employs the statistical procedure of factor analysis in order to delineate syndromes of neuropsychological deficits encountered in these children. The other approach is to divide learning-disabled children according to some specific type of academic problem, for example, children with poor scores on reading versus spelling measures, comparing differences between these two groups on various neuropsychological variables.

The factor analytic approach was first demonstrated by Doehring (1968). In his study, patterns of impairment were examined in children with specific reading disabilities. The clinical population was matched with controls by age, sex, and performance IQ. The latter control may have actually precluded finding some types of dyslexia based upon perceptual–motor disabilities. Children with psychiatric or family problems were excluded. In addition to comparing the control and experimental groups on the individual variables, Doehring (1968) factor-analyzed 79 of the variables included in his study. Two major factors emerged: a reading–spelling factor and a visual–perceptual speed factor. The reading–spelling factor included variables such as spelling achievement, oral spelling, and reading achievement, with negative loadings on many variables requiring visual–perceptual speed. The visual–perceptual speed factor included such items as perceptual speed for numbers, forms, letters, and finger tapping rate on the nondominant hand.

Mattis (1978) obtained three dyslexia syndromes in his sample of 82 children. These included a language disorder syndrome, a speech disarticulation syndrome, and a visual–construction problems syndrome with language intact. He reported much individual variation between subjects within each group. The three syndromes are listed above from highest to lowest percentage of subjects accounted for by each. The three syndromes in total account for 77% of the subjects in this experiment. Mattis, French, and Rapin (1975) used brain-damaged readers, brain-damaged nonreaders, and non-brain-damaged dyslexics in a very similar study. No differences were found between the dyslexics and brain-damaged non-readers on the neuropsychological battery that these authors employed. The language disorder syndrome had high factor loadings on such measures as a Test of Object Naming, the Token Test, the Sentence Repetition Test, and the Speech Sounds Test. The articulation and graphomotor factor had high loadings on the ITPA Sound Blending Subtest and the Benton Visual Retention Test. The visual-spatial-perceptual factor had high loadings on such variables as: verbal IQ (19 points higher than performance IQ); Raven Progressive Matrices (inferior to performance IQ equivalent); and the Benton Visual Retention Test (score at or below borderline level). As these studies indicate the use of brain-damaged controls is important in that it may help control neuropsychological factors associated with dyslexia but that are not causal to it.

Schachter (1976) conducted a factor analysis of neuropsychological test protocols in learning-disabled children, using the Halstead–Reitan. Subjects were not excluded on the basis of intelligence level of profile. With only 43 subjects, 34 variables were factor-analyzed. A large number of neuropsychologically relevant and meaningful factors emerged from the analysis. These included: auditory analysis deficit, spatial relations deficit, motor speed dysfunction, visual–spatial deficit, tactile–sensory deficit, tactile–perceptual deficit, spatial sequencing deficit, and left frontal-temporal brain dysfunction factor. A profile analysis of individual subjects was attempted in order to divide the children into subgroups. Unfortunately, there was so much variability among children that no meaningful subtypes could be derived from this data.

The factor analytic work generally points to the complicated nature of learning problems in children and suggests that neuropsychological research may be able to isolate subtypes for more effective attempts at remediation. A significant difficulty in factor analytic research is a necessity for inclusion of large numbers of subjects. In addition, since some of the deficits associated with reading and learning problems may be developmental lags, it also becomes important to include subjects from various cross sections of the age range. Therefore, an alternative to the cumbersome, factor-analytic research may be the method of composing groups of children on the basis of observed patterns of academic or intellectual strengths and weaknesses, and also on the basis of chronological age. The subgroups may then be tested on neuropsychological measures and compared. This method offers the advantage of using smaller subject samples and comparing children with known differences in age, academic problems, and intellectual profiles, with the intent to determine if they also differ on various measures of neuropsychological abilities.

A number of studies have used the aforementioned method of pattern analysis. Sweeney and Rourke (1978) compared the neuropsychological test performance of children who make phonetically accurate versus phonetically inaccurate spelling errors. The children making phonetically accurate errors differed from normals only on very complex tasks, whereas there were many differences between the inaccurate phonetic spellers and normals. In addition, phonetically inaccurate spelling was associated with WISC verbal IQ being 15 points below performance IQ, with retardation in both spelling and reading.

Adams (1978) selected two groups of learning-disabled children, one with and one without brain dysfunction as diagnosed by medical practitioners. He found that these two groups differed in their ability to benefit from bisensory visual plus tactile training input. The brain-dysfunctional group did benefit from such training, whereas the group without cerebral dysfunction did not, according to these findings.

Naidoo (1972) compared children she defined as being dyslexic, children defined as poor readers, and two control groups on a variety of measures. Reading retardates were worse than spelling-retarded children on tests of reading, whereas spelling retardates had more language and articulation problems. In addition, reading-retarded children did worse than their controls on right–left discrimination tests, whereas this was not the case for spelling-retarded children. Left-handedness was significantly more prevalent in the dyslexic subgroups than in the other groups of subjects.

In a variation of this method of research, Rourke and Finlayson (1975) divided two groups of children on the basis of a pattern of neuropsychological test performance on the Trail Making Test and compared this to their intelligence test profiles. Three groups of children were identified using the Trail Making Test: those with normal performance, those with normal Part A and impaired Part B scores, and those with impairment on both parts of the Trail Making Test. Older children with learning disabilities were the subjects for this inquiry. Rourke and Finlayson (1975) found that subjects with higher verbal than performance IQ did better on Part B of the Trail Making Test, whereas those with higher performance IQ did comparatively better on Part A. Furthermore, subjects with impaired trail making, Part B, performance did poorly on the verbal subtests, whereas those with impaired performance on both trail making tests did poorly on WISC visual–spatial subtests and verbal subtests.

Therefore, it has been demonstrated that the Reitan battery and individual tests from the battery have pointed to similarities between brain-damaged and learning-disabled children. This raises the possibility that subtypes of learning-disabled children may be identified through neuropsychological research. By identifying subtypes, it may be possible for educators to design curricula that meet the special needs of each of these groups. More experimentally oriented neuropsychological research with learning-disabled children has tended to look at one or two phenomena associated with learning disabilities and to study such phenomena in relative depth. This is in contrast to the methods from the Reitan battery tradition.

EXPERIMENTAL NEUROPSYCHOLOGY WITH LEARNING-DISABLED CHILDREN

Neuropsychologists have shown an interest in conducting research into specific deficits encountered in learning-disabled children, such as difficulties on certain verbal tasks, anomalies in the cerebral lateraliztion of language skills, and other phenomena. Much of this research comes from the experimental human neuropsychology school.

The work of Paul Satz has focused on predicting the later occurrence of learning disabilities in very young children. Satz and Friel (1974) originally examined 497 white male kindergarten children on a series of tests. Twenty-two variables were included in their analysis. The tests included the Peabody Picture Vocabulary Test, Finger Tapping Test, Verbal Fluency Test, Embedded Figures, Beery Developmental Test of Visual–Motor Integration, Alphabet Recitation, WISC Similarities, Right–left Discrimination Test, Finger Localization Test, Auditory Discrimination Test, a Dichotic Listening task (with right and left channel recall), and a Finger Localization task. Follow-up examinations were conducted at 2 and 6 years after the initial evaluation.

Satz, Taylor, Friel, and Fletcher (1980) reported on the six-year follow-up from this longitudial study. Early indications of learning problems tended to be on the perceptual tests and tests of sensory integration. With the same children followed up later on, language and formal operations functions were the notable deficits. Satz *et al.* (1980) theorized that learning disabilities occur as a result of a developmental lag in the maturation of the left hemispheric cortex. He distinguishes this from loss of function, which would occur as a result of actual damage or cortical defect. According to this theory, such reading-disabled children should catch up to age peers, although quite slowly.

Some criticism of the Satz and Friel (1974) and Satz *et al.* (1980) studies has been raised on the basis of there having been a ceiling effect on some of the tests (Rourke, 1976). In other words, the tests did not allow for sufficient improvement between initial and follow-up testing to be demonstrated. This would prejudice results in favor of finding a developmental lag versus an ongoing deficit. However, the major contribution of Satz and Friel (1974) and Satz *et al.* (1980) may be the fact that discriminant function analysis of these data led to correct prediction of the outcome of individual children at a 72% hit rate. Using the finger localization, recognition, and discrimination tests, alphabet recitation, Beery Test of Visual-Motor Integration, and Peabody Picture Vocabulary, children were correctly identified as having superior, average, mildly impaired, or severely impaired reading achievement levels 3 years after the initial examination. Satz *et al.* (1980) point out that remediation is probably most effective when given at the period of greatest growth of the cognitive skills underlying reading. Therefore, use of some of the methods described by Satz might allow for this kind of early intervention. However, it should be noted that Satz refers to remediating cognitive skills rather than remediating brain damage. The postulated developmental lag of the left hemisphere is assumed by Satz and Van Nostrand (1973) to mimic brain damage but to be very late in resolving.

Satz and Van Nostrand's (1973) hypothesis that learning disabilities might be due to developmental lag in the maturation of the left hemisphere is one example of the interest that neuropsychologists have developed in the role of hemispheric specialization in learning disorders of children. Anomalies in the expected lateralization of brain function to either the right or left hemisphere have been hypothesized to account for the development of dyslexia and other learning problems.

It has been well established through studies of adults that the left cerebral hemisphere is usually language dominant. Under most circumstances, language functions become primarily processed by the left hemisphere and visual–perceptual functions more dominated by the right hemisphere. Molfese, Freeman, and Palermo (1975) presented auditory stimuli to a selection of subjects ranging from infants to adults (i.e., 1 week old and up) and computed an index of laterality based on the auditory evoked potential that was recorded following stimulation. Even infants gave auditory evoked responses suggestive of greater lateralization of both speech and nonspeech auditory stimuli to the left hemisphere. Thus, the authors have hypothesized that the beginnings of brain lateralization for auditory stimuli seem to occur very early in life. Deficits or developmental lags in the process of lateralizing these brain functions can be assessed through the use of the dichotic listening task.

Studies usng the dichotic listening task with learning-disabled and control children have at times provided evidence suggesting that the learning-disabled (usually reading-disabled) children failed to evidence adequate right ear superiority for language. Springer and Eisenson (1977) found no significant differences with respect to the magnitude of right ear advantage between language-disordered and normal children. However, the language-disordered children in general reported fewer syllables correctly, and the size of the auditory asymmetry was inversely proportional to the severity of the language disorder in the experimental group. In a study demonstrating early lateralization, Kimura (1967) used a sample of children with relatively higher IQs. In her dichotic listening experiment, a right ear superiority for language was demonstrated from age 5 onward in the high IQ group. However, in a sample from lower SES schools, girls showed the right ear superiority by 5 years of age, but boys did not. This was interpreted to indicate that, by testing early enough, it would be possible to show sex differences in the development of this neuropsychological asymmetry.

In a series of experiments reported by Bakker, Teunissen, and Bosch (1976), it was suggested that the nature of the relationship between ear asymmetry and reading ability might be dependent upon the stage at which the child is in the process of learning how to read. Some of the literature that was reported demonstrated that, at 7 to 8 years of age, the best readers could have the smallest differences between ears on the dichotic listening task. In addition, Bakker et al. (1976) showed developmental differences between the asymmetry patterns of boys and girls, indicating that reading proficiency was associated with a right ear advantage in fifth to sixth grade boys and in third grade girls, while either a right or a left ear advantage was associated with reading proficiency in third grade boys and second grade girls. The authors suggested that, in the early stages of learning to read, both hemispheres might possess the capacity to mediate written language, whereas in the later stages only the left hemisphere has the capacity.

This complicated picture of developmental changes in the right ear advantage on dichotic listening tasks has been discussed by Porter and Berlin (1975). Different dichotic tasks can actually assess different levels of language processing. For example, slowly developing mnemonic processes might be tapped by presenting four-digit pairs on each trail, whereas nonsense consonant-vowel pairs may tap phonetic and auditory skills. The levels of processing assessed by certain studies may differ, and each type of language or auditory processing could be lateralized to a different degree or in different hemispheres. For example, Satz, Bakker, Teunissen, Goebel, and Van Der Vlugt (1975) used 34 spoken digit pairs in the Dutch language in their dichotic listening experiment. Children at five age levels—5, 6, 7, 9, and 11 years of age—were included. No significant ear asymmetries were discovered below 9 years of age.

In contrast to this finding, Hiscock and Kinsbourne (1977) instructed their sample of 3-year-olds to listen to one ear for 12 trails and then to the other ear for 12 trails of dichotic digits. The left ear was correct 26% of the time, but the right ear was correct 67% of the trails. In an extension of that study, Hiscock and Kinsbourne (1977) reported that more right-ear intrusion errors were to be found among the samples of right-handed 3- to 5-year-old children. Thus, the right-ear stimulus tended to be reported regardless of the instructions given to the child as to which ear to listen to. Hiscock and Kinsbourne (1977) believed that their results may be due to attentional–perceptual factors.

At this point, methodological differences between studies, as well as sex differences on the dichotic listening task and in the development of ear asymmetry, make it premature to draw conclusions about the role of auditory processing asymmetry in the etiology of learning disorders. However, this area appears to be a promising one for future research, and neuropsychologists must be aware of the possibility that failure to appropriately lateralize certain skills is associated with reading and learning problems.

The equivalent of the dichotic listening task in the visual–perceptual literature is the visual half field experiment. Visual stimuli are presented for very brief durations to the extreme right and left periphery of the visual field. The subject then reports which stimuli he has seen. Gross, Rothenberg, and Schottenfeld (1978) tested normal and reading-disabled children of 10 to 13½ years of age. The reading-disabled group showed a higher threshold for correctly identifying letters in both visual half fields. Much as with the dichotic listening literature, Rourke (1978) suggests that there is no conclusive evidence regarding right and left half field superiorities for verbal versus nonverbal stimuli. However, one might suspect a right visual half field superiority for words in normal readers and perhaps difficulties in establishing the dominance for retarded readers. These patterns would suggest anomalous cerebral dominance in the reading-disabled and left hemispheric advantage for processing visual–verbal signals in normals.

Witelson (1976) has brought forth the view that abnormal right hemispheric specialization might account for some of the phenomena in developmental dyslexia. As mentioned previously, the left hemisphere seems specialized for language in normal persons, whereas the right hemisphere seems to be more dominant for visual and perceptual phenomena. Witelson (1976) devised a dichotomous tactual stimulation task in order to assess hemispheric specialization for tactile perception. In this situation, competing shapes or forms are presented to both hands simultaneously. The shapes are devised so as not to be readily verbally labeled with names. Witelson (1976) found that the left hand is superior with normal boys, thereby suggesting right hemispheric superiority for this task. When verbal labels are easily applied to the shapes, the right hand becomes more proficient. Since reading also involves spatial skills, such as identifying the various letters and the "look" of a word, it is possible that deficits in spatial processing and in hemispheric specialization for spatial processing might be significant in the etiology of reading retardation.

For her investigation, Witelson (1976) selected children with performance IQs equal to or greater than 85 who were at least one and one-half grades retarded in reading achievement. If they were too young to be this retarded in reading, then they had to be absolute nonreaders. Subjects had no detectable brain damage, sensory problems, or emotional disorders. One hundred and thirteen subjects were included, with a six male to one female ratio. One hundred and fifty-six control children were also included, and the age range of both groups was six to fourteen years. Dichotomous shapes were presented and the subjects had to choose the two shapes from an array.

The dyslexics and controls showed no significant differences in overall accuracy on the dichotic shape task. However, the controls had a left-hand superiority while the dyslexics had no superiority, suggesting a deviation from expected hemispheric superiority in that group. Dyslexics had right-hand scores that were better than those in the normal group. This suggested greater left hemispheric spatial processing in the dyslexic group. In the same paper (Witelson, 1976), dichotic tactile letters were presented to both groups of children, who were to orally report the name of the letter in each hand. Normal children did better with the right hand, while dyslexics did better with the left. Witelson (1976) suggests an abnormality in spatial processing and its lateralization in dyslexics in her work. Lack of a left visual half field superiority for recognition of faces, coupled with relative superiority of the left hand on linguistic dichotic tactile forms was interpreted to suggest that dyslexics may use spatial strategies when the test actually uses both linguistic and spatial skills.

Kinsbourne (1975) suggests that both cognitive and attentional processes may be lateralized. He postulates that each hemisphere has its own cognitive and attention mechanisms and that the attention mechanisms are subject to voluntary control. Problems in hemispheric specialization might lead to the attentional deficits found in many learning-disabled children. These processes, according to Kinsbourne's theory, may be due to difficulties in turning on attentional mechanisms necessary for verbal processing as opposed to deficits in higher cognitive processing of verbal material. Far from explaining all learning problems as a result of difficulties in hemispheric lateralization of attention processes, Kinsbourne (1975) also points out that learning-disabled children may have sequencing problems, characterized by relatively low scores on the object assembly and block design subtests of the WISC-R, and translocation errors in spelling (reversing letters or parts of words). Also, Kinsbourne suggests that a form of developmental Gerstmann syndrome may be found in some learning-disabled children. The symptoms of developmental Gerstmann syndrome include dyscalculia, dysgraphia, right–left confusion, and finger agnosia.

Spellacy and Peter (1978) searched for elements of the developmental Gerstmann syndrome in children with dyscalculia. They found that children with dyscalculia could be either good or poor readers and that generally children who might be considered to have developmental Gerstmann syndrome were not a homogeneous group. It should be pointed out that the sample size was very small (only 14) in this study.

Both the clinical and experimental traditions in neuropsychology have contributed to the growing literature on neuropsychology and learning disabilities. One of the principal conclusions that can be drawn from the literature at this stage is that learning-disabled children form an extremely heterogeneous group. Perhaps as larger and better designed factor-analytic studies are conducted, especially ones with longitudinal follow-up, it will be possible to identify different types of learning disabilities and thereby develop more effective educational and neuropsychological remediations. In addition, this type of progress in forming a nosology of learning disabilities would very likely be useful in guiding experimental research into specific deficits. For example, it may be counterproductive to include all types of learning-disabled children in a test of visual half field information processing when perhaps only certain learning-disabled children show difficulties in the cerebral lateralization of visual–verbal information processing. Recommendations for psychoeducational programming on the basis of neuropsychological assessments are discussed later in this chapter.

SENSORY-PERCEPTUAL HANDICAPS AND NEUROPSYCHOLOGY

The study of exceptional children from a neuropsychological viewpoint can be initiated by studying different sensory modalities and their interrelationships. Chalfant and Scheffelin (1969) reviewed some of the early work on central processing problems in children. This approach allows the investigator or the clinician to focus on adaptive functions such as auditory, visual, or tactile processing. In-depth investigation of each of these areas might reveal very discrete problems. Tallal (1976) has studied auditory perceptual problems in language- and learning-disabled children. She reports that language or auditory sequencing problems were first suggested by Orton (1928) as playing a role in communication disorders. In her own work, using nonverbal operant conditioning techniques, Tallal (1976) examined a group of children with developmental dysphasia. These children were impaired in their ability to perceive the temporal order of auditory stimuli when presented rapidly. In addition, they had difficulty in discriminating sound quality. For these dysphasic children, there was no impairment in their abiity to perceive binary visual, nonverbal stimuli as compared to control children.

Tallal's (1976) work also demonstrated that although children with developmental language delays were incapable of processing nonverbal auditory stimuli at rapid rates, they could do so at slower rates of presentation. Tallal (1976) reviewed studies indicating that vowels and certain consonants are processed differently by normal subjects. The most striking deficits in verbal auditory perception of language-delayed children were obtained when stop-consonants like *ba* and *da* were presented, and this deficit was remediated by use of a speech synthesizer to stretch the duration of consonants.

Wilson, Rapin, Wilson, and Van Denburg (1975) examined neuropsychological functioning in children with hearing impairment both with and without brain damage. Motoric and visual performance deficits were frequent among the brain-damaged, hearing-impaired group. Also, this group had lower mean performance IQ (82.8) than the non-brain-damaged (99.3). Results were in the expected directions for presence versus absence of damage, brain-damaged subjects having a lower mean IQ.

Visual components in reading disorders were at one point the focus of neuropsychological investigators, particularly in the work of such pioneers as Strauss and Lehtinen (1947). More recent literature has tended to move into the area of auditory processing and speech and language related deficits, finding only a minority of LD children to have visual–perceptual problems (Denckla & Rudel, 1976). In Denckla and Rudel's (1976) work, a test of childrens' ability to name object drawings was given to dyslexic and nondyslexic neurologically impaired children and to a control group. These researchers found that nondyslexic children with minimal neurological signs made significantly more wrong-name responses than did either normals or dyslexic subjects. Dyslexics made a relatively high proportion of circumlocutions (e.g., describing the picture but not naming it). Dyslexic children, even when giving a wrong name, tended not to be as remote from the object depicted as the nondyslexic, minimal brain dysfunction group. In general, the dyslexic minimal brain dysfunction subjects had greater difficulty in naming pictured objects and longer response latencies when words occurred less than 30 per million in daily usage. The Denckla and Rudel (1976) study is noteworthy for two reasons. First, it is a landmark in the use of a nondyslexic neurologically impaired control group for comparison with the dyslexic, MBD children. Secondly, it represents a reawakening of interest in visual–verbal information processing in work with learning-disabled chidren.

Ocular–motor variables in reading disorders have been studied by Leisman and Schwartz (1976). They report that attentional handicaps, when associated with reading disorders, can have an important visual component. Children with such impairments may show inconsistent patterns of visual scanning and fixating, and a lack of anticipatory saccades, which are the rapid, flickering eye movements that serve to inhibit visual input. Also, children with attention deficits may have an absence of the expectancy wave normally found in computer-averaged EEG records evoked by pairs of visual stimuli. This suggests that the child with an attention–visual handicap may be unable to expect new visual information in an orderly manner. Leisman and Schwartz (1976) believe that the ocular–motor deficits reflect a more basic defect in inhibitory processes rather than being the primary cause of reading impairments.

Research into tactile processing has already been mentioned in the work of Reed (1967a), who studied lateralized finger agnosia and reading achievement. He found that, at 10 years of age, the group making more right-handed finger localization errors were poorer readers than those making left-handed errors. In addition, Witelson's (1976) work on tactile form recognition, with its implications for hemispheric specialization, has been dicussed at length. Reed's (1967a) and Witelson's (1976) researches are complementary in showing that poor readers differ from controls on tests of tactile processing. Specific findings differed in these two studies because of design and subjects' age differences.

Birch and Belmont (1965) began looking into intersensory integration and reading ability. Children from 5 to 12 years of age were tested on a task that required them to create equivalencies between auditory and visual cues. Using a tapping pattern, the children had to select a matching pattern of visual dots. Birch and Belmont (1965) found that this type of integration increased with age and that the most rapid growth was between kindergarten and second grade. This work on intersensory integration seems to have faltered with the untimely death of Dr. Birch. However, according to Birch and Belmont (1965), in order for a child to learn to read, he must establish correspondences between visual cues such as letters and auditory cues so that he can translate letters into spoken sounds and vice versa.

MENTAL RETARDATION AND NEUROPSYCHOLOGY

Mental retardation may be caused by a wide range of agents, including genetic mutation, physical trauma, metabolic disorders, and genetic disease. These etiologies have in common the fact that they all lead to some form of brain dysfunction. Therefore, one could assume that mental retardation should be as fervently studied from the neuropsychological perspective as is learning disability. Unfortunately, difficulties in administering neuropsychological tests to mentally retarded persons, uncertainties in identifying parts of the brain that may have been damaged in mental retardation syndromes (Benton, 1970), and uncertainty regarding differences between malformation of the brain versus other forms of brain damage, have considerably hampered research efforts in the neuropsychology of mental retardation. However, as Benton (1974) notes, the mentally retarded may show specific deficits or deficit patterns in specific etiologies.

Gordon (1977) suggested that the brains of some mentally retarded persons may be anatomically different than the brains of normals because retardation may be caused by agents other than simple damage. The unknown premorbid state of the mentally retarded person's brain makes it difficult to constitute contrast or control groups for research. Gordon (1977) goes on to suggest that a developmental model would be a logical approach for the study of neuropsychology in mental retardation. This would allow for the same tests to be given at different ages in order to observe developmental changes. However, it should be pointed out that it is difficult to devise such tests that would have an effective range of testing with both very young and rather old subjects or with severely retarded as well as normally intelligent subjects (Benton, 1970).

Gordon (1977) notes that a prime focus for neuropsychological investigations into mental retardation can be the bridging of discrepancies between classifications and behavioral data. Neuropsychological testing can lead to fine grain analysis of cognitive, perceptual, motoric, and sensory skills in the mentally retarded, with profiles of these abilities leading to prescriptions for rehabilitation as well as for multiple base-lining, which allow for the documentation of changes in level of functioning.

Some attempts have been made to make standardized neuropsychological tests more useful with mentally retarded clients. Beach and Davis (1966) studied the relationship between IQ level and proficiency in tests of finger agnosia, finger tapping, and fingertip symbol recognition. A linear relationship was found between four IQ levels and both finger agnosia and finger tapping speed, but no relationship was found with fingertip symbol recognition. Charles Matthews (1974) began to develop a set of norms on neuropsychological tests for use with mentally retarded persons. Using the Halstead–Reitan battery, norms were collected for two age ranges and three IQ ranges. Most of the measures in this study had significant correlations with IQ. Matthews (1974) notes that it would be important to extend his normative data by collecting norms according to etiology of retardation and also for mentally retarded children below the age of 9.

Matthews and Reitan (1961) compared the abstraction ability of mentally retarded persons to hospital patients with cerebral lesions. They used the Categories Test, part of Reitan's Neuropsychological Test Battery, as the measure of abstraction. The neurological patients and the mentally retarded persons had equal IQs. It was found that the retardates made significantly more errors than the neurological contrast group. This was likely due to differing ages of onset of the pathological condition that caused the reduced IQs in the two groups. As a follow-up to this study, Matthews and Reitan (1963) attempted to find out if the mentally retarded have less abstraction proportional to other test scores. Again, using the Categories Test as the measure of abstraction, these investigators found that the mentally retarded subjects with poor abstraction ability did better on tests of immediate problem solving, while those with high abstraction ability did better on stored memory tasks. Thus, in working with mentally retarded persons on neuropsychological tests, even a negative finding such as poor abstraction could lead to appropriate recommendations for educational remediation.

Davis and Reitan (1967) used selected items from the Halstead–Wepman Aphasia Screening Test with 80 mentally retarded persons. Level of performance IQ was highly correlated with the number of constructional dyspraxia items failed by the subject. Verbal IQs could be placed in rank order by the number of aphasic symptoms revealed on the Halstead–Wepman. This study lends concurrent validity to the use of aphasia screening items in assessing the retarded.

John Money (1963, 1973) has conducted research into patterns of deficits in individuals with Turner's syndrome, a chromosomal abnormality associated with mental retardation. In one study (Money, 1963), Turner's syndrome patients were compared with victims of Klinefelter's syndrome, another chromosomal abnormality. WISC or WAIS IQ tests were given to all patients and three quotients were obtained. These included verbal comprehension, perceptual organization, and freedom from distractibility quotients. Perceptual organization was low in Turner's syndrome patients, and there was a shift toward the low range of performance IQ in this same group. In further work, Money (1973) summarized studies noting that Turner's syndrome victims often showed deficits in right–left discrimination and on such tests as the Bender–Gestalt and Benton Visual Retention. In his own work, Money (1963, 1973) showed that object assembly and block design subtests were very low in his sample of Turner's syndrome clients, verbal comprehension was high to average, and performance IQs tended to be low. Money suggested that a right parietal dysfunction could account for the pattern of deficits noted above.

Benton (1970) has summarized some of the experimental neuropsychological work with the mentally retarded. Studies of psychomotor functioning, such as those of Money noted above, have pointed to faulty parietal development and/or apraxia in mentally retarded persons with normal neurological exams. Benton (1970) found that the inability to sustain motor acts, which he termed "motor impersistence," was often seen in right hemispheric, acquired brain damage. He demonstrated this phenomenon in some mentally retarded persons even when IQ was taken into account. Benton (1970) noted that these subjects, for the most part, were suffering from the so-called brain-damaged etiologies of mental retardation. Motor impersistence was associated with a poor prognosis for rehabilitation patients. Additional studies summarized by Benton (1970) include examinations of language functions that have shown that some mentally retarded people have specific expressive or receptive language deficits not predicted on the basis of level of intelligence alone. Benton (1970) makes the special point of noting that some of the specific deficits encountered in mental retardation are often overlooked in favor of IQ scores alone. This, of course, does not do justice to the complicated pattern of intellectual strengths and weaknesses that may be found in some, if not all, mentally retarded persons.

NEUROPSYCHOLOGY AND GIFTED CHILDREN

Giftedness has been variously defined as the possession of special talents or of high measured intelligence. As the reader can probably appreciate from the content of previous sections, neuropsychology has largely been concerned with those exceptionalities of childhood that have negative effects on adaptation. Very little has been written in the area of neuropsychology and the gifted.

In a review of the literature on creativity, Araseth (1968) cites no studies on neuropsychology and gifted children. More recently, investigators have turned their attention to patterns of cerebral dominance and the gifted child. Olson (1978) conducted a pilot study in which gifted subjects and their controls were videotaped while being asked questions of verbal versus spatial content. It was found that gifted children, when they were at the Piagetian level of formal operational thought, diverted their gaze to the right when asked verbal content questions and to the left when asked spatial content questions. Unfortunately, the statistics used did not allow for a test of significance. Children at the concrete operational thought level did not show this visual behavior. Olson (1978) failed to report on the number of subjects, their ages, or other characteristics.

Rekdal (1979) based his study on the theory that eyes move in a contralateral direction to the cerebral hemisphere activated by a task. This author proposed that creative thinkers might be identified by patterns of eye movement, and felt that children who move their eyes to the left during thought might be more creative. He speculated that this phenomenon might be used to identify gifted children. Finally, Kershner (1977) compared 10 reading-disabled children to two groups of children who were good readers, those of average intelligence and those who were intellectually gifted. Tachistoscopic presentation of words to the visual half fields showed that poor readers have greater involvement of the left visual half field in reading or identifying words, while good readers were much superior when identifying words in the right visual half field. There was not a statistically significant difference between the gifted versus nonintellectually gifted readers.

With so few studies in the area, it is safe to say that intellectual or creative giftedness has not received much attention in the neuropsychological literature. A greater understanding of the neuropsychology of these children might help us to better understand deficits encountered in children with disabling conditions.

CLASSICAL NEUROLOGICAL HANDICAPS AND NEUROPSYCHOLOGY

For discussion purposes, the author defines such disorders as cerebral palsy, hemiplegia, epilepsy, and traumatic head injury as classical (i.e., readily observable on neurological exam or associated with history of brain insult). Children with such problems may have remediation requirements distinct from those with learning disabilities and/or mental retardation. In addition, their rehabilitation needs may have similarities with those of the retarded and learning disabled. Neuropsychological investigations in this area have not been nearly so frequent as in the area of learning disabilities, but should prove fruitful for future research. This is so because classical neurological conditions are often associated with known neuropathological findings, times of onset, and expected prognoses. This specificity leads to greater clarity in defining variables independent of the neuropsychological status of the child.

As previously discussed at length, the effects of early versus later incurred brain damage in children differ. Early damage is more easily compensated, but there can be a wider variety of deficits following early insult. Later acquired brain damage is usually more specific in its effects, but the deficits are less recoverable and more severe. Related research has focused on relative severity of neuropsychological deficits in different groups of children with presumed brain damage or dysfunction and on differences between chronic and acute brain damage. For example, Selz and Reitan (1979) compared normal, learning-disabled, and brain-damaged children. Eleven of thirteen tests in their neuropsycholgical test battery discriminated between these groups. Mean scores on the tests tended to fall in decreasing order of control group, learning-disabled group, and brain-damaged group. This investigation demonstrated the usefulness of the Reitan tests in discriminating between these three groups.

Klonoff and Low (1974) studied neuropsychological and EEG correlates of three levels of brain dysfunction in two age groups of children. Subjects were divided into acute brain damage, chronic brain damage, and minimal cerebral dysfunction groups, with each of these three categories futher divided into young children and early adolescent subgroups. Six control groups matched by age and sex were also included. IQ levels of the six clinical groups were significantly less than IQs for their matched control groups. Test–retest data was obtained for the neuropsychological variables. For the younger acutely damaged subjects, there was significant improvement on retesting, but their control subjects improved even more. Similar results were obtained for the older acutely damaged subjects. In cases of the younger chronically impaired group, these children never closed the gap between retests. There were striking differences between experimental and control groups here. Specifically, the older chronically brain-damaged subjects showed less improvement at retesting than did the younger chronically impaired children. The younger children with minimal cerebral dysfunction did not differ much from control subjects, while the older minimal cerebral dysfunction group differed even less than the younger group from their respective controls.

Klonoff and Paris (1974) studied immediate, short term, and residual effects of acute head injuries in younger and older children. Retrograde amnesia was found in 15% of the younger group and 22% of the older group, while anterograde amnesia was found in 47% of the younger children and 72% of the older. Academically, the younger group had about the same percentage of school problems, both pre- and post-trauma, while school problems increased in frequency for the older group. Klonoff, Robinson, and Thompson (1969) used discriminant analysis to statistically separate chronic and aute brain syndrome children on the basis of neuropsychological tests and neurological assessments. The Categories Test was the best discriminator between both the acutely and chronically impaired children and their respective controls.

The aforementioned research clearly establishes the validity of neuropsychological assessment in discriminating between different types of brain damage among children. This parallels some of the work done with adults using the Reitan battery and helps set the stage for further research detailing specific patterns of neuropsychological deficits associated with discrete, medically diagnosed conditions.

One example of such research is the work of the Wilsons on cerebral palsy. In one study (Breakey, Wilson, & Wilson, 1974), sensory and perceptual abilities of cerebral palsied children were assessed. Included were 60 spastic, 60 athetoid, and 60 control subjects, ranging in age from 7 to 21 years. It was found that spastic cerebral palsy was associated with more severe deficits and with a greater number of deficits than was athetoid cerebral palsy. A large percentage of both groups of cerebral palsied children had visual defects and visual–perceptual problems. Also included in this study were measures of somato-sensory functioning, including two-point discrimination ability, stereognosis, depth perception, and limb localization. Visual and perceptual deficits appear to interact in this group of children, as determined by significant correlations between them.

Earlier work with this same sample (Wilson & Wilson, 1967a) revealed that both the spastic and athetoid cerebral palsied did more poorly than control subjects in measures of sensitivity to pressure and two point discrimination. The spastic and athetoid groups did not differ from each other significantly. Wilson and Wilson (1967b) found that spastic and athetoid cerebral palsied children did not differ in their ability to recognize objects using tactile and kinesthetic information alone (stereognosis). Identifying objects as being of the wrong size or of the wrong shape were types of errors that decreased as age increased in both groups.

McFie (1961) has done some research on the effects of hemispherectomy on intellectual functioning in cases of infantile hemiplegia. He found that hemispherectomy occurring before 1 year of age does not result in a loss of speech even when the left hemisphere is removed. However, he did find a limit on the level of intelligence in all instances of hemispherectomy. After 1 year of age, patterns of deficit following hemispherectomy approximate those found in adults (i.e., left hemispherectomy and language disorders, right hemispherectomy and spatial problems).

Annett (1973) investigated childhood hemiplegia and its relationships to both speech and intelligence. Speech difficulties were found in over 40% of the right hemiplegic subjects but in only 14% of the left hemiplegic subjects. It should be noted that this group had many more cases of acquired hemiplegia than that of McFie (1961). In cases of right hemiplegia due to brain trauma before 14 months of age, there was a lower incidence of speech problems. When the damage was acquired later, speech difficulties were found in all but one of the cases of left hemiplegia. In both right and left hemiplegics, Annett (1973) found that the more severely impaired the better hand was, the greater was the percentage of speech problems for both groups. It was also found that verbal–performance IQ differences did not differentiate between the right and left hemiplegic groups. When the better hand was unimpaired in a child, there was a slight but consistent performance IQ advantage for both groups. When the better hand was impaired, however, performance IQ went down noticeably.

One area of neurological disorder that has probably not received deserved attention in neuropsychological research is epilepsy and EEG abnormalities. Although epilepsy is normally diagnosed by the neurologist on the basis of behavioral and EEG characteristics of the patient, there are times when both of these forms of evidence are inconclusive. The present author has encountered numerous cases like this in clinical practice, where neuropsychological test batteries have provided evidence for localized brain dysfunction suggestive of possible epileptic foci. The fine grained analysis of brain–behavior relationships made possible by using neuropsychological tests can therefore give evidence of brain dysfunction, which on medical examination may be subclinical or undetectable.

Tymchuk, Knights, and Hinton (1970) investigated neuropsychological test results in children with normal and abnormal EEGs. Both of the EEG groups had no history of brain damage. These groups were compared to a group that had documented brain lesions. Using a neuropsychological test battery, it was found that the group with known lesions obtained the worst scores and the normal EEG group had the best. Of nine tests that showed significant differences only between the two EEG groups, seven indicated that the normal EEG record group performed at a worse level than the abnormal group. Both of these groups of children had been referred for neuropsychological testing because of behavior or school difficulties. This study showed primarily motoric differences between the children generally. These authors cited several studies that gave support for the paradoxical finding of abnormal EEG with behavioral or school problems associated with better test results. This raises the possibility that a prognosis is better if the child has an abnormal EEG in conjunction with a behavior problem.

Hinton and Knights (1966) studied the neurological and psychological characteristics of children with seizures. These authors summarized typical patterns of deficits found in various types of seizures. Although different patterns were found, for example, in *petit mal* versus atypical seizures, *grand mal,* and other forms of epilepsy, some of these same patterns were also found in children with minimal brain dysfunction and no epilepsy. The results were interpreted to indicate that children with seizures not only have brain dysfunction, but the effects of this dysfunction can be assessed by neuropsychological evaluation. The establishment of different patterns of neuropsychological deficits in various forms of epilepsy may be a valuable contribution to classifying children in the absence of positive neurological findings.

Fedio and Mirsky (1969) studied children with temporal lobe or centrencephalic epilepsy. For the group with centrencephalic epilepsy, the primary deficits were in sustained attention and constructional abilities. Children with left temporal lobe seizures had greater difficulty in the learning and recall of verbal material, while those with right temporal lobe seizures had difficulty in learning and recall of nonverbal material such as complex designs and random shapes. Mean IQ fell within the normal range in this sample, and verbal versus performance IQ discrepancies were in the expected directions for lateralization of the epileptic focus.

NEUROPSYCHOLOGY, PSYCHOTHERAPY, AND SPECIAL EDUCATION

Having discussed the various forms of childhood exceptionality and neuropsychological findings, the question remains as to what can be done to benefit the child. In instances of questionable brain dysfunction or of uncertainties regarding the role of emotional versus neurological factors, the neuropsychologist can play a key role. We have already mentioned the example of questionable epilepsy in the absence of neurologic or electroencephalographic findings. In these instances, neuropsychological test data can help to differentiate between purely behavioral disturbances and those based upon cerebral dysfunction. The neuropsychologist, working on an interdisciplinary basis with colleagues in neurology, may then assist the medical personnel in determining whether or not anti-convulsive medications should be tried.

In psychiatric settings, neuropsychological evaluations are also beneficial. A traditional approach has been to use neuropsychological data to help differentiate between functional disorders and organically based disorders. This approach may actually be quite dangerous to the welfare of a child, because often the diagnosis of "brain damage" may lead to a withdrawal of support services. To lay people and inexperienced professionals alike, this label often carries with it implications of hopelessness and poor prognosis. Instead of this state of affairs, neuropsychological data should be employed as a means to place the child in the most appropriate treatment or rehabilitative setting. If the findings are negative in regard to neuropsychological dysfunction, then continued efforts can be made in traditional psychotherapies, behavior therapy, and related treatment modalities.

On the other hand, should there be positive findings for brain dysfunction, it may still be both justified and necessary to continue in psychologically oriented therapy. However, depending upon the type and extent of neuropsychological deficit(s), psychotherapy may be altered to provide greater structure for the patient and to require less insight on his behalf. In addition, certain types of neuropsychological dysfunction can have behavioral effects that closely parallel psychiatric disorders. For example, depression and frontal lobe injury may at times outwardly take similar appearance. In instances similar to these, the reduced cognitive abilities of the brain-damaged individual should be taken into account by the psychotherapist, and an individualized approach to that client may be devised in conjunction with the neuropsychological consultant. In this manner, counseling, psychotherapy, and supportive services may be adapted to the specific needs of patients with brain dysfunction, be they children or adults.

It is of special importance for the neuropsychologist to be aware that very often the diagnosis of brain dysfunction carries with it the stereotype that counseling or psychotherapy would be inappropriate. However, Rutter (1977) reports that severity of brain damage in children is associated with greater number of psychiatric symptoms, as well as lowered IQ and learning problems. Thus, there is probably a greater need for considering brain-dysfunctional children for inclusion in psychotherapy or behavior therapy programs than is commonly thought.

In addition to the contributions that the neuropsychologist can make as consultant to other psychologists, psychiatrists, and mental health workers, direct impact can be made in the area of special education through the formulation of individualized educational plans based upon the child's neuropsychological profile. Kinsbourne and Caplan (1979) have set forth general principles for choosing remedial programs for the learning disabled. The process begins by establishing the child's learning requirements in terms of his current grade equivalent in academic subjects and by detailing his selective strengths and weaknesses. It is in the latter that neuropsychological assessment can make a valuable contribution. As discussed earlier, learning of academic skills such as reading may be interfered with in many different ways because of different kinds of neuropsychological deficits (Luria, 1973). Patterns of neuropsychological deficits are gradually being recognized in the literature (Schachter, 1976; Doehring, 1968; Mattis *et al.*, 1975). The specific neuropsychological strengths and weaknesses should be taken into account in formulating initial recommendations for educational methods.

Kinsbourne and Caplan (1979) suggest that remedial education take advantage of the child's strengths, rather than attack his or her weaknesses. Following this recommendation, children with auditory processing problems should be more effectively instructed, using a curriculum that stresses visual information. The reverse would be true for the child with visual processing problems. In some instances, the learning-disabled child may reveal weaknesses in both the visual and auditory modalities. In such cases, use of tactile–kinesthetic cues might help where applicable. It should be noted that multisensory approaches and environmental enrichment should not flood the child or bombard him with information, as very often children with learning problems also have attentional deficits. Thus, attention should be successively focused on the different modalities where a multisensory approach is needed (Kinsbourne & Caplan, 1979).

Some neuropsychological research may have direct relevance to the formulation of educational recommendations and methods. For example, Bjorklund, Butter, and Wingis (1978) found that haptic training given to fourth grade students led to fewer errors on a match-to-sample visual problem task. The transfer between haptic (i.e., tactile and kinesthetic processing through the hands) training to visual problem solving lends support to some of the multisensory educational methods. Tallal (1976) used a speech synthesizer to stretch the duration of consonants in spoken language. She found that this seemed to help developmentally dysphasic children in their perception of the temporal order of speech. Finally, Adams (1978) found that bisensory input, using visual and tactile modalities, helped the performance of children with cerebral dysfunction on a visual-form recognition task but did not help a control group without cerebral dysfunction.

The principles involved in neuropsychological recommendations for special educational methods have largely evolved out of work with learning-disabled children. However, the principles may be as appropriately employed in working with the mentally retarded, cerebral palsied, and other neurologically impaired children. In all instances, it will be up to educators to insure that children are taught at their current educational level. Repeat neuropsychological evaluations are warranted as a means to obtain data regarding possible changes in the child's neuropsychological status.

In addition to the benefits of more effective and appropriate educational programming that may result from neuropsychological assessment, other factors may come into play. By using more appropriate (i.e., effective) educational strategies, the child should experience a greater number of successes at school. This may prevent or ameliorate poor self-concepts, depression, and lack of motivation or interest in school. In this manner, some of the emotional symptoms that may be seen in learning-disabled, mentally retarded, and otherwise exceptional children can be controlled, if not prevented, through the use of more effective educational methods.

SUMMARY

A survey of neuropsychological research and practices in the area of exceptional children has been presented. The significant contributions of neuropsychology in this area may be summarized as follows: Neuropsychological theory and methods are leading us toward a broader and deeper understanding of the nature of various learning problems. This understanding is not restricted to conceptualizing developmental problems as being due to irreversible brain damage, but also allows us to appreciate the effects of developmental lags. Neuropsychological reports may assist in the provision of both educational and psychotherapeutic services to exceptional children. The rapid expansion of interest and research in the neuropsychology of developmental disabilities is a hopeful sign for deeper understanding and more effective management of the various problems encountered by these children.

REFERENCES

Adams, J. Visual and tactual integration and cerebral dysfunction in children with learning disabilities. *Journal of Learning Disabilities,* 1978, *2,* 197–204.

Annett, M. Laterality of childhood hemiplegia and the growth of speech and intelligence. *Cortex*, 1973, *9*, 4–33.

Araseth, J. D. Creativity and related processes in the young child: A review of the literature. *Journal of Genetic Psychology*, 1968, *112*, 77–108.

Bakker, D. J., Teunissen, J., & Bosch, J. Development of laterality-reading patterns. In R. M. Knights & D. J. Bakker (Eds.), *Neuropsychology of learning disorders: Theoretical approaches.* Baltimore: University Park Press, 1976.

Bannatyne, A. *Language, reading, and learning disabilities.* Springfield, Ill.: Charles C Thomas, 1976.

Beach, A. H., & Davis, L. J. The relationship between intelligence and sensorimotor proficiency in retardates. *American Journal of Mental Deficiency*, 1966, *71*, 55–59.

Benton, A. L. Neuropsychological aspects of mental retardation. *Journal of Special Education*, 1970, *4*, 3–11.

Benton, A. L. Clinical neuropsychology of childhood: An overview. In R. M. Reitan & L. A. Davison (Eds.), *Clinical neuropsychology: Current status and applications.* Washington, D.C.: V. H. Winston, 1974.

Benton, A. L., & Hecaen, H. Steroscopic vision in patients with unilateral cerebral disease. *Neurology*, 1970, *20*, 1084–1088.

Birch, H. G., & Belmont, L. Auditory–visual integration, intelligence and reading ability in school children. *Perceptual and Motor Skills*, 1965, *20*, 295–305.

Bjorklund, D. F., Butter, E. J., & Wingis, L. Facilitative effects of haptic training on children's visual problem solving. *Perceptual and Motor Skills*, 1978, *47*, 963–966.

Boll, T. J. Behavioral correlates of cerebral damage in children aged nine through fourteen. In R. Reitan & L. A. Davison (Eds.), *Clinical neuropsychology: Current status and applications.* Washington, D.C.: V. H. Winston, 1974.

Breakey, A., Wilson, J. J., & Wilson, B. Sensory and perceptual functions in the cerebral palsied. *Journal of Nervous and Mental Disease*, 1974, *158*, 70–77.

Chalfant, J. C., & Scheffelin, M. A. *Central processing dysfunction in children: A review of research.* Washington, D.C.: U.S. Government Printing Office, 1969.

Davis, L. J., & Reitan, R. M. Dysphasia and constructional dyspraxia items, and Wechsler verbal and performance IQs in retardates. *American Journal of Mental Deficiency*, 1967, *71*, 604–608.

Denckla, M. B., & Rudel, R. G. Naming of object-drawings by dyslexic and other learning disabled children. *Brain and Language*, 1976, *3*, 1–15.

Doehring, D. G. *Patterns of impairment in specific reading disability.* Bloomington, Ind.: Indiana University Press, 1968.

Fedio, P., & Mirsky, A. Selective intellectual deficits in children with temporal lobe or centrencephalic epilepsy. *Neuropsychologia*, 1969, *7*, 287–300.

Goldstein, K. The mental changes due to frontal lobe damage. *Journal of Psychology, Neurology, and Psychiatry*, 1936, *17*, 27–56.

Goldstein, K. *After-effects of brain injuries in war.* New York: Grune & Stratton, 1942

Gordon, J. E. Neuropsychology and mental retardation. In I. Bialer & M. Sternlicht (Eds.), *The psychology of mental retardation.* New York: Psychological Dimensions, 1977.

Gross, K., Rothenberg, S., & Schottenfeld, S. Duration thresholds for letter identification in left and right visual fields for normal and reading-disabled children. *Neuropsychologia*, 1978, *16*, 709–715.

Halstead, W. *Brain and intelligence.* Chicago: University of Chicago Press, 1947.

Hinton, G. G., & Knights, R. M. Neurological and psychological characteristics of one hundred children with seizures. *University of Western Ontario Research Bulletin*, 1966, *57.*

Hiscock, M., & Kinsbourne, M. Selective listening in children. Paper presented at meeting of Canadian Psychological Association, Vancouver, 1977.

Kershner, J. Cerebral dominance in disabled readers, good readers, and gifted children: Search for a valid model. *Child Development*, 1977, *48*, 61-67.

Kimura, D. Functional asymmetry of the brain in dichotic listening. *Cortex*, 1967, *3*, 163-178.

Kinsbourne, M. Cerebral dominance, learning, and cognition. In H. R. Myklebust (Ed.), *Progress in learning disabilities* (Vol. 3). New York: Grune & Stratton, 1975.

Kinsbourne, M., & Caplan, P. J. *Children's learning and attention problems*. Boston: Little, Brown, 1979.

Klonoff, H., & Low, M. Disordered brain function in young children and early adolescents: Neuropsychological and electroencephalographic correlates. In R. M. Reitan & L. A. Davison (Eds.), *Clinical neuropsychology: Current status and applications*. Washington, D.C.: V. H. Winston, 1974.

Klonoff, H., & Paris, R. Immediate, short-term and residual effects of acute head injuries in children: Neuropsychological and electroencephalographic correlates. In R. M. Reitan & L. A. Davison (Eds.), *Clinical neuropsychology: Current status and applications*. Washington, D.C.: V. H. Winston, 1974.

Klonoff, H., Robinson, G. C., & Thompson, G. Acute and chronic brain syndromes in children. *Developmental Medicine and Child Neurology*, 1969, *11*, 198-213.

Knights, R. M. *Smoothed normative data on tests for evaluating brain damage in children*. Ottawa, Canada: Carleton University, 1970.

Knights, R. M., & Hinton, G. G. Minimal brain dysfunction: Clinical and psychological test characteristics. *University of Western Ontario Research Bulletin*, 1967, *56*.

Leisman, G., & Schwartz, J. Ocular-motor variables in reading disorders. In R. M. Knights & D. J. Bakker (Eds.), *Neuropsychology of learning disorders: Theoretical approaches*. Baltimore: University Park Press, 1976.

Lenneberg, E. H. *The effect of age on the outcome of central nervous system disease in children*. New York: Wiley, 1967.

Luria, A. R. *The working brain*. New York: Basic Books, 1973.

Matthews, C. G. Applications of neuropsychological test methods in mentally retarded subjects. In R. M. Reitan & L. A. Davison (Eds.), *Clinical neuropsychology: Current status and applications*. Washington, D.C.: V. H. Winston, 1974.

Matthews, C. G., & Reitan, R. M. Comparisons of abstraction ability in retardates and in-patients with cerebral lesions. *Perceptual and Motor Skills*, 1961, *13*, 327-333.

Matthews, C. G., & Reitan, R. M. Relationship of differential abstraction ability levels to psychological test performance in mentally retarded subjects. *American Journal of Mental Deficiency*, 1963, *68*, 235-244.

Mattis, S. Dyslexia: A working hypothesis that works. In A. L. Benton & D. Pearl (Eds.), *Dyslexia: An appraisal of current knowledge*. New York: Oxford University Press, 1978.

Mattis, S., French, J. H., & Rapin, I. Dyslexia in children and young adults: Three independent neuropsychological syndromes. *Developmental Medicine and Child Neurology*, 1975, *17*, 150-163.

McFie, J. The effects of hemispherectomy on intellectual functioning in cases of infantile hemiplegia. *Journal of Neurology, Neurosurgery, and Psychiatry*, 1961, *24*, 240-249.

Molfese, D., Freeman, R. B., & Palermo, D. S. The ontogeny of brain lateralization for speech and nonspeech stimuli. *Brain and Language*, 1975, *2*, 356-368.

Money, J. Two cytogenic syndromes: Psychologic comparisons in intelligence and specific factor quotients. *Journal of Psychiatric Research*, 1963, *2*, 223-231.

Money, J. Turner's Syndrome and parietal lobe functions. *Cortex*, 1973, *9*, 387-393.

Naidoo, S. *Specific dyslexia*. New York: Wiley, 1972.

Olson, M. B. Visual field usage as an indicator of right or left hemispheric information processing of gifted children. *The Gifted Child Quarterly*, 1978, *12*, 243–247.

Orton, S. T. Specific reading disability: Strephosymbolia. *Journal of the American Medical Association*, 1928, *90*, 1095–1099.

Porter, R. J., & Berlin, C. On interpreting developmental changes in the dichotic right ear advantage. *Brain and Language*, 1975, *2*, 186–200.

Reed, H. B. C., Reitan, R. M., & Klove, H. Influence of cerebral lesions on psychological test performance of older children. *Journal of Consulting Psychology*, 1965, *26*, 247–251.

Reed, J. C. Lateralized finger agnosia and reading achievement at ages six and ten. *Child Development*, 1967, *38*, 213–220. (a)

Reed, J. C. Reading achievement as related to differences between WISC verbal and performance IQ's. *Child Development*, 1967, *38*, 835–840. (b)

Reitan, R. M. Psychological effects of cerebral lesions in children of early school age. In R. M. Reitan & L. A. Davison (Eds.), *Clinical neuropsychology: Current Status and Applications*. Washington, D.C.: V. H. Winston, 1974.

Rekdal, C. K. Hemispheric lateralization, cerebral dominance, conjugate saccadic behavior and their use in identifying the creatively gifted. *The Gifted Child Quarterly*, 1979, *23*, 101–108.

Rourke, B. P. Brain–behavior relationships in children with learning disabilities. *American Psychologist*, 1975, *30*, 911–920.

Rourke, B. P. Reading retardation in children: Developmental lag or deficit. In R. M. Knights & D. J. Bakker (Eds.), *Neuropsychology of learning disorders: Theoretical approaches*. Balimore: University Park Press, 1976.

Rourke, B. P. Neuropsychological research in reading retardation: A review. In A. L. Benton & D. Pearl (Eds.), *Dyslexia: An appraisal of current knowledge*. New York: Oxford University Press, 1978.

Rourke, B. P., & Finlayson, M. A. Neuropsychological significance of variations in patterns of performance on the Trail Making Test for older children with learing disabilities. *Journal of Abnormal Psychology*, 1975, *84*, 412–421.

Rourke, B. P., Dietrich, D., & Young, G. Significance of WISC verbal–performance discrepancies for younger children with learning disabilities. *Perceptual and Motor Skills*, 1973, *36*, 275–282.

Rutter, M. Brain damage syndromes in childhood: Concepts and findings. *Journal of Child psychology and Psychiatry*, 1977, *18*, 1–21.

Satz, P., & Friel, J. Some predictive antecedents of specific reading disability: A preliminary two-year follow-up. *Journal of Learning Disabilities*, 1974, *7*, 437–444.

Satz, P., & Van Nostrand, G. Developmental dyslexia: An evaluation of a theory. In P. Satz & C. Ross (Eds.), *The disabled learner*. Rotterdam: University of Rotterdam Press, 1973.

Satz, P., Bakker, D. J., Teunissen, J., Goebel, R., & Van Der Vlugt, H. Developmental parameter of the ear asymmetry: A multi-variate approach. *Brain and Language*, 1975, *2*, 171–185.

Satz, P., Taylor, H. G., Friel, J., & Fletcher, J. Some developmental and predictive precursors of reading disabilities: A six year follow-up. In A. L. Benton & D. Pearl (Eds.), *Dyslexia: An appraisal of current knowledge*. New York: Oxford University Press, 1980.

Schachter, M. *Neuropsychological and social maladjustment patterns in learning disabled children*. Unpublished doctoral dissertaton, The Ohio State University, Columbus, 1976.

Selz, M., & Reitan, R. M. Neuropsychological test performance of normal, learning disabled, and other brain damaged children. *Journal of Nervous and Mental Diseases*, 1979, *167*, 298–302.

Spellacy, F., & Peter, B. Dyscalculia and elements of the developmental Gerstmann Syndrome in school children. *Cortex*, 1978, *14*, 197–206.

Spreen, O., & Gaddes, W. H. Developmental norms for fifteen neuropsychological tests age six to fifteen. *Cortex,* 1969, *5,* 170–191.

Springer, S. P., & Eisenson, J. Hemispheric specialization for speech in language disordered children. *Neurosychologia,* 1977, *15,* 287–293.

Strauss, A., & Lehtinen, L. *Psychopathology and education of the brain-injured child* (Vol. 1). New York: Grune & Stratton, 1947.

Strauss, A., & Werner, H. Comparative psycho-pathology of the brain-injured child and the traumatic brain injured adult. *American Journal of Psychiatry,* 1943, *99,* 835–888.

Sweeney, J. E., & Rourke, B. P. Neuropsychological significance of phonetically inaccurate spelling errors in younger and older retarded spellers. *Brain and Language,* 1978, *6,* 212–225.

Tallal, P. Auditory perceptual factors in language and learning disabilities. In R. M. Knights & D. J. Bakker (Eds.), *Neuropsychology of learning disorders: Theoretical approaches.* Baltimore: University Park Press, 1976.

Teuber, H. L., & Rudel, R. G. Behavior after cerebral lesions in children and adults. *Developmental Medicine and Child Neurology,* 1962, *4,* 3–20.

Trites, R. L. *Neuropsychological test manual.* Ottawa, Canada: Royal Ottawa Hospital, 1977.

Tsushima, W. T., & Towne, W. S. Neuropsychological abilities of young children with questionable brain disorders. *Journal of Consulting and Clinical Psychology,* 1977, *45,* 757–762.

Tymchuk, A. J., Knights, R. M., & Hinton, G. Neuropsychological test results of children's brain lesions, abnormal EEGs and normal EEGs. *Canadian Journal of Behavioral Science,* 1970, *2,* 322–329.

Wilson, B. D., & Wilson, J. J. Sensory and perceptual functions in the cerebral palsied: Pressure thresholds and two-point discrimination. *Journal of Nervous and Mental Diseases,* 1967, *145,* 53–60. (a)

Wilson, B. D., & Wilson, J. J. Sensory and perceptual functions in the cerebral palsied: Stereopsis. *Journal of Nervous and Mental Diseases,* 1967, *145,* 61–68. (b)

Wilson, J. J., Rapin, I., Wilson, B. C., & Van Denburg, F. V. Neuropsychological functions of children with severe hearing impairment. *Journal of Speech and Hearing Research,* 1975, *18,* 634–652.

Witelson, S. F. Abnormal right hemisphere specialization in developmental dyslexia. In R. M. Knights & D. J. Bakker (Eds.), *Neuropsychology of learning disorders: Theoretical approaches.* Baltimore: University Park Press, 1976.

15

Forensic Issues in Clinical Neuropsychology

ELIZABETH A. McMAHON

Psychologists are being called upon increasingly by courts—criminal and civil—to render opinions on aspects of human behavior that have become relevant to judicial proceedings. A small percentage of the professional community adamantly refuses to be involved in any case with legal ramifications. For another group, who find the forensic area extremely stimulating, challenging, and, hopefully, beneficial to the client and society, this area has become the primary focus of their practice. However, most psychologists, especially neuropsychologists, will find themselves at one time or another on the witness stand swearing to tell "the truth, the whole truth, and nothing but the truth."

This chapter will address those issues felt to be most pertinent in the process that culminates in that telling of "the whole truth." But first, the legal framework within which the process takes place will be described, indicating the similarities, differences, and terminologies of the criminal and civil spheres, and a brief overview will be given of the history of clinical psychology in general vis-à-vis the developing case law.

Then, the areas of interaction for neuropsychologists will be delineated, with the specific questions to which they are asked to respond, looking first at the criminal sphere and then the civil—especially personal injury litigation. The issues will be explored in terms of three facets or tasks: the determination of dysfunction, the determination of the effect of the dysfunction upon the individual, and the determination of prognosis. Finally, some reflections and recommendations will be

---

ELIZABETH A. McMAHON • Private practice, Gainesville, Florida 32601.

offered for neuropsychologists who interact with the legal profession, especially with regard to reports, privileged communication, advocacy, and consultation.

Before beginning, however, a word of explanation. Having written in this general area previously, although assuming readers from somewhat different fields, there is a considerable amount of overlap. Some of the material on the history of psychology within the judicial system and the interaction with the criminal sphere is also part of a chapter in a text on forensic psychiatry (Smith, in press). Most of the section concerning personal injury evaluation—the dysfunction, the effects of the dysfunction, and the prognosis—and the sample courtroom dialogue appeared in a previous chapter as well (McMahon & Satz, 1981).

After reviewing the material, the decision was made that, except for minor editing and incorporating a number of more recent studies, no attempt would be made to alter what had been written. The reasons for this are two: either the material itself is factual/historical, or it expresses the views of this author regarding how neuropsychologists should conduct themselves vis-à-vis the legal arena and why—views based on training and several years of experience, views that have not changed since they were previously enunciated.

All trial law is divided into two parts—criminal and civil. "Criminal law is that branch or division of law that treats of crimes and their punishments" (Black, 1968, p. 449). Civil law is "an adversary proceeding of declaration, enforcement, or protection of a right, redress, or prevention of a wrong. . . . [It is] every action other than a criminal action" (Black, 1968, p. 312). Although any trial, hearing or negotiation—whether criminal or civil—is an adversary proceding and all have the same essential structure, there are some important differences in terminology and rules of procedure.

First, the similarities: any adversary proceeding consists of two sides, each represented by an attorney. There is always a liability issue to be decided and, perhaps, a second issue to be weighed. The decisionmaker or trier of fact is the jury or the judge, if a jury is not present.

Next, the differences: In a criminal action, the two sides consist of the State, represented by the prosecutor or state's attorney, and the defendant who is accused of a crime or statutory infraction, represented by defense counsel. The issues to be decided are liability—did the defendant, in fact, commit that act which is alleged?—and then, possibly an issue of his/her responsibility for the behavior. The trier of fact is mandated to reach a decision on the basis that the evidence presented leads to a given conclusion "beyond and to the exclusion of every reasonable doubt"—that is, beyond the degree of doubt that would be formed in the mind of "a reasonable man."

In a civil action, the two sides consist of the plaintiff—the one who is claiming the protection of a right, redress, or prevention of a wrong—and the defense, who may be an individual, a private business, a public corporation, a government organization, or any other legal entity. The issues to be decided are liability (has a right been abridged or would it be if a particular event were to occur) and damages. Damages have to do with the redress of a wrong that has been determined to have occurred, and are essentially two types: (1) actual or compensatory—the "real, substantial and just damages, or the amount awarded to a complaintant in compensation for his actual and real loss or injury"; and (2) exemplary or punitive:

> Damages on an increased scale, awarded to the plaintiff over and above what will barely compensate him for his . . . loss, where the wrong done to him was aggravated by circumstances of violence, oppression, malice, fraud, or wanton and wicked conduct on the part of the defendant, and are intended to solace the plaintiff for mental anguish, lacertion of his feeling, shame, degradation, or other aggravations of the original wrong, or else to punish the defendant for his evil behavior or to make an example of him. (Black, 1968, p. 467)

Finally, the trier of fact is mandated to reach a decision on the basis of the "preponderance of evidence"—meaning that the evidence presented by one side is weightier than that presented by the opposing side.

This is no more than a "bare bones" description of the two major divisions of trial law. The Report of the Task Force on the Role of Psychology in the Criminal Justice System (1978) has stated: "Psychologists who work in the criminal justice system, as elsewhere, have an ethical obligation to educate themselves in the concepts and operations of the system in which they work" (1978, p. 405). Because of the serious ramifications of reports and testimony—and the resulting decisions—for the parties involved, professionally and ethically it is incumbent upon the psychologist to apprise him/herself of the relevant legal issues, questions, criteria, and so forth, for each case with which he/she is involved. This point will be addressed more fully below.

HISTORY

Turning now to a brief look at the historical context of psychologists in the courtroom, three points need to be made at the outset. One, case law has spoken to the issue of the role of clinical psychologists in general in the courtroom rather than to the subspecialty of clinical neuropsychologists. Two, most of the case law with regard to psychologists as expert witnesses has been in the field of criminal law. And three, there are few published cases in point relative to psychologists. However, as Louisell (1955) pointed out 25 years ago: "Of course the paucity of published cases involving psychologists as expert witnesses is not a certain indication of the extent to which they presently are functioning as such in the trial courts" (p. 238).

Generally, cases have focused on the psychologist's competence to assess/diagnose insanity. Thus, in *People v. Hawthorne* (1940), one of the earliest reported decisions, the trial court sustained an objection to a psychologist as an expert on this issue. In its reversal, the appellate court stated it did not think that the psychologist's

> ability to detect insanity is inferior to a medical man whose experience along such lines is not so intensive (p. 23). . . . There is no magic in particular titles or degrees and, in our age of intense specialization, we might deny ourselves the use of the best knowledge available by a rule that would immutably fix the educational qualifications to a particular degree. (p. 25)

Two of the earliest federal court cases involving psychological testimony were somewhat notorious. The treason trial of *U.S. v. Chandler* (1947) and the second trial of Alger Hiss (*U.S. v. Hiss*, 1950) both allowed psychologists to offer expert opinions—in the former regarding insanity and in the latter regarding the psychopathic personality.

A 1954 tort case, *Hidden v. Mutual Life Insurance Company* (1954), concerned the permanent disability clauses of two life insurance policies. The trial court excluded the testimony of a psychologist with considerable experience in his field on the grounds that he was not qualified as an expert in the area of disabling nervous conditions. However, on appeal the court held that

> the uncontradicted testimony tended to show that the expert was qualified in his field by academic training and by experience and also that the objective tests which he described, although perhaps not well known to the general public, were recognized as helpful by medical experts. (p. 821)

In most cases where the psychologist's competence to offer expert tetimony has been litigated, it has been decided in favor of the psychologist (*In Re Masters*, 1944; *Watson v. State*, 1954; *State v. Donahue*, 1954; *People v. McNichol*, 1950; *Doherty v. Dean*, 1960). In a few cases, it has not. In some of these, the issue itself was challenged (*State v. Gibson*, 1954; *Dobbs v. State*, 1935; *People v. Spigno*, 1957), and in others the credentials of the particular psychologist were the reason for the objection (e.g., *State v. Padilla*, 1959). Where the issue has been challenged, the contention has revolved around the qualifications of psychologists to testify as expert witnesses in matters of mental and emotional pathology and, more narrowly, their qualifications to testify as to their conclusions rather than being limited to reciting test results.

The landmark case of *Jenkins v. U.S.* (1962) aired this entire question thoroughly. In this instance, with insanity being the sole defense to three criminal charges, the trial court instructed the jury to disregard the testimony of three defense psychologists on the grounds that a psychologist is not competent to give an opinion as to mental disease or defect. The appellate court reversed the decision, remanded the case for a new trial, and ruled in favor of psychologists as expert witnesses. The government then filed a petition for a rehearing before the entire appellate court with the point of law being the validity of the expert testimony of psychologists.

Amicus curia briefs were filed by both the American Psychological Association and the American Psychiatric Association. Subsequently, the United States Court of Appeals for the District of Columbia Circuit sitting *En Banc* rendered a 7–2 opinion upholding the view that psychologists may qualify as experts in matters relating to the existence and effects of mental disorders under certain standards. The court held in part:

> The critical factor in respect to admissibility is the actual experience of the witness and the probable probative value of his opinion. The trial judge should make a finding in respect to the individual qualifications of each challenged expert. Qualifications to express an opinion on a given topic are to be decided by the judge alone. The weight to be given any expert opinion admitted in evidence by the judge is exclusively for the jury. They should be so instructed. (Hock & Darley, 1965, p. 650)

The holding in the Jenkins case names the exclusion of testimony by a qualified psychologist on this issue reversible error, and most subsequent cases have followed or affirmed the holding. While the majority of these cases deal with criminal matters, Redmount (1974) points out that "the psychological issues and evaluations in mental disturbance or disorder in tort matters are very similar and sometimes identical" (p. 82). For example, in a frequently cited case, *Reese v. Naylor* (1969), an action for personal injuries arising from an automobile accident, the court held that

> a clinical psychologist once qualified as an expert witness by reason of education, training, and experience is competent to testify as to his diagnosis of a person's mental condition based on the use of the devices and techniques ordinarily resorted to by such practitioners. (p. 490)

AREAS OF INTERACTION

What, then, are the points of interaction—between a neuropsychologist and the judicial system—that might lead to being qualified as an expert witness? First of all, it should be emphasized that, with the exception of a malpractice suit, it is extremely rare that neuropsychologists have anything to contribute with regard to the liability phase of a proceeding—that is, did a given act occur or is a given individual at fault for an event? Those are issues of fact and almost always outside the purview of professional opinion. Where we can offer assistance is in the areas of responsibility, damages, comprehension of proceedings, and so forth.

Within the criminal sphere, most frequently the questions relate to competency to stand trial and/or insanity at the time of the offense. However, there are several other very challenging points that are sometimes raised, such as an individual's ability to comprehend the Miranda Warning and knowledgeably waive his right to counsel and/or remain silent, the validity of a reported confession, the likelihood of a specific degree of intent, the presence of factors that might bear on mitigation of sentencing, and the ability of a defendant to understand the ramifications of plea negotiations.

A word of caution is in order. It is extremely rare that the neuropsychological examination, in and of itself, can respond to any of these questions completely, or that cortical dysfunction is a total explanation or sufficient, by itself, for a defense. Certainly there are instances in which it is a major contributing factor, but an individual may evidence severe brain dysfunction and still not meet the legal criteria associated with the issues enumerated above. In most cases, the eventual conclusion is based on considerations in addition to the dysfunction itself—for example, the type of trial that can be anticipated, the ability of the attorney to assist a client through the process, the sophistication of the requisite intent, the setting and circumstances in which rights were waived or a confession was given, and so on.

Consider, for example, the question of competency to stand trial. A young man who was accused of arson and homicide was found to have severely impaired perceptive and expressive language functioning. He could, in the quiet and solitude of his cell or an interview room, "discuss" the facts of the event and various aspects of his case with his attorney. However, the examiner was of the opinion that he could not comprehend the proceedings of a complex and highly emotionally charged trial process, could not challenge prosecution witnesses adequately, and could not testify in his own defense—especially under pressure.

Again, a young man who had suffered repeated cortical insults with resulting language deficits was subjected to intense questioning by four people over a period of several hours. Unable to perceive the subtle varations in wording and nuances in meaning, undoubtedly enhanced by his childlike desire to please others, he eventually confessed to a homicide that he most probably did not commit. The Miranda Rights formula, as presently worded, requires a fifth-grade level of comprehension of the spoken word in order to understand it fully. Some defendants do not have this due to mental retardation, educational deprivation, and/or cortical deficits in the areas of language processing functions. If they are also unsophisticated with respect to arrest and booking procedures, they may consent unknowingly to a situation that will place them in legal jeopardy later.

But, one must be most careful. There are individuals who are extremely limited cognitively, and who might well be incompetent to manage their financial affairs satisfactorily, or even their life generally, but who are competent to proceed through the judicial system. The reason for this is that, because of their lifestyle and their history, they have had a great deal of contact with law enforcement and the courts. Therefore, the area in which they are perhaps *most* competent is that of criminal justice. They still might not be able to understand a fast-paced jury trial, but they are perfectly competent to enter into plea negotiations and may be able even to participate in a nonjury trial.

When functioning within the sphere of criminal law, one must be absolutely certain of the legal standards/criteria that are being used with regard to competency, insanity, mitigating circumstances for sentencing, and so forth. For example, the standard used for insanity in federal courts, the American Law Institute standard, is different from the M'Naughten Rule, which is used in most state courts. Even with the standard firmly in mind, there are times when the opinion is a very difficult one to render and is given only after hours of anguished deliberation.

For example, a young man had been involved in an accident wherein he sustained a major head injury. Subsequent to this, he evidenced a severe posttraumatic syndrome in addition to the cortical dysfunction, and both he and others related various and consistent personality changes. During the period of recovery, he allegedly killed an acquaintance. After an intensive evaluation of his neuropsychological and personality functioning, interviews with his parents, and then repeat interviews with him, it was the examiner's opinion that, although he was still evidencing cortical deficits, he did not meet the criteria for legal insanity. By the same token, it was also the examiner's opinion that the entire tragic event would never have occurred had it not been for the head injury. Thus, in this particular instance, the data was useful to the trier-of-fact only with regard to the question of mitigation of sentencing.

Again, the neuropsychologist is not as frequently involved in criminal matters as in civil. This is not to say that criminal defendants are not neuropsychologically impaired—many of them are. Because the highest incidence of head injuries occurs in young adult males, which is also the group most frequently charged with criminal acts, it stands to reason there would be a considerable overlap. But, as mentioned earlier, cortical dysfunctioning is rarely, if ever, a total defense or a complete explanation—not that it is impossible, only that it is extremely rare.

The area of trial law where the neuropsychologist has, perhaps, the most to offer the trier-of-fact is that of civil law—most especially the three broad areas of (1) Workman's Compensation, (2) disability determination, and (3) personal injury litigation. While both Workman's Compensation hearings and disability— or, conversely, competency—determinations are adversary proceedings, they are usually less formal than a trial and the issues are more narrowly formulated. In Workman's Compensation cases, the questions generally focus on the nature and extent of the injury, whether it is permanent or temporary, and, if the individual cannot return to his/her former employment, what, if any, type of retraining is feasible. However, the examination that is required to respond to these questions competently is essentially the same as that for disability determination and personal injury litigation and will be discussed later.

In disability/competency determinations, the possibility of issues is myriad—

from competency to manage one's own financial and daily living affairs to competency to continue or return to the practice of one's profession (e.g., law, medicine, dentistry, education, commercial flying, to name a few). Needless to say, such evaluations can never be conducted in a vacuum. The examiner must have *extensive* information concerning the tasks the client is expected to perform, the level of decision making that is required, the stresses and pressures that accompany these duties, and so forth. Certainly a decision that results in a license being revoked or reinstated or a member of the judiciary being suspended or returned to the bench—with all the implications and ramifications that this holds for the individual as well as for the scores of people who will be affected—demands the maximum amount of data obtainable.

The third broad area of civil law—personal injury litigation—is the most cogent for the forensic neuropsychologist and the arena where they will most frequently be found. It is that area calling for the fullest presentation of the client— strengths as well as weaknesses—and where the psychologist has the opportunity and obligation to render the most extensive picture of any deficits, how they affect the individual, and what is a reasonable prognosis. This is not to imply that such issues are of no concern in Workman's Compensation and disability hearings. They are, and one must be prepared to address them. But they are not and cannot be the primary focus. That is, what effect a deficit that interferes with professional goals may have on the overall functioning of the individual must be of secondary import when the individual is, for instance, a neurosurgeon and the question concerns his competency to practice!

In personal injury litigation, by contrast, such issues are extremely important, comprise a major portion of the "damages" phase of a trial, and may, in fact, be the area where the clinical neuropsychologist's expertise is most unique and valuable to the court. Thus, one can conceptualize the tasks of the neuropsychologist as being three: (1) determination of the dysfunction; (2) determination of the effect of the dysfunction; and (3) determination of the prognosis and/or a plan of rehabilitation.

DETERMINATION OF THE DYSFUNCTION

What is necessary to the determination of the dysfunction itself? There are at least three major requirements for addressing this task. First is a thorough knowledge of neuroanatomy and higher human brain functioning. The relationship between the brain and behavior is highly complex and intricate, and much of it yet remains beyond our present understanding. But certain broad principles have been delineated and are particularly useful. For example, it has been established that mental processes, defined in behavioral terms, are the result of different functional brain systems working in concert with each other (Luria, 1973). By the same token, discrete mental operations may be disrupted by lesions confined to circumscribed functional brain systems. Further, "there is seldom an isomorphic relationship between cerebral structure and behavior . . . age, maturation, learning, and personality variables all mediate the behavioral manifestations of brain damage" (Wedding & Gudeman, 1980, p. 33). Thus, one must be thoroughly grounded in the anatomy of the brain as well as in how complex adaptive behaviors are affected by other processes and how they may be altered following injury or disease to the brain.

A second requirement is premorbid data. One cannot responsibly assess brain dysfunction in a vacuum—one cannot assess a loss or a deficit without knowing the premorbid level of functioning, without knowing what abilities were present before the alleged loss occurred. Frequently, premorbid data can be obtained from records, particularly school records that often contain results of previous IQ or achievement testing as well as academic grades, employment records, and military records. If these are not available, one can often estimate these data from an initial interview with inquiries concerning highest grade completed in school, type and length of employment, hobbies, leisure time activities, reading material, and so on. Also, information should be sought from family members, employers, co-workers, and other appropriate persons. Whatever the source, such premorbid data are essential—both for comparative purposes to assess loss and for the purpose of formulating a prognosis. One must, at the same time, be *most* cautious regarding selfserving statements and evaluate carefully the compatibility of independently rendered accounts of the client's premorbid level of functioning—especially where litigation is pending.

A third crucial element is, of course, the test battery itself. Whether one uses a standard battery or one modified for specific tasks, the purposes are the same— the understanding of neuropsychological deficits and the validity of these test/ pattern signs. Also the battery must utilize standardized procedures for data collection and include tasks that assess a broad sample of behavior. As Lezak (1976) points out, any battery must meet the criteria of suitability, practicality, and usefulness.

> A suitable battery provides an examination that is appropriate to the patient's needs, whether they call for a baseline study, differential diagnosis, rehabilitation planning, or any other type of assessment. . . . A practicable battery is relatively easy to administer and has inexpensive equipment. . . . A useful battery provides the information the examiner wants. (p. 439)

By the same token, a battery is only a tool and is only as good as the examiner employing it. As stated above, the evaluation must include tests that are valid and an examiner who is sufficiently trained to interpret these tests within the broader context of adaptive functioning. As brought out by Wedding and Gudeman (1980):

> Test behavior, in the hands of a *skilled* and *experienced* psychologist, can be pieced together in such a way as to provide considerable information concerning the nature of the process occurring in cases of brain damage (e.g., multiple sclerosis, vascular disorders, trauma, etc.) the site of neoplastic lesions, and the acuteness or chronicity of the disorder. (p. 32, emphasis added)

In order to accomplish this, the investigation must begin with a general evaluation of various aspects of mental activity and then proceed to a more focused assessment of specific neuropsychological functions. Based on the pattern that emerges in the more general, preliminary examination, the investigator must attempt to identify both broad and specific impairments, if any, and to delineate ways in which the patient may be circumventing these impairments. Functions that remain intact should, of course, be pointed out also. Additional tests—supplemental to one's basic battery—may be needed to tease out such information. Needless to say, this step is more complex and demands more flexibility, individualization, and qualitative diagnostic acumen. The ultimate goal, here, is the identification of impairment, how it is manifested in behavior, and how it may affect other mental and adaptive processes.

The need for extensive evaluation and thorough documentation of each of these points cannot be stressed too strongly, especially where they are a matter of legal issue. In clinical practice, we frequently accept the notion of a need for treatment without demanding a great deal of supporting data—the hypothesis being that such treatment will most probably be helpful to the patient and least probably harmful. This hypothesis, however, does not apply to the legal field. Where issues of liability, responsibility, damages, and monetary compensation are at stake, the court has the right as well as the obligation to demand a more stringent degree of probability accompanying opinions from those experts who are proposing both the presence of deficits and the need for treatment. Therefore, one is required to document extensively whatever deficits may be present and whatever treatment is recommended.

Another point to be considered is the time of the examination. If the question relates to the presence of damage and the immediate ramifications to the patient, then the examination should be conducted as early in the posttrauma period as possible. Also at this time, there may be the request and/or opportunity to provide a treatment plan to facilitate rehabilitation. Furthermore, one has a baseline from which to measure recovery. However, in view of the fact that resolution of brain trauma continues for a period of 18 to 24 months, it is *most* important to refrain from any statements regarding permanent/residual deficits until after such time has elapsed. Then, a reevaluation is needed for prognostic purposes, taking several broader issues into account. This will be discussed more thoroughly in the section on prognosis.

One final note: Occasionally, the evaluator will subsequently become the primary therapist. Should this occur, two points need to be kept in mind. One is the need for detailed notes regarding progress in treatment, obstacles, events that facilitate or retard the recovery process, and so forth. If the case is still in litigation, these are all pertinent issues to which one will be required to respond. Because civil suits often take three to five years to reach trial or settlement, it would be foolish to attempt to rely on one's memory for the information. Secondly, in therapy, many facets of the patient's life that are extraneous to the legal issues may arise. These can present points of confusion with regard to confidentiality (to be discussed in the final section). One solution may be to have a colleague serve as the therapist while the evaluator remains cognizant of and ultimately responsible for that portion relating to rehabilitation from the actual trauma.

DETERMINATION OF THE EFFECT OF THE DYSFUNCTION

As stated above, it is in personal injury litigation that broader questions are entertained—questions relating to what a particular impairment *means* to this particular individual, how it affects the quality of his/her life and overall functioning, what effect it has upon family members, and so on. It is here that the clinical neuropsychologist orchestrates data from many sources to present to the court as complete a picture as possible of the client as an individual—with strengths and weaknesses, neuropsychological and psychological. As so cogently stated by Wedding and Gudeman (1980); "The most exquisite method of determining the location of a tumor will not reveal the extent of functional deficit nor will it assist in determining what training methods will be most beneficial in helping the brain-injured individual" (p. 33).

In order to address oneself to these broader issues, one must have a thorough knowledge of and familiarity with the principles of personality development, psychopathology, and adjustment. All too frequently, psychologists from nonclinical disciplines have been observed rendering opinions regarding neuropsychological deficits without attempting to integrate these findings into the broader context of personality dynamics and damages. Failure to consider these more extensive issues could render a disservice not only to the court, which must rule on legal points, but to the patient, who must cope with the handicaps caused by the trauma.

What appears to be, essentially, the same deficit incurred by two individuals may, in fact, have very different ramifications for each. For example, two young men of approximately the same age each sustained left temporal lobe contusions— one as a result of an automobile accident and the other as a result of an accident at work in which he was struck by a falling tree. Neurological studies were similar on each, and they both evidenced similar patterns of deficits on the neuropsychological evaluation. However, the first individual was a very bright young man with college degrees in Philosophy and English. He evidenced a "catastrophic reaction" to the verbal dysfluency that accompanied his verbal memory loss and Brocca's aphasia. The other young man, by comparison, had dropped out of school at the first opportunity and had subsequently established an excellent employment history as a manual laborer. His residual difficulties in verbal memory and expressive speech were inconsequential, in his view, and his only concern was to return to work at the earliest permissible date.

While this example is a dramatic one, the principle is applicable across cases: Each individual reacts to a deficit uniquely. This uniqueness is a function of his/ her personality structure, prior adjustment, level of aspiration, coping skills, defense mechanisms, past experiences, present situations, support systems, and so forth—each of which *must* be explored and evaluated in order to assess the context in which the specific deficit occurs. Thus, there is no such thing as a neuropsychological evaluation, *per se,* with rare exception. Rather, the task is to evaluate a *person* who has experienced an injury that may be specific or general, mild or severe, keeping in mind that his/her reaction to the deficit is only partially dependent on the type and severity of the trauma itself.

Of equal importance with the test material as a source of data is the psycho-diagnostic interview, not only with the patient but also with family and/or others who can shed light on both past and current functioning. Certainly one looks first to the patient for an explanation of how an injury has affected his/her life, and frequently much information is available at this level—but not always. For instance, a young man who, following an automobile accident, suffered such severe residual antereograde memory loss that he described his life as "waking up to a brand new world every morning," was unable to express (retrieve) the full impact of this condition on his current life situation.

A related area that requires considerable caution and thorough investigation is that of severe right hemisphere trauma. These patients will frequently state they are "okay" or "much better"—even with obvious physical disabilities—when, in fact, they behave emotionally in a "zombie" or childlike manner in their interactions with others. Thus, while some individuals overendorse or exaggerate problems, others underendorse or deny them. Nevertheless, these aspects, although perhaps not as quantifiable, are most important when one is assessing damages in personal injury litigation, and they must be thoroughly explained.

A brief word is in order concerning the phenomenon of the posttraumatic syndrome, which is commonly seen following head trauma. This symptom complex—characterized by depression, memory impairment, emotional lability, excessive fatigue, and irritability—is highly controversial with respect to its occurrence and its etiology. Adverse premorbid personality traits and low intellectual capacity have been implicated in explaining, at least in part, some of the symptoms. However, there seems to be no clear relation between the pattern of symptoms and the severity of the brain injury. Thus it is not surprising to find considerable speculation and continual controversy with regard to underlying causation, with organic and psychological factors alternately gaining the greater attention. As Trimble (1981) observes:

> There is often great difficulty in reality in demonstrating a cause and effect relationship between accident and injury symptoms, and usually all that can be shown is some statistical relationship of increased probability between two factors, certain proof being unattainable. Since . . . there is little definitive knowledge of the origins of neurosis, it is not surprising that proof of the relationship between trauma and consequent neurosis is often a matter of vigorous argument. The fact that causality in law has a different emphasis from scientific causality leads to the illogical position that although cause–effect relationships are theoretically universal, judicial causation differs from one country to the next, implying that causality is relative to the country in which a person lives and not related to material phenomena. (pp. 131–132)

In addition, there is a concept in law known as the "cracked vase" principle, the thrust of which is that one "takes the victim as he finds him." Therefore, in personal injury litigation, and especially with respect to such issues as the post-traumatic syndrome, the neuropsychologist is frequently queried as to whether a given symptom is evidenced by an individual to a greater or lesser degree as a result of his/her prior level of functioning. This, again, points out the necessity for premorbid data. However, there are cases in which, even with such data, it is most difficult, or perhaps impossible, to offer an opinion on this question. At such times, the expert should not hesitate to inform the court that he/she does not know, and why, or to couch his/her opinion in whatever conditions, qualifications, or probability statements are needed to reflect the lack of certainty.

Another issue often addressed in personal injury litigation is that of mental pain and suffering or mental pain and anguish—a confusing area in which multiple definitions of the word "pain" are used. Schribner (in Hoffman, 1975) defines pain, medically, as a "localized sensation of distress or agony, caused by stimulation of particular sensory nerve endings" (p. 279), generally associated with tissue damage. Although the quality of the sensation is essentially subjective in nature, it is recoverable under general damages and Workman's Compensation. A neuropsychologist can speak *only* to *report* of pain by the patient and the effect that perception has on the patient's life. Neuropsychologists are *not* competent to speak to the presence of pain itself, its compatibility with the injury, it's severity, and so forth. That is within the purview of the medical profession only.

Mental pain and anguish is generally viewed, psychologically, as stress—"the effects of external influences upon the human mind and body" (Wasmuth, 1957, p. 7). As such, it may occur independent of any physical injury—in fact, independent of any impact—and is assessable by psychological, rather than neuropsychological, techniques. Mental anguish, then, is essentially a legal form and is defined as follows:

> When connected with a physical injury . . . includes both the resultant mental sensation of pain and also the accompanying feelings of distress, fright and anxiety. In other connections, and as a ground for damages or an element of damages, it includes the

mental suffering resulting from the excitation of the more poignant and painful emotions, such as grief, severe disappointment, indignation, wounded pride, shame, public humiliation, despair, etc. (Black, 1968, p. 137)

As with physical pain and suffering, the area of mental pain and anguish or stress is an extremely difficult one to assess, and there is a great deal of latitude for false testimony. In some states, there has been an effort to reduce what are considered abuses in this area by removing the issue entirely from consideration in litigation resulting from automobile accidents. At the same time it seems that it is being put forth increasingly in malpractice suits, in litigations concerning expected level of safety provided when an assault/rape has occurred, and in the myriad of incidents in which the Delayed Stress Response Syndrome of the Viet Nam veterans has been thought to be a factor.

On the one hand, there are fairly consistent sequelae to any perceived loss, whether of a loved one, an aspect of self-concept, employment, status, physical or mental ability, level of functioning, and so on. The presence and extent of these sequelae are assessable by psychological methods. On the other hand, they do tend to abate somewhat with the natural course of events and, therefore, the closer in time to the traumatic event that the patient can be evaluated, the better able the psychologist is to speak to these effects. Any consideration of permanency would, of course, require a later examination.

Here, again, it is necessary to note the disparate ways in which patients with unilateral brain injury react. The depression and agitation often experienced by those with left hemisphere lesions are most obvious. By contrast, those with right hemisphere lesions are less likely to evidence signs of emotional distress. If anything, these patients more commonly reveal a lack or denial of affect, which is striking in view of the cognitive deficits that often exist (Gasparrini, Satz, and Heilman, 1978; Heilman and Valenstein, 1980; Ley & Bryden, 1978). The signs of emotional distress are more readily observed in the families of these patients than in the patients themselves. The neuropsychologist must be prepared to explain how damages in this latter instance might be parodoxically present.

A final note with regard to the issue of pain and suffering concerns those cases in which the spouse of a seriously injured individual files a joinder suit for damages as a result of his/her loss of consortium. In such cases, the neurosychologist must be prepared to address not only the question of behavioral impairment and how it affects the patient, if at all, but also how it affects one's ability to offer "company, cooperation, affection, and aid. . . . in every conjugal relation" (Black, 1968, p. 382) to one's spouse. It is not infrequent in cases involving severe head trauma, often followed by prolonged loss of consciousness, that residual, permanent deficits involve not only cognitive and motoric functions but dramatic personality changes as well. In such cases, spouses describe their homelife as, "It is like having another child in the house." Assessment of the psychological effect of this type of situation upon the spouse is a very real part of the neuropsychologist's role in personal injury litigation.

Finally, mention should be made of two possible complicating factors—hysteria and malingering. As described by Alarcon (1973), the "changing faces" of hysteria have moved from the gross somatic symptoms, unexplainable on an organic basis, to the simulation of finer psychiatric symptoms. The comment has been made that 40 years ago, hysterical patients walked into the courtroom on crutches; now they walk in with a bottle of Valium. In any event, hysteria is still the "great simulator."

However, several essential features of hysteria can be delineated: (1) a discrepancy between symptoms as reported and the findings on examination; (2) "the presence of signs which cannot originate from nervous system disease or trauma; (3) patterns of disorder that plainly arise from mental dispositions . . . (and) reflect the subject's notions about his bodily arrangements and functions" (Walshe in Woolsey & Goldner, 1976, p. 301); and (4) a frequent lack of anxiety or concern regarding the physical disability itself. Points three and four require a particular explanation by means of a thorough psychological evaluation and diagnostic interview to determine if the patient has a personality structure that would give rise to hysterical symptoms, and to ascertain if there is any element of secondary gain—financial, emotional, or social.

In conjunction with this, an excellent article by Stern (1977) addresses the interaction of the lateralization of lesions and the presence of conversion reactions. He puts forth the hypothesis that the right hemisphere is particularly involved in the mediation of affectively or motivationally determined somatic symptoms. While not suggesting that hysteria is present only in conjunction with right hemisphere damage, it does appear that there is a high incidence in cases of right-sided lesions.

Hysterical conversion is viewed by the courts as a reasonable sequel to injury. However, a point very frequently raised is the extent to which the particular act or event for which the plaintiff is seeking redress is, in fact, a proximate cause of the disability. The alternative explanation is that the plaintiff's present condition is, to a greater extent, due to a pre-existing weakness. This latter alternative is supported to some degree by the fact that only a small percentage of physical injury victims actually develop psychological sequelae. Again, the need for premorbid data, in order to address this issue, is paramount. By the same token, even the identifiable presence of a predisposition does not relieve the defendant of responsibility since, as stated above, one must "take the victim as he finds him."

If distinguishing between true symptoms and hysteria is difficult, distinguishing between hysteria and malingering approaches the impossible. Malingering

> includes the simulation of diseases or disability which is not present; the much commoner gross exaggeration of minor disability; the conscious and deliberate attribution of a disability to an injury or accident that did not in fact cause it, for personal advantages. (Miller & Cartlidge, 1972, p. 580)

Conscious and deliberate are the big terms here. It has even been said that the hysteric deceives him/herself unconsciously, while the malingerer deceives others with conscious intent. One finds the dual issues of degree of consciousness and context (possible social, emotional, or financial gain) discussed repeatedly in both the psychological and legal literature on this point. However, since gain, or the anticipation of it, is present in both hysteria and malingering, the two issues, in practice, reduce to one: To what extent is gain a conscious, primary reinforcer of the simulation, or is it an unconscious, secondary reinforcer?

An interesting article by Heaton, Smith, Lehman, & Voyt (1978) reports that "intentional malingerers" were distinguishable from true head-trauma patients on the basis of a "blind reading" of the neuropsychological test battery and MMPI profiles by clinical neuropsychologists to the maximum extent of 20% above chance level. The authors have provided some preliminary evidence for certain neuropsychological test patterns and MMPI profiles that should cause the clinician to be somewhat wary—and doubly so if they are both obtained from a client who is in the process of litigation.

Of course, responsible psychologists do not perform "blind readings" of any data for any purpose where decisions are being made regarding potential clients. While the authors do discuss the fact that the clinicians did not have access to much of the background information usually available in a clinical setting, they further omitted one of the clinician's most important sources of data—his/her own interview of, observations of, and interactions with the patient. It is often at this juncture that one begins to sense that the subjective complaints and objective findings are not consistent.

As Miller and Cartlidge (1972) point out, malingering is viewed differently by different examiners: as evidence of mental illness itself; as an expression of the examiner's moral condemnation of the patient; or as a valid and separate psychological entity. They state that the particular view frequently appears to be a function of experience. Certainly, those neuropsychologists who are involved in the psycholegal sphere are more than familiar with the "feigning" of injury and/or defect that complicates personal injury cases.

Yet, one must be most cautious. Feigning is still very difficult to diagnose, and one should be *most* certain before rendering such an opinion. As Larson (1970) emphasizes, "A heavy burden must be placed upon the party that alleges malingering" (p. 1257); due to the imperfect state of medical knowledge and the harm of a mistaken finding—"it deprives the individual of compensation and publicly labels him a liar and a cheat" (p. 1257). It may also deny the plaintiff much needed treatment, for the courts tend not to view such treatment as recoverable damage and may deny or reduce jury awards when it views simulation as intentional.

Whether or not examiners suspect hysteria or malingering, they should always be ready to address the issue on the witness stand as, inevitably, it will arise. It will be brought up either as an affirmative allegation, demanding a response and supporting data, or in the form of a request to explain why the examiner is of the opinion that one or the other condition can be ruled out. If the examiner suspects either, and/or until both can be comfortably ruled out, the evaluation may have to be more extensive and tailor-made to tease out the needed data, for all of the reasons stated above.

DETERMINATION OF THE PROGNOSIS

Having determined the nature of the dysfunction itself and how that particular deficit affects a particular individual, the neuropsychologist must now turn to the question of prognosis—what can be predicted for this patient in terms of future functioning? Included in that question are issues of the extent of recovery itself, the residual effects that may remain, expectations of the patient and the family, and so forth. In view of the fact that cerebral damage continues to resolve for a period of 18 to 24 months, especially in young adults, there should certainly be no statement regarding permanent or residual deficits before that recovery period has elapsed. And, almost without exception, attorneys themselves are unwilling to settle a case or take it to court until after this time, if permanency is an issue.

At that point—of settlement or litigation—a reexamination of the patient should be made. One is then in a position to render an opinion on the current, and probably permanent, status of the patient regarding level of recovery; further treatment that may be needed; expectations for the future, and so on. By obtaining data from two points in time, the examiner can not only observe the damages that have occurred, but also has a basis for projecting a probable course of future events.

Again, in addition to one's own observations and test data and the client's report, the examiner should have input from family members, keeping in mind that the patient may understate or overstate his/her extent of recovery. As brought out above, an understatement most often occurs in conjunction with hysteria or malingering or, in some instances, when the client is genuinely unaware of improvements because of preoccupation with the deficits that remain. In contrast, those who overstate their recovery are individuals who tend to have difficulty accepting their resulting limitations or whose deficits preclude an accurate self-assessment of their situation.

In any event, when permanent damage is present, the neuropsychologist must be prepared to discuss the probable future level of functioning, what treatment or retraining may be beneficial, what level of care and protection may be needed, what changes have or may occur in family relationships and activities, the advisability and availability of various treatment modalities and/or resources for care, costs involved, and similar items. Many of these issues may need to be addressed with contingencies (e.g., as long as family members can provide care, and then when they are no longer able to do so; if public/governmental resources are adequate, and if they are not and private ones must be sought).

It is not unusual to be asked to design a comprehensive plan for the rehabilitation and/or care of a client—from minimum requirements to the "best of all worlds"—taking into account several possible alternatives. Such a plan may be needed for a short period of time or may cover a life expectancy that projects another 40 or 50 years. One must be careful, in such instances, not to go beyond one's area of expertise but to consult with professionals in the specific areas (e.g., speech, physical, or occupational therapists, nutritionists, vocational counselors, economists) or suggest that the attorney do so.

FUTURE TRENDS

Where does clinical neuropsychology appear to be heading in the forensic area? Unquestionably, neuropsychologists are being called upon by attorneys and the judiciary with increasing frequency to evaluate clients and to offer opinions. Those jurists in the area of civil litigation, particularly personal injury, are becoming more and more familiar with procedures such as neuropsychological test batteries, as well as becoming more confident in the clinician's ability to assess deficits, predict future functioning, and delineate treatment needs. "This skill becomes especially critical in trauma cases (e.g., automobile or industrial accident litigation) where it is desired that recompense be proportional to damage" (Wedding & Gudeman, 1980, p. 34).

While the largest area of interaction is still personal injury, and while the opinions all relate to cortical dysfunctioning, the particular issues involved encompass an ever broader and more fascinating spectrum of behavior. In addition to the questions addressed in criminal and civil litigation mentioned earlier, neuropsychologists have been involved in cases which centered around such issues as: a hospital's failure to conduct a proper examination of a young girl following a suicide attempt, resulting in severe anoxia; a projected plan to address the lifetime needs of a brain-injured infant; an institution's possible 45 years' unlawful detention of an individual who could have lived in the community in a less restrictive environment; a rehabilitation plan for a retarded child who was injured by another retarded child while being transported on a school bus; the ability of an individual who had sustained severe head injuries to testify validly against his alleged assailants; an allegation of intent to defraud the federal government against someone who prepared income tax returns for small businesses; the possible role of temporal lobe epilepsy, alcohol psychosis, and specific learning disability in the commission of crimes such as homicide, armed robbery, and burglary. These particular instances are enumerated only to give a flavor of the myriad questions for which neuropsychological data and opinions may be requested.

There are those such as Wedding and Gudeman (1980) who predict that, with the increasing use of CAT scanners, neuropsychologists will not be called upon as frequently as in the past to answer the same types of questions. In their opinion, the "CAT technique is rapid, noninvasive, and more accurate than traditional neurodiagnostic and neuropsychological measures" (p. 31). Thus, the question of the location of suspected brain lesions is better answered by that technique than by neuropsychological test data, especially in a medical setting.

By contrast, Snow's (1981) recent study compared the frequency of abnormal results in 102 patients classified as brain damaged, normal, or equivocal on the basis of final medical diagnosis using neuropsychological and neurodiagnostic procedures. He found that: "The Impairment Index (from the Halstead–Reitan Neuropsychological Test Battery) was more sensitive to brain damage than any neurodiagnostic measure, yet no more likely to call patients in the other two groups abnormal than CT or EEG" (p. 22).

In any event, when utilized in forensic practice, the specific questions are somewhat different from those that are most commonly posed in a medical setting. Furthermore, in personal injury litigation, there are usually *reams* of medical records, and the injury itself is well documented from a physiological viewpoint. The questions then have to do with behavioral sequelae, overall effect on the individual, prognosis, treatment, and so forth. While the question of brain dysfunction may arise initially in civil litigation, it most often does so in the criminal sphere. In either area, if sufficient data are presented to the court, it is usually willing to order any other procedures that the neuropsychologist may request in order to explore further or rule out certain conditions.

While Wedding and Gudeman (1980) are of the opinion that neuropsychologists will be asked to isolate the location of brain lesions less frequently in the future—and this is already true in the forensic area—they predict that clinicians will be asked to specify the extent of cortical dysfunction in particular cases and make inferences regarding prognosis.

> It is our opinion that what distinguishes clinical neuropsychologists from their peers in the neurosciences is their research skill and their training as accurate and systematic observers of human behavior . . . we feel that the proper role of the clinical neuropsychologist lies in precise delineation of those behavioral deficits that are the sequelae of brain damage and the development and execution of training programs for remediation of those deficits. (p. 34)

FURTHER REFLECTIONS

Having addressed areas in which law and clinical neuropsychology interface, having stated what training and experience has dictated is the manner in which examinations should be conducted and why, and having cautioned regarding some of the pitfalls and issues that demand particular concern, attention will now be given, briefly, to a few of the more practical matters that arise for anyone functioning within this interface.

It would be extremely beneficial for any psychologist who intends to engage in forensic work to take a few courses in law, especially constitutional law, procedure, and advocacy. The reason for this is as follows: Psychologists and attorneys come from *very* different training backgrounds. The manner in which they are taught to approach a problem, how they are taught to seek a solution, even the identification of the problem itself—or at least the priority of issues involved—is different. The framework in which they have been taught to carry out their functions—cooperative vs. adversarial—is different.

As forensic psychologists, we are operating in the legal professional's "ball park." It is an immense help if we can acquire a working understanding of the game and the rules by which it is played. We are immeasurably more comfortable ourselves when we have a grasp of the structure within which we are performing, and our assistance to the court and the attorneys is enhanced a hundredfold. One finds that, with such understanding, expectations are much more realistic and negative experiences are virtually nonexistent.

But the responsibility is even more grave than simply for our own comfort and efficacy in a particular case. Recommendation four of the Report of the Task Force on the Role of Psychology in the Criminal Justice System (1978) states: "Psychologists who work in the criminal justice system, as elsewhere, have an ethical obligation to educate themselves in the concepts and operations of the system in which they work" (p. 1105). Shah (1975) states it even more emphatically:

> [Psychologists] who work in forensic or legal settings, or those who choose to function in situations requiring involvement with the legal system, have a clear and definite responsibility to become properly informed about the relevant legal issues, questions, and criteria pertaining to their roles and functions. . . . Acquiring a sound and accurate understanding of the relevant issues must be viewed as a *professional* and *ethical requirement.* (p. ix, emphasis in original)

A second issue concerns reports. A psychologist involved in a legal case needs a clear understanding concerning to whom reports are to be rendered. If the evaluation is being conducted subsequent to a court order, the report is most frequently sent to the court and is then available to both attorneys. However, there are now exceptions to this in some states when the Office of Public Defender is involved. When the psychologist is called in by a private attorney, as is the case in personal injury litigation, the report is rendered *exclusively* to him/her unless there has been a prior stipulation. What occurs after the report has been submitted is contingent upon not only the content of the report itself but also the legal strategy that the attorney is employing in the case. It is important to maintain close contact and consultation with the attorney who initiated the referral, should any further involvement be required.

One should devote care and attention to the report, never slighting its comprehensiveness or underestimating its effectiveness. It is not unusual for a case to be settled out of court, for both attorneys to stipulate to a complete issue, or for entire recommendations to be read into the record and ordered on the basis of a thorough and well enunciated report. In such instances, the report has saved a great deal of time, effort, money, and sometimes the psychological wellbeing of the parties involved.

The licensing statutes of most states delineate quite clearly those instances in which confidentiality is automatically waived. In general, they consist of any legal or administrative cause in which the client puts forth his/her mental status as a factor to be considered. However, one needs to be conversant with the particular rulings that are holding in any given case and/or jurisdiction, as well as with their limitations and exceptions. This cannot be emphasized too strongly—for the sake of the client and for the protection of the psychologist serving as an expert witness. Furthermore, one needs to be most familiar with the APA Rules of Ethics in order to make an educated decision should one ever be confronted with the choice of confidentiality versus contempt of court.

A fourth issue is that of opinion. As Schofield (1956) so well stated it:

> The law requests not a statement of fact but an opinion. . . . It would be helpful to potential experts . . . to understand correctly the nature of opinion. An opinion is a state of information intermediate to ignorance and omniscience . . . essentially a statement of probability . . . a statement of some degree of conviction is based upon an appraisal of probability. (p. 4)

The expert's education, training, and experience, and the data he/she has collected in the instant case—on a subject considered to be "beyond the ken of the average layman"—are the bases for the court's determination that he/she may offer such an opinion or statement of probability, *in the absence of fact.*

Fifth is the issue of advocacy. Hopefully, the psychologist who enters the legal arena does so as an independent and impartial professional for the purpose of offering an opinion that will aid the trier of fact in reaching a decision, with absolutely no investment in the outcome. The role of every attorney is to be the best possible advocate for his client. The role of the psychologist is to observe, evaluate, infer, conclude, and recommend on the basis of psychological data. The two roles are very different and should *never* be confused: "Mental health professionals should be careful not to go beyond their data and offer personal, social, and moral judgments in the guise of scientific judgments" (Morse, 1978, p. 391). Again, quoting Schofield (1956):

> "If the attorney can in any way establish that the expert witness has become personally involved, that he has obviously selected, distorted, or extrapolated his data so as to support or deny the point in dispute, he can reduce greatly his influence on the jury. (p. 2)

Furthermore, the expert makes him/herself liable for a legal charge of perjury and/or an ethics charge before the APA.

The sixth issue of concern is consultation. Increasingly, neuropsychologists are being asked to render an opinion—occasionally in the courtroom but more frequently in consultation with an attorney—regarding particular case strategy, the reasonableness of the financial redress being sought in damages, the adequacy of another professional's evaluation, the soundness of the conclusions, the rationale of the recommendations, what literature might support or negate those conclusions, and so forth. Any psychologist functioning within the legal sphere needs to be aware of the fact that there will probably be more than one "expert," that his/her professional expertise is most likely going to be reviewed by one or more professional peers. Such a consultative role is frequently being sought by attorneys even to the point of asking for assistance in preparing cross-examination questions for the other "experts" (i.e., the strengths and weaknesses of their credentials, examination, conclusions, and so on).

Finally, there is courtroom testimony. The following is a brief format of what could be considered "typical" in personal injury litigation cases. After having been sworn in, the witness is asked to state his/her name, address, and occupation or profession. Then questions will follow such as: "Please tell the jury what your educational background is." "Please tell the jury what your professional experience has been." "To what, if any, professional organizations do you belong?" "What, if any, articles have you published in this field?" "Have you ever appeared as an expert witness in any jurisdiction prior to this time?" There may or may not be any further initial questions; if there are, they will most probably address the psychologist's further expertise in some area felt to be especially germane to the case at hand.

Following this, the opposing counsel is given the opportunity to question the witness concerning credentials and expertise. Sometimes this is done and sometimes it is not. In either event, the attorney who called the psychologist will eventually "tender" the witness to the court as an expert in his/her particular field. The court may or may not accept the witness as an expert, although it usually does.

Assuming that it does, the direct examination begins, conducted by the attorney who subpoenaed the psychologist, and would proceed approximately as follows:

> ATTORNEY A: Dr. X, in your practice of psychology, have you had an occasion to see one John Doe?
> DOCTOR X: Yes, I have.
> ATTORNEY A: Where and on what date or dates did you see him?
> DOCTOR X: In my office on June 11 and 12, 1979.
> ATTORNEY A: By whom was Mr. Doe referred to you?

DOCTOR X: By your office (*or whoever is the referral source*).

ATTORNEY A: And for what purpose was he referred to you?

DOCTOR X: To assess his current psychological and neuropsychological functioning.

ATTORNEY A: How long did the examination take?

DOCTOR X: The complete evaluation took approximately 1½ hours.

ATTORNEY A: Doctor, would you tell the jury what the evaluation consisted of; describe the evaluation for the jury.

At this point, the psychologist should explain each of the tests and procedures used and their purpose, in layman's terms and in sufficient detail so that the jury will have some comprehension of what transpired during the evaluation, and why, without getting bored with irrelevant or overly technical minutiae.

ATTORNEY A: And what did you find with regard to Mr. Doe as a result of your examination?

This is now the psychologist's opportunity to present Mr. John Doe to the jury as an individual with whatever strengths and weaknesses he possesses. This is accomplished most effectively by using the pattern stated above (i.e., starting with the narrower picture of any deficits that may be present and proceeding to the broader picture of what these mean to him as an individual and how they have affected his life). Juries both attend and retain more when this information is presented in narrative form rather than in a series of questions and answers between the attorney and the witness.

ATTORNEY A: Doctor, do you have any idea as to how Mr. Doe might have sustained these deficits?

DOCTOR X: I was informed that he had been in an automobile accident in March of 1976, and I examined the records of his hospitalization subsequent to that incident.

ATTORNEY A: And, in your opinion, are Mr. Doe's present deficits compatible with the injury he received in that accident.

DOCTOR X: Yes, they are.

ATTORNEY A: Doctor, do you have an opinion as to the permanency of Mr. Doe's condition?

DOCTOR X: Yes, I do.

ATTORNEY A: And what is that opinion?

DOCTOR X: It is my clinical opinion, based on a reasonable degree of psychological certainty (*or probability*), that Mr. Doe's condition is permanent.

ATTORNEY A: Doctor, why do you feel his condition is permanent?

DOCTOR X: Because of his age, the extent of his injuries, the length of time since the accident, and the amount of progress that he has made during the intervening months (*explaining the effect of each of these*).

At this time, depending on the case itself, there may be questions regarding the need for psychotherapy, special living arrangements, special conditions should family not be available as caretakers, and so forth. The psychologist should be prepared to respond to these plus any other issues unique to the particular case.

ATTORNEY A: Thank you, Doctor, I have no further questions. Your witness.

The possibilities for cross-examination are far too numerous to attempt examples. However, it does have to be restricted to material covered in the direct examination. An attorney may want to do several things on cross-examination: question the adequacy of the examination and/or of the particular techniques used; raise doubt in the jurors' minds regarding the certainty with which conclusions can be drawn from the evaluation; downplay the severity of the deficits and their effect upon the individual's life; stress any compensating factors; question the opinion of permanency; and, of course, raise the issue of malingering or at least hysterical overlay. As in all cases, the psychologist should be both honest and cautious—stating where he/she thinks hysteria may be present or saying, "While that is always a possibility, I do not think it is present in this case because. . . ."

One needs to remember *not* to become defensive. It is the opposing attorney's role to dilute the expert witness's testimony, but this is not a personal attack on the witness. If, in any way, the jury begins to acquire an "erroneous" view of John Doe and his condition, it is up to Attorney A to rectify this on re-direct examination. Nevertheless, we are all advocates for and invested in our own opinions. If one wishes to function within the legal arena, one must be prepared to have one's thoughts, ideas, and philosophies challenged as well as one's opinions, conclusions, and recommendations. While not necessarily pleasant, neither is such a state of affairs necessarily negative. One would hope that it makes each of us who are subject to challenge think our positions through more carefully. Each of us needs to be very aware of his/her bias—so aware that it will not be a handicap—in order to function more effectively within the legal sphere.

Two final notes with regard to the role of a witness: First, testimony should always be directed to the jury or to the judge if there is no jury, but not to the attorney. The jury, or judge, is the trier-of-fact, and our purpose in being in the courtroom is to offer them additional information—including our opinions—on which to make their decision. The role of the attorney at that time is simply to facilitate the conveyance of the information we have to offer within the bounds of the rules of procedure and evidence.

Second, the importance of pretrial conferences with the attorney who is calling the psychologist to testify cannot be stressed too strongly. During such conferences certain areas should be covered thoroughly (e.g., the expert's credentials, what the attorney will ask on direct examination, in what manner the expert is most comfortable testifying, exactly what the expert's response will be to any equivocal or doubtful issues, what the expert is legally forbidden to relate, what questions can be anticipated on cross-examination, and what are the strengths and weaknesses of the testimony). A discussion of these and other issues is absolutely mandatory in order to maximize the expert's effectiveness and minimize the chance of "unexpected" disaster.

As Costello (1981) points out in a valuable article on "do's and don'ts" of direct examination:

> Experts play a most important part in the presentation of evidence, either for the defendant or the plaintiff, particularly in complicated, involved negligence cases. . . . The expert's part in the trial should never be underestimated. Therefore, due consideration should be given in preparing him to testify in court. (p. 21)

In almost every instance, the attorney will arrange a meeting for the purpose of this preparation but if, for some reason, he/she does not, the psychologist should insist upon it.

CONCLUSION

Although much of what has been stated has been factual, historical, and scientific data, much has also been opinion. Two attitudes regarding the field of forensic/clinical neuropsychology have been stressed: caution and excitement.

The reason for caution is very well stated by Morse (1978):

> Most lawyers regard mental disorders as arcane and disturbing phenomena that are beyond their comprehension and are understood by only a few highly trained experts. Lawyers therefore tend to defer to mental health experts and mental health law decisions are often based more on mental health reasoning or conclusions than on legal reasoning. Thus, it behooves mental health professionals to tread cautiously in court since their influence may be immense. What is adequate science for the clinic, lab, or classroom may not be adequate science for the court in which the result may be the deprivation of fundamental rights. (p. 391)

The reason for the excitement is the fact that forensic neuropsychology is a most stimulating and challenging speciality. It is an area with uncalculated ramifications for our clients, our society, and our profession, provided that we are prepared for that challenge—not just adequately, but to the greatest degree possible.

LEGAL CITATIONS

Dobbs v. State 191 Ark 236, 85 SW2d 694. (1935)
Doherty v. Dean 337 SW2d 153. (1960)
Hidden v. Mutual Life Insurance Co. 217 F2d 818, 78 ALR2d 921. (1954)
In Re Masters 216 Minn 553, 13 NW2d 487, 158 ALR 1210. (1944)
Jenkins v. U.S. 113 App DC 300, 307 F2d 637. (1962)

People v. Hawthorne 293 Mich 15, 291 NW 205. (1940)
People v. McNichol 100 Cal App2d 554, 224 P2d 21. (1950)
People v. Spigno 156 Cal App2d 279, 319 P2d 458. (1957)
Reese v. Naylor 222 S2d 487. (1969)
State v. Donahue 141 Conn 656, 109 A2d 364. (1954)
State v. Gibson 15 NJ 384, 105 A2d 1, 42 ALR2d 1461. (1954)
State v. Padilla 66 NM 289, 347 P2d 312, 78 ALR2d 908. (1959)
U.S. v. Chandler 72 Fed Supp. 230. (1947)
U.S. v. Hiss 185 F2d 822. (1950)
Watson v. State 161 Tex Crim 5, 273 SW2d 879. (1954)

REFERENCES

Alarcon, R. D. Hysteria and hysterical personality: How come one without the other? *Psychiatric Quarterly,* 1973, *47,* 258–275.
Black, H. C. *Black's law dictionary* (Rev. 4th ed.). St. Paul, Minnesota: West Publishing, 1968.
Costello, J. M. The direct examination of the expert witness. *For the Defense,* 1981, *23,* 2–24.
Gasparrini, W., Satz, P., & Heilman, K. Hemispheric asymmetrics of affective processing as determined by the MMPI. *Journal of Neurology, Neurosurgery, and Psychiatry,* 1978, *41,* 470–473.
Heaton, R. K., Smith, H. H., Lehman, R., & Voyt, A. T. Prospects for faking believable deficits on neuropsychological testing. *Journal of Consulting and Clinical Psychology,* 1978, *46,* 892–900.
Heilman, K., & Valenstein, E. Emotional disorders resulting from central nervous system dysfunction. *Geriatrics,* 1980, *35,* 77–86.
Hoch, E. L., & Darley, J. G. A case at law. *American Psychologist,* 1965, *20,* 623–654.
Hoffman, M. The medico-legal significance of pain and suffering. *South Texas Law Journal,* 1975, *15,* 279–288.
Larson, A. Mental and nervous injury in Workman's Compensation. *Vanderbilt Law Review,* 1970, *23,* 1243–1263.
Ley, R. G., & Bryden, M. P. *Hemispheric differences in processing emotions and faces.* Unpublished manuscript, 1978.
Lezak, M. D. *Neuropsychological assessment.* New York: Oxford University Press, 1976.
Louisell, D. W. The psychologist in today's legal world. *Minnesota Law Review,* 1955, *39,* 235–272.
Luria, A. R. *The working brain: An introduction to neuropsychology.* New York: Basic Books, 1973.
McMahon, E. A., & Satz, P. Clinical neuropsychology: Some forensic applications. In S. B. Filskov & T. J. Boll (Eds.), *Handbook of clinical neuropsychology.* New York: Wiley, 1981.
Miller, H., & Cartlidge, N. Simulation and malingering after injuries to the brain and spinal cord. *Lancet,* 1972, *1,* 580–585.
Morse, S. J. Law and mental health professionals: The limits of expertise. *Professional Psychology,* 1978, *9,* 389–399.
Redmount, R. S. The use of psychologists in legal practice. *The Practical Lawyer,* 1974, *20,* 29–91.
Report of the Task Force on the Role of Psychology in the Criminal Justice System. *American Psychologist,* 1978, *33,* 1099–1113.
Schofield, W. Psychology, law, and the expert witness. *American Psycholgist,* 1956, *11,* 1–7.
Shah, S. Forward. In A. Stone, *Mental health and the law: A system in transition.* Washington, D.C.: U.S. Government Printing Office, 1975.
Smith, S. N. (Ed.). *Textbook of forensic psychiatry.* New York: Medical Examinations Publishing, in press.

Snow, W. G. A comparison of frequency of abormal results in neuropsychological vs. neurodiagnostic procedures. *Journal of Clinical Psychology,* 1981, *37,* 22–28.

Stern, D. B. Handedness and the lateral distribution of conversion reactions. *Journal of Nervous and Mental Disorders,* 1977, *164,* 122–128.

Trimble, M. R. *Post-traumatic neurosis: From railway spine to the whiplash.* New York: Wiley, 1981.

Wasmuth, C. E. Medical evaluation of mental pain and suffering. *Cleveland-Marshall Law Review,* 1957, *6,* 7–16.

Wedding, D., & Gudeman, H. Implications of computerized axial tomography for clinical neuropsychology. *Professional psychology,* 1980, *11,* 31–35.

Woolsey, R. M., & Goldner, J. A. The medical–legal ramifications of hysteria. *California Western Law Review,* 1976, *12,* 299–330.

16

Sex Differences in Neuropsychological Functioning

RICHARD J. BROWNE

Throughout most of recorded history, there was relatively little confusion and doubt regarding the basic differences between men and women. Not only were the physiological and structural differences viewed as apparent, they were also considered to be enduring and immutable. This view also extended into the areas of aptitudes, temperament, abilities, and intelligence (Maccoby & Jacklin, 1974). Today, while the physiological and structural differences for the most part continue undisputed (Money & Ehrhardt, 1972), the certainty regarding what aptitudes, temperament, abilities and intellect are concomitants of which sex has been brought under close scrutiny.

In the past 20 years a burgeoning growth of studies on the nature and extent of neuropsychological differences between the sexes has been witnessed (Maccoby & Jacklin, 1974). The pupose of this chapter will be to present information regarding the nature and limits of neuropsychological differences between males and females as it is known to date. The chapter's focus will be in three primary areas—neuroanatomy, spatial ability, and verbal ability.

NEUROANATOMY

Cerebral dominance means simply that one hemisphere of the brain is more responsible for certain functions than the other. This concept was not widely

RICHARD J. BROWNE ● Neuropsychology Laboratory, McGuire Veterans Administration Medical Center, Richmond, Virginia 23249.

accepted before the 1860s although as Benton and Joynt (1960) have noted, the relationship between aphasia and brain function was made much before this period.

Today it is generally believed that language, musical skills, emotionality, spatial abilities, recognition of faces, and handedness are related to hemispheric dominance. What did not follow so readily was the evidence to indicate a neurological substrate within the cortex for these various functions and abilities. As recently as 1962 von Bonin expressed the opinion that the evidence for anatomical differences between right and left hemispheres was not adequate enough to account for the functional differences. Since 1968, however, a number of studies have been published that have been contrary to von Bonin's view. Geschwind and Levitsky (1968) examined 100 adult human brains that were obtained at autopsy and were free of "significant" pathology. They reported that the planum temporale (a portion of the speech cortex) was one-third longer on the left side in 65% of the brains, longer on the right in 11%, and equal in 24%. They reasoned that since about 90% of the general adult population is left hemisphere dominant for speech, their cases must have consisted of a large majority of subjects who were also left hemisphere dominant for speech. These findings have subsequently been confirmed in other studies (Chi, Dooling, & Gilles, 1977; Galaburda, LeMay, Kemper, & Geschwind, 1978; Galaburda, Sanides, & Geschwind, 1978; Wada, 1969; Wada, Clarke, & Hamm, 1975; Witelson & Pallie, 1973).

Witelson and Pallie (1973) raised the question as to when in the course of ontogenetic development did this hemispheric asymmetry first become manifest. Is the asymmetry the result of environmental factors or due to an innate biological factor? In order to shed light on this question, they examined 16 adult brains and 14 infant brains (11 of whom were neonates). The range in age for the infant specimens was 1 day to 3 months, with a median age of 12 days. All of the specimens were free of neurological disease. The investigators found that both sets of measures showed the left planum was significantly larger than the right for the adult and the infant groups. In both groups the left plana were larger in over 80% of the cases. The left–right difference in the neonates was proportionately as large as in the adults.

Of direct relevance to this chapter, the authors compared the female neonate specimens with those of the males. They had to reduce the size of the male group to make the ages comparable. With 5 specimens in each group, the investigators found that the left planum was significantly larger than the right in the female group but not significantly larger in the male group.

Wada et al. (1975) examined normal brains from 100 adults and 100 infants. The age range for the adult brains was 17 to 96 years, with a mean age of 69. The infant age range was from the 19th gestational week to the 18th postnatal month with a mean age of 48 weeks. A larger planum was found more often on the left ($N = 28$) as compared to the right ($N = 7$) in adults as well as infants (11L:1R). In 9 infant and 8 adult specimens no planum was noted on the right side. In 10 adult and 12 infant specimens the right planum was larger than the left. There were 32 infant and 8 adult brains that were approximately equal on left and right. Using a right/left ratio to indicate the size of the right planum as a percentage of the left, these researchers were able to directly compare the adult and infant specimens. The ratio indicated that the asymmetry was greater in adults than in infants. They speculated from this that possibly the left planum develops to a relatively larger size with age. They also noted a trend for infant male plana to be larger on both sides and adult male plana to be larger on the left, but this was not significant. In the adult specimens the females were more likely than the males to have a reversed asymmetry $(R > L)$. This was significant $(p < .05)$.

Thus, Wada *et al.* (1975) results confirmed earlier studies (Geschwind & Levitsky, 1968; Witelson & Pallie, 1973) that showed asymmetry of the temporal planum in adults and also provided confirmatory evidence of a similar difference in infant brains (Witelson & Pallie, 1973). The finding of approximately 90% of the cases in both adult and infant group having larger left than right temporal planum is consistent with the presumed incidence of speech lateralization to the left cerebral hemisphere. The larger right planum found in adult but not infant females raises the possibility of a sex and developmental difference.

Chi, Dooling, and Gilles (1977) examined 207 fetal brains ranging in gestational age from 10 to 44 weeks. In 54% of the fetal brains the temporal plane was larger on the left than on the right side. Given such early indications of temporal planum asymmetry, which supported earlier studies, the possibility may be entertained that a neural substrate underlies the process of lateralization of speech and language function. Contrary to earlier studies, Chi *et al.* (1977) did not find any differences between male and female fetuses.

Gallaburda, Sanides *et al.* (1978) were concerned that the observed cortical asymmetries may result from differences in the folding of the two hemispheres and not from differences in brain structure. If this were the case, then one would have to question the presumed relationship between the asymmetries and language function. They thus set out to measure the distinctive cellular areas of the auditory regions of the brain using 4 normal adult specimens. They looked at the auditory area of the cortex and went beyond the limits of the planum, which earlier studies had not done. They found the left planum to be larger than the right in three of the four cases, with the percentage range being 37% to 200%. The fourth specimen's right planum was larger by 13%. They suspected this was due to measurement error. The temperoparietal cortex (area Tpt) was larger on the left in all four cases, with the difference ranging from 626% larger to only 14% larger (the 14% difference was considered to be in the range of measurement error). The Tpt and planum asymmetries are comparable in the four cases. Their results are similar to findings of the earlier studies and add evidence to the notion that an anatomical substrate for language functioning exists in the left hemisphere.

In summary, the studies conducted so far have been primarily concerned with determining the existence of anatomical asymmetries between right and left cerebral hemispheres which might then lend support to the assumption that a neural substrate underlies the functional lateral asymmetries that have been reported quite consistently in the literature. The studies cited above, specifically Witelson and Pallie (1973) and Wada *et al.* (1975) indicate that there may also be sex differences in the distribution and extent of these asymmetries. Such differences suggest that females, as opposed to males, have significantly larger left plana than right, at least in the neonatal period. The asymmetry between left and right plana in adult males and females is greater than it is in infancy, with the left usually being larger. Female adults also seem more likely to have reverse asymmetry of the plana (R >L) than male adults, and the latter group has a tendency to have a larger left plana. Given the limitations of the studies upon which these findings are based, the results should be viewed as tentative but certainly worthy of further exploration. Greater elucidation of neuroanatomical sex differences may well provide a basis for explaining some of the sex differences in neuropsychological performance that will be cited in the remainder of this chapter.

SPATIAL ABILITY

Maccoby and Jacklin (1974), in their book on sex differences, remarked that spatial ability is an area in which consistent sex differences have been observed. The term itself has been defined in a number of ways. Guilford and Lacey (1947), for example, referred to an ability to mentally rotate objects, to fold and unfold patterns, and to be able to appreciate the relative changes of these objects and patterns in space. They also referred to an ability to appreciate the arrangement of stimuli within a visual pattern. Thurstone (1950) perceived that these factors were involved with visual orientation in space. The first factor he described as an ability to identify an object when it was received from different angles. The second was an ability to imagine the movement of parts or elements within a total configuration, and the third an ability to think about spatial relations when the observer's body orientation is an essential part of the problem.

The similarities in these early descriptions have led to numerous tests being devised to measure and evaluate these spatial abilities. Much of this early work originated in factor analytic studies of intellectual functioning. McGee (1979) noted that recent factor analytic studies have attempted to describe and define the nature of the various subskills involved in spatial abilities. He felt that they fairly conclusively demonstrated that there are at least two spatial factors, one of which can be called visualization and the other, orientation. The former seems to involve the mental manipulation and rotation of objects and the ability to appreciate the relative changes of these objects in space after such rotation and manipulation. This is compatible with the second factor described by Thurstone. Orientation has to do with the ability to appreciate the arrangement of stimuli within a visual pattern and with the first and third factors described by Thurstone.

The spatial abilities literature is most persistent in its findings that males tend to be superior to females (Anastasi, 1958; Buffery & Gray, 1972; Maccoby & Jacklin, 1974; Sherman, 1971; Smith, 1964). It has been indicated, however, that approximately 25% of women do score above the mean of males on psychometric tests of spatial ability (Bock, 1973).

Waber (1976) examined both verbal and spatial performance and lateralization of linguistic processing as they related to sex and maturational rate. She sampled 80 early and late maturing adolescents at two age levels. The females were 10 and 13 years old while the males were 13 and 16 years old. She found that early maturers, regardless of sex, scored better on verbal than on spatial tasks and that late maturers scored better on spatial than verbal tasks. She also found that early maturers were less lateralized for speech perception than late maturers. Waber concluded that the sex differences in verbal and spatial abilities may have quite different etiologies and that the rate of maturation may have a very significant role in the organization of higher cortical functions.

Visualization Ability

Mental Rotation

The Differential Aptitude Tests (DAT) are widely used in the educational and vocational counseling of students in grades 8 through 12. One of its tests, Space Relations, requires the subject to mentally construct a three-dimensional object from a visually displayed, two-dimensional flat pattern. After having done so, the subject has to select the correct three-dimensional objects from a choice of four visually displayed alternatives. The process involved in the completion of this test is very much akin to the descriptions of Guilford and Lacey (1947) and Thurstone (1950) and can be referred to as a visualization ability. It has consistently been demonstrated that males outperform females (Flanagan, Dailey, Shaycoft, Gorham, Orr, Goldberg, & Neyman, 1961; Hartlage, 1970; Vandenberg, Stafford, & Brown, 1968). Stafford (1961) obtained similar results by presenting his subjects with two-dimensional representations of three-dimensional figures, which were in the form of blocks. The young males he tested were superior in performance to the females.

Shephard and Metzler (1971) reported a study in which they presented subjects with two-dimensional representations of three-dimensional figures produced by a computer. One of these representations had been rotated with respect to the other. They found that the time it took the subjects to make a decision whether or not the two representations were the same or different (except for rotation) was linearly related to the degree of rotation involved. Therefore, it appeared that the task was measuring the time it took for the subject to make the appropriate mental rotations. Metzler and Shepard (1974) noted that their female subjects showed longer overall reactions times and the slope of the reaction time functions tended to be steeper (i.e., slower rates of mental rotation) than did their male subjects. (It should be pointed out, however, that the authors had not intended to examine sex differences. Their studies only involved a few subjects who had been preselected for good spatial ability.)

Bryden and Tapley (1976) performed two studies using the mental rotation task. The first was to determine if a sex difference existed with an adult population (Metzler and Shepard had used college students). Their study differed from Shepard and Metzler (1971) in that they used actual three-dimensional objects rather than pictures. One of the experimental conditions involved actual physical rotation of the object, and another involved a mental rotation. They discovered that in the mental rotation condition the women showed a trend toward slower reaction times. Accuracy decreased from the physical rotation condition to the mental rotation condition with the women displaying a greater decrement between the two conditions.

In their second study, Bryden and Tapley (1976) tried to more accurately observe the nature of the sex differences. To do this, they manipulated the angle of rotation in 30° increments from 0° to 180°. Photographs were taken and slides made of the objects used in the first study, at the specified degrees of rotation. They were presented to the subjects in pairs, with the object on the left always being shown at 0°. Supporting Shepard and Metzler (1971), they found that the mean response time increased linearly with the degree of rotation. Accuracy scores indicated that men were more accurate than women and that accuracy decreased in a linear fashion with the degree of rotation. They asked subjects, after the study, to describe their approaches to the task. They labelled two of the approaches as "visual–holistic," which referred to a literal mental rotation of the objects, and two other approaches as "verbal–analytic," which involved a counting of blocks. Of the classifiable subjects, 73% of the men and 47% of the women claimed a visual–holistic strategy ($p < .10$). There was no apparent reationship between performance and strategy.

Tapley and Bryden (1977) performed a follow-up study in which they again looked at sex differences in the performance of a mental rotation task and the influence of strategy on that performance. They administered to 20 male and 20 female college students the Spatial Relations subtest of the Differential Aptitude Test, the Paivio Imagery Test, and the Standardized Road Map Test of Direction Sense. The Paivio Imagery Test is an 86-item, true–false questionnaire that provides a verbal/imagery ratio. A low score indicates that the subject's general method of thinking is very visual. A high score indicates the method is highly verbal. They then used copies of the original Shepard and Metzler (1971) figures as stimuli.

The figures were paired (100 total) into equal numbers of same and different pairs for each of the 0°, 40°, 80°, 120°, and 160° rotations. The subjects were presented the stimuli tachistoscopically and had to decide whether the items in the pair were the same or different. The authors found two sex differences. Men were more accurate than women, and men had shorter reaction times than women. The authors also observed that accuracy was related to the degree of rotation. The rate of rotation and accuracy correlated with the Spatial Relations Test and the Road Map Test, suggesting to the authors that some general spatial factor may be relevant to both measures (rate and accuracy). Men who used visual imagery had a more rapid rate of mental rotation than those who used verbal mediation. This relationship was not found with the women. They found that spatial men (as measured by the Spatial Relations Test) were somewhat better visual imagers, while spatial women were better verbal imagers. Contrary to their first two studies, this study revealed, via post-experiment interviews, that as many men as women used some form of verbal mediation in performing the task. Strategy again did not have any relationship with performance.

Vandenberg and Kuse (1978) have developed a paper-and-pencil test of spatial visualization based upon the original stimuli of Shepard and Metzler (1971). They called the test "Mental Rotations," after the name used by Shepard and Metzler to describe the cognitive process that they felt is involved in the performance of their task. DeFries and Wilson and their associates (DeFries, Ashton, Johnson, Kuse, McClearn, Mi, Rashad, Sandenberg, & Wilson, 1976; Wilson, DeFries, McClearn, Vandenberg, Johnson, & Rashad, 1975) and McGee (1978) have demonstrated sex differences using this test. Again the males performed better than the females, although not always significantly.

Mathematical Ability

Hills (1957) found relatively high correlations between performance in college math and two tests of spatial ability. He found very low correlations between the same performance and verbal reasoning tests. His subjects were 148 college students, and the tests had been taken from the Guilford-Zimmerman Aptitude Survey. Bennett, Seashore, and Wesman (1974) found high correlations between performance in geometry and the Space Relations Test of the Differential Aptitude Test Battery. Smith (1960) found that grades in arithmetic and algebra correlated less highly with tests of spatial ability than did grades in geometry. Saad & Storer (1960) found that fifth grade males had greater comprehension and appreciation of concepts and principles in geometry than did their female classmates. It would appear that male superiority is most evident in coursework that has a strong spatial component (i.e., geometry), whereas the superiority is less evident in those courses that do not (i.e., arithmetic and algebra).

This view is consistent with Benbow and Stanley (1980), who feel that achievement in and aptitude toward mathematics is due to a superior male mathematical ability and possibly also to greater male ability in spatial tasks. They reached their conclusions based on exhaustive data on mathematical aptitude they had gathered during a study of mathematically precocious youth during the period 1972 to 1979. During this time they had conducted six talent searches to find seventh and eighth graders who scored in the upper 2% to 5% on standardized mathematics achievement tests. The approximately 10,000 children, 43% of whom were girls, were administered the verbal and mathematics sections of the Scholastic Aptitude Tests (SAT). The investigators argued that the mathematics portion is designed to measure mathematical reasoning ability and that at these grade levels, students have not been formally taught the principles that underlie mathematics problems. Thus, if a student can solve these problems, he or she must have some unusual ability.

For each talent search, the boys and girls did equally well on the verbal section of the SAT. However, on the mathematical section a sex difference in favor of the boys was found for each talent search. Even though all the students were within the 5th percentile in mathematical reasoning ability, on the average the boys performed better than did the girls in each talent search. The investigators did not consider the observed sex differences to be the result of differential training in mathematics. They presumed that at the seventh-grade level, all the students had taken essentially the same number and type of math courses in their academic programs. This presumption was supported by the finding that in one of the talent searches there was no difference between boys and girls in their participation in special mathematics programs. The conclusions drawn by the investigators were that a number of hypotheses could account for the consistent sex differences in mathematical ability. Their preference was to relate the superior male mathematical ability to greater male ability in spatial tasks.

Orientation Ability

Field Dependence—Field Independence

Witkin and his colleagues have consistently found sex differences on measures of field dependence–field independence (Witkin, Dyk, Faterson, Goodenough, & Karp, 1962; Witkin, Lewis, Hertzman, Machover, Meissner, & Wapner, 1954). The two tests most associated with this concept are the Rod and Frame Test and the Embedded Figures Test. The Rod and Frame Test requires that the subject adjust a luminated rod to true vertical while the rod is inside a luminated square frame. This is done while the frame and/or the subject himself is tilted. Sex differences on this test have been reported as early as 5 to 10 years of age (Graves & Koziol, 1971; Keogh & Ryan, 1971; Maccoby & Jacklin, 1974; Witkin, Goodenough, & Karp, 1967). From adolescence upward, the superior male performance has been amply documented (Bogo, Winget, & Gleser, 1970; Fiebert, 1967; Saarni, 1973; Schwartz & Karp, 1967; Silverman, Bucksbaum, & Stierlin, 1973; Witkin *et al.*, 1962, 1967).

The Embedded Figures Test requires that the subject look at a simple geometrical shape and then, with that shape in memory, try to locate it in a complex geometrical figure. Witkin *et al.* (1954) considered this test a measure of cognitive differentiation or field dependence. The sex differences on the Embedded Figures Test are not seen as early as they are in the Rod and Frame Test. No differences between males and females, 5 to 10 years of age, were found in speed or accuracy of performance (Graves & Koziol, 1971; Keogh & Ryan, 1971; Maccoby & Jacklin, 1974; Witkin *et al.*, 1954). In the adolescent years, superior male performances are fairly reliable (Fiebert, 1967; Schwartz & Karp, 1967; Witkin *et al.*, 1967), and there is abundant evidence of this same superiority in adulthood (Bennett, 1956; Goodnow, 1962; Schwartz & Karp, 1967).

Witkin (1949, 1950) has claimed that sex difference in spatial ability is an example of a more general sex difference in analytic ability or field dependence. Sherman (1967), however, has argued that the sex difference in field dependence is due to a spatial component in Witkin's tests and not to their analytic component. There is some evidence in favor of her position. Gardner, Jackson, and Messick (1960) found a correlation of .53 between the Embedded Figures Test and the Spatial Orientation Test from the Guilford–Zimmerman Aptitude Survey. A .35 correlation was found between the Rod and Frame Test and the Spatial Orientation Test. Witkin, Birnbaum, Lomonaco, Lehr, and Herman (1968) found no difference between males and females on nonvisual analogues to the Embedded Figures Test. Similarly, Hyde, Geiringer, and Yen (1975) found that males and females performed comparably when spatial ability differences are eliminated in field dependence. Factor analysis has demonstrated a convergence of standard spatial abilities tests and measures of field dependence (Gardner *et al.*, 1960; Hyde *et al.*, 1975).

Thus it would appear that the spatial component, as measured in the Rod and Frame Test and in the Embedded Figures Test, is a significant factor in the emergence of sex differences. As a result, Harris (1978) cautions against overinterpreting sex differences on the Rod and Frame and the Embedded Figures tests. These tests are usually referred to as measures of field independence and field dependence. When sex differences on these tests are found, conclusions are drawn that females are field dependent, global in their thinking, and cognitively undifferentiated, while males are described as field independent, analytical, and cognitively differentiated. Harris (1978) emphasizes a point previously made (Sherman, 1967) that most tests of field dependence have strong visuospatial components and thus the male superior performance is to be expected. However, interpretation of these results as evidence for a general cognitive style is not warranted because other measures of field dependence that do not contain a spatial component do not elicit sex differences.

Directional Sense

Berry (1966) compared the Eastern Canadian Eskimos of Baffin Island with members of the Temne tribe of Africa on various perceptual and spatial tasks. The environments, daily experiences, and life habits of these two groups are very different. The eskimos (both men and women) are hunters who must travel widely in their search of food. Berry reasoned that they needed to have a keen spatial ability that would take into account the various subtleties and nuances of their essentially featureless environment. The Temne tribespeople, on the other hand, are primarily farmers, and while their environment is richer in flora and fauna, the Temne do not need to traverse their environs to any significant degree in search of food.

Berry felt that these cultural differences should be reflected in these peoples' performances on tests such as Kohs Blocks, Morrisby Shapes, and the Embedded Figures Test. His results indicated that the spatial abilities of the Eskimos as measured by these tests were in all instances superior to the spatial abilities of the Temne tribespeople. Within the Temne group the men performed better than the women, but there were no sex differences within the Eskimo group. Thus it would appear that frequent traversing of one's environment may enhance the development of spatial abilities. Support for this view comes from a study by Munroe & Munroe (1968) of the children of the Logoli tribe in Africa. They observed that the males tended to wander farther from the village than did females. These researchers found that the females performed more poorly than the males on Block Design and on a measure designed to evaluate the subject's ability to appreciate and construct diagonals.

Witkin et al. (1962) found that children who were given greater freedom of movement and less restriction in their play and leisure activities performed in a superior fashion on the Rod and Frame Test and the Embedded Figures Test than did children who were more restricted and less free. Again a sex difference was noted in favor of males.

Wolf (1973) asked a number of physicians and their spouses if they had difficulty identifying right and left. He obtained responses from 408 men and 382 women. He found that 17.5% of the women and 8.8% of the men indicated that they experienced frequent confusion in right–left orientation. Bakan & Putnam (1974) tested 400 undergraduate students (123 male right-handed, 228 female right-handed, 28 male left-handed, and 21 female left-handed) on a measure of right–left discrimination and the Culver Lateral Discrimination Test. Handedness was determined by which hand the subject wrote with. The subjects were presented with 32 slides, each of which contained a human body part. The subject was instructed to look at the picture and decide whether the body part was left or right. The authors found that, regardless of handedness, males were superior to females. For right-handed subjects ($N = 351$) the difference was statistically significant ($p < .001$), while for left-handed subjects ($N = 49$) the difference was not significant. The differences between right- and left-handed subjects were not significant. Corballis & Beale (1976) have proposed that right–left discrimination is related to the development of hemispheric functional asymmetry. They reason further that females' poorer performance on right–left discrimination tasks suggests a less functional asymmetry for women.

Money, Alexander, and Walker (1965) administered the Road Map Test of Direction Sense to 1,000 children between the ages of 7 and 18 years. On this test the subject is required to look at a schematic outline map of several city blocks and follow a standard route. The subject imagines the route taken and verbalizes the direction of each turn (left or right). At all ages males performed better than females, but these differences were not always significant.

Porteus (1918, 1924) was seeking an alternative to verbal measures of intelligence. He wanted to assess those aspects of intelligence he felt had practical social utility. He called them foresight and planning capacity. In order to do this he developed his Maze Tests. On these tests the subject is required to trace with a pencil the shortest path from the entrance to the exit of a maze. There is no time limit, and the subject cannot lift his pencil from the paper. The mazes have varying levels of difficulty. He discovered repeatedly with large groups of subjects that males consistently outperformed females on these mazes (Porteus, 1965). Keogh (1971) demonstrated that males who were required to produce a particular pattern by walking were able to benefit from visual clues, while women were not able to benefit.

Piagetian Tests

Tuddenham (1970) developed a number of tasks to try to assess quantitatively some of Piaget's principles of cognitive development. A number of these tasks have varying degrees of spatial ability requirements. One such task has the subject look at several photographs of a farm and then choose which one represents the farm view from a particular perspective or vantage point. On a task using geometrical forms, the subject is asked to select from several pictures of flat patterns the one that, if folded, would result in simple three-dimensional form. On another task, the subject is required to construct buildings from blocks by following house plans. On each of these tasks, the mean score for males was higher than it was for females.

The Water Level task is used to evaluate the principle that the level of a still liquid is always horizontal regardless of the tilt of the container that holds the liquid (Piaget & Inhelder, 1956). In most studies of this principle, subjects are usually shown drawings of various containers tilted at different angles and are asked to draw a line representing the liquid level for each container. Or they are shown containers with lines already drawn and are asked if the liquid level would behave in this manner. According to Piaget and Inhelder (1956) this principle should be mastered by the age of 12 years. However, this has been found to be more true for males than for females (Liben, 1973; Thomas, 1971; Thomas, Jamison, & Hummel, 1973). Even among college populations and older adults, males again are superior in performance to females (Kelly & Kelly, 1977; Maxwell, Croake, & Biddle, 1975; Munsinger, 1974; Rebelsky, 1964; Walker & Krasnoff, 1978; Willemsen & Reynolds, 1973). Thomas (1971) and Kelly and Kelly (1977) have found that fully half of their female subjects are not able to perform the task accurately. Harris (1978) argued that the consistently inferior performance of females relative to males on this task is due to the spatial requirements of the task. Geisinger and Hyde (1976) looked at the relationship between errors on the Water Level task and a spatial orientation test. They found significant negative correlations for both sexes. Males were again superior to females on both tasks, but when spatial orientation skills were statistically covaried out, the sex differences were eliminated.

Conservation

There are other Piagetian tasks that seem to require spatial abilities as well as logical skills. These are tasks of conservation of number, distance, length, and area. The research in this respect is generally not consistent with regard to sex differences. Harris and Allen (1971) presented 18 first-graders (9 males; 9 females) with a conservation of length task. Sticks of equivalent length were presented randomly to the subjects in a horizontal or a vertical alignment, and they were asked to determine, with and without displacement, whether the sticks were the same length. No difference between males and females was obtained. Gruen and Vore (1972) matched familial retarded children from three different mental age levels—5, 7, and 9 years—for mental age and chronological age with normal children. The subjects were evaluated for conservation of number, continuous quantity (water), and weight. Since the subjects were not matched for sex, uneven splits of males and females occurred in certain groups. For the groups in which relatively even splits occurred, no sex differences were noted.

In those studies where sex differences were observed, the males have been shown to be statistically superior on conservation tasks. Goldschmid (1967) studied different types of conservation and their relation to age, sex, I.Q., mental age, and vocabulary. The conservation tasks included substance, weight, continuous and discontinuous quantity, number, area, distance, length, and 2-dimensional and 3-dimensional space. The subjects were 102 children in first and second grades, some of whom were emotionally disturbed. Among the normal children (38 males and 38 females) it was found that males performed statistically on a higher level on 2 of 10 conservation tasks. Goldschmid (1967) found no significant differences between males and females with respect to their age, IQ, or vocabulary. Goldschmid (1967) hypothesized that the sex difference may have been due to the males having greater "opportunity to manipulate objects and perceive them after different transformations than girls do" (p. 1240).

Tuddenham (1970) tested approximately 500 children in kindergarten and the first four grades of school over a 6-year period. On tests of conservation of mass, volume, length, number, and area, he found that "boys do slightly better than girls, . . . but most correlations with sex are insignificant" (p. 65).

VERBAL ABILITIES

Techniques for Studying Brain Lateralization

Cerebral laterality in individuals with surgically intact brains is studied by the use of techniques that allow for the presentation of test stimuli selectively to each hemisphere. The basis for such a procedure is that the central projections from peripheral sensory receptors are primarily to the opposite side of the brain. For example, the right half of each eye sends information to the left hemisphere. The right half of both eyes input the left hemisphere, while the left halves input the right hemisphere. This allows one to determine the performance capacity of each hemisphere and, finally, how the hemispheres interact with each other.

On tests using the visual modality, the subject is required to fixate on a central point. Then visual stimuli are presented to a hemisphere by exposure in the opposite visual field. One can then present peripheral stimuli simultaneously in both fields, by presenting stimuli randomly in either the right or left peripheral field, by monitoring eye movements, or by presenting a simultaneous identification task in the center of the field (Gazzaniga, 1970).

On tests employing the auditory modality, the stimuli are presented to a specific hemisphere by simultaneously stimulating both ears with different stimuli. Each ear sends connections to both hemispheres. However, when different stimuli are presented simultaneously, the connections to the opposite (contralateral) hemisphere predominate (Mononen & Seitz, 1977; Zaidel, 1976).

Investigation of the tactile modality is performed by presenting stimuli selectively to each hemisphere by stimulating the contralateral side of the body. For example, each hand is first touched separately to determine whether the blindfolded subject can accurately respond to the stimulation. Once this has been established, then bilateral simultaneous stimulation is interspersed with unilateral stimulation. A normal subject will be able to accurately respond to the unilateral and the bilateral stimulation. Subjects with lateralized brain lesions will often be able to respond accurately to the unilateral stimulation, but when presented with the bilateral simultaneous stimulation, they may fail to respond to the hand contralateral to the damaged hemisphere (Reitan & Davison, 1974).

There are a number of assumptions about functional asymmetry that are evident when these techniques are employed with subjects having intact brains. One is that the projection of the sensory inputs is primarily to the contralateral hemisphere. Another is that the processing of inputs is done in one specialized hemisphere. A third assumption is that there is some decay and also delay of information transmission along the pathway from the peripheral receptor to the nonspecialized contralateral hemisphere and then across to the specialized hemisphere. Thus, the identification of stimuli is a function of the primary receptive cortical area, the interhemispheric connections, and the specialized association area.

There are a number of other techniques that are employed in assessing brain function. One is the use of scalp EEG electrodes to record brain activity at various sites while the subject is performing some task (Donchin, Kutas, & McCarthy, 1977; Doyle, Arnstein, & Galin, 1974; Galin & Ornstein, 1972; Kocel, Galin, Ornstein, & Merrin, 1972). Another technique is to evaluate metabolic activity in various parts of the brain by taking measures of regional blood flow (Lassen, Ingvar, & Skinhøj, 1978). Electrical conductance of the skin and the observation of initial eye movements when the subject is first presented with a task are other approaches to the assessment of brain function (Bakan, 1969; Gruzelier, 1973; Gruzelier & Hammond, 1976; Gruzelier & Venables, 1974; Gur, Gur & Harris, 1975).

Right–Left Hemisphere Differences

It is well documented that, from a neuropsychological perspective, the cerebral hemispheres are asymmetrically organized. Nonverbal stimuli are generally processed by the right hemisphere and verbal stimuli are processed by the left hemisphere (Milner, 1975; Mountcastle, 1962). This has been extensively documented in aphasia research (e.g., Goodglass & Quadfasel, 1954; Hecaen & DeAjuriaguerra, 1964; Hecaen & Sauguet, 1971; Roberts, 1969; Subirana, 1958; Zangwill, 1960). It has also been demonstrated by Wada and Rasmussen (1960) and Milner and her colleagues (Milner, Taylor, & Sperry, 1968) using intracarotid sodium amytal injections to determine the cerebral hemisphere that controls speech. This asymmetry has also been demonstrated using EEG techniques (Dumas & Morgan, 1975; Galin & Ellis, 1975; Low, Wada, & Fox, 1973; Moore, 1979; Ray, Morell, Frediani, & Tucker,1976; Rebert & Mahoney, 1978; Robbins & McAdam, 1974; Tucker, 1976). It has also been observed with dichotically or monaurally presented stimuli (Bakker, 1970; Doehring, 1972; Kimura, 1967; Milner *et al.*, 1968; Simon, 1967) as well as in tachistoscopic recognition studies (Bryden, 1970; Zurif & Bryden, 1969).

Sex Differences

A number of investigators have attributed the observed superiority of the right ear in processing verbal stimuli to the dominance of the left hemisphere for language functions (Geschwind, 1968; Kimura, 1961, 1963; Satz, 1972). While this view is generally accepted and amply documented, much of the original work in the area of hemispheric asymmetry was performed using adult males as subjects. The concern about possible sex differences in hemispheric functioning has only more recently been reflected in the literature (McGlone, 1977).

The studies of intact brains have supported the position of less complete lateralization of verbal and nonverbal functions in females as compared to males (Hannay & Malone, 1976a, 1976b; Kimura, 1961; Remington, Krashen, & Harshman, 1974). Evidence of this difference has also been documented in studies of males and females with unilateral brain damage (Lansdell, 1961, 1962; Lansdell & Urbach, 1965; McGlone, 1977; McGlone & Davidson, 1973; McGlone & Kertesz, 1973). The evidence for asymmetry differences for verbal tasks between men and women is not as consistent as the evidence for asymmetry differences for nonverbal tasks (Brust, Shafer, Richter, & Brunn, 1976; Lansdell, 1961, 1962, 1968, 1973; McGlone & Kertesz, 1973). In some instances sex differences in hemispheric asymmetry have not been found (Bryden, 1965; Hannay & Boyer, 1978; Moore, 1979).

Developmentally, the age at which sex differences in hemispheric lateralization of verbal abilities appears is an issue that has not been completely resolved. In terms of right versus left ear differences without regard to sex, a right ear superiority for verbal stimuli has been found in 3- to 12-year olds (Berlin, Hughes, Lowe-Bell, & Berlin, 1973; Borowy & Goebel, 1976; Kimura, 1963; Knox & Kimura, 1970; Nagafuchi, 1970). On the other hand, Bakker and Appelboom (1973) did not find a significant ear asymmetry until 9 to 10 years of age. These authors also noted an increase in asymmetry consistent with an increase in age. Kimura (1963) & Nagafuchi (1970) found that their youngest subjects displayed a greater ear asymmetry, a finding in contradiction to Bakker and Appelboom (1973). A number of studies have supported the notion that ear asymmetry develops at an earlier age in females than in males (Bryden, 1970; Kimura, 1967; Nagafuchi, 1970). Again, there are a number of studies that have not found sex differences (Bakker & Appelboom, 1973; Borowy & Goebel, 1976; Kimura, 1963; Knox & Kimura, 1970). Maccoby and Jacklin (1974) in their review concluded that there are certain distinct phases that both sexes go through as they grow and develop verbal skills. The first phase, they suggested, occurs early, before the age of 3. Males catch up to females by age 3 and the differences are minimal until about 10 or 11 years of age, when girls start to outperform boys fairly consistently.

For the most part, the developmental literature on sex differences in functional asymmetry of the cerebral hemispheres is fraught with inconsistencies and contradictions (Marcel, Katz, & Smith, 1974; Witelson, 1976). McGlone (1978) offers several explanations to account for this. One has to do with the problem of obtaining reliable and valid data from children using the techniques described earlier. Another problem involves the differential brain maturation rates between boys and girls (see also Buffery & Gray, 1972). McGlone (1978) takes this issue of maturation a step further and suggests that verbal, spatial, and sensory-motor systems may develop differentially, both with respect to each other and with respect to sex.

As noted earlier, Waber (1976) has found that the rate of physical maturation affects verbal and spatial abilities and also is related to the degree of language lateralization. Knox and Kimura (1970) presented verbal and nonverbal tasks dichotically to males and females who were between the ages of 5 and 8. They observed that both groups exhibited equivalent ear difference scores. However, males were found to correctly identify significantly more nonverbal sounds than girls. In one part of the study they also found that, with a group of preschool children, males were superior to females in identifying animal sounds nondichotically. This suggests earlier development of the right hemisphere for processing nonverbal sounds in males. Rudel, Denckla, and Spalten (1974) taught 80 right-handed children (40 males, 40 females), aged 7 to 14, to read 12 Braille letters by touch, using a paired associates method. Even though language is involved, both sexes performed better using the left hand. This left-hand superiority in Braille reading was found to be achieved relatively late in the course of development, and at different ages for males and females. At age 7 to 8, females were found to be significantly more efficient in Braille reading using their right hand. It was not until age 13 to 14 that the left hand emerged superior. The males however, displayed a significant left-hand superiority at age 11. The authors hypothesized that later development of left hand superiority in Braille reading for females may reflect greater utilization of language strategies on their part.

Witelson (1976) attempted to assess the extent of specialization of the right hemisphere for spatial processing using a test procedure that seemingly reduces the likelihood that a left hemisphere verbal–analytic strategy would be employed by the subjects. She tested 200 right-handed children, ranging in age from 6 to 13 years. There were 25 subjects of each sex within each 2-year interval. The test procedure required that each subject palpate simultaneously two different meaningless shapes for 10 seconds, using the index and middle fingers of each hand. The shapes were not available for viewing during this time. The subject was then required to select the two shapes from a visual display containing such shapes.

Witelson (1976) found that males, but not females, obtained significantly more correct left- than right-handed scores. The difference between hand scores was found to be significant even for the youngest subgroup of boys. Witelson concluded that the superiority of the left hand on this task reflected a superiority of the right hemisphere for spatial processing. She also indicated that while males displayed an apparent lateralization of the spatial process at age 6, females with no difference between scores for each hand actually were bilaterally represented for spatial processing, at least until adolescence. She suggested that for at least one aspect of cognition–spatial processing, the same neural structures in males and females may have different functions or, conversely, the same cognitive process may be mediated by different neural structures in males and females.

Studies of infants have not provided support for this model, however. Entus (1977) employed a paradigm that involved the presentation of a dichotic stimulus pair contingent on sucking activity of her infant subjects. Discrimination of the stimulus change was inferred from the recovery of sucking of experimental babies relative to that of controls. The stimuli were consonant–vowel syllables and the note "A" played on four musical instruments. There were 48 babies (24 males and 24 females) who participated. She found the recovery of sucking was greater in response to a stimulus change in the right ear when the stimulus was a consonant–vowel syllable. When music was the stimulus, greater recovery occurred following stimulus change in the left ear. Thus, even though the infants displayed a pattern of lateral asymmetry, no significant sex differences were found.

Molfese, Freeman, and Palermo (1975) compared auditory evoked responses (AER) from the temporal regions of both cerebral hemispheres of infants (4 males, 4 females) in response to speech and nonspeech acoustic stimuli. They found left hemisphere AER's were larger in amplitude than right hemisphere AER's to speech stimuli. For the nonspeech stimuli, the AER's in the right hemisphere were of a larger amplitude. No sex differences were reported.

Best and Glanville (1976) studied the relationship between musical stimuli and change in cardiac rate for 12 infants. No sex differences were noted in this study. These three studies suggest that while functional asymmetry of the cerebral hemispheres are noted very early in life, sex differences are not apparent.

MODELS OF HEMISPHERIC LATERALIZATION

A number of models have been proposed to account for sex differences in neuropsychological functioning. One espouses the position that there is greater right hemisphere specialization in males. It assumes that since males demonstrate, early in life, a superior spatial ability, then the right hemisphere must develop earlier and faster in males than females. Support for this position has come from a number of sources (Knox & Kimura, 1970; Rudel *et al.*, 1974; Witelson, 1975).

However, studies of infants have not provided support for this model (Best & Glanville, 1976; Entus, 1977; Molfese *et al.*, 1975). These studies suggest right hemisphere specialization for spatial abilities but find that the degree of specialization is comparable for males and females.

A second model is one proposed by Buffery and Gray (1972) in which they claim that earlier and greater lateralization in females facilitates verbal ability, and also that bilateral representation of spatial abilities in males facilitates the expression of this ability. There is some marginal support for this position to be found in the anatomical studies of Wada *et al.* (1975) and Witelson & Pallie (1973). Wada *et al.* (1975) noted greater asymmetry in the frontal areas of female brains than in male brains, while Witelson and Pallie (1973) noted that the temporal planum was significantly larger on the left in female infant brains but not in male infant brains. The assumption is that these anatomical differences reflect earlier and greater lateralization of language function in females. There is neuropsychological evidence for this model. Girls have been known to speak words first and have larger vocabularies than boys (Morley, 1957; Nelson, 1973). McCarthy (1930) also found girls' speech to be more comprehensible than that of boys.

Contrary evidence is found with the studies of Best and Glanville (1976), Entus (1977), and Molfese (1977). While their infant subjects demonstrated a right ear advantage for speech sounds, no differences between males and females were noted. Further nonsupport for the Buffery and Gray (1972) model is found in the study by Knox and Kimura (1970), where there were no right–left ear differences between boys and girls on a digit recognition task. Thus, there is some evidence to support this model, but other evidence exists that tends to negate its appropriateness and utility.

Another flaw in this model (Harris, 1978) is the lack of empirical evidence to suggest that bilateral hemispheric representation of spatial abilities is important for the expression of those abilities. Also there is a clear lack of evidence that spatial abilities are bilaterally represented more in the male than the female. There is also a lack of adult studies that suggest greater language lateralization in females. The differences in language functioning between males and females in their early years may reflect the maturational advantage females have over males during this period (Taylor, 1969).

Harris (1978) discussed a third model, which argues that the male is initially less lateralized. Then, over time, the degree of lateralization between the sexes becomes comparable, and finally the male attains a greater degree of lateralization for language. The female, on the other hand, is left with bilateral representation of language. This bilateral representation of language interferes with the expression of spatial abilities and, consequently, the female is not able to perform in this area as well as the male. Levy (1969), although she was not specifically concerned with sex differences, proposed a similar model that says, in effect, "this hemisphere ain't big enough for both of us". She proposed that the left hemisphere is specialized for analytic, verbal activities, while the right hemisphere is specialized for synthetic, nonverbal activities. When these activities are localized within the same hemisphere, the analytic and synthetic functions conflict to the detriment of the synthetic functions. It should be noted that Levy (1969) proposed this model to account for differences she encountered between left- and right-handed individuals rather than for differences between males and females.

Support for this proposition that females have bilateral representation for language comes from a number of sources (Hannay & Malone, 1976a, 1976b; Lansdell, 1961; Remington *et al.*, 1974). Lansdell (1961) examined men and women who were to undergo unilateral temporal lobectomies using a proverbs test. It follows from this model that since males have language more lateralized in one hemisphere, the impact of surgery, when it is on that hemisphere, should be greater. Thus, the male scores on the proverbs test should be more adversely affected when the surgery is on the language hemisphere. This in fact is what Lansdell (1961) found. The males' performance on the proverbs test declined and the females' performance did not change when the surgery was performed on the language hemisphere.

In another study, Lansdell (1962) evaluated males and females before and after temporal lobe surgery using the Graves Design Judgment Test. This test is a measure of artistic appreciation and purportedly has a spatial component to it. When surgery was performed on the language hemisphere, the males' scores improved and the females' scores declined. The exact opposite occurred when the surgery was done on the nonlanguage hemisphere: the males' scores declined and the females' scores improved. It thus appears that males have greater lateralization of verbal abilities in the left hemisphere, and spatial abilities in the right hemisphere. It alo appears that females may have less lateralization (or more bilateral representation) of these same abilities. In an attempt to account for his findings, Lansdell (1962) proposed that the neural substrates for spatial and verbal abilities in women were intermingled or overlapped, whereas in men he suggested that the neural substrates resided in opposite hemispheres.

In another study McGlone and Kertesz (1973) investigated the effects of unilateral brain damage in 78 adult men and women on an aphasia battery and the Block Design Test from the Wechsler–Bellevue Intelligence Scale. Among the subjects, 35 males and 22 females had left hemispere lesions, while 13 males and 8 females had right hemisphere lesions. They found that patients with left hemisphere lesions did significantly worse on the aphasia test and sigificantly better on the Block Design Test as compared to patients with right hemisphere lesions. Sex differences were not found for the aphasia or block design tests. However, it was noted that the males with right hemisphere lesions tended to perform more poorly on the Block Design Test than the other groups. A significant correlation was found between scores on the aphasia test and the block design test for the females who had left hemisphere lesions. McGlone and Kertesz (1973) concluded that greater functional asymmetry was present in adult male brains as compared to adult female brains. More specifically they concluded that nonverbal functions are more lateralized in men than in women.

McGlone (1977) investigated the possibility of sex differences in the cerebral lateralization of verbal functions using a group of unilateral brain-damaged men and women as well as a group of normal controls. There were 92 patients in all and the age range was from 15 to 70 years. In all cases lesion onset was after the age of 10 years and was due to vascular problems or tumors. There were 32 men and 20 women with left hemisphere lesions and 23 men and 17 women with right hemisphere lesions. All patients were right-handed. They were administered the Minnesota Test for the Differential Diagnosis of Aphasia, the Wechsler Adult Intelligence Scale (WAIS), and the Wechsler Memory Scale. McGlone (1977) discovered that the verbal deficits were dependent not only on the site of the lesion (left or right), but also on the sex of the patient. The various types of language deficits were either minimal or absent in females with left hemisphere lesions. Aphasia resulting from left-sided damage was present three times more often in male patients than in female patients. She subsequently analyzed the data, after having removed the aphasic patients from the left hemisphere group, and she found that the verbal deficits in intellectual and memory tasks were still more prominent in males than females.

Conversely, only the female patients with right hemisphere damage displayed mildly lower verbal intelligence scores relative to the normal controls. She concluded that language functions may well be organized differently within the cortex for men as compared to women. She felt that sex differences may be related to the degree of bilateral language representation and also to the underlying neural organization of verbal abilities within the left hemisphere. The possibility of a different neural organization of language within the left hemisphere between men and women was suggested by the observation that male aphasics were more homogeneous in their scores on expressive and receptive verbal tasks as compared to female aphasics. Also the Verbal IQ subtest profiles differentiated male and female nonaphasics with left-sided damage.

This suggested to McGlone (1977) that the components of verbal intelligence may not have been similarly affected in the males and females. In another publication, McGlone (1978) reported on the Verbal-Performance IQ discrepancies for these same patients. She noted that only the male patients displayed verbal deficits after left-sided lesions, or performance deficits after right-sided lesions. The deficits for the female patients were described as generally "less severe and less specific" (p. 126). Her conclusion was that there is greater functional asymmetry in the brains of right-handed adult males than in right-handed adult females.

Thus the data generally seem to support this model that proposes that males are more lateralized for verbal functions. The data also strongly suggest that males are more lateralized for spatial abilitis as well. However, not all of the studies have been consistent with this model. Kertesz and McCabe (1977) reasoned that if women had bilateral representation of language, then it would be expected that women would show a better rate of recovery from aphasia than men. However, their findings were negative in this regard; their female patients did not display a greater rate of recovery from aphasia than did their male patients.

Hannay and Boyer (1978) found that both their male and female subjects processed linguistic material in the left hemisphere. There were no sex differences in the degree of lateralization demonstrated. In fact, they obtained slightly larger laterality measures for their female subjects. They concluded that there was no difference in the degree of hemispheric asymmetry for visually presented verbal material between men and women. This is in contradiction to conclusions made earlier by the primary author (Hannay & Malone, 1976a, 1976b) to the effect that there is less complete lateralization of function in females.

In order to extract themselves from this dilemma, Hannay and Boyer (1978) reasoned that laterality tasks may not merely measure hemispheric asymmetry. They proposed that such tasks may also serve as indicators of the mode of processing or cognitive strategy being used by the subject. Thus, while all subjects in a group may share the same hemispheric functional asymmetry, when presented with a particular lateralization task, some subjects within the group may employ a verbal strategy, and other subjects may employ a spatial strategy. Such differences, when averaged over the group, may mislead the investigator as he attempts to draw conclusions about the degree of lateralization of function for the particular task. In relation to their own study, Hannay and Boyer (1978) speculated that their tasks differed enough from the earlier studies (Hannay & Malone, 1976a, 1976b) such that they were eliciting different cognitive strategies from their subjects, and were obtaining data that were essentially contradictory in the conclusions that could be drawn from them.

This reasoning has been expressed before. Kimura (1969) had found a right hemisphere superiority for spatial abilities in her male subjects but not in her female subjects. She had suggested that the females may have been using a verbal as opposed to a spatial strategy on the task. Similar arguments were made by McGlone and Davidson (1973). Tucker (1976) had his male and female subjects perform two visual–spatial tasks. Recording of electroencephalographic wave activity was done as the subjects (21 male and 20 female right-handed college students) completed the tasks. Tucker found that when the males performed a visual–spatial task, only their right hemispheres were significantly activated. When the females performed the same task, both of their hemispheres became active. When an analytic visual–spatial task was performed, both sexes seemed to rely on both hemispheres.

Harris (1978) proposed that different developmental histories for males and females might predispose them to employ different strategies during the performance of spatial tasks. Specifically, males would generally rely on right hemisphere processing strategies and females would rely on left hemisphere processing strategies. With this view in mind, Harris reinterpreted the results of studies whose authors had previously concluded were reflecting lateralization differences between males and females. Very cogently Harris demonstrated that the results were also compatible with a preferential processing model. She suggested that treating these data as measures of lateralization differences alone is too narrow and restrictive. Instead, investigators should look to not only the particular hemisphere that is activated in order to appreciate sex differences, but they should also inquire about the type of processing strategy employed by the sexes as well.

Hannay and Boyer (1978) and Harris (1978) both have suggested that the ultimate study to decide the relative merits of a lateralization versus preferential processing model has not been done. They feel that the first step would be to establish which hemisphere is lateralized for speech in groups of normal males and females. The technique that would be most helpful in determining this laterality is the sodium amytal test (Wada & Rasmussen, 1960). Once established, various tasks could be administered that would elicit different processing modes, or would suggest the extent of hemispheric asymmetry. The sodium amytal test, being an invasive procedure, has its risks and is therefore not likely to be used with normal subjects. In lieu of this methodology, Harris (1978) has suggested that a more acceptable procedure would be to continuously monitor hemispheric activity, via cerebral bloodflow and electroencephalography, as normal subjects perform various verbal and spatial tasks. With this type of procedure, closer attention could be focused on the differential activity not only between hemispheres but also between specific regions within each hemisphere.

SUMMARY

Neuroanatomical studies have been primarily concerned with determining the existence of anatomical asymmetries between right and left cerebral hemispheres, which might then lend support to the assumption that a neural substrate underlies the functional lateral asymmetries that have been reported quite consistently in the literature. A few studies have considered whether anatomical differences of the cerebrum might exist between the sexes. These studies are few in number and have employed rather small n's. The results are not definitive by any means, however they do suggest the possibility of sex differences in cerebral anatomy.

In the area of spatial abilities, the consistent tendency is for males to be superior to females. These differences, however, do not always appear until early to late adolescence. When they have been found earlier, the males tend to be superior. The rate of maturation also seems to be important. It has been found that early maturing adolescents, regardless of sex, perform better on verbal than spatial tasks, and with late maturing adolescents, the opposite has been found. It has also been demonstrated that early maturers apparently have more bilateral representation of language than late maturers. Thus the rate of maturation may play a very significant role in the organization of higher cortical functioning.

When males and females are required to mentally construct a three-dimensional object from a visually displayed, two-dimensional flat pattern, males consistently outperform females. The differences, however, may not be due to the nature of the task, but rather the strategy that is used to solve the task. It has been found that females have a greater tendency to employ a verbal-analytic strategy to solve mental rotation tasks, whereas males are more likely to use a visual-holistic strategy. Thus females may rely upon their left hemisphere while males will rely upon their right hemisphere to perform a mental rotation task.

It has been demonstrated that males perform better than females on measures of mathematical ability. These differences have been observed even among grade-school children. It would seem that, at this early age, differential exposure of the sexes to mathematics curricula has not as yet taken place. Therefore the differences in performance between the sexes may be due to differences in cortical functioning. However, other environmental factors have not been adequately studied and thus cannot be ruled out at this time.

In studies of field dependence–field independence, which have used the Rod and Frame Test and the Embedded Figures Test, males have consistently performed in a less field-dependent manner. On the Embedded Figures Test, the sex differences are not noted until the adolescent years, whereas sex differences on the Rod and Frame Test are found as early as 5 years of age. Some speculation has been made about differences between the sexes in general cognitive style based on performances on these tests. Such speculation seems premature and not in appreciation of all the data. It has been shown that when the spatial component of field dependence–field independence measures has been removed, the sex differences in performance are eliminated. Parsimoniously then, the differences found between males and females on the Rod and Frame Test and the Embedded Figures Test reflect the superiority of males on spatial tasks, and nothing more.

Females seem to have more difficulty with right–left discrimination and with following road maps and working mazes. However, the differences have not always been significant.

On tasks designed to assess quantitatively some of Piaget's principles of cognitive development, sex differences have not consistently been found. No differences have been noted on tasks of conservation of length, number, continuous quantity, and weight. However, when sex differences have been observed, males have been found to be superior to females.

Lastly, it has been found that verbal and nonverbal functions in females are less completely lateralized than in males. This has been demonstrated with cerebrally intact subjects as well as with individuals who have unilateral brain damage. However, the evidence for asymmetry differences for verbal tasks between males and females is not as consistent as the evidence for asymmetry differences for nonverbal tasks. Also the age at which sex differences in hemispheric lateralization of verbal abilities occurs has not been completely resolved.

Current methodologies and investigative techniques limit somewhat the scope of the inquiry into the functioning of the cerebral hemispheres. If the history of neuropsychology is any indicator, then it is expected that ingenious devices and tools will be developed that will help elucidate further the principles of brain-behavior relationships. Such devices and tools should allow for the study of problem-solving strategies. A spatially defined task may not elicit from subjects similar strategies. Grouping subjects who employ different strategies to solve a task can wash out important individual differences. More documentation is needed in regard to the question of when do neuropsychological differences in functioning occur beteen males and females. Longitudinal studies will be of great importance in this area. Also, the relationship between exogenous and endogenous factors needs to be explored.

ACKNOWLEDGMENT

The author wishes to express his thanks to Anita Jefferson for her clerical assistance in the preparation of this chapter.

REFERENCES

Anatasi, A. *Differential psychology: Individual and group differences in behavior* (3rd ed.). New York: Macmillan, 1958.

Bakan, P. Hypnotizability, laterality of eye-movements and functional brain asymmetry. *Perceptual and Motor Skills,* 1969, *28,* 927–932.

Bakan, P., & Putnam, W. Right–left discrimination and brain lateralization. *Archives of Neurology,* 1974, *30,* 334–335.

Bakker, D. J. Ear-asymmetry with monaural stimulation: Relations to lateral dominance and lateral awareness. *Neuropsychologia,* 1970, *8,* 103–117.

Bakker, D. J., & Appelboom, E. *The effects of stimulus intensity and recall mode on ear asymmetry subsequent to monaural stimulation.* Research Report No. 732, Department of Developmental and Educational Neuropsychology, Paedologisch Instituut, Amsterdam, 1973.

Benbow, C., & Stanley, J. Sex differences in mathematical ability: Fact or artifact? *Science,* 1980, *310,* 1262–1264.

Bennett, D. H. Perception of the upright in relation to body image. *Journal of Mental Science,* 1956, *102,* 487–506.

Bennett, G. K., Seashore, H. G., & Wesman, A. G. *Manual for the differential aptitude tests: Forms S & T* (5th ed.). New York: The Psychological Corporation, 1974.

Benton, A. L., & Joynt, R. J. Early descriptions of aphasia. *AMA Archives of Neurology,* 1960, *3,* 205–222.

Berlin, C., Hughes, L., Lowe-Bell, S., & Berlin, H. *Dichotic right ear advantages in children 5 to*

13. Paper presented at the International Neuropsychological Society, New Orleans, Louisiana, 1973.

Berry, J. W. Temne and Eskimo perceptual skills. *International Journal of Psychology,* 1966, *1,* 207–229.

Best, C. T., & Glanville, B. B. *A cardiac measure of cerebral asymmetries in infant perception of speech and nonspeech.* Paper pesented at the meeting of the Midwestern Psychological Association, Chicago, 1976.

Bock, R. D. Word image: Sources of the verbal and spatial factors in mental test scores. *Psychometrika,* 1973, *38,* 437–457.

Bogo, N., Winget, C., & Gleser, G. C. Ego defenses and perceptual styles. *Perceptual and Motor Skills,* 1970, *30,* 599–604.

Borowy, T., & Goebel, R. Cerebral lateralization of speech: The effects of age, sex, race, and socioeconomic class. *Neuropsychologia,* 1976, *14,* 363–370.

Brust, J., Shafer, S., Richter, R., & Brunn, B. Aphasia in acute stroke. *Stroke,* 1976, *7,* 167–174.

Bryden, M. P. Tachistoscopic recognition, handedness, and cerebral dominance. *Neuropsychologia,* 1965, *3,* 1–8.

Bryden, M. P. Laterality effects in dichotic listening: Relations with handedness and reading ability in children. *Neuropsychologia,* 1970, *8,* 443–450.

Bryden, M. P., & Tapley, S. M. *Sex differences in mental rotation.* Paper presented at the annual meeting of the Canadian Psychological Association, Toronto, 1976.

Buffery, A. W. H., & Gray, J. H. Sex differences in the development of spatial and linguistic skills. In C. Ounstead & D. C. Taylor (Eds.), *Gender differences: Their ontogeny and significance.* London: Churchill, 1972.

Chi, J. G., Dooling, E., & Gilles, F. Left–right asymmetries of the temporal speech areas of the human fetus. *Archives of Neurology,* 1977, *34,* 346–348.

Corballis, M., & Beale, I. L. *The psychology of left and right.* New York: Lawrence Erlbaum Associates, 1976.

DeFries, J. C., Ashton, G. C., Johnson, R. C., Kuse, A. R., McClearn, G. E., Mi, M. P., Rashad, M. N., Sandenberg, S. G., & Wilson, J. R. Parent–offspring resemblance of specific cognitive abilities in two ethnic groups. *Nature,* 1976, *261,* 131–133.

Doehring, D. G. Ear-asymmetry in the discrimination of monaural tonal sequences. *Canadian Journal of Psychology,* 1972, *26,* 106–110.

Donchin, E., Kutas, M., & McCarthy, G. Electrocortical indices of hemispheric utilization. In S. Harnad, R. W. Doty, L. Goldstein, J. Joynes, & G. Krauthamer (Eds.), *Lateralization in the nervous system.* New York: Academic, 1977.

Doyle, J. C., Arnstein, R. E., & Galin, D. Lateralization of cognitive mode: II. EEG frequency and analysis. *Psychophysiology,* 1974, *11,* 567–578.

Dumas, R., & Morgan, A. EEG asymmetry as a function of occupation, task, and task difficulty. *Neuropsychologia,* 1975, *13,* 219–228.

Entus, A. K. Hemispheric asymmetry in processing of dichotically presented speech and nonspeech stimuli by infants. In S. J. Segalowitz & F. A. Gruber (Eds.), *Language development and neurological theory.* New York: Academic, 1977.

Fiebert, M. Cognitive styles in the deaf. *Perceptual and Motor Skills,* 1967, *24,* 319–329.

Flanagan, J. C., Dailey, J. T., Shaycoft, M. F., Gorham, W. A., Orr, D. B., Goldberg, J., & Neyman, C. A., Jr. *Counselor's technical manual for interpreting test scores* (Project Talent, Palo Alto, California). Boston: Houghton Mifflin 1961.

Galaburda, A., LeMay, M., Kemper, T., & Geschwind, N. Right–left asymmetries in the brain. *Science,* 1978, *199,* 852–856.

Galaburda, A., Sanides, F., & Geschwind, N. Human brain. *Archives of Neurology,* 1978, *35,* 812–817.

Galin, D., & Ellis, R. Asymmetry in evoked potentials as an index of lateralized cognitive processes: Relation to EEG alpha asymmetry. *Neuropsychologia*, 1975, *13*, 45–50.

Galin, D., & Ornstein, R. Lateral specialization of cognitive mode: An EEG study. *Psychophysiology*, 1972, *9*, 412.

Gardner, R. W., Jackson, D. N., & Messick, S. J. Personality organization in cognitive controls and intellectual abilities. *Psychological Issues*, 1960, *2*, (Whole No. 8).

Gazzaniga, M. *The bisected brain*. New York: Appleton-Century-Crofts, 1970.

Geisinger, E. R., & Hyde, J. Sex differences on Piaget's water level task: Spatial incognito. *Perceptual and Motor Skills*, 1976, *42*, 1323–1328.

Geschwind, N. Neurological foundations of language. In H. R. Mylkebust (Ed.), *Progress in learning disabilities: I.* New York: Grune & Stratton, 1968.

Geschwind, N., & Levitsky, W. Human brain: Left–right asymmetries in temporal speech region. *Science*, 1968, *161*.

Goldschmid. M. L. Different types of conservation and non-conservation and their relation to age, sex, IQ, MA, and vocabulary. *Child Development*, 1967, *38*, 1229–1246.

Goodglass, H., & Quaddfasel, F. A. Language laterality in left-handed asphasics. *Brain*, 1954, *77*, 521–548.

Goodnow, R. Cited in H. A. Witkin, R. B. Dyk, G. E. Faterson, D. R. Goodenough, & S. A. Karp, *Psychological differentiation*. New York: Wiley, 1962.

Graves, M. F., & Koziol, S. Noun plural development in primary grade children. *Child Development*, 1971, *42*, 1165–1173.

Gruen, G. E., & Vore, D. A. Development of conservation in normal and retarded children. *Developmental Psychology*, 1972, *6*, 146–157.

Gruzelier, J. Bilateral asymmetry of skin conductance orienting activity and levels in schizophrenics. *Biological Psychology*, 1973, *1*, 21.

Gruzelier, J., & Hammond, N. Schizophrenia: A dominant hemisphere temporal–limbic disorder? *Research Communications in Psychology, Psychiatry, and Behavior*, 1976, *1*, 33.

Gruzelier, J., & Venables, P. Bimodality and laterality asymmetry in skin conductance orienting activity in schizophrenics: Replication and evidence of lateral asymmetry in patients with depression and disorders of personality. *Biological Psychology*, 1974, *8*, 55.

Guilford, J. P., & Lacey, J. I. *Printed classification tests, A.A.F* (Aviation Psychological Progress Research Report No. 5). Washington, D.C.: U.S. Government Printing Office, 1947.

Gur, R. E., Gur, R. C., & Harris, L. J. Cerebral activation as measured by subjects' lateral eye movements is influenced by experimenter location. *Neuropsychologia*, 1975, *13*, 35–44.

Hannay, H. J., & Boyer, C. L. Sex differences in hemispheric asymmetry revisited. *Perceptual and Motor Skills*, 1978, *47*, 315–321.

Hannay, H. J., & Malone, D. R. Visual field effects and short-term memory for verbal material. *Neuropsychologia*, 1976, *14*, 203–209.(a)

Hannay, H. J., & Malone, D. R. Visual field recognition memory for right-handed females as a function of familial handedness. *Cortex*, 1976, *12*, 41–48.(b)

Harris, L. J. Sex differences in spatial ability: Possible environment, genetic, and neurological factors. In M. Kinsbourne (Ed.), *Asymmetrical function of the brain*. Cambridge: Cambridge University Press, 1978.

Harris, L. J., & Allen, T. W. The effects of stimulus alignment on children's performance in a conservation-of-length problem. *Psychonomic Science*, 1971, *23*, 137–139.

Hartlage, L. C. Sex-linked inheritance of spatial ability. *Perceptual and Motor Skills*, 1970, *31*, 610.

Hecaen, H., & DeAjuriaguerra, J. *Left-handedness*. New York: Grune & Stratton, 1964.

Hecaen, H., & Sauguet, J. Cerebral dominance in left handed subjects. *Cortex*, 1971, *7*, 19–48.

Hills, J. R. Factor analyzed abilities and success in college mathematics. *Educational Psychological Measurement*, 1957, *17*, 615–622.

Hyde, J. S., Geiringer, E. R. & Yen, W. On the empirical relation between spatial ability and sex differences in other aspects of cognitive performance. *Multivariate Behavioral Research*, 1975, *10*, 289-301

Joynt, R. R. & Benton, A. L. The memoir of Marc Dax on aphasia. *Neurology*, 1964, *14*, 91.

Kelly, J. T., & Kelly, G. N. Perception of horizontality by male and female college students. *Perceptual and Motor Skills*, 1977, *44*, 724-726.

Keogh, B. K. Pattern copying under three conditions of an expanded spatial field. *Developmental Psychology*, 1971, *4*, 25-31.

Keogh, B. K., & Ryan, S. R. Use of three measures and field organization with young children. *Perceptual and Motor Skills*, 1971, *33*, 466.

Kertesz, A., & McCabe, P. Recovery patterns and prognosis in aphasia. *Brain*, 1977, *100*, 1-18.

Kimura, D. Cerebral dominance and the perception of verbal stimuli. *Canadian Journal of Psychology*, 1961, *15*, 166-171.

Kimura, D. Speech lateralization in young children as determined by an auditory test. *Journal of Comparative and Physiological Psychology*, 1963, *56*, 899-902.

Kimura, D. Functional asymmetry of the brain in dichotic listening. *Cortex*, 1967, *3*, 163-178.

Kimura, D. Spatial localization in left and right visual fields. *Canadian Journal of Psychology*, 1969, *23*, 445-458.

Knox, C., & Kimura, D. Cerebral processing of nonverbal sounds in boys and girls. *Neuropsychologia*, 1970, *8*, 227-237.

Kocel, K., Galin, D., Ornstein, R. E., & Merrin, E. L. Lateral eye movement and cognitive mode. *Psychonomic Science*, 1972, *27*, 223-226.

Lansdell, H. The effect of neurosurgery on a test of proverbs. *American Psychologist*, 1961, *16*, 448.

Lansdell, H. A sex difference in effect of temporal-lobe neurosurgery on design preference. *Nature*, 1962, *194*, 852-854.

Lansdell, H. Effect of extent of temporal lobe ablations on two lateralized deficits. *Physiology and Behavior*, 1968, *3*, 271-273.

Lansdell, H. Effect of neurosurgery on the ability to identify popular word associations. *Journal of Abnormal Psychology*, 1973, *81*, 255-258.

Lansdell, H., & Urbach, N. Sex differences in personality measures related to size and side of temporal lobe ablations. *Proceedings of American Psychological Association*, 1965.

Lassen, N., Ingvar, D., & Skinhøj, E. Brainfunction and blood flow. *Scientific American*, 1978, *239*, 62-71.

Levy, J. Possible basis for the evolution of lateral specialization of the human brain. *Nature*, 1969, *224*, 614-615.

Liben, L. S. *Operative understanding of horizontality and its relation to long-term memory*. Paper presented at Biennial Meetings of the Society for Research in Child Development, Philadelphia, 1973.

Low, M. D., Wada, J. A., & Fox, M. Electroencephalographic localization of conative aspects of language production in the human brain. *Transactions of the American Neurological Association*, 1973, *98*, 129-133.

Maccoby, E. E., & Jacklin, C. N. *The psychology of sex differences*. Stanford, Calif.: Stanford University Press, 1974.

Marcel, T., Katz, L., & Smith, M. Laterality and reading proficiency. *Neuropsychologia*, 1974, *12*, 131-139.

Maxwell, J. W., Croake, J. W., & Biddle, A. P. Sex differences in the comprehension of spatial orientation. *Journal of Psychology*, 1975, *91*, 121-131.

McCarthy, D. *The language development of the preschool child* (Institute of Child Welfare Monograph Series No. 4). Minneapolis: University of Minnesota Press, 1930.

McGee, M. G. Effects of training and practice on sex differences in Mental Rotation Test scores. *Journal of Psychology,* 1978, *100,* 87-90.

McGee, M. G. Human spatial abilities: Psychometric studies and environmental, genetic, hormonal, and neurological influences. *Psychological Bulletin,* 1979, *86,* 889-918.

McGlone, J. Sex differences in the cerebral organization of verbal functions in patients with unilateral brain lesions. *Brain,* 1977, *100,* 775-793.

McGlone, J. Sex differences in functional brain asymmetry. *Cortex,* 1978, *14,* 122-128.

McGlone, J., & Davidson, W. The relation between cerebral speech laterality and spatial ability with special reference to sex and hand preference. *Neuropsychologia,* 1973, *11,* 105-113.

McGlone, J., & Kertesz, A. Sex differences in cerebral processing of visuospatial tasks. *Cortex,* 1973, *9,* 313-320.

Metzler, J., & Shepard, R. N. Rotation of tri-dimensional objects. In R. L. Solso (Ed.), *Theories in cognitive psychology: The Loyola Symposium.* New York: Wiley, 1974.

Milner, B. Psychological aspects of focal epilepsy and its neurosurgical management. In D. Purpura, J. K. Penry, & R. Walter (Eds.), *Neurosurgical management of the epilepsies (Advances in neurology,* Vol. 8). New York: Raven, 1975.

Milner, G., Taylor, L. B., & Sperry, R. W. Lateralized suppression of dichotically presented digits after commisural section in man. *Science,* 1968, *161,* 184-185.

Molfese, D. L. Infant cerebral asymmetry. In S. J. Segalowitz & F. A. Gruber (Eds.), *Language development and neurological theory.* New York: Academic, 1977.

Molfese, D. L., Freeman, R. B., Jr., & Palermo, D. S. The ontogeny of brain lateralization for speech and nonspeech stimuli. *Brain and Language,* 1975, *2,* 356-368.

Money, J., & Ehrhardt, A. *Man and woman, boy and girl.* Baltimore: Johns Hopkins University Press, 1972.

Money, J., Alexander, D., & Walker, H. T., Jr. *A standardized road map test of direction sense.* Baltimore, Md.: Johns Hopkins University Press, 1965.

Mononen, L. J., & Seitz, M. R. An AER analysis of contralateral advantage in the transmission of auditory information. *Neuropsychologia,* 1977, *15,* 165-173.

Moore, W. H., Jr. Alpha hemispheric asymmetry of males and females on verbal tasks: Some preliminary results. *Cortex,* 1979, *15,* 321-326.

Morley, M. E. *The development and disorders of speech in childhood.* London: Livingstone, 1957.

Mountcastle, V. *Interhemispheric relations and cerebral dominance.* Baltimore: Johns Hopkins Press, 1962.

Munroe, R. L., & Munroe, R. H. *Space and numbers: Some ecological factors in culture and behavior.* Paper presented at the workshop of the Maberere Institute of Social Research, New York, 1968. (Cited in L. J. Harris, Sex differences in spatial ability: Possible environmental, genetic, and neurological factors. In J. M. Kinsbourne (Ed.), *Asymmetrical function of the brain.* Cambridge: Cambridge University Press, 1978.)

Munsinger, H. Most California college women already know that the surface of still water is always horizontal. *American Journal of Psychology,* 1974, *87,* 717-718.

Nagafuchi, M. Development of dichotic and monaural hearing abilities in young children. *Acta Otolaryngologica,* 1970, *69,* 409-415.

Nelson, K. Structure and strategy in learning to talk. *Monograph of the Society for Research in Child Development,* 1973, *38* (1-2, Serial No. 149).

Piaget, J., & Inhelder, B. *The child's concept of space.* New York: Humanities press, 1956.

Porteus, S. D. The measurement of intelligence: 653 children examined by the Binet and Proteus tests. *Journal of Educational Psychology,* 1918, *9,* 13-31.

Porteus, S. D. *Guide to Porteus Maze Test.* Vineland, N.J.: The Training School, 1924.

Porteus, S. D. *Porteus maze tests: Fifty years' application.* Palo Alto, Calif.: Pacific Books, 1965.

Ray, W. J., Morell, M., Frediani, A. W., & Tucker, D. Sex differences and lateral specialization of hemispheric functioning. *Neuropsychologia,* 1976, *14,* 394.

Rebelsky, F. Adults' perception of the horizontal. *Perceptual and Motor Skills*, 1964, *19*, 371–374.

Rebert, C. S., & Mahoney, R. A. Functional cerebral asymmetry and Performance III. Reaction time as a function of task, hand, sex, and EEG asymmetry. *Psychophysiology*, 1978, *15*, 9–15.

Reitan, R., & Davison, L. *Clinical neuropsychology: Currect status and applications.* New York: Wiley, 1974.

Remington, R., Krashen, S., & Harshman, R. A possible sex difference in the degree of lateralization of dichotic stimuli. *Journal of the Accoustical Society of America*, 1974, *55*, 434.

Robbins, K. I., & McAdam, D. W. Interhemispheric alpha asymmetry and imagery mode. *Brain and Language*, 1974, *1*, 189–193.

Roberts. L. Aphasia. apraxia, and agnosia in abnormal states of cerebral dominance. In P. J. Vinken & G. W. Bruyn (Eds.), *Handbook of clinical neurology* (Vol. 4). Amsterdam: North-Holland, 1969.

Rudel, R. G., Denckla, M. B., & Spalten, E. The functional asymmetry of Braille letter learning in normal sighted children. *Neurology*, 1974, *24* 733–738.

Saad, L. G., & Storer, W. O. *Understanding in mathematics.* Edenburgh, Scotland: Oliver and Boyd, 1960.

Saarni, C. I. Piagetian operations and field independence as factors in children's problem-solving performance. *Child Development,* 1973, *44*, 338–345.

Satz, P. Pathological left-handedness: An explanatory model. *Cortex,* 1972, *8*, 212–235.

Schwartz, D. W., & Karp, S. A. Field dependence in a geriatric population. *Perceptual and Motor Skills,* 1967, *24*, 495–504.

Shepard, R. N., & Metzler, J. Mental rotation of three dimensional objects. *Science,* 1971, *171*, 701–703.

Sherman, J. A. Problem of sex differences in space perception and aspects of intellectual functioning. *Psychological Review,* 1967, *74*, 290–299.

Sherman, J. A. *On the psychology of women: A survey of empirical studies.* Springfield, Ill.: Charles C Thomas, 1971.

Silverman, J., Bucksbaum, M., Stierlin, H. Sex differences in perceptual differentiation and stimulus intensity control. *Journal of Personality and Social Psychology,* 1973, *25*, 309–318.

Simon, J. R. Ear preference in a simple reaction-time task. *Journal of Experimental Psychology,* 1967, *75*, 45–55.

Smith, I. M. The validity of tests of spatial ability as predictors of success on technical courses. *British Journal of Educational Psychology,* 1960, *30*, 138–145.

Smith, I. M. *Spatial ability: Its educational and social significance.* London: University of London, 1964.

Stafford, R. E. Sex differences in spatial visualization as evidence of sex-linked inheritance. *Perceptual and Motor Skills,* 1961, *13*, 428.

Subirana, A. The prognosis in aphasia in relation to cerebral dominance and handedness. *Brain,* 1958, *81*, 415–425.

Tapley, S. M., & Bryden, M. P. An investigation of sex differences in spatial ability: Mental rotation of three-dimensional objects. *Canadian Journal of Psychology,* 1977, *31*, 122–130.

Taylor, D. C. Differential rates of cerebral maturation between sexes and between hemispheres. *Lancet,* 1969, *2*, 140–142.

Thomas, H. *The development of water-level representation.* Paper presented at Biennial Meetings of the Society for Research in Child Development, Minneapolis, 1971.

Thomas, H., Jamison, W., & Hummel, D. D. Observation is insufficient for discovering that the surface of still water is invariantly horizontal. *Science,* 1973, *181*, 173–174.

Thurstone, L. L. *Some primary abilities in visual thinking* (Report No. 59). Chicago: University of Chicago Psychometric Laboratory, 1950.

Tucker, D. M. Sex differences in hemispheric specialization for synthetic visuospatial functions. *Neuropsychologia,* 1976, *14*, 447–454.

Tuddenham, R. D. A Piagetian test of cognitive development. In W. B. Dockrell (Ed.), *On Intelligence: The Toronto Symposium on Intelligence.* London: Methuen, 1970.

Vandenberg, S. G., & Kuse, A. R. Mental rotations: A group test of three-dimensional spatial visualization. *Perceptual and Motor Skills,* 1978, *47,* 599–604.

Vandenberg, S. G., Stafford, R. E., & Brown, A. The Lousiville twin study. In S. G. Vandeberg (Ed.), *Progress in human behavior genetics.* Baltimore: John Hopkins Press, 1968.

Von Bonin, G. Anatomical asymmetries of the cerebral hemispheres. In V. B. Mountcastle (Ed.), *Interhemispheric relations and cerebral dominance.* Baltimore: Johns Hopkins Press, 1962.

Waber, D. P. Sex differences in cognition: A function of maturation rate? *Science,* 1976, *192,* 572–574.

Wada, J. Interhemispheric sharing and shift of cerebral speech function. *Excerpta Medica International Congress Series,* 1969, *193,* 296–297.

Wada, J., & Rasmussen, J. Intracarotid injection of sodium amytal for the lateralization of cerebral speech dominance. *Journal of Neurosurgery,* 1960, *17,* 266–282.

Wada, J., Clarke, R., & Hamm, A. Asymmetry of temporal and frontal speech zones in 100 adult and 100 infant brains. *Archives of Neurology,* 1975, *32,* 239–246.

Walker, J. T., & Krasnoff, A. G. The horizontality principle in young men and women. *Perceptual and Motor Skills,* 1978, *46,* 1055–1061.

Willemsen, E., & Reynolds, B. Sex differences in adults' judgments of the horizontal. *Developmental Psychology,* 1973, *8,* 309.

Wilson, J. R., DeFries, J. D., McClearn, G. E., Vandenberg, S. G., Johnson, R. C., & Rashad, M. N. Cognitive abilities: Use of family data as a control to assess sex and age difference in two ethnic groups. *International Journal of Aging and Human Development,* 1975, *6,* 261–276.

Witelson, S. F. *Age and sex differences in the development of right hemispheric specialization for spatial processing as reflected in a dichotomous tactual stimulation task.* Paper presented to Society for Research in Child Development, Denver, 1975.

Witelson, S. Sex and the single hemisphere: Right hemisphere specialization for spatial processing. *Science,* 1976, *193,* 425–427.

Witelson, S., & Pallie, W. Left hemisphere specialization for language in the newborn. *Brain,* 1973, *96,* 641–646.

Witkin, H. A. Sex differences in perception. *Transactions of the New York Academy of Sciences,* 1949, *12,* 22–26.

Witkin, H. A. Individual differences in case of perception of embedded figures. *Journal of Personality,* 1950, *19,* 1–15.

Witkin, H. A., Birnbaum, J., Lomonaco, S., Lehr, S., & Herman, J. L. Cognitive patterning in congenitally blind children. *Child Development,* 1968, *39,* 768–786.

Witkin, H. A., Dyk, R. B., Faterson, G. E., Goodenough, D. R., & Karp, S. A. *Psychological differentiation.* New York: Wiley, 1962.

Witkin, H. A., Goodenough, D. R., & Karp, S. A. Stability of cognitive style from childhood to young adulthood. *Journal of Personality and Social Psychology,* 1967, *7,* 291–300.

Witkin, H. A., Lewis, H. B., Hertzman, M., Machover, K., Meissner, P. B., & Wapner, S. *Personality through perception.* New York: Harper & Row, 1954.

Wolf, S. M. Difficulties in right–left discrimination in a normal population. *Archives of Neurology,* 1973, *29,* 128–129.

Zaidel, E. Language, dichotic listening, and the disconnected hemispheres. In D. O. Walters, L. Rogers, & J. M. Finzi-Fried (Eds.), *Conference on human brain function.* Los Angeles: University of California at Los Angeles, Brain Research Information Publication Office, 1976.

Zangwill, O. *Cerebral dominance and its relation to psychological function.* London: Oliver and Boyd, 1960.

Zurif, E. G., & Bryden, M. P. Familial handedness and left–right differences in auditory and visual perception. *Neuropsychologia,* 1969, *7,* 179–188.

17

Education and Credentialing Issues in Neuropsychology

MANFRED J. MEIER

This chapter is intended to provide the interested undergraduate and early graduate student in psychology a basis for examining the options and making a decision to pursue a course of graduate or postdoctoral study in clinical neuropsychology. A brief outline of the conditions that have determined the content and direction of this rapidly evolving specialty will be used to identify the need for relevant educational models and adequate credentialing criteria. It is proposed that the effective choice of a curricular path in clinical neuropsychology will be facilitated by establishing an historical frame of reference and an appreciation of the rather intricate and complexly determined course the field of clinical neuropsychology has taken over the past three decades. The resulting diversification of interests and approaches has led to considerable refinement of theories of brain function and a rich data base for understanding brain-behavior relationships and for clinical application. Acceleration of research and clinical activity over the past decade now promises to move clinical neuropsychology beyond the diagnostic domain and into new roles of rehabilitation, agency and institutional consultation, and consumer education. Educational preparation for such an expansion of professional roles will necessarily require more educational program options and the articulation of credentialing criteria for ensuring the quality of clinical practice. Thus, this chapter will attempt to identify the determinants of the identity of

MANFRED J. MEIER ● Neuropsychology Laboratory, Department of Neurosurgery, University of Minnesota Medical School, Minneapolis, Minnesota 55455.

this evolving specialty and examine the educational options for developing effective professional competencies and for fostering the clinical research productivity necessary for a vital specialty. Such a discussion requires consideration of the clinical and experimental basis of the specialty and the need to blend these components in educational preparation for a strong professional role. In turn, requirements of this role would then be translated into terms that would make it possible to verify the nature and level of the associated competencies through appropriate credentialing mechanisms.

The development of a new specialty such as clinical neuropsychology provides an excellent opportunity to relate curriculum content to professional practice in a more systematic way than has characterized the traditional specialty areas of professional psychology in the past. Like the traditional specialty areas of clinical, counseling, school and industrial psychology, the professional roles and competencies of the specialty have evolved on an ad hoc, unsystematic basis as a result of applied roles and consumer needs that have been identified outside the academic environment. Sometimes, fortuitous environmental and historical circumstances played a predominant role as evidenced by clinical psychology that evolved during World War II in response to an accentuated need for assessment and psychotherapeutic services, a need that the medical specialty of psychiatry could not meet. Such precursors of specialty development may not favor the orderly development of effective curricula or the establishment of external credentialing procedures for defining and evaluating professional practice. Curriculum development may then be determined by events that may not produce an optimal or systematic course of specialty evolution. Although the contrast may not be as sharp as the argument requires, it seems reasonable to expect that clinical neuropsychology, considered from the standpoint of its historical development, is in an advantageous position to design competency-based curricula and to establish the necessary linkage between educational preparation and external credentialing procedures. Clinical neuropsychology may well be in a position to provide a model for more systematic specialty development and, thereby, assist the American Psychological Association in implementing criteria for new specialties.

HISTORICAL PERSPECTIVE

Clinical neuropsychology has become a broad and definitive activity area with numerous lines of intra- and interdisciplinary development. More extensive accounts of the events that have determined the growth of clinical neuropsychology have been reviewed earlier (Costa, 1976; Meier, 1974). The most relevant history focuses on the past three decades and involves activities in clinical psychology, experimental psychology, and behavioral neurology. Clinical psychologists have long attempted to establish efficient predictors of central nervous system involvement based on single tests (Spreen & Benton, 1967). This rather limited assessment emphasis was derived largely from the fact that clinical psychologists were working in psychiatric settings during the 1940s when much of the research on single tests was done. The primary clinical issue involved was the differentiation of organic from functional disorders in such settings where patients with focal cerebral lesions rarely appeared.

Ward Halstead in the late 1940s and his protégé Ralph Reitan in the early 1950s recognized a need to extend the quantitative test approach to the question of presence and location of focal cerebral lesions, to the differentiation of focal from diffuse lesions, and to the identification of pseudoneurologic behavioral changes of a functional origin. The empirical analysis of neuropsychological deficits associated with focal lesions required a multivariate approach, a requirement that was recognized by Halstead and elaborated by Reitan in a now well known series of clinical investigations. Their work was significant in many respects, of course, but is noteworthy for the fact that it reflects the early contribution of physiological and experimental psychologists to the investigation of clinical problems. They were among the first to apply quantitative behavioral measurements in the neurological setting, and they brought the skills of the cognitive and physiological psychologist to the assessment of brain-behavior relationships in humans. Interestingly, their battery also incorporated procedures that had been developed by the nineteenth century European neurologists and some twentieth century American neurologists (Bender, 1952; Denny-Brown, Meyer, & Horenstein, 1952) for the evaluation of sensory suppression phenomena, hemispatial neglect, and visual field impairments.

Except for these contributions, American neurology had not contributed heavily to the neurology of behavior. Much of the interest in cerebral localization was to be found in the work of Europeans such as Broca, Liepmann, Dejerine, and more recently Critchley and Hécean (Luria, 1966). Halstead and Reitan appeared to have been filling a void created by the relative neglect of behavioral phenomena, at least at the level of formal evaluation, on the part of most American neurologists. The Halstead–Reitan approach thereby enjoyed remarkable success in the 1950s and 1960s and became the foundation for the assessment role for clinical psychologists in medical settings.

In the meantime, American neurologists were reminded in 1965 of the rather rich and extensive clinical observations of the nineteenth century European neurologists. Their observations focused primarily on language disorders of focal origin, which had been relatively disregarded by American neurology until Geschwind (1965) attempted to integrate the nineteenth century European behavioral neurology literature. His exhaustive review not only had a major impact on the development of behavioral interests among American neurologists but also affected the course and direction of research of psychologists of both clinical and experimental persuasion. For example, the Boston Aphasia Diagnostic Examination

(Goodglass & Kaplan, 1972) provided a formal instrument for applying behavioral neurological principles to the evaluation of focal language disorders.

Another less clinical avenue of research that bears on neuropsychological theory and on varying styles of application of professional practice can be found in the work of experimental, physiological, cognitive, and developmental psychologists with special populations such as cerebrovascular accidents, brain tumors, focal epilepsies, and penetrating missile wounds. Foremost among these were Arthur Benton at the University of Iowa, Brenda Milner at McGill University, Hans-Lucas Teuber at the Massachusetts Institute of Technology, and Alexander Ramonovitch Luria at Moscow University. These investigators were grounded more firmly in the basic science of psychology and were concerned with conceptual elaboration and verification as well as with clinical application in the design of their research. As a consequence, they were able to introduce many methods that had not been systematically investigated in the context of direct clinical application (Meier, 1974).

RELATIONSHIP BETWEEN CLINICAL, EXPERIMENTAL, AND NEUROLOGICAL INFLUENCES

Perhaps the most deliberate integration of experimental and clinical concepts and methods in clinical neuropsychology can be found in the work of Arthur Benton and A. R. Luria. These investigators established early that clinical research could contribute to our understanding of brain function while also yielding applicable techniques for assessment and prediction of clinical phenomena (Benton, 1967; Luria, 1966). Their work is being recognized for its virtually total synthesis of each of the converging lines of historical development of clinical neuropsychology, and it provides the basis for the design of curriculum models for the continued vitality and growth of the specialty. The clinical and experimental channels can now claim a distinct contribution to our history. Proceeding now from the confluence of these channels, it seems reasonable to assert that a new specialty is emerging within professional psychology, and that this specialty is distinguishable from traditional clinical psychology.

That we are now confronted with major expansion and growth of the specialty is evidenced by the formation of new journals and organizations to process an expanding clinical and research agenda. In the absence of a mechanism within the American Psychological Association in the 1960s and 1970s, a group of clinical neuropsychologists formed the International Neuropsychological Society (INS) in 1966. The expansion of clinical research in neurological settings and the enhancement of behavioral neurology and experimental neuropsychology through the INS resulted in an interdisciplinary organization, which consisted primarily of clinical and experimental psychologists but also included the entire range of disciplines interested in brain-behavior relationships, including behavior neurologists, audiologists, speech pathologists, psycholinguists, special educators, neurosurgeons, psychiatrists and physiatrists. Nevertheless, the INS remained the primary organization for clinical neuropsychologists who began in the late 1970s to explore educational and professional issues (Costa, 1976; Meier, 1977).

The INS formed a Task Force on Education, Accrediatation and Credentialing, which has been identifying the issues to be addressed in designing curricula and in defining the competencies of the specialty (Meier, 1979). Although the INS is made up of a number of disciplines and remains primarily a scientific organization, it became the primary source of expertise for identifying professional roles and standards. Acknowledging that the role and identity of clinical neuropsychology should be dealt with through appropriate psychological organizations, the INS Task Force encouraged the formation of a Steering Committee to bring educational and credentialing issues to the American Psychological Association. In this direction, the Steering Committee petitioned the clinical neuropsychological community to form a new division of the APA. Strong support was established, and the new Division of Clinical Neuropsychology (Division 40) was formed in 1979. This Division has now identified a group of psychologists who would represent that division on a joint Task Force on Education, Accreditation and Credentialing, the responsibility for which would now be shared between Division 40 and INS (the joint Div 40/INS Task Force). There is now in place a mechanism for processing these issues and for guaranteeing that the educational and professional standards for the specialty will follow a rational and systematic course. Thus, we appear to be at the threshold of significant new opportunities for achieving specialty status within APA and for making substantive educational programs available to students in the future.

CHANGING STYLES OF NEUROPSYCHOLOGICAL APPLICATION

This brief review portrays the general foundations of the specialty. It attributes the recent growth in professional activity in clinical neuropsychology to the research productivity of a heterogenous group of clinical and experimental psychologists as well as behavioral neurologists. These interests and knowledge areas should be incorporated into the definition of specific competencies and the identification of particular curricular requirements for transmitting those competencies. Where an effective partnership exists between the clinical and experimental interests of a growing specialty, it seems reasonable to expect that a lag will arise between current professional applications and the increasing body of knowledge being generated by the field. There may also be a lag between the development of effective professional application and the provision of educational opportunities in graduate psychology programs. Considered superficially, such conditions may appear to be detrimental to the growth of the field. Closer analysis suggests that these are healthy conditions that may become unhealthy only if this lag is allowed to persist. In this direction, the new Division 40 of APA and the INS may now be in a position to foster realistic growth by creating change in the academic departments, the clinical training centers, and the various credentialing boards that may become involved with this specialty. Such change could also be facilitated by organizations not directly or intensively involved in these developments to date, such as the National Academy of Neuropsychologists, a professional group without extensive linkages to the academic arena.

The nature of the specialty is expected to become increasingly variegated and already includes differing styles of neuropsychological application (Golden, 1980; Kaplan, 1980a, 1980b). Golden has extended the multivariate approach to the methods of Luria in an attempt to quantify the entire range of variables observed in higher cortical dysfunction. Kaplan has demonstrated the effectiveness of qualitative observations in clinical assessment and in improved understanding of the neuropsychological processes that are affected by brain lesions and become involved in adjusting to or compensating for neuropsychological deficits. Such differences in approach may well generate controversy in the field. They are a healthy aspect of growth if resolved within the neuropsychological community in a goal-oriented manner and, thereby, promote change rather than become divisive. It is proposed that the diversity within neuropsychology, as evidenced in the contribution of the many factions that are contributing to the growth of the specialty, promises to make this a leading specialty with enormous potential for serving the consumer and for providing career development paths for interested graduate students.

As indicated above, the growth and professional activity of clinical neuropsychology can be attributed to the activities of both clinically and experimentally oriented individuals. As experimental neuropsychologists develop new applications, it is reasonable to expect that they will become more committed to applied work. Clinical neuropsychologists have been the primary contributors to the expansion of professional activity. However, there is a clear trend toward clinical involvement on the part of experimentally trained people who have managed to find more attractive job market conditions in neurological and rehabilitation settings.

Since their educational backgrounds are primarily in cognitive, physiological, experimental, and developmental psychology, they have introduced an analytic emphasis to clinical application. This contribution to clinical practice should be recognized for its intrinsic value and not perceived as a threat. Experimental psychologists, by virtue of their skills in analyzing psychological processes and the stimulus conditions that may interact with pathophysiological processes to determine the outcomes of neurological involvement, may be in a position to improve clinical psychological assessment and establish a technology of remediation and intervention. Such an interaction between scientific and professional interests and the increased overlap among clinical and experimental interests may ultimately provide the major basis for improving the quality of professional neuropsychological services. The process-oriented style of neuropsychological application may be more effective interprofessionally since experimental neuropsychologists appear well accepted in the neurological setting.

Neurologists, neurosurgeons, physiatrists, and psychiatrists recognize that the psychological processes underlying behavioral changes that result from central nervous system involvement may be of even greater importance in clinical decision making and strategy formation than the identification and localization of lesions. Modern neuroradiographic techniques have reduced the impact of the fixed test battery approach of clinical neuropsychologists in the neurological setting. Because it is highly unlikely that clinical neuropsychology can justify its existence over the long term on the basis of a diagnostic role alone, it would appear to be maladaptive to emphasize the fixed test battery approach over more analytic, process-oriented approaches to psychological assessment, since the latter may potentially yield more for defining rehabilitation strategies and designing specific behavioral therapies.

The concern with process and the theoretical bases of behavioral change distinguishes the experimental and clinical interests in the field and appears to account for much of the growth of the specialty beyond clinical description and quantification of behavioral consequences of brain lesions. The latter emphasis may well yield to a new set of roles derived from the former and, therefore, should be acknowledged in any educational program. The current status of clinical neuropsychology and the rich mixture of orientations, content areas, methods, and clinical problems provides a remarkable foundation for designing predoctoral curricula, postdoctoral training programs, or clinical internships directed at clinical neuropsychological competencies. The credentialing mechanisms of the future, such as licensure or board certification, should address the various competencies that are merging in the field and make provision for their assessment and validation.

ASSESSMENT: POINT OF DEPARTURE FOR EDUCATIONAL PLANNING

The characteristic role of the clinical neuropsychologist has been the identification, description, and multivariate quantification of psychological deficits associated with central nervous system involvement. The fixed test battery approach has been directed at the detection and localization of cerebral and subcortical lesions. Formulation of rehabilitation strategies and specific interventions and consultation to the patient and families and the provision of counseling or educational activities have not been central to the fixed battery approach, yet it will no doubt remain the central concern of some training programs, particularly those that conform with Model I, and to some extent Model II (these are described later). More recent applications of this approach show promise for improving predictive validity and may also shorten testing and professional time and thus reduce cost to the consumer. Recent applications are also hoped to improve rehabilitation strategy formation and planning (Golden, 1980).

Further innovation in clinical neuropsychological assessment may be anticipated in the future by means of approaches that combine the qualitative process analysis with the more quantitative test battery approach that has characterized the specialty (Kaplan, 1980a, 1980b; Lezak, 1976). A predominantly qualitative approach might be utilized to design a one-hour screening procedure for establishing the presence and location of a lesion and to differentiate focal from diffuse involvement. The screen would also identify impairments that deserve further study by means of exacting quantitative procedures. This second phase of a combined qualitative/quantitative assessment model would require perhaps an additional hour of testing time. A third hour could then be devoted to the introduction of highly individualized assessment of those processes that have been identified in phases I and II of the assessment for the purpose of rehabilitation strategy formulation. An array of specific interventions can be envisioned that would be addressed to the modification of the behavior changes associated with differing psychological processes underlying the neuropsychological deficits. Preliminary efforts to develop an assessment model that would incorporate both qualitative and quantitative observations is underway. This effort will be guided by the joint Div 40/INS Task Force to integrate the various approaches and interest groups within the specialty and, therefore, has potential of serving as a unifying mechanism as well as a basis for relating clinical neuropsychology to general psychology and behavioral neurology.

It can be seen that neuropsychology as a specialty requires a scientist/practitioner educational model and is likely to become a recognized new specialty within the family of psychological specialties in American psychology. Appropriate new training programs are already beginning to emerge at the predoctoral, internship, and postdoctoral levels. The growth of these programs is slow but deliberate.

MAJOR OPTIONS IN CAREER DEVELOPMENT

With the direct role that clinical psychology has played in the development of clinical neuropsychology, it is reasonable to establish a neuropsychological emphasis in the curriculum of traditional clinical programs. The same argument could be applied to a program in counseling psychology, for example, since those students frequently seek careers in rehabilitation settings where neuropsychological assessments are frequently done. A relevant group of didactic courses and practicum experiences within the clinical psychology curriculum could be sufficient to establish a competency in clinical neuropsychology. However, those curricula are already crowded with competing contents and orientations and may not have sufficient time or adequate faculty for this purpose. While faculty with expertise in clinical neuropsychology are being recruited by some clinical programs, most of the relevant expertise is available in the health sciences centers that have neuropsychology laboratories with a productive research and clinical record. There is now evidence of increased concern with clinical neuropsychological assessment in the curriculum of many clinical psychology programs, but the nature and quality of these components has not been established (Golden & Kuperman, 1980).

While this may not be an optimal way to obtain training in clinical neuropsychology, it remains perhaps the most accessible, certainly at a predoctoral level, and should therefore be considered. It is not the purpose of this chapter to provide specific recommendations and guidelines for selecting a particular program since there are insufficient data to make such recommendations. Instead, the role of this training model will be considered as the most feasible under current conditions. Nevertheless, clinical psychology training programs may not provide the necessary background in neurological sciences to establish a definitive competency in clinical neuropsychology. The curriculum may be sufficiently crowded to preclude adequate preparation in physiological and cognitive psychology. The necessary clinical practicum training for applying psychological science or for integrating neurosciences content in clinical practice may not be adequate. The emphasis of such programs is necessarily upon psychiatric populations, community mental health, and psychotherapy. Also, these programs are available to a relatively narrow range of students whose expressed interest is in traditional clinical psychology. This makes such programs relatively inaccessible to students whose undergraduate background and early graduate interest involve physiological and cognitive psychology, the areas that may become increasingly important for the growth of clinical neuropsychology in the future.

This state of affairs introduces distinct barriers to the rational flow of interested graduate students into clinical neuropsychology and is stimulating some academic departments to establish distinct predoctoral programs in neuropsychology (Sheer, 1978). These programs are in the early stages of development and are essentially untested for educational quality or for their relevance to particular student needs and interests. The Div 40/INS Task Force is conducting a survey of these programs and will be defining evaluative criteria for accreditation purposes in the future. In the meantime, the graduate student is advised to examine available educational options and utilize the services of the various organizations involved in the neuropsychological arena by joining them as a student member and by approaching their officers and committee chairpersons for the most current information. Those who have already completed training in a traditional professional specialty or in experimental or physiological psychology are encouraged to explore postdoctoral training opportunities. These are likely to develop at a more rapid pace and become the most important training vehicle for clinical neuropsychologists for a number of reasons:

1. Most clinical, counseling, or school psychology programs may be unable to provide adequate preparation in clinical neuropsychology in the foreseeable future.
2. The cost and political barriers to developing a complete predoctoral curriculum are sufficiently high to preclude the feasibility of obtaining the necessary institutional support for such programs.
3. The Div 40/INS Task Force on Education, Accreditation and Credentialing has been focusing on one year of supervised postdoctoral experience or three years of unsupervised experience in a neurological setting as the entry level for clinical neuropsychology.

Whether in pursuit of pre- or postdoctoral training, the student may benefit from a review of the major training models available. Some of these have been presented elsewhere (Meier, 1981) but are updated and include a fifth model, which is likely to be introudced some time during the 1980s as a new option.

PREDOCTORAL EDUCATIONAL MODELS FOR CLINICAL NEUROPSYCHOLOGY

There are at least five conceivable ways in which definitive training in clinical neuropsychology might be obtained:

I. Subspecialization within a traditional applied curriculum such as clinical or counseling psychology
II. A minor or interdepartmental supporting program in neuropsychology and clinical neuroscience
III. An integrated scientist/practitioner curriculum.
IV. A coordinated graduate curriculum with separate PhD and PsyD degrees
V. A clinical neuropsychology major or track within an integrated clinical neurosciences PhD degree program

The choice of a particular educational model for designing an individual curriculum will depend upon the available options in a given institutional setting. These options remain rather limited in most settings so that the student must negotiate an effective curriculum even when the available resources are adequate for obtaining a full complement of training in neuropsychology. As training programs emerge, the range of available options should include variants of these models with the possible exception of Model IV, which is likely to remain an unavailable ideal in the foreseeable future. It is described here in order to underscore the need to distinguish between scientific and clinical competencies and to identify the requirements for achieving expertise in each domain.

It is assumed in all these models that the core knowledge for clinical neuropsychology involves content in both psychological and neurological sciences and requires an institutional setting in which both a department of psychology and a health sciences center with strong neurosciences activities are available. This combined knowledge base in psychology and neurological sciences is necessary to develop the core and the terminal competencies necessary for functioning as a clinical neuropsychologist. The doctoral level of preparation is considered essential for competing in the marketplace insofar as virtually all neuropsychologists in the field today have a doctorate and the necessary preclinical preparation in psychology and neurology is sufficiently extensive to add substantially to the requirements of an existing applied psychology program.

The models contraindicate the efficacy of the free-standing professional school as a setting in which an appropriate program can be provided. This consideration leads directly to some variant of the scientist/practitioner model as the basis for preparing doctoral level personnel for this specialty. Subdoctoral personnel will likely be developed for more limited technological roles to be carried out under the supervision of the doctoral level scientist/practitioner. Technical roles are already being implemented by individuals at the baccalaureate and masters level so that there should be ample opportunity for meaningful, but more limited, clinical roles at those levels. This will depend on the thorough testing of the evolving competencies and technologies so that they can be selectively transferred to beginning and intermediate level personnel who would then extend the capability of the doctoral level individual. Extender or support personnel already exist but have not been trained formally. For the most part, they have received inservice training in neuropsychology laboratories after obtaining a baccalaureate degree in psychology, sometimes even at the subbaccalaureate level.

Model I: Subspecialization in a Traditional Applied Curriculum Such as Psychology

As indicated above, the typical clinical psychology curriculum is already quite crowded with content and practicum requirements. Most students are doing 5 to 6 years of graduate work to complete those requirements. It is also widely known that those curricula tend to be relatively weak in clinical neuropsychology although some training is now being provided in many programs. The product of the typical clinical program is not expected to have highly refined competencies in any area but is encouraged to pursue such refinement on a postdoctoral basis, either through experience or through formal postdoctoral training activities. Thus, the goal of such programs is to prepare a generalist who is then assumed to be sufficiently based in psychological knowledge to pursue further competency development through experience or postdoctoral training (Peterson, 1976).

Eligibility for examination by theAmerican Board of Professional Psychology for the various traditional psychological specialties requires such an extended period of postdoctoral experience, although the essential external credential, the state license, is usually available within two years. Such generalists are regarded as equally competent in research and in service roles since the training programs have been derived from the scientist/practitioner model developed at the Boulder Conference (Raimy, 1947). This scientist/practitioner model has been the basis for training professional psychologists for many years, until the introduction of the professional degree concept and the corresponding attempt to differentiate between scientific and professional roles in predoctoral educational preparation (Korman, 1974). Because the traditional applied programs are committed to developing a generalist, they neither attempt to develop technical skills nor professional competencies at the level being embraced by the neuropsychological community, at least as evidenced by the Div 40/INS Task Force and the recent expansion of knowledge and competency potential of this specialty.

For these reasons, clinical programs do not provide a ready avenue for definitive competency development. However, they continue to provide the primary access to the field and are beginning to welcome and sometimes even solicit students with neuropsychological interests. A major advantage for the student is the availability in the clinical psychology curriculum of opportunities to develop a professional role identity as well as the basic foundations in behavioral science necessary to function as a neuropsychologist. The student is still required to secure the necessary foundation in the clinical neurosciences and needs to obtain access to courses in clinical neurology, neuroanatomy, neurophysiology, neuropathology, special diagnostic techniques, and conferences on neurosurgery and rehabilitation medicine to develop the necessary conceptual basis for clinical practice.

Whether or not a given clinical psychology program will accommodate the needs of the student interested in clinical neuropsychology will depend on the particular department and faculty involved. The student is forced to make a careful assessment of these background conditions before even applying. Competition for slots in a clinical psychology program, it should be emphasized, is quite remarkable in most departments with strong health sciences linkages. Even if admitted to the program, the student may find that much of the curriculum is not directly related to his or her interests and that, therefore, an incongruency may be present that introduces conflict, uncertainty, and discomfort.

For the student coming out of experimental, physiological, cognitive, or developmental psychology, prospects for admission to the program may be minimal or the student may be inadequately prepared for a clinical curriculum. Such individuals would be well advised to pursue doctoral preparation in their interest area, following a straight scientific preparation model, and then seek formal post-doctoral training to establish clinical competencies in neuropsychology. There is clearly a double bind for the experimental/physiological student insofar as professional preparation is quite advantageous for securing work in neurological settings while individual potential for contributing to the field in the future is greatly enhanced by scientific training. The pursuit of formal postdoctoral studies is probably more realistic and beneficial for such students under present academic circumstances.

Model II: A Minor or Interdepartmental Supporting Program in Neuropsychology and Clinical Neurosciences

This model provides a compromise solution to the dilemma posed for both clinical and nonclinical students when pursuing studies in clinical neuropsychology through a traditional clinical psychology curriculum. Most graduate programs in psychology require a minor or an interdepartmental supporting program outside the major department. This model simply utilizes the available time for extra-departmental requirements and provides courses and practica for scientific or for professional role development as appropriate. The advantage for the graduate student is that the graduate major does not define the supporting program. This means that students in any traditional applied curriculum or in a basic behavioral sciences curriculum may begin to develop either clinical or scientific competencies in neuropsychology at the predoctoral level.

This model assumes the availability of an established neuropsychology program in a medical school and appropriate relationships between the department of psychology and of the basic and clinical neurosciences departments. The necessary linkage is provided by neuropsychologists in medical schools, although the amount of time and resources they can provide for the student requires careful examination before a supporting program arrangement is negotiated. The more serious the student, the more elaborate the supporting program is likely to become. This may necessitate adding a year or more to the graduate curriculum. The resulting curriculum plan may approach Model III, which calls for a comprehensive predoctoral curriculum in clinical neuropsychology. A typical Model II curriculum would include courses or conferences in neuroanatomy, clinical neurology and neurosurgery, clinical neuropsychological assessment, behavioral neurology, and specialized radiographic and electrophysiologic techniques in the neurological setting. This model has been relatively effective at the University of Minnesota, where students in clinical psychology, physiological psychology, cognitive psychology, speech pathology, and school psychology have availed themselves of neuropsychological and medical resources provided through the neuropsychology laboratory and the departments of neurosurgery, neurology, and psychiatry.

The purpose of such a program is to provide the equivalent of one year of postdoctoral training in clinical neuropsychology for individuals who have had no more than casual exposure to neuropsychology in their graduate program. Thus, properly designed, Model II can provide the necessary training for meeting what is anticipated to become the entry level requirements for clinical practice in the future. This claim, however, would apply more to clinical than nonclinical graduate students unless the latter had adequate coursework in clinical interviewing, abnormal psychology, descriptive psychopathology, and professional ethics— courses not readily provided within the framework of a minor or supporting program. Nonclinical students would then require access to those courses in their parent department, namely, the department of psychology.

Some medical school psychology programs may have such courses. Medical students and medical specialty residents may have higher priority so that they may be incompletely accessible for psychology graduate students. The interested graduate student should exercise caution in the evaluation of these resources since they may not favor completion of the combined curriculum in a reasonable period of time. An interdepartmental supporting program can also provide the context in which the PhD dissertation is produced and, thus, may help provide adequate predoctoral preparation in clinical neuropsychology.

Model III: Integrative Scientist/Practitioner Curriculum for the PhD Degree

The scientist/practitioner model was introduced by the Shakow report (1947) and the Boulder Conference to combine preparation for clinical research skills and for clinical proficiencies of the specialty of clinical psychology. While there have been many problems associated with reaching this combined educational goal in clinical psychology, there appears to be considerable enthusiasm for this model among clinical neuropsychologists (Meier, 1981). As applied to clinical neuropsychology, the model would not yield a generalist but would prepare a specialist with broad general background in both behavioral and neurological sciences. Even proponents of professional degree programs in psychology acknowledge the validity of the scientist/practitioner model when applied to a PhD in a specialized area of substantive content and depth (Peterson, 1976). Thus, clinical neuropsychology may be one of the more apt examples of an area in which the scientist/practitioner model might well flourish. The overall goal of such a program would be the production of highly competent professionals who function within clearly defined boundaries of professional role functioning and clinical research.

This specialized PhD model has not been widely adopted, partly because of resistance by the departments of psychology to add applied programs and partly because the funding climate for federal training grants has become unfavorable. Arthur Benton's program at the University of Iowa has approximated this model, but he has done so largely through the clinical program which is somewhat atypical in that a PhD in clinical is awarded without an internship, and there is considerable flexibility within the curriculum for obtaining training in clinical neuropsychology. Attempts are underway to develop a Model III program at the University of Houston (Sheer, 1978) and the University of Victoria (Costa, 1979). A comprehensive educational evaluation of the existing programs, however, has not been reported in the literature.

The general goal of this model, therefore, is systematic preparation for functioning in professional as well as scientific roles. If successful, the model would produce individuals who are currently effective in their professional functioning and who have the scientific expertise to produce the necessary research for the future growth of the specialty. The success of the model depends on the feasibility of developing both sets of competencies, an achievement that may be limited to relatively few exceptional and dedicated individuals. The Model III curriculum calls for extensive preparation in psychology and the neurological sciences. It is appropriate to distinguish between the knowledge base that precedes competency formation, the essential or core competencies that might apply to any scientist/practitioner in psychology, and the terminal competencies that characterize the specialty.

The curriculum outline in Table 1 provides a guide for the interested graduate student in designing a definitive curriculum. During the precompetency phase, an attempt is made to differentiate between required and elective courses, the latter being selected on the basis of individualized needs assessments. There would appear to be sufficient flexibility to accommodate individual interests. The proposed outline assumes that the necessary new courses during Phase 2 (core competency development) would be made available by neuropsychologists on the faculty, whether they work directly in the department of psychology or in a neuro-

Table 1
Curriculum Outline: Model III

Precompetency Phase (Years 1–2)	
Psychological science	Elective subset (15 credit hours)
Required (30 quarter credit hours)	Behavior analysis and modification
Cognitive psychology	Learning disorders
Psychological measurement	Psychopharmacology
Individual differences	Psychophysiology
Human learning and memory	Behavior genetics
Physiological psychology	Psycholinguistics
Abnormal psychology	Personality
Life-span developmental psychology	
Descriptive psychopathology	
Experimental design and statistics	

(*continued*)

Table 1 (*Cont.*)

Precompetency Phase (Years 1–2)

Neurological science
    Required (12 quarter credit hours)
        Functional neuroanatomy
        Clinical neurology/neurosurgery
        Behavioral neurology
        Specialized diagnostic technologies

Elective subset (6 credit hours)
    Clinical neurophysiology
    Clinical neuropharmacology
    Neuropathology
    Neurolinguistics
    Biophysics

Core Competency Development Phase (Years 2–3)

Scientific and professional roles in neuropsychology (15 quarter credit hours)
    Sociology of professionalization
    Ethics of research and professional practice
    Preparation of grant requests
    Grants management
    Scientific and professional role survey
    Proseminar: Assessment, intervention in clinical neuropsychology
    Selection of terminal competencies and goals
Core competency establishment (15 quarter credit hours)
    Interviewing methods and practica
    Problem- and goal-oriented records and goal attainment scaling
    Research project design
    Clinical project design: Assessment and intervention
        Assessment
            Application of selected neuropsychological test batteries
            Analysis of individual cognitive processes
        Intervention (2 required—one from each group)

Group A	Group B
Cognitive therapy	Behavior therapy/situational depression
Behavior analysis/modification	Rational/emotive psychotherapy
Psychophysiological procedures	

Terminal Competency Refinement Phase (Years 3–4)

Implementation of research study
Implementation of clinical projects
Literature review for dissertation project
Design and initiation of dissertation project

Competency Evaluation Phase (Year 5)

Assessment
    Performance review of representative cases
    Boardlike examination of clinical projects
Intervention
    Boardlike examination of clinical projects
Research
    Present research study at scientific/professional meeting
    Present literature review at faculty/student colloquium
    Final oral exam based on dissertation

psychology laboratory of a health sciences center. In the absence of a wide selection of existing programs, the student is forced to negotiate these additional courses and may need to assume the role of change agent in the departmental setting. Thus, while this may become a working model for training clinical neuropsychologists in the future, the student who would pursue a definitive curriculum at this time is faced with the reality problems associated with the existing lag between knowledge base and program availability.

Model IV: Coordinated Graduate Curriculum with Separate PhD and PsyD Components

Model IV does not exist nor is it likely to exist in the foreseeable future. Therefore, the model can be characterized as an ideal involving educational goals that are too expansive for realistic attainment under present or immediate future conditions. Model III already constitutes a compromise with the ideal presented by Model IV but is a much more realistic alternative for consideration at this time. The Model IV coordinated graduate curriculum calls for the differentiation of the scientist and professional competency domains into separate curricular designs. While distinct, the designs do overlap so that the student would be pursuing both degrees simultaneously. Tables 2 and 3 provide curriculum outlines for the PhD and PsyD components, respectively.

This approach to curriculum coordination is seen in alternated form in some clinical departments of medical schools where medical specialty residents can pursue a PhD in a clinical department (as contrasted with a basic science department such as anatomy or physiology) while completing residency training. In such instances the credits obtained for clinical training are applied toward the PhD degree. Additional coursework, preliminary examinations, and a dissertation are added to the residency to complete a basis for a PhD in, for example, neurology. The individual then terminates with both the MD and the PhD degree. The latter is not usually as rigorous a curriculum as would be found, for example, in a basic science department or in the department of psychology.

What this ideal is designed to accomplish is a stronger guarantee that both the professional and the scientific components of academic preparation are fully attained. Separation of the curricula also makes it possible for an individual to pursue one or the other competency domain. This would permit the production of basic scientists who have no inclination to become clinicians. As applied to clinical neuropsychology, the PsyD would not be available as an option, independently of the PhD. Model IV would be of interest perhaps to those few individuals who develop an early commitment to an academic career but wish to establish an unequivocal and identifiable set of clinical competencies. The two curricula can be seen to overlap particularly at the preprofessional and core competency levels. Model IV, therefore, provides an option to pursue a PhD without clinical com-

Table 2

Curriculum Outline: Model IV PhD Component

Integrated Prescientist/Professional Phase (Years 1–2)

Psychological science

    Required (40 quarter credit hours)   Elective subset (25 credit hours)

        Cognitive psychology   Behavior analysis and

        Psychological measurement   modification

        Individual differences   Learning disorders

        Human learning and memory   Psychopharmacology

        Physiologcal psychology   Psychophysiology

        Abnormal psychology   Behavior genetics

        Life-span developmental psychology   Psycholonguistics

        Descriptive psychopathology   Personality

        Experimental design and statistics

Neurological science

    Required (15 quarter credit hours)   Elective subset (9 credit hours)

        Functional neuroanatomy   Clinical neurochemistry

        Clinical neurology/neurosurgery   Clinical neurophysiology

        Behavioral neurology   Neuropathology

        Specialized diagnostic technologies   Neurolinguistics

                                      Clinical neuropharmacology

---

Core Competency Phase (Years 2–3)

Research as a scientific and professional role (9 credit hours)

    Sociology of professionalization

    Ethics of research with human subjects

    Scientific roles/problems in neuropsychology

    Preparation of grant requests

    Grants management

    Proseminar: Assessment, intervention

Core competency phase (24 credit hours)

    Interviewing methods and practica

    Goal attainment scaling

    Experimental design exercise

    Field study design exercise

    Theory and methodology underlying core competencies

    Preliminary written/oral examinations

Terminal Competency Refinement Phase (Year 3)

Implementation of experiment

Implementation of field study

Literature review of selected topic: Normal population

Literature review of selected topic: Pathological population

Design and initiate dissertation project

Competency Evaluation Phase (Year 4)

Present experimental or field study at scientific meeting

Present literature reviews at faculty/student colloquium

Complete dissertation

Final oral exam based on dissertation

Table 3
Curriculum Outline: Model IV PsyD Component

Integrated Prescientist Professional Phase (Years 1–2)

Psychological science

Required (30 quarter credit hours)
Cognitive psychology
Psychological measurement
Individual differences
Human learning and memory
Physiological psychology
Abnormal psychology
Life-span developmental psychology
Descriptive psychopathology

Elective subset (15 credit hours)
Experimental design and statistics
Behavior analysis and
modification
Learning disorders
Psychopharmacology
Psychophysiology
Rehabilitation psychology
Behavior genetics
Psycholinguistics
Personality

Neurological science

Required (12 quarter credit hours)
Functional neuroanatomy
Clinical neurology/neurosurgery
Behavioral neurology
Specialized diagnostic technologies

Elective subset (6 credit hours)
Clinical neurochemistry
Clinical neurophysiology
Neuropathology
Neurolinguistics
Clinical neuropharmacology

Core Competency Phase (Years 2–3)

Professionalization and role definition (15 credit hours)
Sociology of professionalization
Professional roles in neuropsychology
Ethics and professional standards
The professional as a consumer of research
Proseminar: Assessment, intervention, consultation, education
Tentative selection of terminal competencies
Core competency establishment (30 credit hours)
Interviewing methods and practica: Interpersonal process recall
Definition of clinical problems and history-taking
Problem- and goal-oriented records and goal attainment scaling
Audit, quality assurance, and services system evaluation
Theory and methodology underlying core competencies

Terminal Competency Refinement Phase (Years 4–5)

Assessment (modular design—Three selected competency areas)
Traditional and innovative neuropsychological batteries
Cognitive processes, including automated applications
Test construction exercise
Intervention (modular design—Three selected competency areas)
Two of the following
Cognitive therapy (e.g., learning and mnestic disorders)
Behavior modification—individual, group, or institutional context
Psychophysiological procedures
One of the following
Rational/emotive psychotherapy
Behavior therapy/situational depression

(*continued*)

Table 3 (*Cont.*)

Terminal Competency Refinement Phase (Years 4–5)

Consultation (modular design—Two settings)
    Schools
    Forensic applications
    Long-term care institutions
    Social security and vocational agencies
    Rehabilitation unit
Consumer education (modular design—Two contexts)
    Individual and family support system
    Media project
    Other health professionals
    Hospital information and education service

Competency Evaluation Phase (Year 5)

Boardlike professional examination
    Written
    Oral
Terminal objectives of competency—Determined modules
    Assessment: Performance review of representative cases
    Intervention: Performance review of representative cases
    Consultation: Performance review of representative cases
    Education: Performance review of representative cases

petency development or to add clinical competency development as a distinctly different pursuit. Although as yet unrealistic, the model has the virtue of helping to define appropriate postdoctoral training programs for people who have a PhD in psychology but may not have any previous clinical training, as well as people with previous clinical training and some limited research preparation who now wish to develop stronger research competencies. Thus, Phases 3 and 4 of the Model IV curriculum could be packaged into a 1- or 2-year postdoctoral program as appropriate. These phases would then be defined in terms of continuing education units or certificates of achievement, rather than degrees, for licensure of board certification purposes.

Model V: Clinical Neuropsychology Track of an Integrated Neurosciences PhD Degree Program

Another possible option for academic career preparation in neuropsychology involves a more direct relationship between the various neurosciences departments in a medical school and a department of psychology. There appear to be no instances of this model in operation, but the increased priority of neurosciences activities within health sciences centers may favor the development of an interdisciplinary PhD program in the neurosciences with specialization in one or another of the tracking disciplines. Thus, an integrated neurosciences PhD program might have specialty tracks in the basic sciences such as neuroanatomy, neurophysiology, neurochemistry, or experimental neuropsychology, or in the clinical sciences such as neurology and clinical neuropsychology. A consortium of departments would provide a core neurosciences curriculum from which specialized tracks can flow. The one major advantage of such a program would be the availability of an inter-disciplinary faculty and a coordinated basic behavioral and neurological sciences curriculum.

There is a general value that favors the possible development of such pro-grams in the future, namely, that the neurosciences constitute the last and the largest frontier of scientific activity and knowledge in the health sciences. Not only the neurosciences as a group but even neuropsychology can now be identified as an interdisciplinary enterprise. Educational innovations that would bring faculty and students of these various disciplines together to define and explore problems jointly might well lead to advances in knowledge in each area that would exceed expectancy based on traditional curriculum goals. Applying such a model to a neuropsychology track might involve an elaboration of the neurological sciences prescientific competency development phase of Model IV. Thus, the student would obtain the usual extensive preparation in psychology but would then embark on a core precompetency development curriculum in the neurosciences before entering the research competency development phase. A problem for most psychology students with a more intensive neurosciences curriculum than that pro-vided in Model IV or Model III is the need for basic biological sciences prepa-ration as a prerequisite for the neurosciences core curriculum. Thus, this model would probably not be workable for students who did not have coursework in basic anatomy, physiology, biochemistry, and biophysics. Such coursework would be difficult to make up at the graduate level and would need to be built into the student's undergraduate curriculum. In essence, the model requires that the stu-dent pursue a premedical undergraduate curriculum with a major in psychology, the latter slanted toward the experimental, cognitive, physiological and develop-mental content areas. A limited version of such a curriculum may be available through Model II with an expanded interdepartmental supporting program and with adequate subbaccalaureate preparation in basic biological sciences. In any case, there is already discussion among the faculty of some of the larger health sciences centers about the feasibility of an integrated neurosciences curriculum with provision for disciplinary tracking. The tracking procedure is essential to guarantee that competencies will be developed that can be validated and reviewed by existing accreditation and credentialing mechanisms.

Very few areas lend themselves to interdisciplinary treatment of this kind. Analogous attempts outside the neurosciences context have been only marginally successful, probably as a result of the blurring of disciplinary lines and the result-ing dilution of the curricular components of individual disciplines. The tracking design would eliminate most of the problems associated with interdisciplinary curricula but, obviously, calls for a rather ambitious academic goal structure for the degree. As in the case of Model IV, only the most dedicated and qualified students would be admitted to such an ambitious program. Nevertheless, it is necessary to consider such options because they are the most likely to produce advanced scientific personnel to ensure the continued vitality and growth of neuropsychology.

CONCLUSION

The expansion of knowledge and application in clinical neuropsychology over the past three decades is leading to recognition of clinical neuropsychology as a new specialty in applied psychology. The foundations of clinical neuropsychology are now well established and appear suitable for the development of educational programs in accord with the scientist/practitioner model. The growing community of clinical neuropsychologists is becoming sufficiently organized to define the educational requirements for productive scientific and clinical roles. The specialty appears to have reached a point in its evolution where educational and credentialing issues can be processed effectively in the interests of the specialty and the public.

Formal educational programs are beginning to emerge at the predoctoral, internship, and postdoctoral levels. An attempt has been made in this chapter to provide guidelines for the design of predoctoral curricula as examplified in five models for curriculum design. These guidelines are intended to assist the interested undergraduate or graduate student in planning a curriculum and identifying institutions and settings in which adequate training in neuropsychology might be obtained. Elements of these varying models can also be converted into terms that relate to specialized internships or postdoctoral fellowships in clinical neuropsychology as these begin to be available. Some reference was made to the directions the specialty is likely to follow in the future and the need for establishing a closer relationship between educational programming and the external credentialing procedures that are likely to evolve for validating clinical and research competencies.

A key consideration not included in this analysis is the availability of academic and clinical positions in clinical neuropsychology. Precise information about job market conditions is not available at this time, although there is a general consensus in the clinical neuropsychological community that fully trained graduates are having no difficulty finding employment in health sciences centers, community hospitals, and private clinics. The Veterans Administration remains a strong employer of neurospychologists, although current policies clearly favor individuals trained in the APA-approved clinical psychology program. As the Division of Clinical Neuropsychology of the American Psychological Association and the International Neuropsychological Society move cooperatively toward the establishment of curriculum guidelines and competency definitions, the specialty seems likely to meet the APA criteria for specialty status. This would strengthen the representation of Division 40 in APA by permitting participation in the projected National Commission on Education and Credentialing in Psychology. If established, this commission will formulate uniform guidelines and criteria for training and credentialing in the various specialties within psychology in the future. As one of the first new specialties, clinical neuropsychology, it is hoped, will demonstrate how innovation in education can produce a more effective clinical scientist/professional, following a competency-based approach.

REFERENCES

Bender, M. B. *Disorders in perception.* Springfield, Ill.: Charles C Thomas, 1952.
Benton, A. L. Constructional apraxia and the minor hemisphere. *Confinia Neurologica,* 1967, *29,* 1–16.
Costa, L. D. Clinical neuropsychology: Respice, adspice, prospice. Presidential address, International Neuropsychological Society, Toronto. In *The INS Bulletin,* Ann Arbor, March 1976.
Costa, L. D. Personal communication, 1979.
Denny-Brown, D., Meyer, J. S., & Horenstein, S. The significance of perceptual rivalry resulting from parietal lobe lesion. *Brain,* 1952, *75,* 434–471.
Geschwind, N. Disconnexion syndromes in animals and man. *Brain,* 1965, *88,* 237–294; 585–644.
Golden, C. J. *Luria–Nebraska neuropsychological test battery: A qualitative and quantitative approach.* Presented at the American Psychological Assocation meeting, Montreal, September 1980.
Golden, C. J., & Kuperman, S. K. *Training opportunities in neuropsychological diagnosis at APA approved internship settings.* Presented at the American Psychological Association meeting, Montreal, September 1980.
Goodglass, H., & Kaplan, E. *The assessment of aphasia and related disorders.* Philadelphia: Lea and Febiger, 1972.
Kaplan, E. *Qualitative analysis of neuropsychological impairment.* Presidential address, International Neuropsychological Society, San Francisco, February 1980. (a)
Kaplan, E. *The case for the qualitative approach to neuropsychological assessment.* Presented at the American Psychological Assocation meeting, Montreal, September 1980. (b)
Korman, M. National conference on levels and patterns of professional training in psychology: The major themes. *American Psychologist,* 1974, *29,* 441–449.
Lezak, M. D. *Psychological assessment.* New York: Oxford University Press, 1976.
Luria, A. R. *Higher cortical functions in man* (B. Haigh, Trans.). New York: Basic Books, 1966. (Originally published, Moscow: Moscow University Press, 1962.)
Meier, M. J. Some challenges for clinical neuropsychology. In R. M. Reitan & L. A. Davison (Eds.), *Clinical neuropsychology: Current status and applications.* Washington, D.C.: V. W. Winston, 1974.
Meier, M. J. *Credentialing of neuropsychological role competencies.* Symposium on Professionalization of Selected Neuropsychological Roles, International Neuropsychological Society meeting, Santa Fe, 1977.
Meier, M. J. *Interim progress report: INS Task Force on Education, Accreditation and Credential-*

ing. Presented at the annual meeting of the International Neuropsychological Society, New York, February 1979.

Meier, M. J. Education for competency assurance in human neuropsychology: Antecedents, models and directions. In S. B. Filskov & T. J. Boll (Eds.), *Handbook of clinical neuropsychology.* New York: Wiley/Interscience, 1981.

Peterson, D. R. Need for the doctor of psychology degree in professional psychology. *American Psychologist,* 1976, *31,* 792–798.

Raimy, V. C. *Training in clinical psychology (Boulder Conference).* Englewood Cliffs, N.J.: Prentice Hall, 1947.

Shakow, D. In M. R. Harrower (Ed.), *Training in clinical psychology: Minutes of the first conference.* New York: Josiah Macy, 1947.

Sheer, D. E. *Survey of training programs.* Symposium (0777), Professional Issues and Educational Directions in Human Neuropsychology, American Psychological Association meeting, Toronto, 1978.

Spreen, O., & Benton, A. L. Comparative studies of some psychological tests for cerebral damage. *Journal of Nervous and Mental Disease,* 1967, *140,* 323–333.

APPENDIX

Neuroanatomy: Basic Concepts

It is not the intent nor within the scope of this book to discuss neuroanatomy in any detail. The reader is referred to the many available texts on neuroanatomy if more information is necessary or simply desired. The concepts below are intended for individuals with no background in this area and cover some basic terms necessary for the understanding of the text in some sections of this book.

The brain is divided into two halves most commonly called the *cerebral hemispheres.* The hemispheres are separated by a fissure known as the *longitudinal fissure.* The two hemispheres are called the *right and left hemisphere.* In general, each hemisphere controls the *contralateral* (opposite) side of the body for motor and sensory function. Thus, the left hemisphere is responsible for most of the tactile and motor functions of the right side of the body, the input from the right ear, and the input from the right half of each eye, while the right hemisphere is largely responsible for the same functions on the left side. It should be noted, however, that this division is not perfect. Especially for auditory and tactile modalities, as well as motor skills, there is also some control of each side of the body from the *ipsilateral* hemisphere, that is, the one on the same side of the body.

Each hemisphere is subdivided into several *lobes.* The most anterior areas (roughly behind the forehead) of the brain form the *frontal lobes,* the areas responsible for executive functions of the brain (coordinating and planning behavior) as well as motor skills. Somewhat more to the rear as well as lower in the three-dimensional structure of the brain, roughly above the ears, are the *temporal lobes.* These structures are responsible for auditory input and analysis. More posterior are the *parietal lobes,* which are responsible for the input and analysis of somatory sensory information (touch, feedback from the joints and muscles, and so on) as well as many higher cognitive skills that require the integration of different sensory modalities. These skills include most academic skills such as reading, as well as the understanding of complex and abstract forms of language and the ability to do such things as name objects. Finally, the very most posterior area of the brain is the *occipital lobe*, which is responsible for the input and analysis of visual information.

The type of analyses that occurs in each hemisphere is somewhat different. Although theorists disagree on the exact nature of these differences, on a practical level this results in the left hemisphere analyzing verbal material and responsible for related skills, while the right hemisphere is primarily responsible for a variety of nonverbal material such as visual spatial skills and musical abilities. In general, the left hemisphere is referred to as the *dominant hemisphere* because of its control over verbal abilities, while the right hemisphere is usually called *nondominant*. However, in about 4% of all right-handed people and up to 30% of all left-handed people, the relationships described above are reversed and the right hemisphere becomes the dominant, verbal hemisphere. In other cases, there is mixed dominance in which the hemispheres share more equally the control of verbal abilities. Studies of brain anatomy have indicated that the dominant hemisphere is generally larger than the nondominant hemisphere, especially in the temporal lobe area, which is responsible for the auditory analysis of spoken speech. It has been theorized that the degree of size difference between the hemispheres may be a clue to how well verbal skills are lateralized (present) in a single hemisphere. (See Chapter 16 on sex differences, for example.)

Below the surface of the brain, within the hemispheres, are *subcortical* (below the cortex, the outer layer) structures important for emotions, levels of arousal, the transmittal of information from the sense organs of the body to the cortex and the areas described above, and the transmittal of motor commands from the frontal lobes to the muscles of the body. Injury to some of these areas may cause death by interfering with such basic processes as breathing, or it can cause partial or complete losses of consciousness. Structures included within the subcortical areas include the *thalamus, hypothalamus, basal ganglia, limbic system, brain stem, pons, medulla, midbrain, cerebellum,* and numerous other structures.

Author Index

Subject Index